Novel Approaches in Chemotherapy

Novel Approaches in Chemotherapy

Edited by Sebastian Young

hayle medical

New York

Hayle Medical,
750 Third Avenue, 9th Floor,
New York, NY 10017, USA

Visit us on the World Wide Web at:
www.haylemedical.com

ISBN: 978-1-63241-839-5

Cataloging-in-Publication Data

Novel approaches in chemotherapy / edited by Sebastian Young.
p. cm.
Includes bibliographical references and index.
ISBN 978-1-63241-839-5
1. Cancer--Chemotherapy. 2. Chemotherapy. 3. Cancer--Treatment. I. Young, Sebastian.
RC271.C5 N68 2020
616.994 061--dc23

Table of Contents

Preface

This book has been an outcome of determined endeavour from a group of educationists in the field. The primary objective was to involve a broad spectrum of professionals from diverse cultural background involved in the field for developing new researches. The book not only targets students but also scholars pursuing higher research for further enhancement of the theoretical and practical applications of the subject.

Chemotherapy is a form of chemical drug therapy that is used to destroy rapidly growing cells of a body. It is a systemic therapy as it affects the whole body. It is primarily used in the treatment of cancer. However, it can also be used in the treatment of immune system disorders, such as rheumatoid arthritis or lupus. It lowers the number of cancer cells in the body, reduces metastasis, shrinks the tumor and reduces symptoms. When cancer is at an advanced stage, chemotherapy is used to relieve pain and symptoms. It can be delivered directly into the tumor to a specific part of the body through localized treatment, or administered orally, topically or in single shots. Due to its systemic nature, chemotherapy drugs target the cells in the blood, lining of the intestinal tract, the skin and the hair as well as where fast growing cells reside. This leads to side effects such as diarrhea, fatigue, mouth sores, easy bruising and bleeding, dry mouth, neuropathy, infections, memory problems, etc. Though many of these symptoms subside after conclusion of the treatment, damage to internal organs may also be incurred. This book elucidates new techniques and applications of chemotherapy in a multidisciplinary manner. It includes some of the vital pieces of work being conducted across the world, on various topics related to chemotherapy and oncological medicine. As this field is emerging at a rapid pace, the contents of this book will help the readers understand the modern concepts and applications of the subject.

It was an honour to edit such a profound book and also a challenging task to compile and examine all the relevant data for accuracy and originality. I wish to acknowledge the efforts of the contributors for submitting such brilliant and diverse chapters in the field and for endlessly working for the completion of the book. Last, but not the least; I thank my family for being a constant source of support in all my research endeavours.

Editor

1

Computed Tomography (CT) Perfusion as an Early Predictive Marker for Treatment Response to Neoadjuvant Chemotherapy in Gastroesophageal Junction Cancer and Gastric Cancer

Martin Lundsgaard Hansen[1]*, Eva Fallentin[1], Carsten Lauridsen[1,2], Ian Law[3], Birgitte Federspiel[4], Lene Bæksgaard[5], Lars Bo Svendsen[6], Michael Bachmann Nielsen[1]

1 Department of Radiology, Rigshospitalet, Copenhagen, Denmark, 2 Bachelor's Degree Programme in Radiography, Department of Technology, Metropolitan University College, Copenhagen, Denmark, 3 Department of Clinical Physiology, Nuclear Medicine and PET, Rigshospitalet, Copenhagen, Denmark, 4 Department of Pathology, Rigshospitalet, Copenhagen, Denmark, 5 Department of Oncology, Rigshospitalet, Copenhagen, Denmark, 6 Department of Surgical Gastroenterology, Rigshospitalet, Copenhagen, Denmark

Abstract

Objectives: To evaluate whether early reductions in CT perfusion parameters predict response to pre-operative chemotherapy prior to surgery for gastroesophageal junction (GEJ) and gastric cancer.

Materials and Methods: Twenty-eight patients with adenocarcinoma of the gastro-esophageal junction (GEJ) and stomach were included. Patients received three series of chemotherapy before surgery, each consisting of a 3-week cycle of intravenous epirubicin, cisplatin or oxaliplatin, concomitant with capecitabine peroral. The patients were evaluated with a CT perfusion scan prior to, after the first series of, and after three series of chemotherapy. The CT perfusion scans were performed using a 320-detector row scanner. Tumour volume and perfusion parameters (arterial flow, blood volume and permeability) were computed on a dedicated workstation with a consensus between two radiologists. Response to chemotherapy was evaluated by two measures. Clinical response was defined as a tumour size reduction of more than 50%. Histological response was evaluated based on residual tumour cells in the surgical specimen using the standardized Mandard Score 1 to 5, in which values of 1 and 2 were classified as responders, and 3 to 5 were classified as nonresponders.

Results: A decrease in tumour permeability after one series of chemotherapy was positively correlated with clinical response after three series of chemotherapy. Significant changes in permeability and tumour volume were apparent after three series of chemotherapy in both clinical and histological responders. A cut-off value of more than 25% reduction in tumour permeability yielded a sensitivity of 69% and a specificity of 58% for predicting clinical response.

Conclusion: Early decrease in permeability is correlated with the likelihood of clinical response to pre-operative chemotherapy in GEJ and gastric cancer. As a single diagnostic test, CT Perfusion only has moderate sensitivity and specificity in response assessment of pre-operative chemotherapy making it insufficient for clinical decision purposes.

Editor: Ramasamy Paulmurugan, Stanford University School of Medicine, United States of America

Funding: The authors acknowledge financial support from Poul Lundbeck and wife Fund and Civil engineer Johs. E. Ormstrup and wife Grete Ormstrup Fund. The funders had no role in study design, data collection and analysis, decision to publish, or preparation of the manuscript.

Competing Interests: The authors have declared that no competing interests exist.

* E-mail: mlundsgaard@dadlnet.dk

Introduction

Computed Tomography (CT) perfusion can visualise changes in tumours vascular physiology, and could thereby potentially provide a biomarker for therapeutic response to chemotherapy [1–8]. With the advent of multidetector row CT scanners and improved image reconstruction methods, larger structures and entire organs can be analysed in a single CT perfusion study. Potentially, CT perfusion could supplement CT or PET/CT imaging as a one-stop modality for cancer staging and therapy assessment in cancer imaging.

In patients with locally advanced esophageal cancer, gastro-esophageal junction (GEJ) cancer and gastric cancer perioperative chemotherapy improves overall and progression-free survival as confirmed by several randomised trials and meta-analyses [9–11]. Accordingly, a regimen of 9 weeks of chemotherapy prior to surgery is now included in the Danish national guidelines and is a standard treatment in our institution. The individual response to chemotherapy varies between 30 and 60% depending on evaluation methods [12–15] based either on histological or clinical response. The consequence to patients not responding to treatment is a delay in their definitive surgical treatment.

Moreover, it is important to identify non-responders, as continuous chemotherapy carries a risk of on-going progression, non-curability, side effects to chemotherapy and costs related to ineffective chemotherapy. To optimise and individualise treatment an imaging modality predicting or assessing treatment response at an early time point after treatment start would, thus, be of great value.

Our hypothesis was that a reduction in perfusion parameters could predict treatment response of pre-operative chemotherapy. To address this hypothesis changes in CT perfusion parameters in GEJ and gastric cancer during preoperative chemotherapy were measured and analysed for correlation with both clinical and histological response.

Materials and Methods

Patients

From October 2011 to January 2013 thirty consecutively admitted patients with biopsy confirmed adenocarcinoma at the gastro-esophageal junction or in the stomach were included in the study after being considered potentially resectable at a multidisciplinary tumour (MDT) conference and offered preoperative chemotherapy. Exclusion criteria were: allergy to contrast material, impaired renal function, and patient unfitness for chemotherapy. Of these thirty patients, one patient completed only the first scan and one patient was excluded from the study due to motion artefacts appearing in all three perfusion scans. The remaining 28 patients constituted the study group (24 males, 4 females, median age 65, range 44–79). Twenty-six patients underwent all three scans as described below. One patient was excluded from the third scan due to elevated serum creatinine levels, and one patient did not undergo the second scan due to hardware failure, leaving 27 patients for evaluation after one series of chemotherapy and 27 for presurgical responses. The diagnostic workup consisted of an upper endoscopy with biopsy, CT of the chest and abdomen combined with ultrasound of the neck and/or PET-CT for tumour staging, and after MDT conference a diagnostic laparoscopy to rule out peritoneal carcinomatosis. Patients with locally advanced tumour (T2– T4), with or without lymph node involvement (N0– N3) and no distant metastases (M0) were included. Methods and results are presented according to the REMARK recommendations for biomarker studies [16] - see supplementary Checklist S1.

Ethics

The research protocol was approved by the Committees on Biomedical Research for the Capital Region of Denmark (protocol number H-1-2010-132). All patients gave oral and written informed consent according to the Helsinki II Declaration.

Perfusion CT

All CT perfusion examinations were performed using a 320-detector row CT scanner (Aquilion ONE, Toshiba Medical Systems, Ohtawara, Japan). The study protocol consisted of three perfusion scans: baseline (median 8 days before starting chemotherapy, range 3–37 days), after the first cycle of chemotherapy (median 20 days, range 18–31 days) and - before surgery - after three cycles of chemotherapy (median 79 days, range 61–102 days). The last scan was performed at a median of 6 days before surgery (range 1–21 days).

Each patient was instructed to fast 2-hours prior to the CT examination, and was given 500 mL of water just prior to the CT perfusion study to distend the stomach for better visualisation of the tumour. The anticholinergic, hyoscine butylbromide, was administered (20 mg, *I.V.*) as a gastrointestinal motility inhibitor. An abdominal strap was placed around the patient to reduce movement and to encourage shallow breathing during the examination.

An area of 12–16 cm which covered the extent of the tumour was selected, and this area was used for all subsequent scans. A 16–18-gauge catheter was placed in the antecubital vein for administration of contrast material. Twenty mL of non-ionic contrast material (Omnipaque 350; GE Healthcare) was used as a test-bolus (single slice acquisition, 1-second intervals for 20 seconds) to determine the initial delay from contrast administration to arrival in the aorta. The arrival of contrast was visually determined and the delay for the CT perfusion scan was set to assure the acquisition of 2 full scan volumes without contrast material in the dynamic sequence.

The CT perfusion scan protocol consisted of 19 consecutive volumes divided into 3 phases: The first phase consisted of 11 volumes at 2 second intervals, a second phase of 6 volumes at 3 second intervals, and a third phase of 2 volumes at 5 second intervals. The first volume scan started between 7.5 and 13.5 seconds after contrast administration, and the total acquisition time ranged from 55 to 60 seconds. The contrast volume ranged from 30 to 40 mL, dependant on patient bodyweight (below 50 kg: 30 mL, between 50 and 79 kg: 35 mL, above 80 kg: 40 mL) followed by a saline flush of 30 mL. The injection rate varied from 5 to 8 mL/s, so that the overall contrast injection time never exceeded 5 seconds. The image acquisition used the following parameters: 100 kV, 100 mA, 0.5 s/rotation time, fixed table position, and 0.5 mm reconstruction.

Image Post Processing and Analysis

Images were reconstructed using AIDR 3D (Adaptive Iterative Dose Reduction, Toshiba Medical Systems, Japan). All datasets were corrected for motion using a non-rigid registration algorithm on the scan console (Toshiba). The volume containing the peak aortic enhancement was selected as a reference phase for motion correction. In two cases, the two late volumes were scanned at a different table position, and could therefore not be included in the motion correction.

The reconstructed, motion-corrected datasets were transferred to a stand-alone workstation (Vitrea 6.3, Vital Images, Toshiba Medical Systems, Minnetonka, USA) for post-processing. For data analysis, the input artery was selected by placing a 100 mm^2 circular Region of Interest (ROI) in the centre of the abdominal aorta and a second ROI was placed in the tumour. Parametric perfusion maps were generated with the following perfusion parameters: Arterial flow (tissue perfusion measured in $mL \cdot min^{-1} \cdot 100\ g^{-1}$), blood volume (measured in $mL \cdot 100\ g^{-1}$) and permeability (measured as k^{trans} in $mL \cdot min^{-1} \cdot 100\ g^{-1}$). Based upon consensus between two radiologists, a free-hand ROI was drawn around the tumour-border on slices containing visible tumour and these circumscribed areas were utilized to define tumour volume using a sculpt-tool. Care was taken to exclude esophageal and gastric lumen and surrounding tissue. A ROI was also drawn on baseline scans in healthy appearing gastric tissue.

Treatment

Patients were Scheduled for Three Cycles of Chemotherapy Preoperatively. after Completion of the Study, Patients Were Scheduled for Postoperative Chemotherapy, in Accordance with the MAGIC Study [10]. Each 3-Week Cycle Consisted of Epirubicin (50 Mg per Square Meter of Body-Surface Area) Intravenously on Day 1, Cisplatin (60 Mg per Square Meter) Or Oxaliplatin (130 Mg per Square Meter on Day 1) Intravenously on Day 1, Combined with Peroral Capecitabine (500 Mg per Square Meter Twice Daily) Continuously for 21 Days. Substituting Cisplatin with Oxaliplatin Has Proven to Be Non-Inferior and Was Considered an Alternative Regimen [17]. before and during Each Cycle of Treatment, a Full Blood Analysis Was Obtained Including Serum Creatinine Level. If Myelosuppression Or Thrombocytopenia Was Observed, Cycle 2 Or Cycle 3 Was Postponed until Normalisation of the Blood Count. Patients Were Closely Monitored for Side Effects during Chemotherapy and Modifications of the Dose Were Made Based on Observed Toxicity. Treatment Changes and Decisions Were Made Blinded for Any Changes Measured Using CT Perfusion. One Patient Did Not Start the Third Series of Chemotherapy Due to Side Effects. This Patient Was Later Classified as Both a Clinical and a Histological Responder.

Surgery

In patients with tumour at the gastro-esophageal junction an Ivor-Lewis Esophagectomy with extended D1+ lymphadenectomy was performed. In patients with a stomach tumour a complete gastrectomy was performed. One patient (tumour at the gastro-esophageal junction) was not resected due to local tumour growth invading the pancreas and was because of this classified as a clinical nonresponder without histological grading.

Clinical and Histological Response Evaluation

Responses were evaluated both clinically and histologically. Investigators performing the evaluations were blind to patient outcome and results of the imaging studies. For the clinical response evaluation, the endoscopic imaging and tumour length, measured with a straight endoscope at the level of the incisors, before chemotherapy was compared with the macroscopic measurements of tumour in the surgical specimen – taking tumour shrinkage of 10% due to fixation into account [18]. Patients with a tumour length reduction of more than 50% were classified as clinical responders. For the histological response evaluation, all surgical resection specimens were evaluated by a single experienced pathologist and the tumour response was graded according to a score established by Mandard et al [19]. Patients with no or a few scattered small tumour areas (regression score 1 and 2) were classified as responders. Patients with larger residual tumour areas (regression score 3,4 and 5) were classified as non-responders – see Figure 1A and 1B.

Tumour perfusion parameters at baseline were compared with perfusion parameters from normal gastric tissue. Changes between tumour perfusion parameters at baseline and the second, and third scans, were calculated using the following formulas, respectively, where brackets represent a perfusion measure:

$$\%\ early\ changes = \frac{[Baseline]-[2scan]}{[Baseline]} \cdot 100\%$$

$$\%\ late\ changes = \frac{[Baseline]-[3scan]}{[Baseline]} \cdot 100\%$$

Statistics

All statistical tests were performed using SPSS (version 20, IBM, USA). Perfusion parameters at baseline and at the third scan were compared between responders and nonresponders using Mann-Whitney U-test. Changes in tumour perfusion between first and second scans, and changes between first and third scans were compared between groups based on response type using univariate logistic regression. Comparisons of tumour tissue perfusion and normal gastric tissue perfusion was performed by using a Wilcoxon signed-rank test. A 2-sided p-value below 0.05 was considered statistically significant. A Receiver Operating Characteristic (ROC) analysis was made to determine the optimal diagnostic cut-off value for changes in perfusion parameters in regards of sensitivity and specificity for predicting clinical response.

Results

Baseline Values, Clinical and Histological Response

Of the 28 patients available for clinical response evaluation, 13 were classified as clinical responders and 15 were classified as nonresponders. One patient was not resected due to local tumour growth invading the pancreas and was because of this classified as a clinical nonresponder. Based on histological examination, eight cases (Mandard score 1 and 2, complete or subtotal regression) were classified as responders and 19 cases (Mandard score 3, 4 and 5) were classified as nonresponders. Table 1 summarises statistical results of baseline scanning of clinical responders and nonresponders. There were no significant statistical differences between the two groups at baseline. With regard to the histological response evaluation, the responding patients had significantly smaller tumours ($p<0.05$). Table 2 summarises differences in clinical and histological response evaluation. Comparison of tumour tissue

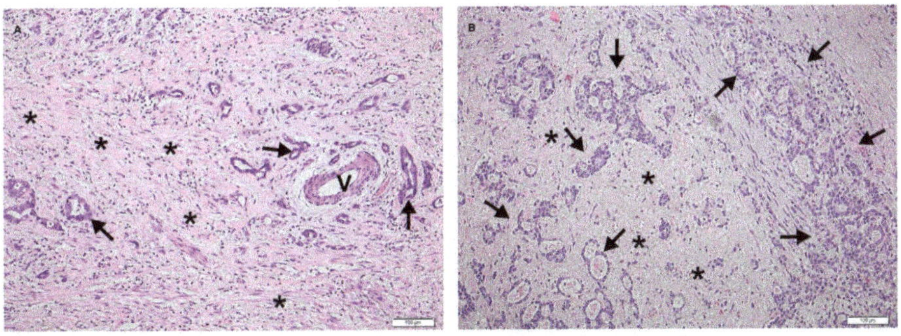

Figure 1. Illustration of histological response evaluation using Mandard score. A) Tumour regression grade 2 (Mandard). Few, scattered residual cancer areas (arrows) separated by fibrosis (*). One tumour area is surrounding a vessel (V) and another tumour area is seen to the left. This patient was a histological responder. B) Tumour regression grade 4 (Mandard). Residual cancer areas (arrows) outgrowing fibrosis (*). This patient was a histological nonresponder.

Table 1. Baseline perfusion parameters and tumour volume.

	Clinical Nonresponders (n = 15)	Clinical responders (n = 13)	p-value
Arterial flow mL·min^{-1}·100g^{-1}	107.4 (96.5–146.0)	116.1 (84.5–140.8)	p = 0.79
Blood volume mL·100g^{-1}	6.7 (4.1–7.5)	6.3 (3.4–9.6)	p = 0.90
Permeability (k^{trans}) mL·min^{-1}·100g^{-1}	25.2 (20.9–34.9)	28.9 (23.0–30.3)	p = 0.79
Tumour volume mL	34.3 (22.7–59.9)	30.8 (9.8–51.6)	p = 0.25

Meassurements for clinical responders and non-responders. Values are medians and interquartile range in parentheses.

perfusion and perfusion measured in normal gastric tissue revealed a significantly higher perfusion in tumour versus gastric tissue (116.0 mL·min^{-1}·100 g^{-1} versus 77.2 mL·min^{-1}·100 g^{-1}, $p < 0.01$).

Clinical Response: Changes in Perfusion Parameters and Tumour Volume after First Series of Chemotherapy

Figure 2 and 3 illustrate a clinical responder and a clinical nonresponder. Figure 4 illustrates a comparison of changes in tumour size and perfusion parameters from baseline to the first series of chemotherapy based on clinical response. A logistic regression analysis showed that response probability was positively correlated to a decrease in tumour permeability (p = 0.03). Eighteen out of 27 (67%) patients had decreases in permeability between baseline and after the first series of chemotherapy, whereof 11/13 (85%) were clinical responders and 7/14 (50%) were clinical nonresponders. This difference was not statistically significant (p = 0.10, Fisher's exact test). There were no significant changes in arterial flow, blood volume or tumour volume size when comparing responders to nonresponders.

Using ROC analysis (Figure 5), a cut-off value of more than 25% reduction in tumour permeability yielded a sensitivity of 69% and a specificity of 58% for predicting response after the first series of chemotherapy.

Clinical Response: Changes in Perfusion Parameters and Tumour Volume between Baseline and following 3 Series of Chemotherapy

After three series of chemotherapy, the probability of responding was correlated with a decrease in tumour permeability (p = 0.03). A decrease in tumour volume was also positively correlated with response (p = 0.01). The absolute change in blood volume was positively correlated with response (p = 0.03), but not in percentage change (p = 0.08).

Table 3 summarises changes in perfusion parameters and tumour volume after the first series of chemotherapy and after three series of chemotherapy.

Histological Response: Changes in Perfusion Parameters and Tumour Volume during Treatment

The logistic regression analysis showed that the probability of a histological response increased with a reduction in permeability (p = 0.03) and in tumour volume (p = 0.03) between baseline scan and after third series of chemotherapy. Changes in arterial flow and blood volume were not significant (p = 0.39 and p = 0.89, respectively). We observed no significant changes after the first series of chemotherapy in arterial flow (p = 0.39), blood volume (p = 0.42), permeability (p = 0.20), or tumour volume (p = 0.25). Comparison of perfusion parameters and tumour volume of the

Table 2. Clinical versus histological response.

	Clinical Nonresponders (n = 15)	Clinical Responders (n = 13)
Histological response (n = 27)		
Mandard 1		4
Mandard 2	1	3
Mandard 3	1	3
Mandard 4	8	2
Mandard 5	4	1
Not resected	1	
Tumour t-staging at baseline		
≤T2	1	5
= T3	12	7
= T4	2	1

Clinical response compared to histological response (Mandard Score 1 to 5) and tumour stage based on CT evaluation before chemotherapy.

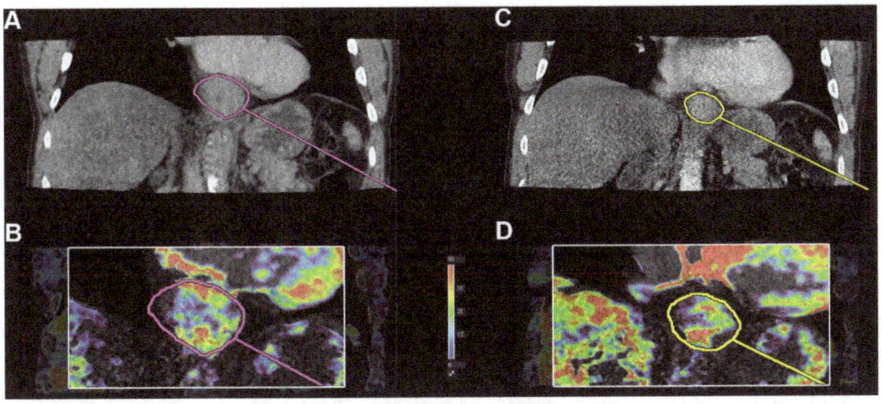

Figure 2. CT perfusion images of a clinical responder. Permeability k^{trans} parametric map in a clinical responder with a reduction in permeability between baseline and the first series of chemotherapy. **A+B)** Before chemotherapy ($k^{trans} = 32.1$ mL·min^{-1}·100 g^{-1}) **C+D)** After first series of chemotherapy ($k^{trans} = 23.9$ mL·min^{-1}·100 g^{-1}). Perfusion measures are averages from the entire tumor volume. The image illustrates perfusion measured in a reconstructed coronal plane which is possible with volume perfusion.

preoperative scan with histological response showed a significant difference in permeability between histological responders and nonresponders ($p<0.05$), as demonstrated by clinical response. Likewise, responding patients had significantly smaller tumours than non-responding patients ($p<0.01$). There were no statistically significant differences in blood volume ($p = 0.31$) and arterial flow ($p = 0.43$) (Figure 6).

One-year Follow up for Recurrence of Disease

Within the first year after inclusion 8 out of the 27 resected patients (30%) had recurrence of disease. Four of these 8 were clinical responders after surgery (4 out of all 13 clinical responders = 31%) and 1 was a histological responder (1 out of all 8 histological responders = 13%).

Discussion

The main finding of this study was that there was a positive correlation between a decrease in tumour permeability (k^{trans}) after one series of chemotherapy (three weeks) and treatment response after three series of chemotherapy measured by clinical response. This correlation appeared before significant changes in tumour volume were detectable in the scans. Patients with a histological response had a significantly lower tumour permeability compared to nonresponding patients. To our knowledge, this is the first longitudinal study using CT perfusion as a method to measure early response to pre-operative chemotherapy in GEJ and gastric cancer.

Perfusion is the delivery of blood through the vascular bed and can be estimated using different kinetic models. The basis of CT perfusion is the transport of a contrast material by blood flow through the intravascular space, and subsequently, the distribution

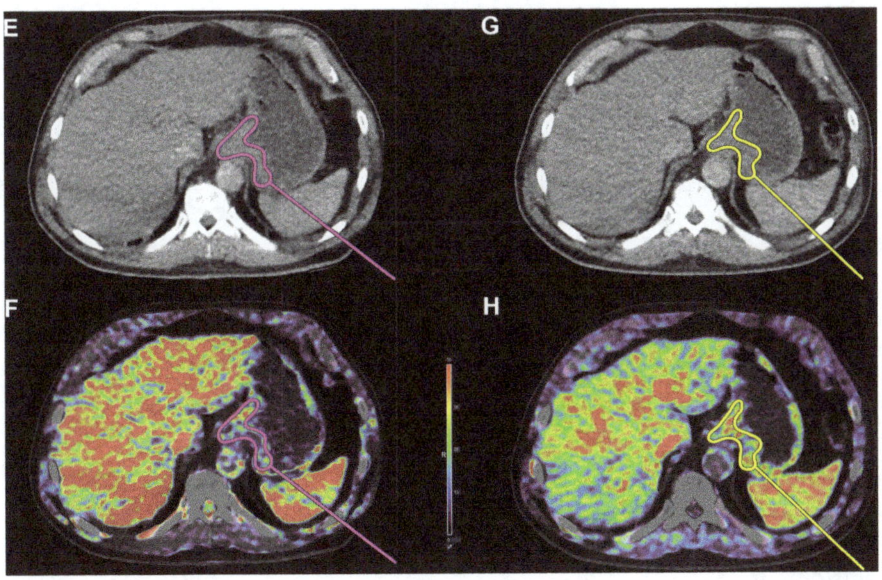

Figure 3. CT Perfusion images of a clinical nonresponder. Permeability k^{trans} in a clinical nonresponder. An increase in k^{trans} is observed. **E+F)** Before chemotherapy ($k^{trans} = 13.7$ mL·min^{-1}·100 g^{-1}) and **G+H)** After first series of chemotherapy ($k^{trans} = 21.0$ mL·min^{-1}·100 g^{-1}). Perfusion measures are averages from the entire tumor volume.

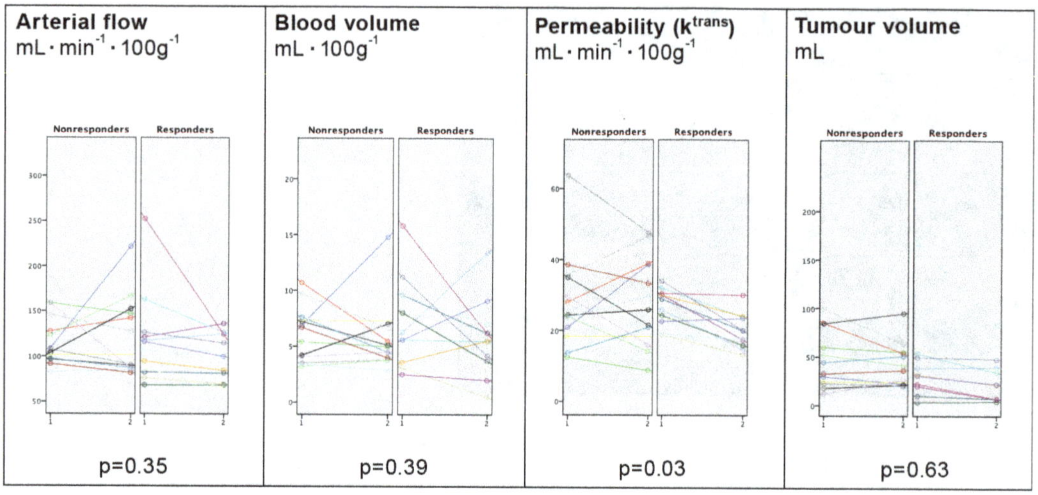

Figure 4. Early changes in perfusion parameters and tumour volume in clinical responders. Changes from baseline to first follow-up scan after first series of chemotherapy for the 27 cases available for early follow up evaluation. Each case is illustrated with a line between the baseline and the second scan. All values are in absolute numbers.

of the contrast material between the intravascular and extravascular interstitial space [20,21]. Previous studies using CT perfusion in esophageal and gastric cancer have found a significant correlation with blood volume [22–24] and permeability surface area product [22], and histological evaluation of micro vessel density [22–24] and Vascular Endothelial Growth Factor (VEGF) expression [25]. Likewise, Satoh et al. [26] found a negative correlation between tumour perfusion and stromal density. Makari

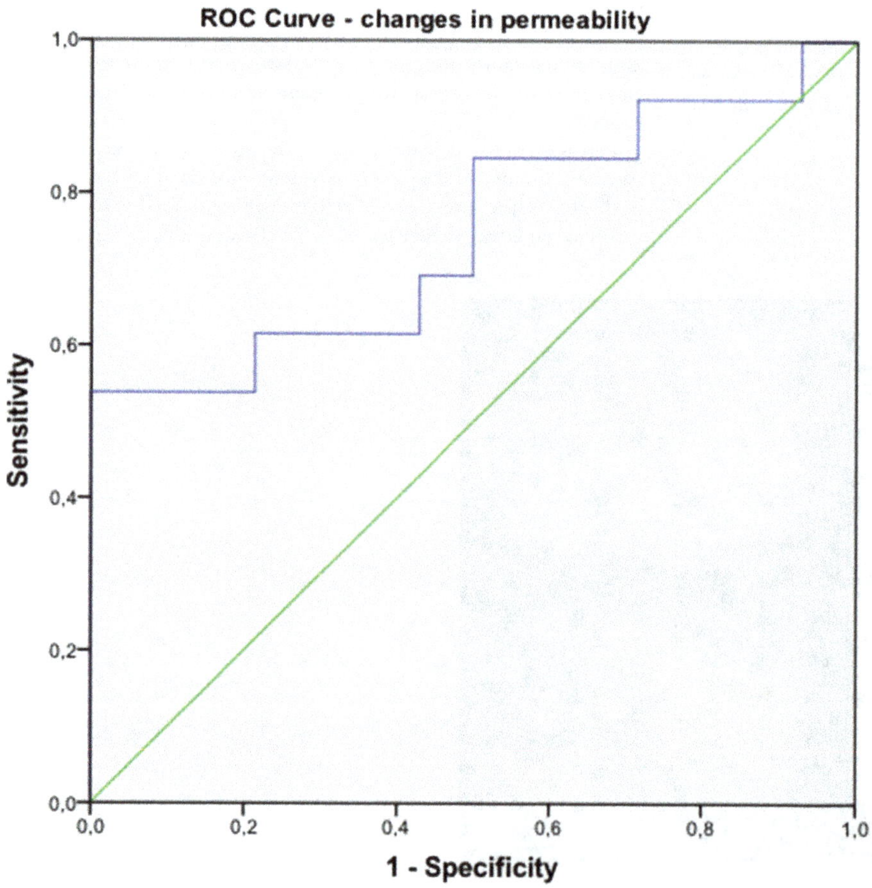

Figure 5. ROC analysis. ROC curve with a cut-off value of 25% reduction in permeability between baseline and early follow up scan. Area under curve is 0.74 (Confidence interval 0.55–0.93).

Table 3. Changes in perfusion parameters and tumour volume during preoperative chemotherapy.

	Clinical Nonresponders			Clinical Responders			Statistics*			
	Baseline	1. series	3. series	Baseline	1. series	3. series	After 1st series		After 3rd series	
							OR	p-value	OR	p-value
Arterial flow	107.4	91.6	102.3	116.1	100.2	88,1	0.992	p = 0.35	0.990	p = 0.31
$mL \cdot min^{-1} \cdot 100g^{-1}$	[96.5; 146.0]	[86.5; 148.4]	[81.1; 121.8]	[84.5; 140.8]	[75.5; 125.9]	[61.0; 103.6]	CI (0.973–1.010)		CI (0.972–1.009)	
		−7%	*−12%*		*−9%*	*−25%*	0.982	p = 0.23	0.986	p = 0.32
		[−13%; 22%]	*[−27%; 7%]*		*[−20%; 0%]*	*[−30%; −11%]*	CI (0.953–1.012)		CI (0.959–1.014)	
Blood volume	6.7	5.1	5.0	6.3	5.5	3.4	0.886	p = 0.39	0.699	**p = 0.03**
$mL \cdot 100g^{-1}$	[4.1; 7.5]	[4.0; 6.7]	[3.7; 8.0]	[3.4; 9.6]	[3.5; 6.6]	[2.5; 5.2]	CI (0.740–1.125)		CI (0.506–0.966)	
		−9%	*−15%*		*−27%*	*−47%*	1.002	p = 0.56	0.982	p = 0.08
		[−34%; 21%]	*[−49%; 20%]*		*[−41%; −3%]*	*[−10%; −67%]*	CI (0.995–1.010)		CI (0.962–1.002)	
Permeability (k^{trans})	25.2	28.4	26.9	28.9	20.1	16.3	0.880	p = **0.03**	0.881	**p = 0.03**
$mL \cdot min^{-1} \cdot 100g^{-1}$	[20.9; 34.9]	[19.8; 38.9]	[18.3; 32.4]	[23.0; 30.3]	[15.5; 23.8]	[11.3; 20.1]	CI (0.786–0.985)		CI (0.786–0.987)	
		+2%	*+1%*		*−30%*	*−43%*	0.964	p = **0.03**	0.962	**p = 0.03**
		[−31%; 37%]	*[−30%; 18%]*		*[−41%; −3%]*	*[−53%; −16%]*	CI (0.933–0.996)		CI (0.930–0.996)	
Tumour volume	34.3	38.9 **	38.8	30.8	21.8	11.4	0.987	p = 0.63	0.916	p = **0.03**
mL	[22.7; 59.9]	[21.0; 54.2]	[14.7; 54.7]	[9.8; 51.6]	[7.1; 38.3]	[5.5; 23.0]	CI (0.947–1.033)		CI (0.846–0.991)	
		−14%	*−10%*		*−29%*	*−56%*	0.992	p = 0.47	0.947	p = **0.01**
		[−37%; 13%]	*[−33%; 18%]*		*[−43%; −1%]*	*[−73%; −47%]*	CI (0.970–1.014)		CI (0.910–0.987)	

Perfusion parameters and tumour volume before, after first series of chemotherapy and after third series of chemotherapy grouped by clinical response. Reported values are median values and interquartile range.
*Odds ratio and 95% confidence intervals are reported on both absolute changes and changes in percentage using logistic regression. Significant p-values are highlighted.
**Although the median is higher after first series of chemotherapy versus baseline, the median change is negative.

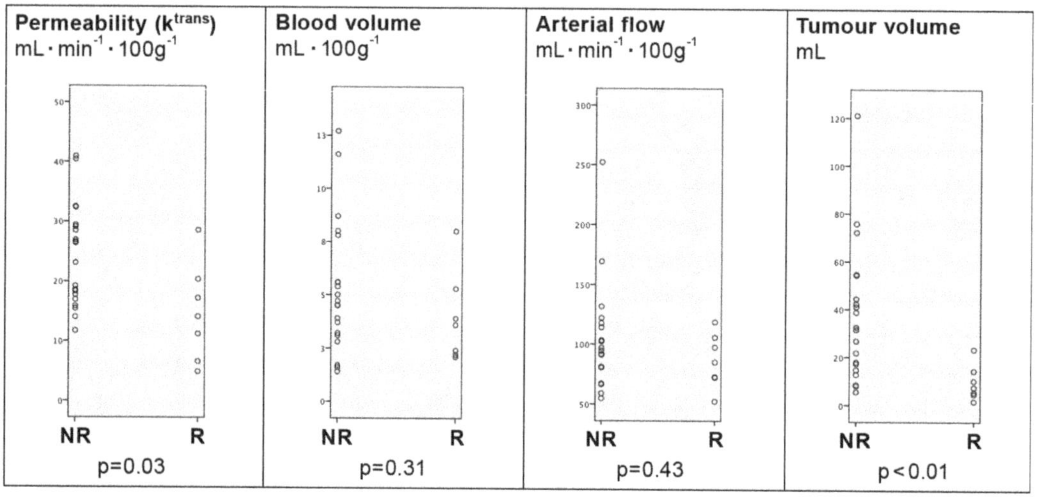

Figure 6. Pre-operative scan and histological response based on Mandard Score. Correlation between perfusion parameters pre-operatively and histological response. n = 27.

et al. [27] examined changes in tumour perfusion before and after chemo-radiation in esophageal squamous cell carcinoma and found a positive correlation between perfusion changes and tumour size reduction. Our baseline perfusion measures are in the same range as some studies [22,28], and differs from other studies [24,25]. The analysis software used in this study is based on two kinetic models: the maximum slope method to estimate tissue perfusion and Patlak method to estimate both blood volume and permeability (k^{trans}), which is the rate constant for transfer between the intravascular and extravascular (interstitial) spaces. The lack of standardisation of CT perfusion protocols, and implementation of kinetic models complicate direct comparison of values between studies.

The first adoptions of the CT perfusion technique were limited to single slice studies. With the use of a 320-detector row CT scanner it is possible to cover 16 cm in a single gantry rotation, thereby improving the temporal resolution compared to a helical scan [29]. A 16 cm coverage enables correction for motion in all three planes, which allows a free-breathing scan protocol, and makes three-dimensional volume perfusion measurements possible [30]. We observed a significant correlation between a reduction in permeability and response to chemotherapy. It has been shown, that cisplatin inhibits the expression of growth factors e.g. in ovarian cancer cells [31,32] and as growth factors are important for angiogenesis in tumour growth, this inhibition could explain some of the observed reductions in permeability. Previous longitudinal studies using CT perfusion of colorectal cancer [7,8] have demonstrated a significant post-therapeutic reduction in blood volume (84 and 91 days, respectively), but these studies did not examine any differences in changes between responders and nonresponders. A post-therapeutic reduction in blood volume has been demonstrated in lung cancer [33,34], in blood flow in liver metastasis after 3 weeks [4,35] and in blood volume in animal models of hepatic tumours [36,37]. Our study did not show any early changes in blood volume, but the reduction was significant in absolute numbers after three series of chemotherapy (table 3).

The clinical response rate in our study was 46% (13/28), which is comparable to those of other response evaluation studies of esophageal and gastric cancer [15]. Not all patients exhibiting a clinical response also demonstrated a histological response. Despite a significant reduction in tumour volume, some regions of tumour might display groups of viable tumour cells, which would classify the patient as a non-responder based on histopathological grading. Histopathological evaluation of regression is considered a gold standard for response evaluation and is clearly associated with survival (34). In our study, only 1 out of 8 patients with histological response had recurrence within the first year, whereas 4 out of 13 patients with clinical response had recurrence. This indicates, that response evaluation based on tumour size reduction is unreliable. The clinical utility of histopathological grading is however limited to modifying only the postoperative, adjuvant therapy.

Other imaging modalities have been used for response assessment of preoperative chemotherapy for adenocarcinomas in the esophagus and at the gastroesophageal junction. Studies using Positron Emission Tomography (PET) with fludeoxyglucose (FDG) as tracer [13,14] have demonstrated a larger reduction in FDG uptake in responding versus nonresponding tumours after 14 days of neoadjuvant chemotherapy. The MUNICON-1 trial [38] indicated that chemotherapy can be discontinued at an early stage in metabolic nonresponders without compromising the prognosis. MUNICON-2 [39] showed that the addition of neoadjuvant radiotherapy in metabolic nonresponders did not lead to an improvement of their poor prognosis, thus showing that early non-response indicates dismal tumour biology. The MUNICON trials thus illustrated the feasibility of a PET-response-guided treatment algorithm. However, larger, randomised trials are needed. A large fraction of gastric cancers are also found to be non-FDG-avid and PET has been proven not as informative in the evaluation of early response to chemotherapy [40,41]. The advantages of CT perfusion compared to PET-FDG are the great availability of scanners, the easy handling of contrast material, and the possibility of adding vascular physiological measures to already existing diagnostic protocols. CT perfusion could also be applied in a combination with PET/CT imaging.

There are some limitations to our study. First, our study sample is small and the data presented should be interpreted with this in mind. Secondly, albeit GEJ and gastric cancer arise from the same epithelial cells, they are located at different sites in the gastrointestinal tract, with possible different outcome to treatment. There is consensus on treating the cancers in the same peri-operative setting, and the MAGIC trial [10] and a study by Ychou et al. [9] confirms no difference in outcome between esophageal and gastric cancer. Thirdly, cancers in the gastrointestinal tract are difficult tumours to visualise with high resolution imaging technology. The organs are affected both extrinsically by respiratory and cardiac movement, and intrinsically due to peristalsis and varying distension of the lumen. We compensated for some of these factors by applying motion correction to the dataset and administering a motility inhibitor. Fourthly we included all patients with both GEJ and gastric cancer eligible for perioperative chemotherapy and made no selection bias on tumour size. The tumour sizes in our study were smaller compared to other studies with response evaluation [13,38]. Lastly, our clinical response evaluation is based on tumour size reduction. There is evidence of histological response evaluation as predictor of recurrence and overall survival, whereas validation on tumour size reduction (clinical response) lacks. Our 1-year follow up indicates a higher frequency of recurrence among clinical responders compared to histological responders.

In conclusion, our study found a positive correlation between an early decrease in tumour permeability (k^{trans}) after one series of chemotherapy and the response after three series of chemotherapy, based on tumour size reduction. A cut-off value with a reduction in permeability of more than 25% gives a sensitivity of 69% and a specificity of 58% after one series of chemotherapy, which makes the diagnostic quality moderate and insufficient as a single discriminatory test. With regards to histological response, our study finds significantly lower permeability in responding tumours compared to non-responding after three series of chemotherapy, but not after the first series of chemotherapy. Histological response evaluation seems better than clinical response to estimate the risk of recurrence of disease.

Acknowledgments

Radiographers Tina Bock-Pedersen, Beth Reimer and Jane Ellingsgaard are thanked for technical assistance. Statistician Ulla B Mogensen, Department of Biostatistics, University of Copenhagen is thanked for statistical assistance.

Author Contributions

Conceived and designed the experiments: MLH EF LB BF LBS MBN. Performed the experiments: MLH EF LB BF LBS. Analyzed the data: MLH EF CL IL BF LBS. Wrote the paper: MLH EF CL BF IL LB LBS MBN.

References

1. Li Z-P, Meng Q-F, Sun C-H, Xu D-S, Fan M, et al. (2005) Tumor angiogenesis and dynamic CT in colorectal carcinoma: radiologic-pathologic correlation. World J Gastroenterol 11: 1287–1291.
2. Hayano K, Okazumi S, Shuto K, Matsubara H, Shimada H, et al. (2007) Perfusion CT can predict the response to chemoradiation therapy and survival in esophageal squamous cell carcinoma: Initial clinical results. Oncology Reports 18: 901–908.
3. Koyasu S, Isoda H, Tsuji Y, Yamamoto H, Matsueda K, et al. (2012) Hepatic arterial perfusion increases in the early stage of severe acute pancreatitis patients: evaluation by perfusion computed tomography. Eur J Radiol 81: 43–46.
4. Jiang T, Kambadakone A, Kulkarni NM, Zhu AX, Sahani DV (2012) Monitoring response to antiangiogenic treatment and predicting outcomes in advanced hepatocellular carcinoma using image biomarkers, CT perfusion, tumor density, and tumor size (RECIST). Invest Radiol 47: 11–17.
5. Fournier LS, Oudard S, Thiam R, Trinquart L, Banu E, et al. (2010) Metastatic Renal Carcinoma: Evaluation of Antiangiogenic Therapy with Dynamic Contrast-enhanced CT1. Radiology 256: 511–518.
6. D' Assignies G, Couvelard A, Bahrami S, Vullierme M-P, Hammel P, et al. (2009) Pancreatic endocrine tumors: tumor blood flow assessed with perfusion CT reflects angiogenesis and correlates with prognostic factors. Radiology 250: 407–416.
7. Bellomi M, Petralia G, Sonzogni A, Zampino MG, Rocca A (2007) CT Perfusion for the Monitoring of Neoadjuvant Chemotherapy and Radiation Therapy in Rectal Carcinoma: Initial Experience. Radiology 244: 486–493.
8. Sahani DV, Kalva SP, Hamberg LM, Hahn PF, Willett CG, et al. (2005) Assessing tumor perfusion and treatment response in rectal cancer with multisection CT: initial observations. Radiology 234: 785–792.
9. Ychou M, Boige V, Pignon J-P, Conroy T, Bouché O, et al. (2011) Perioperative chemotherapy compared with surgery alone for resectable gastroesophageal adenocarcinoma: an FNCLCC and FFCD multicenter phase III trial. J Clin Oncol 29: 1715–1721.
10. Cunningham D, Allum WH, Stenning SP, Thompson JN, Van de Velde CJH, et al. (2006) Perioperative Chemotherapy versus Surgery Alone for Resectable Gastroesophageal Cancer. New England Journal of Medicine 355: 11–20.
11. Sjoquist KM, Burmeister BH, Smithers BM, Zalcberg JR, Simes RJ, et al. (2011) Survival after neoadjuvant chemotherapy or chemoradiotherapy for resectable oesophageal carcinoma: an updated meta-analysis. Lancet Oncol 12: 681–692.
12. Van Hagen P, Hulshof MCCM, van Lanschot JJB, Steyerberg EW, Henegouwen MI van B, et al. (2012) Preoperative Chemoradiotherapy for Esophageal or Junctional Cancer. New England Journal of Medicine 366: 2074–2084.
13. Weber WA, Ott K, Becker K, Dittler H-J, Helmberger H, et al. (2001) Prediction of Response to Preoperative Chemotherapy in Adenocarcinomas of the Esophagogastric Junction by Metabolic Imaging. JCO 19: 3058–3065.
14. Wieder HA, Ott K, Lordick F, Becker K, Stahl A, et al. (2007) Prediction of tumor response by FDG-PET: comparison of the accuracy of single and sequential studies in patients with adenocarcinomas of the esophagogastric junction. Eur J Nucl Med Mol Imaging 34: 1925–1932.
15. Chen Y, Pan X, Tong L, Shi Y, Chen T (2011) Can 18F-fluorodeoxyglucose positron emission tomography predict responses to neoadjuvant therapy in oesophageal cancer patients? A meta-analysis. Nuclear Medicine Communications November 2011 32: 1005–1010.
16. McShane LM, Altman DG, Sauerbrei W, Taube SE, Gion M, et al. (2005) REporting recommendations for tumour MARKer prognostic studies (REMARK). Br J Cancer 93: 387–391.
17. Cunningham D, Starling N, Rao S, Iveson T, Nicolson M, et al. (2008) Capecitabine and Oxaliplatin for Advanced Esophagogastric Cancer. New England Journal of Medicine 358: 36–46.
18. Siu KF, Cheung HC, Wong J (1986) Shrinkage of the esophagus after resection for carcinoma. Ann Surg 203: 173–176.
19. Mandard A-M, Dalibard F, Mandard J-C, Marnay J, Henry-Amar M, et al. (1994) Pathologic assessment of tumor regression after preoperative chemoradiotherapy of esophageal carcinoma. Clinicopathologic correlations. Cancer 73: 2680–2686.
20. Lundsgaard Hansen M, Norling R, Lauridsen C, Fallentin E, Bæksgaard L, et al. (n.d.) Computed Tomography (CT) Perfusion in Abdominal Cancer: Technical Aspects. Diagnostics 2013, 3, 261–270.
21. Lee T-Y, Purdie TG, Stewart E (2003) CT imaging of angiogenesis. Q J Nucl Med 47: 171–187.
22. Song T, Shen Y-G, Jiao N-N, Li X-H, Hu H-T, et al. (2012) Esophageal Squamous Cell Carcinoma: Assessing Tumor Angiogenesis Using Multi-Slice CT Perfusion Imaging. Dig Dis Sci 57: 2195–2202.
23. Yao J, Yang Z-G, Chen H-J, Chen T-W, Huang J (2010) Gastric adenocarcinoma: can perfusion CT help to noninvasively evaluate tumor angiogenesis? Abdom Imaging. 2011 Feb;36(1):15–21.
24. Chen T-W, Yang Z-G, Li Y, Li Z-L, Yao J, et al. (2009) Quantitative assessment of first-pass perfusion of oesophageal squamous cell carcinoma using 64-section MDCT: initial observation. Clinical Radiology 64: 38–45.
25. Chen T -W, Yang Z-G, Chen H-J, Li Y, Tang S-S, et al. (2012) Quantitative assessment of first-pass perfusion using a low-dose method at multidetector CT in oesophageal squamous cell carcinoma: Correlation with VEGF expression. Clinical Radiology 67: 746–753.
26. Satoh A, Shuto K, Okazumi S, Ohira G, Natsume T, et al. (2010) Role of Perfusion CT in Assessing Tumor Blood Flow and Malignancy Level of Gastric Cancer. Digestive Surgery 27: 253–260.
27. Makari Y, Yasuda T, Doki Y, Miyata H, Fujiwara Y, et al. (2007) Correlation between tumor blood flow assessed by perfusion CT and effect of neoadjuvant therapy in advanced esophageal cancers. Journal of Surgical Oncology 96: 220–229.
28. Motosugi U, Ichikawa T, Sou H, Morisaka H, Sano K, et al. (2012) Multi-organ perfusion CT in the abdomen using a 320-detector row CT scanner: Preliminary results of perfusion changes in the liver, spleen, and pancreas of cirrhotic patients. European journal of radiology. 2012 Oct; 81(10):2533–7.
29. Goh V, Liaw J, Bartram CI, Halligan S (2008) Effect of Temporal Interval Between Scan Acquisitions on Quantitative Vascular Parameters in Colorectal

Cancer: Implications for Helical Volumetric Perfusion CT Techniques. AJR 191: W288–W292.

30. Ng QS, Goh V, Klotz E, Fichte H, Saunders MI, et al. (2006) Quantitative Assessment of Lung Cancer Perfusion Using MDCT: Does Measurement Reproducibility Improve with Greater Tumor Volume Coverage? AJR 187: 1079–1084.
31. Duyndam MCA, van Berkel MPA, Dorsman JC, Rockx DAP, Pinedo HM, et al. (2007) Cisplatin and doxorubicin repress Vascular Endothelial Growth Factor expression and differentially down-regulate Hypoxia-inducible Factor I activity in human ovarian cancer cells. Biochemical Pharmacology 74: 191–201.
32. Zhong X-S, Liu L-Z, Skinner HD, Cao Z, Ding M, et al. (2007) Mechanism of vascular endothelial growth factor expression mediated by cisplatin in human ovarian cancer cells. Biochemical and Biophysical Research Communications 358: 92–98.
33. Tacelli N, Santangelo T, Scherpereel A, Duhamel A, Deken V, et al. (2013) Perfusion CT allows prediction of therapy response in non-small cell lung cancer treated with conventional and anti-angiogenic chemotherapy. Eur Radiol 23: 2127–2136.
34. Fraioli F, Anzidei M, Serra G, Liberali S, Fiorelli A, et al. (2013) Whole-tumour CT-perfusion of unresectable lung cancer for the monitoring of anti-angiogenetic chemotherapy effects. The British Journal of Radiology 86: 20120174.
35. Kim DH, Kim SH, Im S-A, Han S-W, Goo JM, et al. (2012) Intermodality comparison between 3D perfusion CT and 18F-FDG PET/CT imaging for predicting early tumor response in patients with liver metastasis after chemotherapy: preliminary results of a prospective study. Eur J Radiol 81: 3542–3550.
36. Ma G-L, Bai R-J, Jiang H-J, Hao X-J, Dong X-P, et al. (2012) Early changes of hepatic hemodynamics measured by functional CT perfusion in a rabbit model of liver tumor. Hepatobiliary Pancreat Dis Int. 2012 Aug 15; 11(4):407–11.
37. Stewart EE, Sun H, Chen X, Schafer PH, Chen Y, et al. (2012) Effect of an angiogenesis inhibitor on hepatic tumor perfusion and the implications for adjuvant cytotoxic therapy. Radiology 264: 68–77.
38. Lordick F, Ott K, Krause B-J, Weber WA, Becker K, et al. (2007) PET to assess early metabolic response and to guide treatment of adenocarcinoma of the oesophagogastric junction: the MUNICON phase II trial. The Lancet Oncology 8: 797–805.
39. Zum Büschenfelde CM, Herrmann K, Schuster T, Geinitz H, Langer R, et al. (2011) (18)F-FDG PET-guided salvage neoadjuvant radiochemotherapy of adenocarcinoma of the esophagogastric junction: the MUNICON II trial. J Nucl Med 52: 1189–1196.
40. Mukai K, Ishida Y, Okajima K, Isozaki H, Morimoto T, et al. (2006) Usefulness of preoperative FDG-PET for detection of. Gastric Cancer 9: 192–196.
41. Ott K, Herrmann K, Schuster T, Langer R, Becker K, et al. (2011) Molecular imaging of proliferation and glucose utilization: utility for monitoring response and prognosis after neoadjuvant therapy in locally advanced gastric cancer. Ann Surg Oncol 18: 3316–3323.

2

IGFBP3 Methylation is a Novel Diagnostic and Predictive Biomarker in Colorectal Cancer

Lucia Perez-Carbonell[1], Francesc Balaguer[2], Yuji Toiyama[1], Cecilia Egoavil[3], Estefania Rojas[3], Carla Guarinos[4], Montserrat Andreu[5], Xavier Llor[6], Antoni Castells[2], Rodrigo Jover[7], C. Richard Boland[1]*, Ajay Goel[1]*

1 Division of Gastroenterology, Department of Internal Medicine, Charles Sammons Cancer Center and Baylor Research Institute, Baylor University Medical Center, Dallas, Texas, United States of America, **2** Gastroenterology Department, Hospital Clinic, CIBERehd, IDIBAPS, University of Barcelona, Barcelona, Spain, **3** Department of Pathology, Hospital General Universitario de Alicante, Alicante, Spain, **4** Research Unit, Hospital General Universitario de Alicante, Alicante, Spain, **5** Gastroenterology Department, Hospital del Mar, Barcelona, Spain, **6** Department of Medicine and Cancer Center, University of Illinois at Chicago, Chicago, Illinois, United States of America, **7** Unidad de Gastroenterología, Hospital General Universitario de Alicante, Alicante, Spain

Abstract

Background and Aim: Aberrant hypermethylation of cancer-related genes has emerged as a promising strategy for the development of diagnostic, prognostic and predictive biomarkers in human cancer, including colorectal cancer (CRC). The aim of this study was to perform a systematic and comprehensive analysis of a panel of CRC-specific genes as potential diagnostic, prognostic and predictive biomarkers in a large, population-based CRC cohort.

Patients and Methods: Methylation status of the *SEPT9, TWIST1, IGFBP3, GAS7, ALX4 and miR137* genes was studied by quantitative bisulfite pyrosequencing in a population-based cohort of 425 CRC patients.

Results: Methylation levels of all genes analyzed were significantly higher in tumor tissues compared to normal mucosa ($p < 0.0001$); however, cancer-associated hypermethylation was most frequently observed for *miR137* (86.7%) and *IGFBP3* (83%) in CRC patients. Methylation analysis using the combination of these two genes demonstrated greatest accuracy for the identification of colonic tumors (sensitivity 95.5%; specificity 90.5%). Low levels of *IGFBP3* promoter methylation emerged as an independent risk factor for predicting poor disease free survival in stage II and III CRC patients (HR = 0.49, 95% CI: 0.28–0.85, p = 0.01). Our results also suggest that stage II & III CRC patients with high levels of *IGFBP3* methylation do not benefit from adjuvant 5FU-based chemotherapy.

Conclusion: By analyzing a large, population-based CRC cohort, we demonstrate the potential clinical significance of *miR137* and *IGFBP3* hypermethylation as promising diagnostic biomarkers in CRC. Our data also revealed that *IGFBP3 hyper*methylation may serve as an independent prognostic and predictive biomarker in stage II and III CRC patients.

Editor: Hassan Ashktorab, Howard University, United States of America

Funding: The present work was supported by grant R01 CA72851 and CA181572 from the National Cancer Institute, National Institutes of Health and funds from the Baylor Research Institute. Lucia Perez-Carbonell is a recipient of a 2012 post-doctoral grant from Fundación Alfonso Martín Escudero. Francesc Balaguer is a recipient of a grant from the Instituto de Salud Carlos III (PI10/00384). CIBEREHD is funded by the Instituto de Salud Carlos III. Carla Guarinos is a recipient of a grant from the Generalitat Valenciana (Vall+D Acif/2010/018). The funders had no role in study design, data collection and analysis, decision to publish, or preparation of the manuscript.

* Email: ajay.goel@baylorhealth.edu (AG); rickbo@baylorhealth.edu (CRB)

Introduction

Colorectal cancer (CRC) is one of the most common cancers in Western countries, and is the second leading cause of cancer-related deaths in adults [1]. Accumulating evidence indicates that epigenetic changes play an essential role in the pathogenesis of CRC. Aberrant DNA methylation represents one of the most studied epigenetic alteration, and it is well understood that tumor suppressor genes are frequently silenced by methylation of CpG islands which commonly reside in the 5′ regions of approximately half of all human genes [2,3,4]. Transcriptional silencing of tumor suppressor genes has emerged as an important step in the step-wise process of colorectal carcinogenesis. Epigenetic alterations, particularly DNA hypermethylation, can be used for the early detection of premalignant lesions, including adenomatous polyps in the colon, and is present in the non-neoplastic tissues adjacent to adenomatous polyps and cancers in the colon [5,6]. In addition to their use as diagnostic biomarkers, epigenetic changes show promise as determinants of cancer prognosis, as well as biomarkers for response to specific chemotherapies [7,8].

In CRC, systematic genome-wide approaches have identified several genes that show tumor-specific promoter hypermethylation

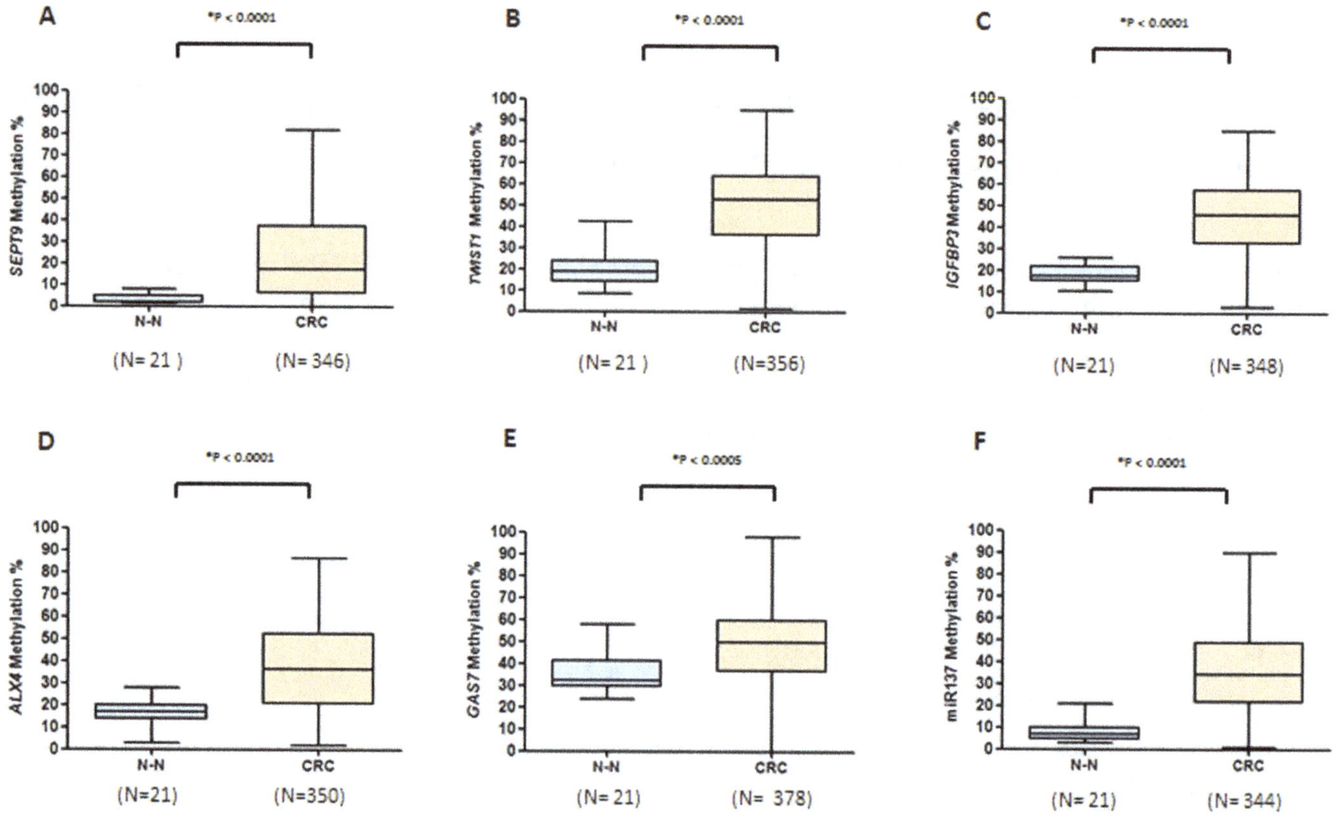

Figure 1. Comparison between levels of methylation in primary tumors vs. normal colonic mucosa. Bisulfite pyrosequencing results for methylation of *SEPT9* (A), *TWIST1* (B), *IGFBP3* (C), *ALX4* (D), *GAS7* (E) and *miR137* (F) genes comparing normal mucosa from healthy controls (N–N) and primary tumors from CRC patients.

that can potentially be developed into clinically relevant diagnostic, prognostic and predictive biomarkers. In the context of CRC, several such biomarkers have recently been described as potentially promising diagnostic biomarkers, including: *SEPT9* (Septin 9), a member of the septin family involved in cytokinesis and cell cycle control [9,10,11]; *ALX4* (Homeobox protein aristaless-like 4), a transcription factor involved in skull and limb development [12,13]; *TWIST1* (Twist homolog 1), an antiapoptotic and prometastatic transcription factor [14,15]; *IGFBP3* (Insulin-like grown factor binding protein 3), a member of the insulin-like growth factor binding protein family [16]; *GAS7* (growth arrest-specific 7), which plays a putative role in neuronal development [17,18]; and *miR137*, a non-coding microRNA which is embedded in a CpG island [17,19,20,21]. However, to date, none of these methylation markers have undergone a systematic validation in a large cohort of CRC patients to fully ascertain their potential as clinically useful diagnostic, prognostic or predictive biomarkers. For this reason, we aimed at exploring the diagnostic, prognostic and predictive value of *SEPT9, TWIST1, ALX4, IGFBP3, GAS7*, and *miR137* promoter hypermethylation in a large, well-characterized, population-based CRC cohort. Furthermore, we examined associations between the methylation status of individual markers and their combination with the clinicopathological features in these primary CRCs, and for the first time report that *IGFBP3* hypermethylation is a promising diagnostic and predictive biomarker in CRC patients.

Material and Methods

Patients

This study included 425 CRC patients that were enrolled as part of the Epicolon-I project, which is a population-based trial of CRC as described previously [22,23,24]. Since this study aimed to determine the prognostic and predictive potential of methylation biomarkers, the patient specimens included in this study were randomly selected from a previously described cohort of patients for whom follow-up data were available [7,25,26]. Demographic, clinical, and tumor-related characteristics of probands, as well as a detailed family history, were obtained using a previously established questionnaire [22]. Clinicopathological and molecular features of patients included in those studies are described in **Table S1.** The study was approved by the ethics committee of all participating hospitals in the EPICOLON cohort (Hospital 12 de Octubre, Madrid; Hospital Clinic, Barcelona; Hospital Clínico Universitario, Zaragoza; Hospital Cristal-Pinor, Complexo Hospitalario de Ourense; Parc de Salut Mar, Barcelona; Hospital Donostia, CIBERehd, University of Country Basque, San Sebastian; Hospital General Universitario de Alicante; Hospital General de Granollers; Hospital General de Vic; Hospital General Universitario de Guadalajara and Fundación para la Formación e Investigación Sanitarias Murcia; Hospital General Universitario de Valencia), and written informed consent was obtained from each patient. The promoter methylation status of six genes (*SEPT9, TWIST1, IGFBP3, GAS7, ALX4* and *miR-137*) was analyzed in all 425 CRC patients, as well as in normal colonic mucosa from 21 healthy individuals with a normal colonoscopy.

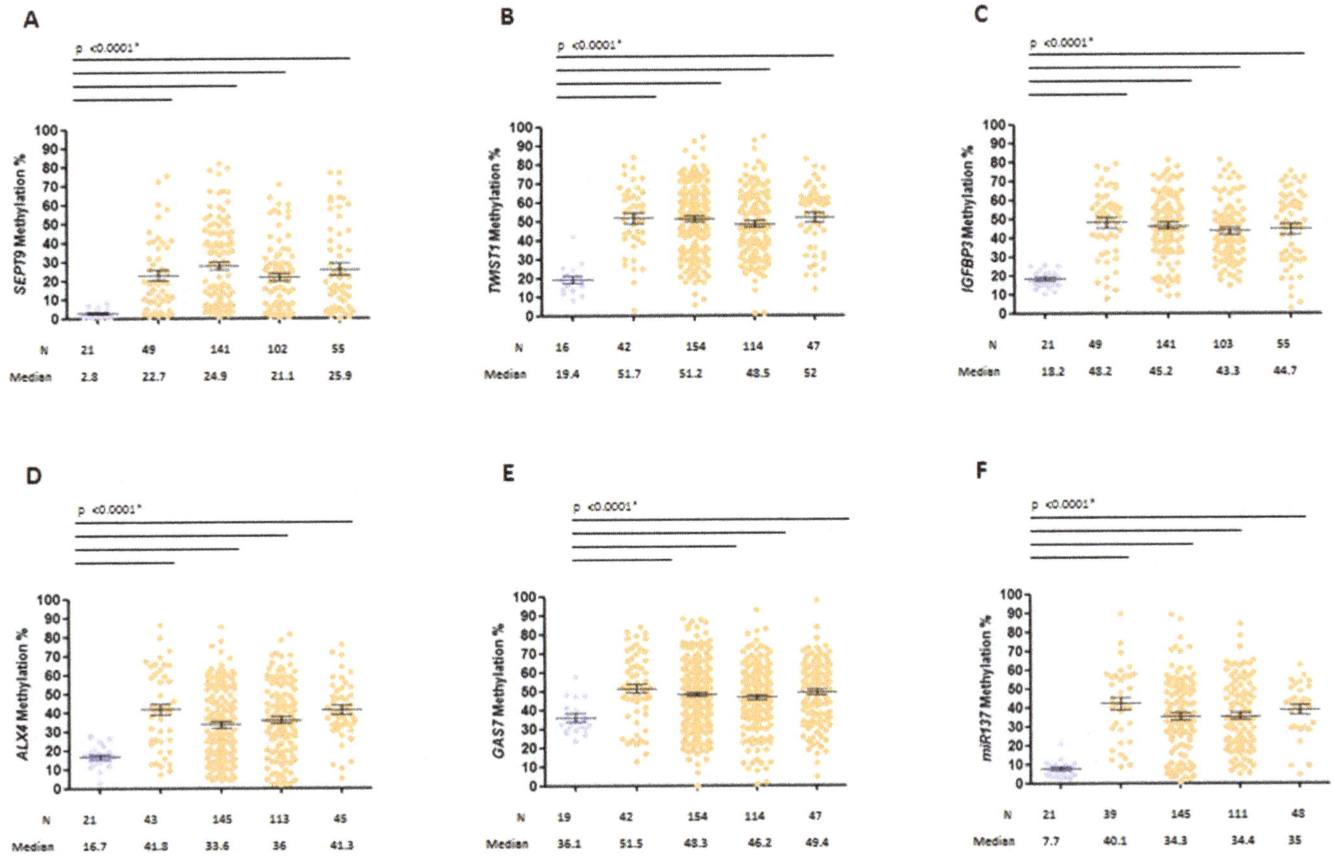

Figure 2. Levels of methylation in normal colonic mucosa and crc tumors from all tnm stage patients. Bisulfite pyrosequencing results of methylation of *sept9* (a), *twist1* (b), *igfbp3* (c), *alx4* (d), *gas7* (e) and *mir137* (f) comparing normal mucosa from healthy patients (n-n) and primary tumors from crc patients of all tnm stages i–iv. n (number of subjects); median of methylation (%).

DNA extraction and bisulfite modification

Genomic DNA was extracted from paraffin-embedded tumor tissue (FFPE) specimens in the Epicolon-I study. Under supervision of the study pathologist, tissue sections were carefully examined, tumor-enriched regions identified and carefully dissected for DNA extraction. Following paraffin removal by xylene, DNA was isolated using QiaAmp DNA Mini kits, as per the manufacturer's instructions (Qiagen, Valencia, CA). The resultant genomic DNA was modified with sodium-bisulfite using the EZ Methylation Gold Kit (Zymo Research, Orange, CA).

DNA Methylation analysis

Bisulfite pyrosequencing was performed for quantitative methylation analysis as previously described (**Figure S1**) [7,25,26].

Table 1. Performance Characteristics Of Methylation Markers For The Identification Of Colorectal Cancer.

Gene(s)	Sensitivity (%)	Specificity (%)	PPV (%)	NPV (%)	Accuracy (%)
SEPT9	70.5	95.2	99.6	16.4	65.8
TWIST1	75.6	93.8	99.6	14.7	69.3
IGFBP3	83.0	100.0	100.0	26.3	83.0
GAS7	42.9	94.4	99.4	7.3	37.3
ALX4	61.1	100.0	100.0	13.4	61.6
miR137	87.8	90.5	99.3	31.1	78.3
miR137+*IGFBP3*	95.5	90.5	99.3	59.4	86.0
TWIST1+IGFBP3	92.2	90.5	99.3	45.2	82.7
***TWIST1*+miR137**	92.8	85.7	98.9	45.0	78.5
miR137+IGFBP3+TWIST1	98.7	93.3	99.3	87.5	92.0

PPV, Positive Predictive Value; NPV, Negative Predictive Value.

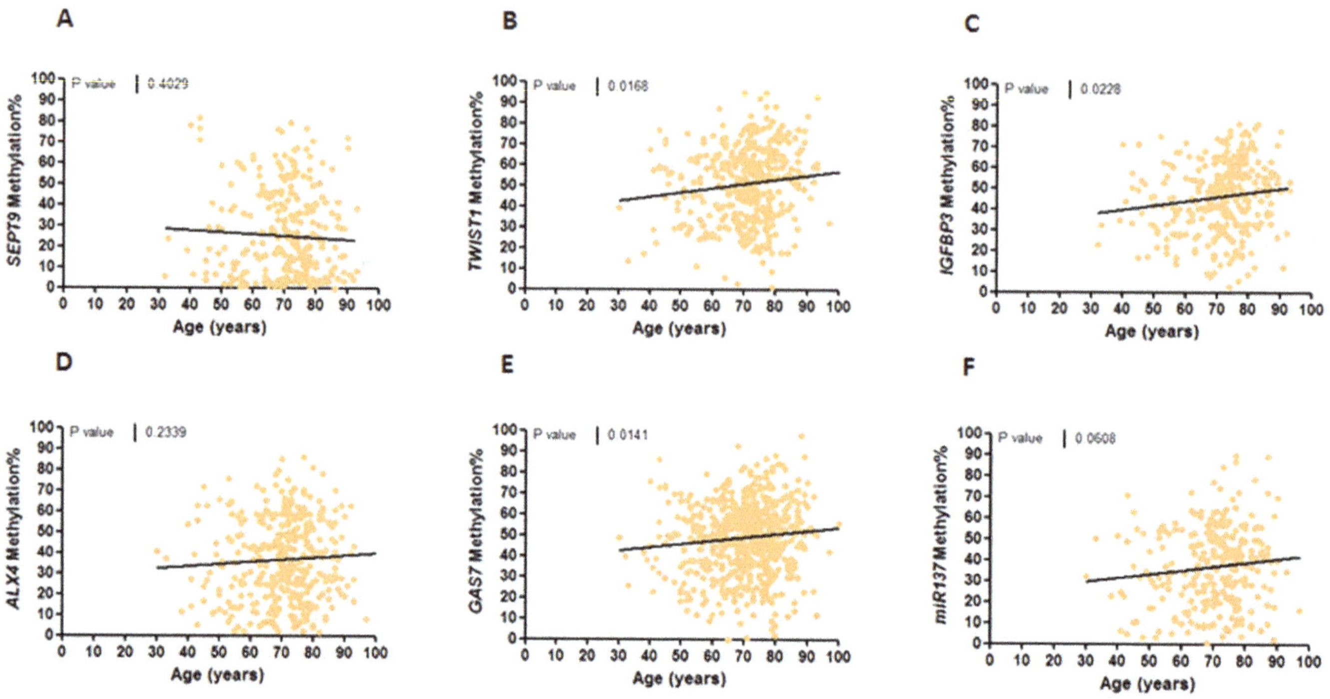

Figure 3. Correlation between primary tumor methylation and age of the crc patients. linear regression analysis comparing tumor methylation of *sept9* (a), *twist1* (b), *igfbp3* (c), *alx4* (d), *gas7* (e) and *mir137* (f) vs age of crc patients (years).

Primers used were designed using the PyroMark 1.0 design software, and pyrosequencing assays were run on the bisulfite-modified DNA (**Table S2 and Information S1**). Mean percentage methylation for all the CpG sites in each assay was calculated for each gene/marker. Methylation cut-off values were determined for each marker based on the average methylation levels observed in normal colonic mucosa from healthy individuals +2 standard deviations. Additional confirmatory methylation analysis for *IGFBP3* was also undertaken by a quantitative MSP (qMSP) assay for the promoter/exon1 CpG island using the primers and PCR conditions as previously described [27].

CpG Island Methylator Phenotype (CIMP) and Microsatellite Instability (MSI) status

The CIMP status of the CRC samples from the Epicolon-I cohort was previously determined using bisulfite pyrosequencing of the CIMP markers *CACNAG1*, *SOCS1*, *RUNX3*, *NEUROG1*, and *MLH1*, as reported previously [7]. A CRC was considered CIMP-positive if at least 3/5 promoters were methylated [7]. Microsatellite instability (MSI) testing was performed using BAT26 and NR24 quasimonomorphic markers as previously described [28]. Tumors were classified as MSI-positive when either marker was mutated, and were deemed microsatellite stable (MSS) when neither marker demonstrated any evidence for genetic instability.

BRAF mutation

Presence of the *V600E BRAF* mutation in CRC samples was detected using TaqMan probes and an ABI Prism 7500 sequence detection system (Applied Biosystems, Foster City, CA), with allelic discrimination, as previously described [29].

Statistical Analysis

Continuous variables are reported as mean + standard deviation (SD), while categorical variables are cited as frequency or percentages. Statistical differences of baseline characteristics between groups were analyzed using the χ^2 test for categorical data, followed by application of Yates' correction and the Mann-Whitney U test for quantitative data analysis. The primary outcomes of this study were overall survival (OS) and disease-free survival (DFS). Analyses of both outcomes were performed for the entire CRC cohort, and separately in the subset of stage II and III CRC patients in order to specifically evaluate the effect of methylation status on the prognosis and response to adjuvant chemotherapy. OS was defined as the time from enrollment to death, and DFS was defined as the time from enrollment to death from any cause or the first relapse. Data on OS and DFS were censored at 1100 days from the date of cancer diagnosis. CRC tumors were categorized into high and low methylation status groups using Receiver Operating Characteristics curve (ROC) analysis. Kaplan-Meier analysis was performed to estimate the distributions of DFS and OS in stage II and III patients. Survival distributions were compared using the log rank test. A multivariate analysis for determination of hazard ratios for death or tumor recurrence was performed using several variables, including, lymph node metastasis, TNM stage, MMR status, tumor differentiation grade, age and adjuvant chemotherapy. Further analyses were performed using Cox's proportional hazards regression in a stepwise manner to test the effect of methylation status of a given gene/marker with DFS and its interaction with chemotherapy. Hazard ratios and 95% confidence interval (95% CI) for death were computed using Cox survival modeling. All reported p values are two sided, and p values <0.05 were considered significant. All calculations were performed using SPSS 10.0 or GraphPad Prism 4.0 statistical software.

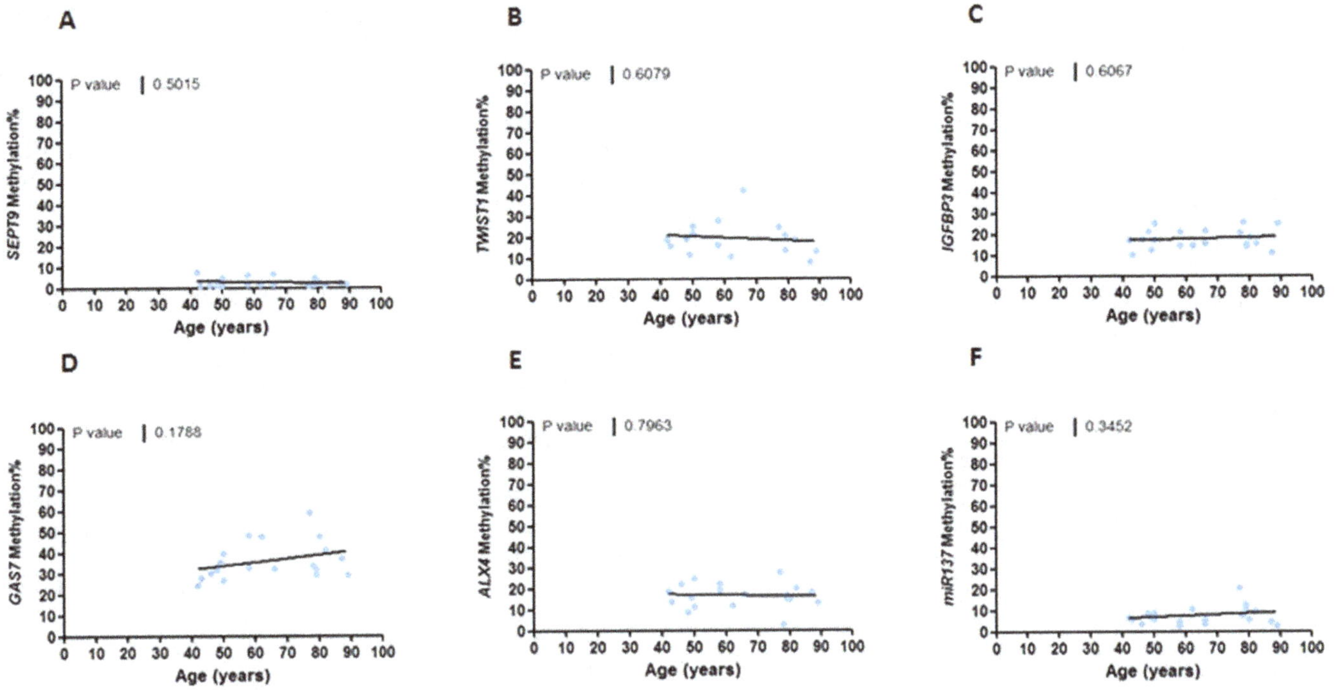

Figure 4. Correlation between colon mucosa methylation and age of healthy controls. linear regression analysis comparing tumor methylation of *sept9* (a), *twist1* (b), *igfbp3* (c), *alx4* (d), *gas7* (e) and *mir137* (f) vs age of the healthy control patients (years).

Results

In our series of 425 CRC cases, the mean ± SD age of the patients was 70.4 ±11 years, and there were more male patients than females (252/425; 60.3%). Of the 425 tumors, 117 (27.9%) were located in the proximal colon, 151 (36.2%) were in the distal colon, and 150 (35.9%) were located in the rectum. Approximately 12.8% of the cases were stage I, 33.7% stage II, 39.7% stage III, and 13.7% stage IV tumors. We found that 35/425 (8.2%) CRCs were MSI, 90/303 (29.7%) were CIMP-positive, and 21/191 (10.9%) harbored a somatic V600E mutation in the *BRAF* gene. As expected, the CIMP-positive phenotype was more frequently associated with MSI and the presence of *BRAF* V600E mutation (22.3% vs. 2.3%, $p<0.0001$ for the MSI phenotype, and 31% vs. 1.5%, $p<0.0001$ for the *BRAF* V600E mutation).

Diagnostic significance of methylation markers in CRC

The mean methylation levels for each gene in primary CRC tissues were: 23.8% for *SEPT9*, 50.5% for *TWIST1*, 44.9% for *IGFBP3*, 50.2% for *GAS7*, 36.5% for *ALX4*, and 35.3% for *miR137*. As shown in **Figure 1**, methylation levels of each gene were significantly higher in CRC versus normal mucosa from healthy subjects ($p<0.0001$ to $p<0.0005$ for all comparisons). These results demonstrate the cancer-specificity for hypermethylation of these genes and establish a rationale for their exploitation as potential diagnostic biomarkers for CRC, considering that all 6 markers demonstrated hypermethylation in all stages of CRCs (**Figure 2**).

In order to assess the performance of each methylation marker individually for CRC diagnosis, methylation results were analyzed as a categorical variable. Accordingly, each gene was classified as methylated when mean methylation levels were higher than 7.1% for *SEPT9*, 35.7% for *TWIST*, 27.5% for *IGFBP3*, 53.5% for *GAS7*, 28.5% for *ALX4*, and 11.9% for *miR137*. Based upon these analyses, the most frequently methylated markers in CRC tissues were the *miR-137* gene (302/344, 87.7%), followed by *IGFBP3* (289/348, 83%), *TWIST1* (269/356, 75.6%), *SEPT9* (244/346, 70.5%), *ALX4* (214/350, 61.1%), and *GAS7* (164/378, 43.3%). To further assess whether a combination of markers would further enhance the diagnostic accuracy of the assay, we analyzed combination marker panels and found that the *miR137+ IGFBP3* combination yielded an diagnostic accuracy of 86%, followed by *TWIST1+IGFBP3* (82.7%) and *TWIST1+miR137* (78.5%). Furthermore, we found that the combination of *miR137+ IGFBP3*+TWIST1 methylation had the highest diagnostic accuracy, 92%, as shown in **Table 1.**

Clinicopathological features associated with methylation biomarkers

We next investigated the relationship between various clinicopathological and molecular features and their association with aberrant methylation of all six genes analyzed in this study. The clinicopathological variables included age, gender, TNM staging and tumor location, and the molecular factors included the MMR status, CIMP phenotype and the *BRAF* mutational status. Tumor location and TNM stages did not associate with the methylation status of any of the gene markers. Curiously, *SEPT9* methylation was significantly associated with male gender ($p<0.05$; **Table S3**). When methylation was analyzed as a continuous variable, we observed a trend for higher methylation of *TWIST1*, *IGFBP3*, *ALX4*, and *GAS7* ($p<0.05$) and older patients with CRC; however, we did not find a positive correlation between normal colonic mucosa methylation in these genes and age in healthy individuals (**Figures 3 & 4**).

Table 2. Molecular features associated with gene methylation in crc patients.

Genes	MSI Status (% methylation)			CIMP Status (% methylation)			*BRAF Mutation (% methylation)*		
	Mean + SD			Mean + SD			Mean + SD		
	MSI	MSS	P-value*	Positive	Negative	P-value*	Mutated	WT	P-value*
SEPT9	20.9 + 18.9	24.5 ± 20.6	NS	24.5 + 20.5	25.3 + 21.4	NS	17.1 + 14.3	23.4 + 20.8	NS
ALX4	34.6 + 20.2	36.6 + 19.5	NS	44.5 ± 17.6	35.8 + 18.3	<0.0001	51.8 + 6.2	35.8 + 17.7	<0.001
TWIST1	40.3 + 51.1	51.0 + 18.5	< 0.05	53.4 ± 17.2	50.2 + 17.2	NS	52.3 + 12.6	51.6 + 17.4	NS
IGFBP3	47.5 + 18.7	44.8 + 17.3	NS	51.4 ± 17.2	43.5 + 17.2	<0.001	54.5 + 13.1	43.7 + 17.7	< 0.05
GAS7	49.9 + 17.9	48.3 + 17.0	NS	56.0 + 10.1	48.6 + 15.5	<0.0001	54.1 + 13.7	49.1 + 15.9	NS
miR137	38.4 + 21.6	35.1 + 17.9	NS	43.1 ± 15.4	34.4 + 17.7	<0.001	42.2 + 14.4	35.4 + 17.7	NS

*Evaluated with student's -t test
SD: Standard deviation; l; mmr: mismatch repair; msi: microsatellite instability; mss: microsatellite stable. Cimp: cpg island methylator phenotype; wt: wild type; ns: no significant.

With regards to molecular associations, *TWIST1* methylation levels were higher in MSS compared to MSI CRCs (51% vs 40.3%; $p<0.05$) (**Table 2**). Methylation of four genes, *ALX4, IGFBP3, GAS7*, and *miR137*, was significantly correlated with CIMP-positive tumors ($p<0.001$). Furthermore, as shown in **Table 2**, CRCs with *ALX4* and *IGFBP3* methylation were more frequently associated with a somatic *BRAF* V600E mutation (13.5% vs. 1.8%, $p<0.05$ for *ALX4*, and 12.4% vs. 0%, $p<0.05$ for *IGBFP3*).

Aberrant hypermethylation of genes and its influence on CRC patient prognosis

The median follow-up for the series of 425 patients included in this study was 1268 days (3.4 years; range 0–2204 days). At the end of the follow-up period, 169 patients had died (39.7%), and the median follow-up for this group was 671±513 days (1.8±1.4 years). Information regarding the cause of death was available in 99 patients; 67.7% (67/99) died due to complications of tumor progression, 18.2% (18/99) died due to complications of chemotherapy, and 14.1% (14/99) succumbed to death from other causes, including post-operative complications. Tumor recurrence was observed in 116/370 patients (31.3%), with a median time duration of 644±448 days (1.7±1.2 years) post-surgery.

To determine the prognostic significance of the methylation status for each gene, all CRCs were categorized into two groups based on their methylation levels (high versus low), and the dose–response relationship between the degree of methylation and event-free survival was examined by ROC curve analysis. Overall, high levels of methylation of the *GAS7* (prognosis cut-off value = 52.62%; high-methylation: 43.3%, low-methylation: 56.7%; χ^2 p = 0.03) and *ALX4* genes (prognosis cut-off value = 25.8%; high-methylation: 67.1%, low-methylation: 32.9%; χ^2 p = 0.005) associated with poor DFS in CRC patients (data not shown). In contrast, low levels of *IGFBP3* methylation demonstrated an association with significantly worse DFS according to unadjusted analysis (prognosis cut-off value = 53.1%; high-methylation: 30.9%, low-methylation: 69.1%; χ^2 p = 0.01; **Figures 5A and B**). Following multivariate Cox regression analysis where multiple variables were analyzed, only low levels of *IGFBP3* methylation emerged as an independent risk factor for poor DFS in stage II and III CRC patients (HR = 0.49, 95% CI: 0.28–0.85, $p<0.01$). Furthermore, the methylation status of the *IGFBP3* gene was the only statistically significant risk factor for stage II CRC, after adjustment for other prognostic factors such as age, adjuvant 5-FU (5-Fluorouracil) chemotherapy or MSI status (HR = 0.28, 95% CI: 0.12–0.70, p = 0.006; **Table 3**).

Aberrant gene hypermethylation and its influence on patient survival following chemotherapy treatment

Chemotherapeutic treatment was given to 257/425 patients (60.5%), mainly using 5FU+leucovorin (236; 91.8% of patients). Among the entire cohort, 315 patients (74.1%) had either a stage II or III disease, and 155 (49.2%) of these received 5FU-based adjuvant chemotherapy. Only 9 stage II and III patients received other chemotherapeutic treatments, and were excluded from further analysis. After a median follow-up of 1221 days (3.3 years), 92 (31.2%) patients with stage II and III showed tumor recurrence, and by the end of the follow-up period, 101 (34.2%) patients from these groups had died.

Adjuvant chemotherapy provided a significant improvement in OS in stage II and III CRC patients compared to patients who did not receive chemotherapy (chemotherapy: 49.1%, no-chemother-

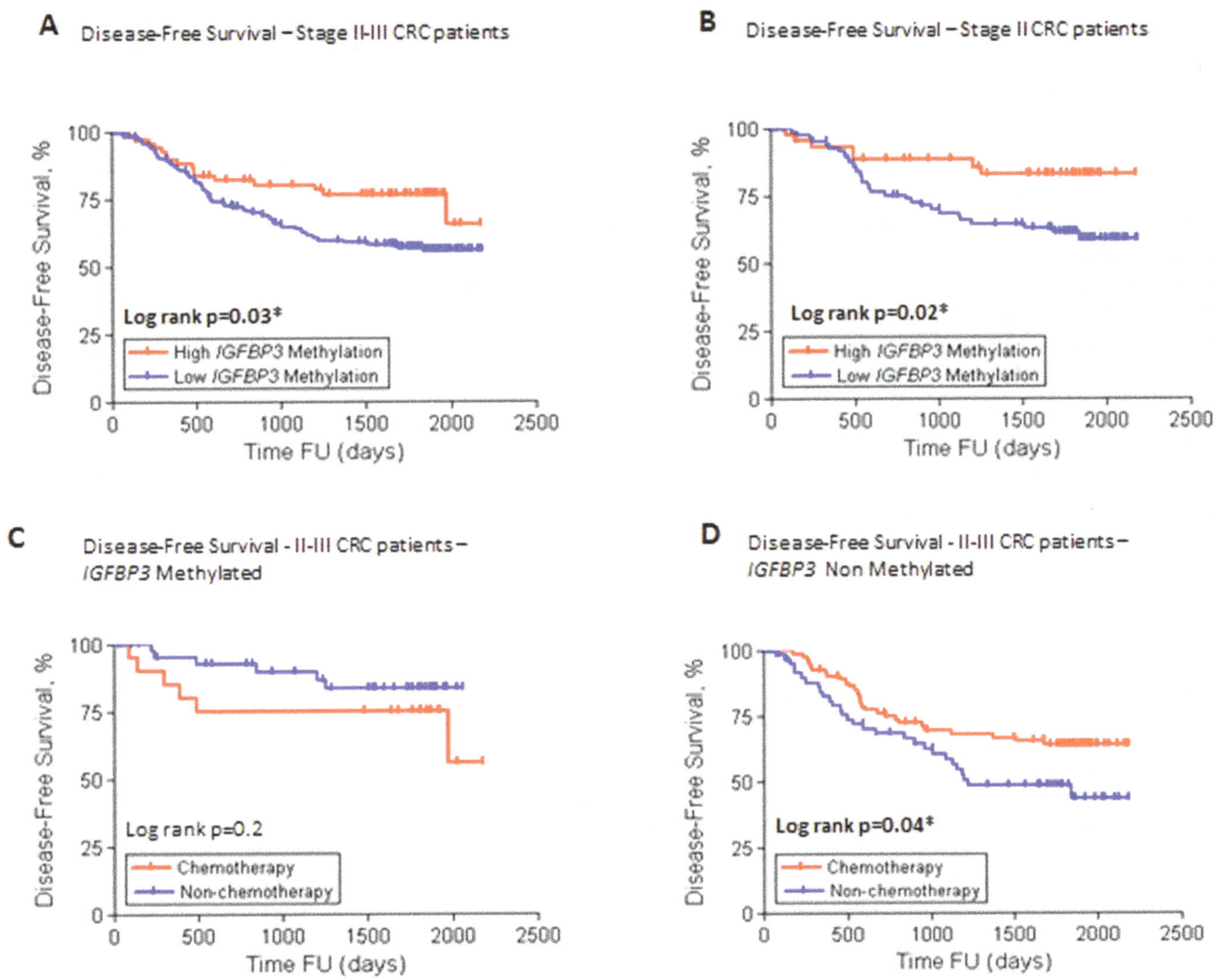

Figure 5. Relationship between igfbp3 methylation and prognostic and predictive response in stage ii and iii crc patients. (a) Disease-free survival of patients with stage ii and iii crc, according to *igfbp3* methylation status (high methylation, n = 73, (30.3%) low methylation, n = 168, (69.7%). (b) Disease-free survival of patients with stage ii disease, according to *igfbp3* methylation (high methylation, n = 45, (32.4%); low methylation, n = 94, (67.6%). (c) Disease-free survival of patients with stage ii and iii disease, in high *igfbp3* methylation tumors based on adjuvant chemotherapy (chemotherapy, n = 20, (22.5%); no chemotherapy, n = 69, (77.5%). (d) Disease-free survival of patients with stage ii and iii disease, in low *igfbp3* methylation tumors according to adjuvant chemotherapy (Chemotherapyc n = 83, (52.7%); NO Chemotherapy, n = 74, (47.2%).

apy: 50.9%; χ^2 p = 0.0001). These differences in OS were also present in multivariate analysis which controlled for age, gender, lymph node metastasis, MMR, and CIMP phenotype status (HR = 0.55, 95% CI: 0.36–0.85, p = 0.007).

Interestingly, among all 6 methylation markers investigated, only *IGFBP3* methylation levels were predictive of the response to 5FU-based chemotherapy. According to our results, patients with low *IGFBP3* methylation levels had longer OS (p = 0.0007) and DFS (p = 0.05) when they received chemotherapy. Conversely, in patients with high *IGFBP3* methylation, adjuvant chemotherapy did not improve OS (p = 0.4) or DFS (p = 0.3; **Figure 5C and D**). Using multivariate Cox regression analysis (**Table 4**), in patients with low-*IGFBP3* methylation, adjuvant chemotherapy independently predicted better OS (HR = 0.49, 95%CI: 0.29–0.80, p = 0.004); however, it did not significantly influence DFS (p = 0.08). On the other hand, MMR status was the only variable that independently predicted OS (p = 0.05) and DFS (p = 0.04) in patients with high *IGFBP3* methylation (**Table 4**). In the patient cohort treated with 5-FU adjuvant chemotherapy, *IGFBP3* methylation status did not independently predict OS and DFS. In contrast, DFS was positively affected by *IGFBP3* methylation status in patients who did not receive adjuvant chemotherapy (HR = 0.41, 95%CI: 0.18–0.91, p = 0.02).

Discussion

In the recent years, a number of promising gene methylation-based diagnostic biomarkers including *SEPT9, TWIST 1, IGFBP3, GAS7, ALX4*, and *miR137* have been proposed for the early detection of colorectal neoplasia. However, the majority of these markers have been confined to initial small-scale discovery

Table 3. Multivariate analysis of disease-free survival based on *IGFBP3* promoter methylation in stage II and III CRC patients.

Stage II and III CRC Patients	Hazard Ratios (HR)	95% CI	P-value
Tumor size (T3/4 vs. T1/2)	1.479	0.46–4.69	0.5
Lymph Node metastasis (Positive vs. Negative)	1.605	1.01–2.54	**0.04**
MMR Status (MSI vs. MSS)	0.739	0.26–2.06	0.5
Differentiation Grade (Poor vs. Well/Moderate)	0.86	0.34–2.16	0.7
IGFBP3 Methylation (High vs. Low)	0.479	0.26–0.87	**0.01**
Stage II CRC Patients	**Hazard Ratios (HR)**	**95% CI**	**P-value**
Age (> Median vs. < Median)	0.774	0.36–1.70	0.5
Serosal invasion (Yes vs. No)	1.485	0.62–3.51	0.3
Chemotherapy (Yes vs. No)	0.61	0.27–1.36	0.2
MMR Status (MSI vs. MSS)	0.612	0.13–2.73	0.5
Differentiation Grade (Poor vs. Well/Moderate)	0.548	0.20–1.47	0.2
IGFBP3 Methylation (High vs. Low)	0.28	0.12–0.70	**0.006**

CI: Confidence interval; mmr: mismatch repair; msi: microsatellite instability; mss: microsatellite stable.

studies, and have not been developed into clinical practice as they have not been systematically validated in large, independent cohorts of CRC patients. In view of this gap in knowledge, we designed this study to confirm the diagnostic potential of these biomarkers, and to ascertain their prognostic and predictive values in CRC. In addition, we were interested in examining the associations between aberrant hypermethylation of these genes and clinicopathological features by analyzing a large, well-characterized, population-based cohort of CRC patients.

Based on our quantitative methylation analysis, all six genes interrogated fulfilled the criteria for potential clinical use as diagnostic biomarkers of CRC. These criteria included: a) the methylation of each gene occurred in a tumor-specific manner; b) the methylation levels of each gene in neoplastic tissues were significantly higher than in normal colonic mucosa; and c) none of the genes showed an age-dependent increase in DNA methylation in normal colonic mucosa [30,31]. Methylation levels of each gene allowed us to classify colorectal tissues as normal or neoplastic. Among all markers investigated, *IGFBP3* and *miR137* methylation levels showed the highest diagnostic accuracy as individual gene markers for the identification of primary CRCs (83% and 78.3%, respectively). This diagnostic accuracy was further improved by combining the methylation status of two gene markers; in particular, the methylation status of *IGFBP3+TWIST1* or *IGFBP3+miR137* had the highest accura-

Table 4. Multivariate analysis of disease-free survival and overall survival in stage ii and iii crc patients and *igfbp3* promoter methylation status.

	DFS			OS		
	HR	95%CI	P-value	HR	95%CI	P-value
High-*IGFBP3* Methylation Group						
Age (>65, vs. <65)	1.697	0.66–4.35	0.3	1.218	0.49–3.02	0.7
Gender (Male vs. Female)	1.802	0.91–3.55	0.08	1.457	0.77–2.74	0.2
MMR Status (MSI vs MSS)	0.371	0.14–0.98	**0.04**	0.391	0.14–1.02	**0.05**
Lymph Node Metastasis (positive vs. negative)	0.666	0.31–1.41	0.3	0.98	0.59–1.66	0.9
CIMP (positive vs. negative)	1.141	0.57–2.26	0.7	1.443	0.74–2.82	0.3
Adjuvant Chemotherapy (yes vs. no)	0.721	0.35–1.47	0.4	0.52	0.25–1.05	0.07
Low-*IGFBP3* Methylation Group						
Age (>65 vs. <65)	0.995	0.45–2.16	0.9	1.135	0.66–1.92	0.6
Gender (Male vs. Female)	0.897	0.6–1.34	0.6	0.901	0.6–1.34	0.6
MMR Status (MSI vs. MSS)	0.65	0.29–1.33	0.2	0.593	0.27–1.26	0.2
Lymph Node Metastasis (positive vs. negative)	1.372	0.91–2.05	0.1	1.429	1.05–1.93	0.02
CIMP (positive vs. negative)	0.828	0.48–1.41	0.5	0.844	0.49–1.43	0.5
Adjuvant Chemotherapy (yes vs. no)	0.655	0.41–1.05	0.08	0.489	0.29–0.80	**0.004**

DFS: Disease-free survival; os: overall survival; hr: hazard ratio; ci : confidence interval; mmr: mismatch repair; msi: microsatellite instability; mss: microsatellite stable; cimp: cpg island methylator phenotype.

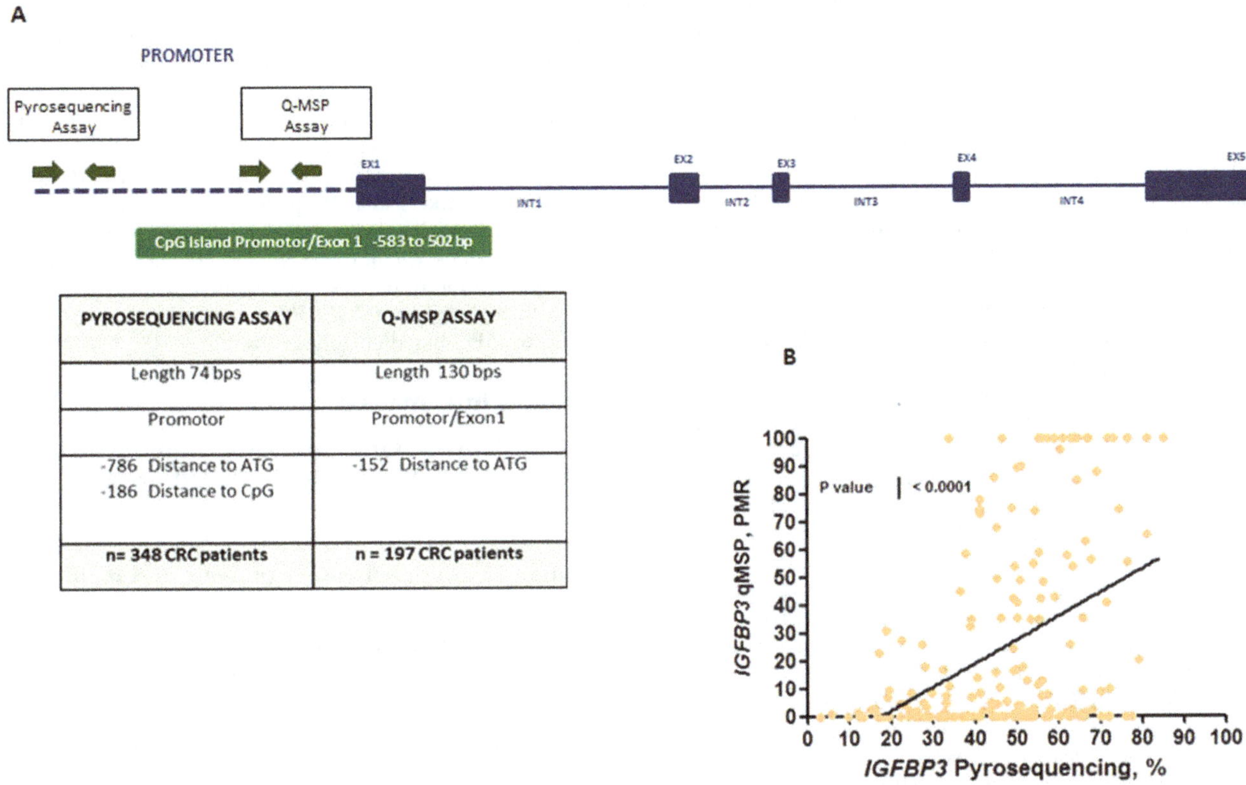

PYROSEQUENCING ASSAY	Q-MSP ASSAY
Length 74 bps	Length 130 bps
Promotor	Promotor/Exon1
-786 Distance to ATG -186 Distance to CpG	-152 Distance to ATG
n= 348 CRC patients	n = 197 CRC patients

Figure 6. Comparison between methylation levels within igfbp3 promoter in crc tissues. (a) Schematic overview of the insulin-like grown factor binding protein 3 (igfbp3) gene. exons are represented by blue boxes, introns with blue lines, and the promoter region by blue dashed lines. the *igfbp3* gene has one cytosine-phosphate-guanine (cpg) island at in the promoter region and exon1 underscoring the potential of modulating gene expression by means of cpg hypermethylation, and this is represented by a green box. we performed two different assays covering both cpgs islands (indicated by green arrows) using two quantitative methods: pyrosequencing and qmsp in order to correlate methylation levels of these two locations. (b) Linear regression analysis comparing *igfbp3* methylation levels by pyrosequencing (% methylation) in 348 patient samples and qmsp (pmr) assays in crc tissues (n = 197).

cy values of 86% and 82.7% respectively, with sensitivity and specificity values > 80%.

We investigated the molecular features associated with tumor methylation levels of these genes. This was of particular interest as molecular classification based on MSI and CIMP status has become increasingly important [32] for its prognostic [33,34,35] and predictive role in CRC patients [7,34,36]. In this study, four of the six genes were positively associated with the CIMP phenotype (*ALX4, IGFBP3, GAS7*, and *miR137*). Furthermore, a positive correlation between *BRAF* V600E mutation and methylation of the *ALX4* and *IGFBP3* genes was associated with CIMP-high in CRC [37,38]. As expected, methylation of the *ALX4* and *IGFBP3* genes was associated with the presence of the *BRAF* gene mutation. *TWIST1* methylation levels were higher in patients with MMR-proficient tumors compared to MSI tumors; however, in our cohort, only a small proportion of CRCs were MMR-deficient (5%), and the correlations between MMR status and methylation markers may have been lost when analyzing the group as a whole.

In stage II and III CRC patients who have undergone potentially curative resection, prognosis depends on disease recurrence, which is primarily associated with distant metastasis. In addition, the benefit from adjuvant chemotherapy, especially for stage II CRC patients has remained an area of controversy and chemotherapeutic resistance remains a major problem in these patients. Therefore, the discovery of novel prognostic and predictive biomarkers that can help identify stage II and III patients that are at high risk of recurrence and metastasis, may improve the current strategy for CRC patient stratification and therapy management. To the best of our knowledge, no previous study has examined the relationship between methylation of the *SEPT9, IGFBP3, TWIST1, GAS7, ALX4*, and *miR137* genes with prognosis in patients with CRC, as well as the ability of these biomarkers to predict response to 5-FU-based adjuvant chemotherapy. Based upon our results in this large, well-characterized population-based cohort, stage II and III CRC patients with low levels of *IGFBP3* promoter methylation had poorer OS and DFS compared to those with high levels of DNA hypermethylation. With regards to response to chemotherapy, when 5-FU based adjuvant chemotherapy was administered to stage II and III CRC patients, only those patients with low levels of *IGFBP3*-methylated tumors were positively affected, resulting in longer DFS and OS times, indicating that the benefit of chemotherapy was limited to this group of CRC patients. Curiously, this effect of *IGFBP3* methylation was independent of CIMP status. Nevertheless it is important to point out that although *IGFBP3* methylation status emerged as the only independent factor that predicted poor DFS probability among stage II CRC patients, additional independent clinical studies are required to prove that *IGFBP3* methylation levels in CRC could represent a potential routine test for prognostication of CRC patients, and in improving the management of patients with localized disease in combination with current clinicopathological and molecular tools.

Other studies have observed a relationship between high levels of *IGFBP3* methylation and poor clinical outcome in lung and ovarian cancers [39,40], and more recently in CRC patients [27]. Discrepant reports using methylation markers may be due to the use of different methodologies and the analysis of different sequence locations within CpG Islands. In this study, we used bisulfite pyrosequencing for methylation analysis, which is a reliable quantitative approach for robust DNA methylation analysis compared to the conventional Methylation Specific PCR (MSP), which lacks the quantification provided by bisulfate pyrosequencing [27,39,40]. In addition, to further ensure the accuracy of our methylation results, we also conducted a quantitative-MSP (qMSP) analysis within the CpG island region previously studied in CRC [41]. As shown in **Figure 6**, we confirmed that our bisulfite pyrosequencing methylation results were positively correlated to the results obtained within the CpG island region previously studied [27,39,40].

Although there are some differences between this study and previously published studies, we believe this work is more robust and comprehensive, as ours employs the largest patient cohort, is population-based, and includes a control group of non-treated CRC patients for comparison. The biological role and timing of *IGFBP3* methylation in CRC is poorly understood; however, recent *in vitro* studies have reported that methylation-induced silencing of *IGFBP3* may lead to significant resistance to cisplatin treatment in lung cancer [42,43]. Conversely, it is also possible that this event is merely a consequence of CIMP, and *IGFBP3* methylation consequently serves as a surrogate marker of this phenotype and may be an important determinant of poor responses to 5-FU-based adjuvant chemotherapy in CRC, as previously shown by our laboratory [7]. It is very likely that *IGFBP3* methylation alone may not provide requisite sensitivity and specificity for a clinically viable test, and inclusion of additional biomarkers may further improve the clinical significance of this biomarker. Although work from our laboratory and other laboratories have previously provided data for the functional role of *miR-137* and *IGFBP3* methylation in colorectal cancer [21,44], additional *in-vitro* and *in-vivo* studies in this regard may further facilitate in gathering a better understanding of the biological roles of these biomarkers in colorectal carcinogenesis.

In summary, this study performed a comprehensive analysis of a large, population-based CRC cohort and clearly highlighted the potential roles of the methylation status of *miR137* and *IGFBP3* as diagnostic biomarkers in CRC patients. In addition, our data revealed that *IGFBP3* promoter methylation serves as an independent prognostic biomarker in stage II and III colorectal cancer patients. Our results also suggest that stage II&III CRC patients with high levels of *IGFBP3* methylation do not benefit from adjuvant 5FU-based chemotherapy.

Supporting Information

Figure S1 Representative pyrograms of methylation markers in the sept9, twist1, alx4, igfbp3, gas7, and mir137.

Information S1 Supplementary patients and methods.

Table S1 Clinicopathological and molecular features of epicolon-i patients.

Table S2 Primer sequences for pyrosequencing.

Table S3 Clinicopathological features associated with gene methylation.

Author Contributions

Conceived and designed the experiments: AG FB LPC AC CRB. Performed the experiments: LPC FB. Analyzed the data: AG LPC YT FB. Contributed reagents/materials/analysis tools: CE ER YT AC CG RJ MA XL. Contributed to the writing of the manuscript: LPC FB AG RJ CRB.

References

1. Smith RA, Cokkinides V, Brooks D, Saslow D, Brawley OW (2010) Cancer screening in the United States, 2010: a review of current American Cancer Society guidelines and issues in cancer screening. CA Cancer J Clin 60: 99–119.
2. Kondo Y, Issa JP (2004) Epigenetic changes in colorectal cancer. Cancer Metastasis Rev 23: 29–39.
3. Ushijima T (2005) Detection and interpretation of altered methylation patterns in cancer cells. Nat Rev Cancer 5: 223–231.
4. Petko Z, Ghiassi M, Shuber A, Gorham J, Smalley W, et al. (2005) Aberrantly methylated CDKN2A, MGMT, and MLH1 in colon polyps and in fecal DNA from patients with colorectal polyps. Clin Cancer Res 11: 1203–1209.
5. Ibrahim AE, Arends MJ, Silva AL, Wyllie AH, Greger L, et al. (2011) Sequential DNA methylation changes are associated with DNMT3B overexpression in colorectal neoplastic progression. Gut 60: 499–508.
6. Regueiro CR (2005) AGA Future Trends Committee report: Colorectal cancer: a qualitative review of emerging screening and diagnostic technologies. Gastroenterology 129: 1083–1103.
7. Jover R, Nguyen TP, Perez-Carbonell L, Zapater P, Paya A, et al. (2011) 5-Fluorouracil adjuvant chemotherapy does not increase survival in patients with CpG island methylator phenotype colorectal cancer. Gastroenterology 140: 1174–1181.
8. Min BH, Bae JM, Lee EJ, Yu HS, Kim YH, et al. (2011) The CpG island methylator phenotype may confer a survival benefit in patients with stage II or III colorectal carcinomas receiving fluoropyrimidine-based adjuvant chemotherapy. BMC Cancer 11: 344.
9. Lofton-Day C, Model F, Devos T, Tetzner R, Distler J, et al. (2008) DNA methylation biomarkers for blood-based colorectal cancer screening. Clin Chem 54: 414–423.
10. He Q, Chen HY, Bai EQ, Luo YX, Fu RJ, et al. (2010) Development of a multiplex MethyLight assay for the detection of multigene methylation in human colorectal cancer. Cancer Genet Cytogenet 202: 1–10.
11. Grutzmann R, Molnar B, Pilarsky C, Habermann JK, Schlag PM, et al. (2008) Sensitive detection of colorectal cancer in peripheral blood by septin 9 DNA methylation assay. PLoS One 3: e3759.
12. Tanzer M, Balluff B, Distler J, Hale K, Leodolter A, et al. (2010) Performance of epigenetic markers SEPT9 and ALX4 in plasma for detection of colorectal precancerous lesions. PLoS One 5: e9061.
13. Ebert MP, Model F, Mooney S, Hale K, Lograsso J, et al. (2006) Aristaless-like homeobox-4 gene methylation is a potential marker for colorectal adenocarcinomas. Gastroenterology 131: 1418–1430.
14. Valdes-Mora F, Gomez del Pulgar T, Bandres E, Cejas P, Ramirez de Molina A, et al. (2009) TWIST1 overexpression is associated with nodal invasion and male sex in primary colorectal cancer. Ann Surg Oncol 16: 78–87.
15. Gort EH, Suijkerbuijk KP, Roothaan SM, Raman V, Vooijs M, et al. (2008) Methylation of the TWIST1 promoter, TWIST1 mRNA levels, and immunohistochemical expression of TWIST1 in breast cancer. Cancer Epidemiol Biomarkers Prev 17: 3325–3330.
16. Kawasaki T, Nosho K, Ohnishi M, Suemoto Y, Kirkner GJ, et al. (2007) IGFBP3 promoter methylation in colorectal cancer: relationship with microsatellite instability, CpG island methylator phenotype, and p53. Neoplasia 9: 1091–1098.
17. Ronneberg JA, Fleischer T, Solvang HK, Nordgard SH, Edvardsen H, et al. (2011) Methylation profiling with a panel of cancer related genes: association with estrogen receptor, TP53 mutation status and expression subtypes in sporadic breast cancer. Mol Oncol 5: 61–76.

18. Kim YH, Lee HC, Kim SY, Yeom YI, Ryu KJ, et al. (2011) Epigenomic analysis of aberrantly methylated genes in colorectal cancer identifies genes commonly affected by epigenetic alterations. Ann Surg Oncol 18: 2338–2347.
19. Bandres E, Agirre X, Bitarte N, Ramirez N, Zarate R, et al. (2009) Epigenetic regulation of microRNA expression in colorectal cancer. Int J Cancer 125: 2737–2743.
20. Silber J, Lim DA, Petritsch C, Persson AI, Maunakea AK, et al. (2008) miR-124 and miR-137 inhibit proliferation of glioblastoma multiforme cells and induce differentiation of brain tumor stem cells. BMC Med 6: 14.
21. Balaguer F, Link A, Lozano JJ, Cuatrecasas M, Nagasaka T, et al. (2010) Epigenetic silencing of miR-137 is an early event in colorectal carcinogenesis. Cancer Res 70: 6609–6618.
22. Pinol V, Andreu M, Castells A, Paya A, Bessa X, et al. (2004) Frequency of hereditary non-polyposis colorectal cancer and other colorectal cancer familial forms in Spain: a multicentre, prospective, nationwide study. Eur J Gastroenterol Hepatol 16: 39–45.
23. Perez-Carbonell L, Ruiz-Ponte C, Guarinos C, Alenda C, Paya A, et al. (2012) Comparison between universal molecular screening for Lynch syndrome and revised Bethesda guidelines in a large population-based cohort of patients with colorectal cancer. Gut 61: 865–872.
24. Moreira L, Balaguer F, Lindor N, de la Chapelle A, Hampel H, et al. (2012) Identification of Lynch syndrome among patients with colorectal cancer. Jama 308: 1555–1565.
25. Jover R, Zapater P, Castells A, Llor X, Andreu M, et al. (2009) The efficacy of adjuvant chemotherapy with 5-fluorouracil in colorectal cancer depends on the mismatch repair status. Eur J Cancer 45: 365–373.
26. Pinol V, Castells A, Andreu M, Castellvi-Bel S, Alenda C, et al. (2005) Accuracy of revised Bethesda guidelines, microsatellite instability, and immunohistochemistry for the identification of patients with hereditary nonpolyposis colorectal cancer. Jama 293: 1986–1994.
27. Yi JM, Dhir M, Van Neste L, Downing SR, Jeschke J, et al. (2011) Genomic and epigenomic integration identifies a prognostic signature in colon cancer. Clin Cancer Res 17: 1535–1545.
28. Xicola RM, Llor X, Pons E, Castells A, Alenda C, et al. (2007) Performance of different microsatellite marker panels for detection of mismatch repair-deficient colorectal tumors. J Natl Cancer Inst 99: 244–252.
29. Benlloch S, Paya A, Alenda C, Bessa X, Andreu M, et al. (2006) Detection of BRAF V600E mutation in colorectal cancer: comparison of automatic sequencing and real-time chemistry methodology. J Mol Diagn 8: 540–543.
30. Toyota M, Ahuja N, Ohe-Toyota M, Herman JG, Baylin SB, et al. (1999) CpG island methylator phenotype in colorectal cancer. Proc Natl Acad Sci U S A 96: 8681–8686.
31. Issa JP (2002) Epigenetic variation and human disease. J Nutr 132: 2388S–2392S.
32. Jass JR (2007) Classification of colorectal cancer based on correlation of clinical, morphological and molecular features. Histopathology 50: 113–130.
33. Wright CM, Dent OF, Barker M, Newland RC, Chapuis PH, et al. (2000) Prognostic significance of extensive microsatellite instability in sporadic clinicopathological stage C colorectal cancer. Br J Surg 87: 1197–1202.
34. Popat S, Hubner R, Houlston RS (2005) Systematic review of microsatellite instability and colorectal cancer prognosis. J Clin Oncol 23: 609–618.
35. Gryfe R, Kim H, Hsieh ET, Aronson MD, Holowaty EJ, et al. (2000) Tumor microsatellite instability and clinical outcome in young patients with colorectal cancer. N Engl J Med 342: 69–77.
36. Ribic CM, Sargent DJ, Moore MJ, Thibodeau SN, French AJ, et al. (2003) Tumor microsatellite-instability status as a predictor of benefit from fluorouracil-based adjuvant chemotherapy for colon cancer. N Engl J Med 349: 247–257.
37. Weisenberger DJ, Siegmund KD, Campan M, Young J, Long TI, et al. (2006) CpG island methylator phenotype underlies sporadic microsatellite instability and is tightly associated with BRAF mutation in colorectal cancer. Nat Genet 38: 787–793.
38. Samowitz WS, Albertsen H, Herrick J, Levin TR, Sweeney C, et al. (2005) Evaluation of a large, population-based sample supports a CpG island methylator phenotype in colon cancer. Gastroenterology 129: 837–845.
39. Wiley A, Katsaros D, Fracchioli S, Yu H (2006) Methylation of the insulin-like growth factor binding protein-3 gene and prognosis of epithelial ovarian cancer. Int J Gynecol Cancer 16: 210–218.
40. Chang YS, Wang L, Liu D, Mao L, Hong WK, et al. (2002) Correlation between insulin-like growth factor-binding protein-3 promoter methylation and prognosis of patients with stage I non-small cell lung cancer. Clin Cancer Res 8: 3669–3675.
41. Hanafusa T, Yumoto Y, Nouso K, Nakatsukasa H, Onishi T, et al. (2002) Reduced expression of insulin-like growth factor binding protein-3 and its promoter hypermethylation in human hepatocellular carcinoma. Cancer Lett 176: 149–158.
42. Cortes-Sempere M, de Miguel MP, Pernia O, Rodriguez C, de Castro Carpeno J, et al. (2013) IGFBP-3 methylation-derived deficiency mediates the resistance to cisplatin through the activation of the IGFIR/Akt pathway in non-small cell lung cancer. Oncogene 32: 1274–1283.
43. Ibanez de Caceres I, Cortes-Sempere M, Moratilla C, Machado-Pinilla R, Rodriguez-Fanjul V, et al. (2010) IGFBP-3 hypermethylation-derived deficiency mediates cisplatin resistance in non-small-cell lung cancer. Oncogene 29: 1681–1690.
44. Borinstein SC, Conerly M, Dzieciatkowski S, Biswas S, Washington MK, et al. (2010) Aberrant DNA methylation occurs in colon neoplasms arising in the azoxymethane colon cancer model. Mol Carcinog 49: 94–103.

3

Meta-Analysis of EGFR Tyrosine Kinase Inhibitors Compared with Chemotherapy as Second-Line Treatment in Pretreated Advanced Non-Small Cell Lung Cancer

Ning Li[1]◈, Lu Yang[2]◈, Wei Ou[1], Liang Zhang[3], Song-liang Zhang[1], Si-yu Wang[1]*

1 Department of Thoracic Surgery, Sun Yat-sen University Cancer Center, Guangzhou, China, 2 Department of Breast Oncology, Sun Yat-sen University Cancer Center, Guangzhou, China, 3 Department of Thoracic Surgery, Tianjin First Center Hospital, Tianjin, China

Abstract

Background: Since efficacy and safety of epidermal growth factor receptor tyrosine kinase inhibitors (EGFR-TKIs) versus chemotherapy in the treatment of patients with pretreated advanced non-small cell lung cancer (NSCLC) remain controversial, we performed a meta-analysis to compare them.

Methods: An internet search of several databases was performed, including PubMed, Embase, and the Cochrane database. Randomized trials that compared an EGFR-TKI with chemotherapy in the second-line setting were included. The outcomes were progression-free survival (PFS), overall survival (OS), objective response rate (ORR), and grade 3–4 toxicities. The PFS, OS for the EGFR mutation-positive (EGFR M^+) and EGFR mutation-negative (EGFR M^-) subgroups were pooled. The pooled hazard ratios (HRs) and odds ratios (ORs) with their corresponding confidence intervals (CIs) were calculated on the STATA software.

Results: Our meta-analysis combined 3,825 patients from 10 randomized trials. Overall, EGFR-TKIs and second-line chemotherapy have equivalent efficacy in terms of PFS (HR, 1.03; 95%CI, 0.87–1.21; P = 0.73; $I^2 = 78.7\%$, $P_{heterogeneity} < 0.001$), OS (HR, 1.00; 95%CI, 0.92–1.08; P = 0.90; $I^2 = 0.0\%$, $P_{heterogeneity} = 0.88$), and ORR (OR, 1.34; 95%CI, 0.86–2.08; P = 0.20; $I^2 = 73.1\%$, $P_{heterogeneity} < 0.001$). However, subgroup analysis based on EGFR mutation status showed that second-line chemotherapy significantly improved PFS (HR, 1.35; 95%CI, 1.09–1.66; P = 0.01; $I^2 = 55.7\%$, $P_{heterogeneity} = 0.046$) for EGFR M^- patients, whereas OS was equal (HR, 0.96; 95%CI, 0.77–1.19; P = 0.69; $I^2 = 0.0\%$, $P_{heterogeneity} = 0.43$); EGFR-TKIs significantly improved PFS (HR, 0.28; 95%CI, 0.15–0.53; P<0.001; $I^2 = 4.1\%$, $P_{heterogeneity} = 0.35$) for EGFR M^+ patients, whereas OS was equal (HR, 0.86; 95%CI, 0.44–1.68; P = 0.65; $I^2 = 0.0\%$, $P_{heterogeneity} = 0.77$). Compared with chemotherapy, EGFR-TKIs led to more grade 3–4 rash, but less fatigue/asthenia disorder, leukopenia and thrombocytopenia.

Conclusions: Our analysis suggests that chemotherapy in the second-line setting can prolong PFS in EGFR M^- patients, whereas it has no impact on OS. EGFR-TKIs seem superior over chemotherapy as second-line therapy for EGFR M^+ patients. Our findings support obtaining information on EGFR mutational status before initiation of second-line treatment.

Editor: Robert K. Hills, Cardiff University, United Kingdom

Funding: The authors have no support or funding to report.

Competing Interests: The authors have declared that no competing interests exist.

* Email: wsysums@163.net

◈ These authors contributed equally to this work.

Introduction

Lung cancer remains the leading cause of cancer death in the world and approximately accounts for 13% of total cases and 18% of total deaths globally [1]. Although patients received standard first-line chemotherapy, most of them progressed ultimately. Docetaxel is considered as standard second-line treatment of advanced non-small-cell lung cancer (NSCLC) [2,3]. Pemetrexed was approved for second-line treatment of advanced NSCLC after findings of a phase III trial by Hanna et al. showed equivalent outcomes. Pemetrexed was associated with few adverse events compared with docetaxel and comparable efficacy [4].

Epidermal growth factor receptor tyrosine kinase inhibitors (EGFR-TKIs, including Erlotinib and Gefitinib) have been approved as second-line therapy [5,6,7]. The BR.21 trial reported prolonged survival with erlotinib compared with placebo (median survival, 7.9 versus 3.7 months) in patients with advanced NSCLC after failure of previous chemotherapy [5].

However, the debate on the selection of EGFR-TKIs or chemotherapy in the second-line setting has heated up, even though several meta-analyses have been performed to address this issue. The editorial in 2012 gave an illustration of this debate [8]. Although the meta-analysis by Qi et al. demonstrated both EGFR-

TKIs and chemotherapy had comparable efficacy in the second-line setting, the potential effect of EGFR mutation status on survival was not analysed [9]. The subsequent comprehensive meta-analysis by Lee et al. showed that an EGFR mutation is a predictive marker of PFS with EGFR-TKIs in all settings, but it included only 5 studies comparing EGFR-TKIs with chemotherapy in the second-line setting [10]. Recently, several trials showed that chemotherapy had superiority in progression-free survival (PFS) over EGFR-TKIs for EGFR mutation-negative (EGFR M^-) patients [11,12,13]. A meta-analysis which included 3 trials in the 2013 ASCO annual meeting demonstrated chemotherapy can improve PFS compared with EGFR-TKIs for EGFR M^- patients [14]. To further investigate the optimal treatment and the role of EGFR mutation status in second-line setting, we performed this meta-analysis to compare the efficacy and safety of EGFR-TKIs versus chemotherapy as second-line treatment for pretreated advanced NSCLC.

Methods

Search Strategy

An internet search of PubMed, the Embase database, the Cochrane Central Register of Controlled Trials database (CENTRAL), the American Society of Clinical Oncology (ASCO), the European Society for Medical Oncology (ESMO) and the World Conference of Lung Cancer (WCLC) was performed in July 2013, via the various combinations of the following terms: "lung cancer", "gefitinib", "erlotinib", "EGFR-TKI", "second-line", "randomized". The language was limited to English. The relevant review articles and meta-analyses concerning the second-line treatment for patients with lung cancer were examined for inclusive trials and were listed.

Selection Criteria

The relevant clinical trials were included if they met the following criteria: (1) they compared an EGFR-TKI with standard second-line chemotherapy (docetaxel or pemetrexed); (2) they were prospective randomized controlled trials (RCTs); (3) enrolled patients were previously treated with platinum compounds; (4) they reported sufficient data for extraction or sufficient data to calculate the effect measure. Two reviewers (L.N. and Y.L.) independently screened each reference to assess their eligibility for inclusion with disagreements settled by the third reviewer (W.SY.) until a consensus was reached.

Data Extraction

Information from studies was extracted independently by 2 researchers (L.N. and Y.L.) and the following data were collected: publication details (such as the first author's last name, year of publication, country in which the study was performed), trial information (such as study design, inclusion criteria, the number of the patients, chemotherapy regimens, type of end point used), patient characteristics (such as age, gender, stage, EGFR mutation status), outcome measures (such as HRs for PFS and OS and their 95%CIs, log-rank test P values, grade 3–4 adverse events). PFS and overall survival (OS) were defined as starting from randomization. The quality of the study was assessed on the Jadad score [15] to assess the trials according to randomization (0–2), appropriate blinding method (0–2), withdrawals and dropouts (0–1). The information extracted by the two researchers achieved excellent consistence.

Statistical Analysis

The analysis was undertaken on an intention-to-treat basis. The results were presented as hazard ratios (HRs) and odds ratios (ORs) with their corresponding confidence intervals (CIs). For time-to-event data, the HRs and their 95%CIs were estimated by the methods proposed by Tierney et al. in the absence of published HRs or their CIs [16]. The summary HRs and their 95%CIs were estimated by a general variance-based method. The drug-related adverse events (AEs) were analyzed as grades 3 or above toxicity according to the National Cancer Institute common toxicity criteria (NCI-CTC) version 3. ORs were computed for dichotomous variables by the methods reported by Mantel and Haenszel [17]. Preplanned subgroup analyses to explore potential effect on PFS, OS based on EGFR mutation status were scheduled. Heterogeneity of the treatment effect between studies was estimated on the Q statistic and the heterogeneity I^2 statistic [18]. If heterogeneity was considered statistically significant, random effects models were used and otherwise fixed effects models were used. Egger's test and Begg's funnel plots were used to check for potential publication bias [19,20]. All the reported P values are 2-sided. STATA (version 12.0) was used for all analyses.

Results

Characteristics of the Included Studies

A total of 10 publications were included in the analysis, of which 6 trials [7,21,22,23,24,25] were identified from previous meta-analyses, 4 trials [11,12,13,26] were identified from internet searching. The flow diagram of our study is shown in Figure 1. Seven trials were reported in full text [7,21,22,23,24,25,26], and the other 3 in conference abstracts [11,12,13]. The total number of randomized patients in these trials was 3825, with 1905 in the EGFR-TKI arm and 1920 in the chemotherapy arm. The total number of randomized patients of each trial ranged from 135 to 1466. None of the 10 included trials were placebo-controlled double-blinded trials and therefore none of them scored Jadad score 4 or above. Eight [7,11,12,22,23,24,25,26] of the 10 trials were phase III RCTs, and the other 2 trials [13,21] were phase II trials. Four trials [21,22,23,24] compared gefitinib and docetaxel, 2 [11,12] compared erlotinib and docetaxel, 2 [13,25] compared gefitinib and pemetrexed, 1 [26] compared erlotinib and pemetrexed, and 1 [7] compared erlotinib and docetaxel/pemetrexed. The baseline characteristics of these studies are listed in Table 1. This meta-analysis followed the guidelines of the Preferred Reporting Items for Systematic Review and Meta-analyses (PRISMA) statement. The PRISMA Flow Diagram and Checklist are shown in Figure S1 and Checklist S1.

Efficacy Analysis Results

All 10 trials reported PFS data. Overall, the pooled hazard ratio for PFS showed that there was no significant difference between an EGFR-TKI and second-line chemotherapy (HR, 1.03; 95%CI, 0.87–1.21; $P = 0.73$, Figure 2). Random effect model was used since heterogeneity across the trials was significant ($I^2 = 78.7\%$, $P < 0.001$).

Data for OS were available from 8 trials [7,12,21,22,23,24,25,26], and the pooled HR for OS showed that there was no significant difference between an EGFR-TKI and second-line chemotherapy (HR, 1.00; 95%CI, 0.92–1.08; $P = 0.90$, Figure 3). Fixed effect model was used since heterogeneity across the trials was not significant ($I^2 = 0.0\%$, $P = 0.88$).

Data for objective response rate (ORR) were available from all 10 trials. The pooled OR for ORR showed that there was no significant difference between an EGFR-TKI and second-line

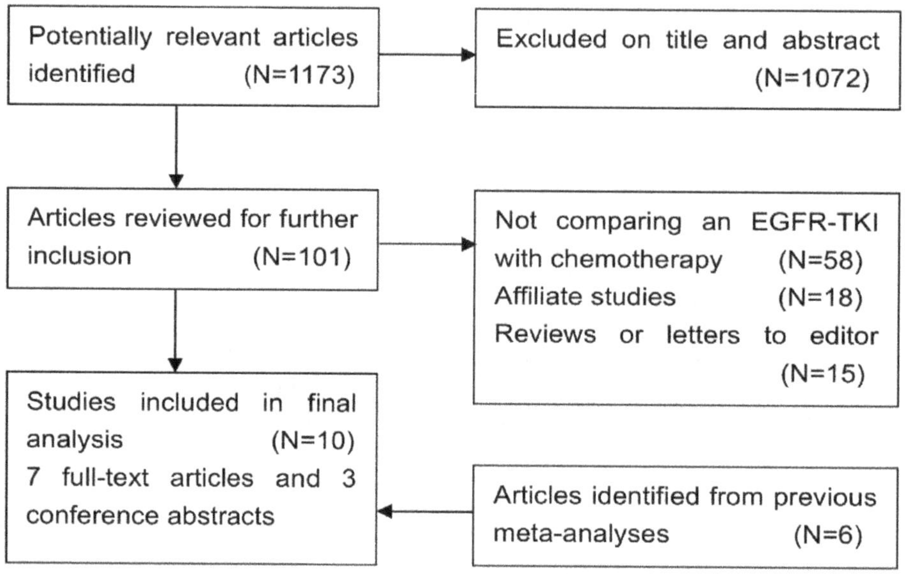

Figure 1. Flow diagram of trial identification process.

chemotherapy (OR, 1.34; 95%CI, 0.86–2.08; P = 0.20, Figure 4). Between-study heterogeneity was significant (I^2 = 73.1%, P< 0.001), and the pooled OR for ORR was performed through random effect model.

Subgroup Analysis Based on EGFR Mutation Status

Six trials [7,11,12,13,22,25] reported HRs for PFS of EGFR M^- lung cancer and 2 [7,22] reported HRs for OS of EGFR M^- lung cancer. Totally, the reported number of EGFR M^- patients was 1119. The pooled HR for PFS and OS showed that there was a significant improvement in PFS for second-line chemotherapy compared with EGFR-TKI therapy for EGFR M^- patients (HR, 1.35; 95%CI, 1.09–1.66; P = 0.01, Figure 5), whereas the OS between them was not significantly different (HR, 0.96; 95%CI, 0.77–1.19; P = 0.69, Figure 5).

Data for PFS of EGFR mutation-positive (EGFR M^+) lung cancer were available from 3 trials [7,22,25] and data for OS of EGFR M^+ lung cancer were available from 2 trials [7,22]. Totally, the reported number of EGFR M^+ patients was 150. The pooled HRs for PFS and OS showed that there was a significant improvement in PFS for EGFR-TKI therapy compared with second-line chemotherapy for EGFR M^+ patients (HR, 0.28; 95%CI, 0.15–0.53; P<0.001, Figure 6), whereas the OS between them was not significantly different (HR, 0.86; 95%CI, 0.44–1.68; P = 0.65, Figure 6).

Toxicity Analysis Results

Drug-related toxicity was described as patient-experienced grade 3–4 toxicity in this analysis. The main toxicities of these trials are listed in table 2. Compared with chemotherapy, EGFR-TKIs led to more grade 3–4 rash (OR, 7.55; 95%CI: 3.97–14.37; P<0.001). Additionally, compared with chemotherapy, a statistically significant decrease in fatigue/asthenia disorder, leukopenia and thrombocytopenia was observed (OR, 0.45; 95%CI: 0.32–0.64; P<0.001; OR, 0.04; 95%CI: 0.01–0.10; P<0.001; OR, 0.25; 95%CI: 0.08–0.83; P = 0.02, respectively). With regard to the risk of grade 3–4 diarrhea, nausea, vomiting, and anemia, equivalent frequencies were found between the EGFR-TKI arm and the chemotherapy arm. The analyses of toxicities were performed on the fixed effect model except for leukopenia (because of heterogeneity).

Publication Bias and Sensitivity Analysis

Egger's test was used to check potential publication bias and the results showed that no evidence of publication bias exists (P = 0.95 for PFS, P = 0.11 for OS and P = 0.73 for ORR). The symmetry Begg's funnel plots indicated that there was no evidence of publication bias in our meta-analysis (Figure S2). Sensitivity analysis indicated that the results of this pooled analysis were not affected by exclusion of a particular trial from the analysis.

Discussion

Standard first-line treatment for advanced lung cancer usually consists of platinum-based doublet chemotherapy, but progression eventually occurs for most patients [27,28]. Available second-line treatment options for patients who have failure of first-line treatment include targeted therapy or further chemotherapy. In the second-line setting, an EGFR mutation status examination was thought to be time-consuming and unnecessary. Recent studies about second-line treatment found that chemotherapy was superior to EGFR-TKIs in PFS for EGFR M^- NSCLC [11,12,13]. Our meta-analysis combined 3825 patients from 10 randomized trials. Our analysis demonstrated that regardless of EGFR mutation status, EGFR-TKIs and second-line chemotherapy had equivalent efficacy for pretreated advanced NSCLC patients. In addition, our analysis demonstrated that in terms of PFS, chemotherapy showed a significant improvement for EGFR M^- patients compared with EGFR-TKIs, and EGFR-TKIs were superior to chemotherapy for EGFR M^+ patients. Overall, these data suggest that obtaining information on EGFR mutational status before initiation of second-line treatment is worth it.

Previously, the meta-analysis by Qi et al. also demonstrated both EGFR-TKIs and chemotherapy had comparable efficacy. However, the potential effect of EGFR mutation status on PFS, OS was not analysed in the analysis [9]. Subsequently, the meta-analysis by Lee et al. investigated the impact of EGFR-TKIs on PFS and OS in NSCLC and showed that an EGFR mutation is a predictive marker of PFS in all settings. However, of the 7 second-

Table 1. Information of trials included in this meta-analysis.

Study/Year	Phase	Country	Therapy	N	Male (%)	Ever smoker (%)	IIIB (%)	IV (%)	EGFR M+ (%)	PFS (mo)	OS (mo)	RR (%)	Jadad score
SIGN, 2006	II	International	Gefitinib	68	30.9	67.6	39.7	60.3	NR	3.0	7.5	13.2	3
			Doc	73	30.1	67.1	43.8	56.2	NR	3.4	7.1	13.7	
INTEREST, 2008	III	International	Gefitinib	733	36.4	79.8	25.0	52.9	15.6	2.2	7.6	9.1	3
			Doc	733	33.4	79.6	28.8	52.3	14.1	2.7	8.0	7.6	
V-15-32, 2008	III	Japan	Gefitinib	245	38.4	71.0	19.2	64.9	NR	2.0	11.5	22.5	3
			Doc	244	38.1	64.3	20.5	61.5	NR	2.0	14.0	12.8	
ISTANA, 2010	III	Korea	Gefitinib	82	32.9	63.4	13.4	86.6	NR	3.3	14.1	28.1	3
			Doc	79	43.0	54.4	17.7	82.3	NR	3.4	12.2	7.6	
TITAN, 2012	III	International	Erlotinib	203	20.6	85.2	20.2	79.8	3.4	1.5	5.3	7.9	3
			Doc/Pem	221	27.6	80.1	23.1	76.9	1.8	2.0	5.5	6.3	
KCSG-LU08-01, 2012	III	Korea	Gefitinib	68	85.3	0	8.8	91.2	23.5	9.0	22.2	58.8	3
			Pem	67	85.1	0	9.0	91.0	25.4	3.0	18.9	22.4	
TAILOR, 2012	III	Italy	Erlotinib	109	29.4	81.7	NR	NR	0	2.4	NR	2.2	3
			Doc	110	33.6	71.8	NR	NR	0	3.4	NR	13.9	
HORG, 2013	III	Greece	Erlotinib	166	18.7	74.7	7.2	92.8	8.1	3.6	8.2	9.0	3
			Pem	166	16.9	77.1	11.4	88.6	9.8	2.9	10.1	11.4	
DELTA, 2013	III	Japan	Erlotinib	150	NR	NR	NR	NR	27.3	2.0	14.8	17.0	3
			Doc	151	NR	NR	NR	NR	40.4	3.2	12.2	17.9	
CTONG0806, 2013	II	China	Gefitinib	81	33.3	59.3	4.9	95.1	0	1.6	NR	13.6	3
			Pem	76	38.2	42.1	13.2	86.8	0	4.8	NR	13.2	

Abbreviations: N, number of patients; IIIB, stage IIIB; IV, stage IV; EGFR M^+, epidermal growth factor receptor mutation-positive; PFS, progression-free survival; mo, month; OS, overall survival; RR, response rate; Doc, docetaxel; Pem, pemetrexed; NR, no report.

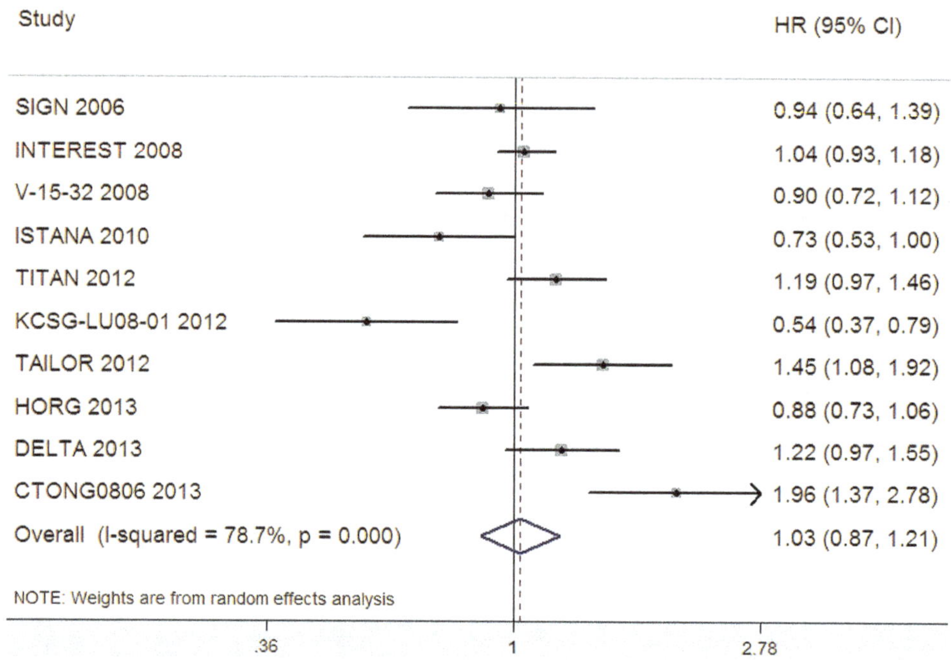

Figure 2. Comparison of PFS between EGFR-TKIs and chemotherapy.

line studies included in their meta-analysis, only 5 studies compared an EGFR-TKI with chemotherapy [10]. A meta-analysis comparing EGFR-TKIs with chemotherapy as second-line therapy for wild-type EGFR lung cancer patients was presented in part at the 2013 ASCO annual meeting and also demonstrated chemotherapy had superiority in PFS over EGFR-TKIs for EGFR M^- patients. However, that meta-analysis only included 3 trials [14]. Our meta-analysis combined 1269 patients with explicit EGFR mutation status. Although the reported number of EGFR M^+ patients was only 150 in these trials and caution should be used when these results are interpreted, our meta-analysis provides information to better the relation of second-line therapy and EGFR mutation status.

Our analysis suggested that PFS favored chemotherapy among pretreated EGFR M^- patients, whereas it favored EGFR-TKIs among those with EGFR M^+ tumors. The possible explanation is that EGFR mutation may be a predictive biomarker for benefit of EGFR-TKIs over chemotherapy beyond first-line treatment. The IPASS trial suggested that the presence of an EGFR mutation is the strongest predictor for benefit of gefitinib in the first-line setting

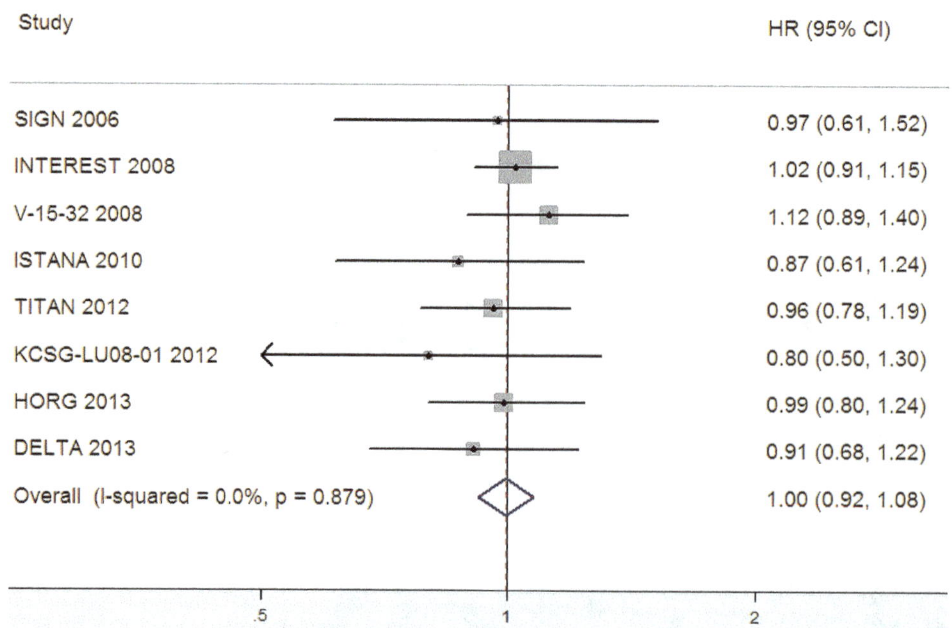

Figure 3. Comparison of OS between EGFR-TKIs and chemotherapy.

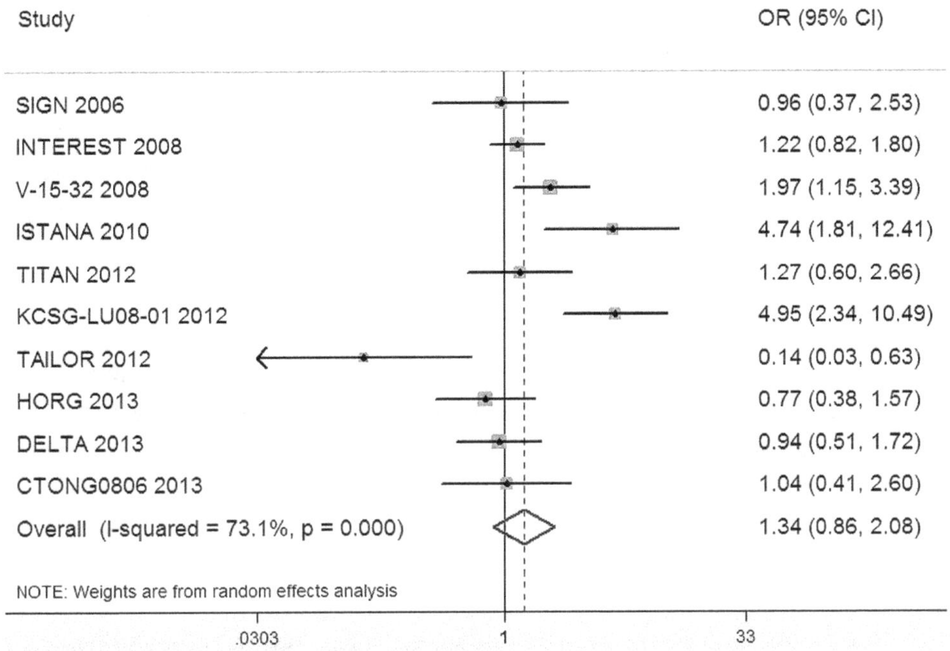

Figure 4. Comparison of ORR between EGFR-TKIs and chemotherapy.

[29]. In IPASS, the PFS benefit of gefitinib was limited to EGFR M^+ patients and gefitinib was associated with poorer PFS than carboplatin–paclitaxel for EGFR M^- patients [30]. The above combined with the results of our study suggests that the predictive value of EGFR mutation may be applied to both first-line and second-line treatment.

In our analysis, the prolonged PFS advantage in different EGFR mutational status didn't translate into an OS advantage. This is mostly because of the high crossover rate after progression. None of these trials prohibited patients from crossing over to the other group. For example, in the INTEREST trial, of the patients in the gefitinib arm, 31% received docetaxel as subsequent therapy, and of the patients in the docetaxel arm, 37% received an EGFR-TKI subsequently [22]. Additionally, in the V-15-32 trial, 36% of patients in the gefitinib arm received subsequent docetaxel, 53% of patients in the docetaxel arm received subsequent gefitinib [23].

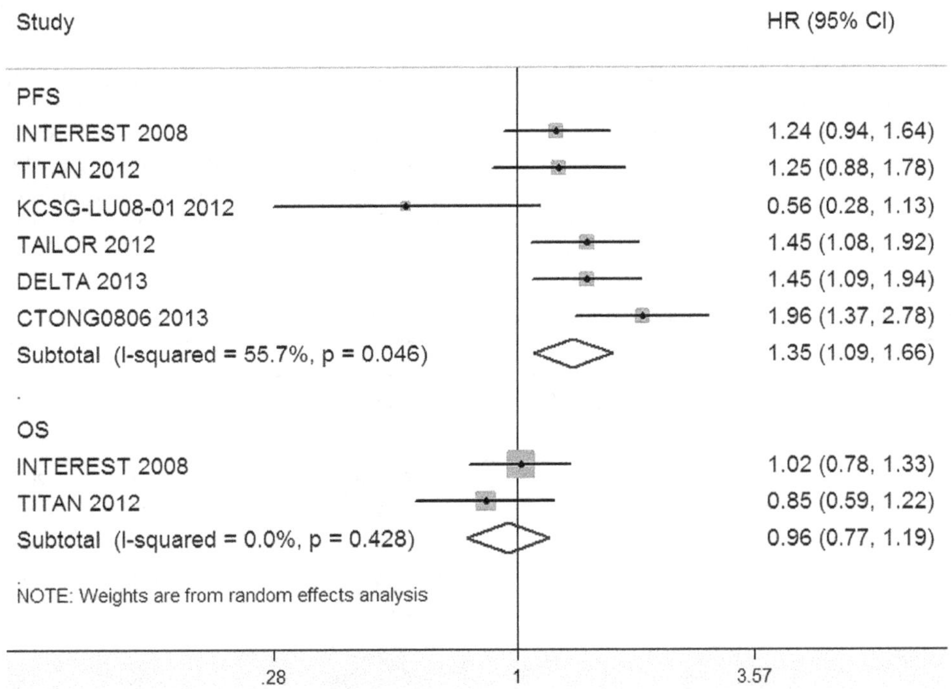

Figure 5. Comparison of PFS and OS between EGFR-TKIs and chemotherapy in subgroup of EGFR M^- patients.

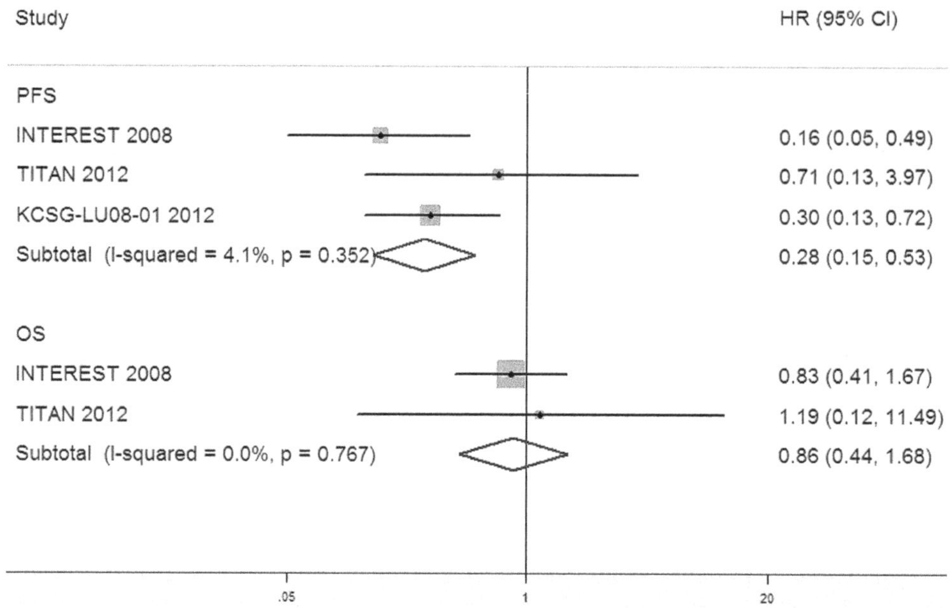

Figure 6. Comparison of PFS and OS between EGFR-TKIs and chemotherapy in subgroup of EGFR M$^+$ patients.

The high crossover rate confounded the interpretation of OS. Since there are more and more active agents emerging in the treatment of NSCLC, a PFS advantage is rarely associated with an OS advantage any more [31,32]. Considering patients' benefit and ethical issues, crossover treatment may be inevitable. So PFS should be deemed as a good end point. More work is still required to demonstrate the impact of PFS on OS.

Regarding grade 3–4 toxicity data, our analysis demonstrated that although EGFR-TKIs produced more rash, they produced less fatigue/asthenia disorder, leukopenia and thrombocytopenia than second-line chemotherapy. Since most of rash can be managed, as far as toxicity profiles are concerned, an EGFR-TKI is favourable. Since the toxicity profiles of EGFR-TKIs are manageable, and the combination of EGFR-TKIs with chemotherapy has shown advantage as first-line treatment [33] and as adjuvant treatment [34], this therapeutic pattern should be explored in this setting.

Several limitations should be noted from this meta-analysis. To begin with, like many other meta-analyses, this is a meta-analysis based on published data as well, so caution should be used when the results are interpreted. Secondly, the assessed EGFR M$^+$ patients were only 150, which restricted our results. Thirdly, the methods for detecting EGFR mutation of these trials were not unified. For example, direct gene sequencing was used to detect EGFR mutation in most trials, while polymerase chain reaction was used in the HORG trial [26]. Different methods have different sensitivity in detecting EGFR mutations. Additionally, several trials were not 100% second-line setting studies, and geographic origin was another concern. Further prospective studies are needed to confirm the best treatment in the second-line setting for advanced NSCLC.

In conclusion, based on this meta-analysis, treatment with chemotherapy can prolong PFS in EGFR M$^-$ patients, whereas has no impact on OS. EGFR-TKIs seem superior over chemotherapy as second-line therapy for EGFR M$^+$ patients. It is worthwhile to obtain information on EGFR mutational status before initiation of second-line treatment. These results, combined

Table 2. Comparison of grade 3–4 toxicities between EGFR-TKIs and chemotherapy.

Grade 3–4 toxicity	Included trials	OR and 95%CI	P value	Heterogeneity	
				I^2	P value
Rash	9	7.55 (3.97, 14.37)	<0.001	26.7	0.21
Diarrhea	9	1.09 (0.68, 1.74)	0.73	0.0	0.61
Fatigue/Asthenia disorder	9	0.45 (0.32, 0.64)	<0.001	4.6	0.40
Nausea	8	0.60 (0.32, 1.13)	0.12	0.0	0.68
Vomiting	8	0.79 (0.37, 1.67)	0.54	0.0	0.65
Anemia	6	0.68 (0.40, 1.14)	0.15	1.6	0.41
Leukopenia	9	0.04 (0.01, 0.10)	<0.001	74.4	<0.001
Thrombocytopenia	5	0.25 (0.08, 0.83)	0.02	0.0	0.53

with the toxicities, should be taken into consideration in the second-line treatment.

Supporting Information

Figure S1 PRISMA Flow Diagram.

Figure S2 Begg's funnel plots of publication bias.

Checklist S1 PRISMA Checklist.

Author Contributions

Conceived and designed the experiments: NL WO SW. Performed the experiments: NL LY. Analyzed the data: NL LY WO. Contributed reagents/materials/analysis tools: LY LZ SZ. Wrote the paper: NL SW.

References

1. Jemal A, Bray F, Center MM, Ferlay J, Ward E, et al. (2011) Global cancer statistics. CA: a cancer journal for clinicians 61: 69–90.
2. Fossella FV, DeVore R, Kerr RN, Crawford J, Natale RR, et al. (2000) Randomized phase III trial of docetaxel versus vinorelbine or ifosfamide in patients with advanced non-small-cell lung cancer previously treated with platinum-containing chemotherapy regimens. The TAX 320 Non-Small Cell Lung Cancer Study Group. J Clin Oncol 18: 2354–2362.
3. Shepherd FA, Dancey J, Ramlau R, Mattson K, Gralla R, et al. (2000) Prospective randomized trial of docetaxel versus best supportive care in patients with non-small-cell lung cancer previously treated with platinum-based chemotherapy. J Clin Oncol 18: 2095–2103.
4. Hanna N, Shepherd FA, Fossella FV, Pereira JR, De Marinis F, et al. (2004) Randomized phase III trial of pemetrexed versus docetaxel in patients with non-small-cell lung cancer previously treated with chemotherapy. J Clin Oncol 22: 1589–1597.
5. Shepherd FA, Rodrigues Pereira J, Ciuleanu T, Tan EH, Hirsh V, et al. (2005) Erlotinib in previously treated non-small-cell lung cancer. The New England journal of medicine 353: 123–132.
6. Thatcher N, Chang A, Parikh P, Rodrigues Pereira J, Ciuleanu T, et al. (2005) Gefitinib plus best supportive care in previously treated patients with refractory advanced non-small-cell lung cancer: results from a randomised, placebo-controlled, multicentre study (Iressa Survival Evaluation in Lung Cancer). Lancet 366: 1527–1537.
7. Ciuleanu T, Stelmakh L, Cicenas S, Miliauskas S, Grigorescu AC, et al. (2012) Efficacy and safety of erlotinib versus chemotherapy in second-line treatment of patients with advanced, non-small-cell lung cancer with poor prognosis (TITAN): a randomised multicentre, open-label, phase 3 study. Lancet Oncol 13: 300–308.
8. Paz-Ares L (2012) Beyond first-line NSCLC therapy: chemotherapy or erlotinib? Lancet Oncol 13: 225–227.
9. Qi WX, Shen Z, Lin F, Sun YJ, Min DL, et al. (2012) Comparison of the efficacy and safety of EFGR tyrosine kinase inhibitor monotherapy with standard second-line chemotherapy in previously treated advanced non-small-cell lung cancer: a systematic review and meta-analysis. Asian Pacific journal of cancer prevention: APJCP 13: 5177–5182.
10. Lee CK, Brown C, Gralla RJ, Hirsh V, Thongprasert S, et al. (2013) Impact of EGFR inhibitor in non-small cell lung cancer on progression-free and overall survival: a meta-analysis. Journal of the National Cancer Institute 105: 595–605.
11. Garassino MC, Martelli O, Bettini A, Floriani I, Copreni E, et al. (2012) TAILOR: A phase III trial comparing erlotinib with docetaxel as the second-line treatment of NSCLC patients with wild-type (wt) EGFR. J Clin Oncol 30, 2012 (suppl; abstr LBA7501).
12. Okano Y, Ando M, Asami K, Fukuda M, Nakagawa H, et al. (2013) Randomized phase III trial of erlotinib (E) versus docetaxel (D) as second- or third-line therapy in patients with advanced non-small cell lung cancer (NSCLC) who have wild-type or mutant epidermal growth factor receptor (EGFR): Docetaxel and Erlotinib Lung Cancer Trial (DELTA). J Clin Oncol 31, 2013 (suppl; abstr 8006).
13. Yang JJ, Cheng Y, Zhao MF, Zhou Q, Yan HH, et al. (2013) A phase II trial comparing pemetrexed with gefitinib as the second-line treatment of nonsquamous NSCLC patients with wild-type EGFR (CTONG0806). J Clin Oncol 31, 2013 (suppl; abstr 8042).
14. Gao GH, Ren SX, Li AW, He YY, Chen XX, et al. (2013) A meta-analysis of comparing EGFR-TKI with chemotherapy as the second-line treatment of NSCLC patients with wild-type EGFR. J Clin Oncol 31, 2013 (suppl; abstr e19166).
15. Jadad AR, Moore RA, Carroll D, Jenkinson C, Reynolds DJ, et al. (1996) Assessing the quality of reports of randomized clinical trials: is blinding necessary? Control Clin Trials 17: 1–12.
16. Tierney JF, Stewart LA, Ghersi D, Burdett S, Sydes MR (2007) Practical methods for incorporating summary time-to-event data into meta-analysis. Trials 8: 16.
17. Kuritz SJ, Landis JR, Koch GG (1988) A general overview of Mantel-Haenszel methods: applications and recent developments. Annu Rev Public Health 9: 123–160.
18. Higgins JP, Thompson SG, Deeks JJ, Altman DG (2003) Measuring inconsistency in meta-analyses. BMJ 327: 557–560.
19. Egger M, Davey Smith G, Schneider M, Minder C (1997) Bias in meta-analysis detected by a simple, graphical test. BMJ 315: 629–634.
20. Begg CB, Mazumdar M (1994) Operating characteristics of a rank correlation test for publication bias. Biometrics 50: 1088–1101.
21. Cufer T, Vrdoljak E, Gaafar R, Erensoy I, Pemberton K (2006) Phase II, open-label, randomized study (SIGN) of single-agent gefitinib (IRESSA) or docetaxel as second-line therapy in patients with advanced (stage IIIb or IV) non-small-cell lung cancer. Anticancer Drugs 17: 401–409.
22. Kim ES, Hirsh V, Mok T, Socinski MA, Gervais R, et al. (2008) Gefitinib versus docetaxel in previously treated non-small-cell lung cancer (INTEREST): a randomised phase III trial. Lancet 372: 1809–1818.
23. Maruyama R, Nishiwaki Y, Tamura T, Yamamoto N, Tsuboi M, et al. (2008) Phase III study, V-15-32, of gefitinib versus docetaxel in previously treated Japanese patients with non-small-cell lung cancer. J Clin Oncol 26: 4244–4252.
24. Lee DH, Park K, Kim JH, Lee JS, Shin SW, et al. (2010) Randomized Phase III trial of gefitinib versus docetaxel in non-small cell lung cancer patients who have previously received platinum-based chemotherapy. Clinical cancer research: an official journal of the American Association for Cancer Research 16: 1307–1314.
25. Sun JM, Lee KH, Kim SW, Lee DH, Min YJ, et al. (2012) Gefitinib versus pemetrexed as second-line treatment in patients with nonsmall cell lung cancer previously treated with platinum-based chemotherapy (KCSG-LU08-01): an open-label, phase 3 trial. Cancer 118: 6234–6242.
26. Karampeazis A, Voutsina A, Souglakos J, Kentepozidis N, Giassas S, et al. (2013) Pemetrexed versus erlotinib in pretreated patients with advanced non-small cell lung cancer: a Hellenic Oncology Research Group (HORG) randomized phase 3 study. Cancer 119: 2754–2764.
27. Schiller JH, Harrington D, Belani CP, Langer C, Sandler A, et al. (2002) Comparison of four chemotherapy regimens for advanced non-small-cell lung cancer. The New England journal of medicine 346: 92–98.
28. Scagliotti GV, De Marinis F, Rinaldi M, Crino L, Gridelli C, et al. (2002) Phase III randomized trial comparing three platinum-based doublets in advanced non-small-cell lung cancer. J Clin Oncol 20: 4285–4291.
29. Fukuoka M, Wu YL, Thongprasert S, Sunpaweravong P, Leong SS, et al. (2011) Biomarker analyses and final overall survival results from a phase III, randomized, open-label, first-line study of gefitinib versus carboplatin/paclitaxel in clinically selected patients with advanced non-small-cell lung cancer in Asia (IPASS). J Clin Oncol 29: 2866–2874.
30. Mok TS, Wu YL, Thongprasert S, Yang CH, Chu DT, et al. (2009) Gefitinib or carboplatin-paclitaxel in pulmonary adenocarcinoma. The New England journal of medicine 361: 947–957.
31. Soria JC, Massard C, Le Chevalier T (2010) Should progression-free survival be the primary measure of efficacy for advanced NSCLC therapy? Ann Oncol 21: 2324–2332.
32. Hotta K, Suzuki E, Di Maio M, Chiodini P, Fujiwara Y, et al. (2013) Progression-free survival and overall survival in phase III trials of molecular-targeted agents in advanced non-small-cell lung cancer. Lung Cancer 79: 20–26.
33. Mok TS, Wu YL, Yu CJ, Zhou C, Chen YM, et al. (2009) Randomized, placebo-controlled, phase II study of sequential erlotinib and chemotherapy as first-line treatment for advanced non-small-cell lung cancer. J Clin Oncol 27: 5080–5087.
34. Wang SY, Ou W, Li N, Sun HB, Zhang L, et al. (2013) Pemetrexed-carboplatin adjuvant chemotherapy with or without gefitinib in resected stage IIIA-N2 non-small cell lung cancer harbouring EGFR mutations: A randomized phase II study. J Clin Oncol 31, 2013 (suppl; abstr 7519).

4

A Retrospective Analysis of Incidence and its Associated Risk Factors of Upper Urinary Tract Recurrence following Radical Cystectomy for Bladder Cancer with Transitional Cell Carcinoma: The Significance of Local Pelvic Recurrence and Positive Lymph Node

Sung Han Kim[1], Hyung-Kook Yang[2], Jung Hoon Lee[3], Eun-Sik Lee[3]*

1 Department of Urology, National Cancer Center, Goyang, Gyanggi, Korea, **2** Department of Epidemiology and Statistics and Cancer Policy Branch of the National Cancer Control Research Institute, National Cancer Center, Goyang, Gyanggi, Korea, **3** Department of Urology, Seoul National University Hospital, Seoul, Seoul, Korea

Abstract

Objective: The aim of this study is to examine the incidence and risk factors of upper urinary tract recurrence (UUTR) following radical cystectomy (RC) in bladder cancer and to evaluate its relationship with neobladder (Neo) or ileal conduit (IC).

Materials and Methods: All clinicopathologic parameters and perioperative parameters of 311 patients who underwent RC with either Neo or IC by a single surgeon from 1999 to 2012 were retrospectively included in this study. Patients with a history of renal surgery, concomitant UUTR, or a histopathology of non-transitional cell carcinoma were excluded. For statistical analyses of predictive risk factors of UUTR, a multivariate analysis was performed with known risk factors of UUTR, including type of urinary diversion with significance defined as $P < 0.05$.

Results: During the median follow-up period of 53 months, 143 (46.0%) IC and 168 (54.0%) Neo were performed, resulting in 11 (3.5%) cases of UUTR (Neo 7 and IC 4) after RC and all patients then underwent nephroureterectomy. No significant differences in incidence and overall survival in UUTR were observed according different types of urinary diversion (p = 483), and the prognosis for survival of Neo was insignificantly better than that of IC (5-year overall survival 78% vs 74%, respectively, p>0.05). Higher number of positive lymph nodes (HR 9.03) and the presence of pelvic local recurrence (HR 7286.08) were significant predictive factors of UUTR (p<0.05).

Conclusion: This study reports a UUTR rate of 3.5%, and positive lymph nodes and presence of local recurrence at the pelvis as important risk factors. No significant differences in incidence and survival were observed between Neo and IC.

Editor: Syed A. Aziz, Health Canada and University of Ottawa, Canada

Funding: The authors have no support or funding to report.

Competing Interests: The authors have declared that no competing interests exist.

* E-mail: eslee@snu.ac.kr

Introduction

Approximately 20–30% of cases of bladder cancer (BC) are reportedly found at muscle-invasive status at initial presentation and even 20–50% of early detected superficial BC also progressed to invasive, with a loco-regional recurrence rate of 5–15% during follow-ups [1,2]. For muscle-invasive or frequently recurred BC, radical cystectomy (RC) with urinary diversion of either neobladder or ileal conduit is a standard treatment, and upper urinary tract recurrence (UUTR) is another important issue during postoperative follow-ups. However, because incidence of UUTR following RC for BC is relatively rare, ranging between 0.74% and 6.4%, and prognosis is poor, with median survival within 24 months after development, and with late occurrence until nine years after RC, the characteristics and clinical course of UUTR have not yet been fully defined and the different follow-up strategy of evaluating upper urinary tract has still been discussed [3–10]. Various risk factors for UUTR have been reported, such as age, nuclear grade, stage, multifocality, histology, a positive margin of urethra or ureter, lymph nodal positivity, and the presence of carcinoma in situ (CIS) [3,6,7,11–14]. Therefore, prediction of an increased likelihood of UUTR and its risk factors is important in order to define the strategy for monitoring during follow-up [9,10,12].

In this study, we reviewed our computerized RC Database Registry in order to examine the incidence and clinical course of UUTR after RC and to determine its predictive risk factors. In addition, the relationship between the incidence of UUTR and the different types of urinary diversion of RC was also evaluated.

Materials and Methods

Of the 366 RC patients treated for primary BC since 1992, the records of 311 patients who underwent RC with 168 orthotopic (neobladder) or 143 non-orthotopic (ileal conduit) urinary diversion by a single surgeon (ESL) between April 1999 and December 2012 were reviewed. Patients were censored at last follow up or date of death due to BC and other causes according to the cancer database in the Korean National Insurance Health Statistics, where all cancer patients in Korea should be automatically registered and followed up until death. No deaths or UUTR were detected among patients who were lost to follow-up or transferred to another hospital because of the accessibility of distance. Minimum follow up period for living patients was one year. Indications for RC included muscle invasive BC, CIS refractory to Bacillus Calmette-Guerin intravesical therapy, recurrent multifocal high grade superficial BC refractory to transurethral resection, and large superficial papillary BC with severe comorbidities without muscle invasive at initial transurethral section, but not enough to perform multiple transurethral operations. We excluded patients who underwent palliative cystectomy for control of bleeding and pain relief, who had a previous history of renal surgery before RC as well as concomitant UUTR at RC, who had no history of postoperative follow-up at our institution, or who had non-transitional cell carcinoma on final pathologic specimen of bladder at RC.

UUTR was defined as any abnormal findings of occurred and proven cancer recurrence in radiography, endoscopy, or pathology along the upper urinary tract [7]. Cancer recurrence and pathological staging, including UUTR and RC specimens, were staged and graded according to the TNM classification (TNM), the World Health Organization system (WHO), and American Joint Committee on Cancer criteria (AJCC) [15–17]. Nephroureterectomy (NU) was also graded, pathologically staged with histology. All preoperative and postoperative pathological studies were reviewed by pathologists. In addition, the mode of clinical manifestation and method of diagnosis, time to recurrence, type of therapy, and clinical outcomes were collected retrospectively by chart reviews.

Preoperative Evaluation

Preoperative evaluation included cystoscopy, washing cytology, transurethral resection of bladder tumor and/or bladder biopsy with anesthesia, upper urinary tract (UUT) imaging with excretory urography (EXU) or intravenous pyelography (IVP) and/or enhanced abdominal computed tomography (CT), and chest X-ray. Some patients underwent further metastatic evaluation, including whole-body bone scan (WBBS), chest CT, and/or positron emission tomography-CT (PET-CT), as clinically indicated.

Additional treatment

Neoadjuvant or adjuvant chemotherapy was administered based on the decision of the surgeon. The indication for neoadjuvant chemotherapy was those patients suspicious for whether single nodal positive or microscopically extravesical extended states on imaging studies and cytoscopic findings with endoscopically resected specimens. The indication for adjuvant chemotherapy was routinely recommended for all node-positive advanced or newly developed metastatic patients at our institute, except for those who were medically intolerant or who refused this treatment. Most patients with neoadjuvant chemotherapy received two to four cycles of a combination of gemcitabine and carboplatin/cisplatin (GC/GP) according to the functional status of their kidney. Most patients with adjuvant chemotherapy received a combination of GC/GP or methotrexate, vinblastine, doxorubicin, and cisplatin (MVAC) until no response. The cycles and combination of chemotherapeutic agents for neoadjuvant and adjuvant chemotherapy were performed according to the extent of coverage by the national insurance policy, tumor response, and general performance status including underlying disease such as chronic kidney disease with an estimated glomerular filtration rate less than 60 mL/min/1.72 m^2.

Operative procedure

RC was completed, including routine serial intraoperative frozen section examination of the ureters above the crossing iliac vessels and/or the urethra until the resection was clear. These results determined the need for subsequent resection of the proximal ureter, NU, and urethrectomy. Redundant ureter excised at the time of ureteroenteric anastomosis constituted the final specimen. Lymph node dissection and its extent of dissection (none, limited, standard, and extended lymph node dissection [LND]) were completed according to surgeon decision that any nodal involvements during preoperative imaging work ups or intraoperative suspicious lymph nodal enlargements, or clinical tumor stages were indicated for performance of LND. The extent of LND was determined according to previous reports [18,19].

Postoperative follow-up protocol

The follow-up schedule was determined according to the pathology of the RC specimen. Patients with pT2 or lower without nodal involvement underwent follow-up examinations every 3–6 months for two years after RC, and then every 6–12 months. Patients with pT3-4 or nodal positive underwent follow-up examinations every three months after RC. Regular follow-up examinations included physical examination, blood chemistry studies, complete blood count, urinary analysis and cytology, chest X-ray and EXU or IVP or enhanced abdominal CT. Further imaging, including retrograde ileography, was performed if recurrence was suspected based on unexplained symptoms or clinical concern. In the absence of recurrence for five years after RC, the interval between examinations was extended based on the decision of the surgeon in consideration of tumor pathology with intraoperative disease states and clinical severity. Patients diagnosed with UUTR underwent metastatic evaluation, including abdominal CT, chest X-ray, and WBBS or PET.

Statistical measures

For the statistical analysis, all clinicopathologic parameters and perioperative parameters were considered. Statistical analyses were performed by an experienced medical statistician (HK.Y) using independent t-test and Mann-Whitney t-tests for numerical variables and Chi-square and Fisher's exact tests for categorical variables to compare the UUTR incidences between different urinary diversions of RC. Multivariate model was performed by logistic regression analysis among variables found to be both clinically and statistically significant in univariate analysis.

To define clinical prognosis of survival and recurrence with their associated risk factors for UUTR, the Kaplan–Meier method, log–rank test, and Cox proportional hazards model were applied using SPSS 18.0 (SPSS Inc., Chicago, USA). Two-sided statistical analyses were performed and significance was defined as $P < 0.05$.

Ethics statement

An ethics committee and an institutional review board (IRB) of Seoul National University Hospital approved computerized RC Database Registry was used to report clinical outcomes of UUTR after RC for primary BC (IRB No. H1208-081-422). All the patients participated in his study did provide verbal informed consent and the ethics committees/IRB approved this consent procedure and the exemption of written informed consent.

Results

The median age of 311 patients was 64.0 (46–86) years old with a median follow-up period of 53.0 (13-207) months. Male (88.7%) was more predominant than female (11.3%). For types of urinary diversion, 143 IC (46.0%) and 168 Neo (54.0%) were performed. Intravesical, neoadjuvant, and adjuvant chemotherapies were administered for 64 (20.5%) (4 GC and 60 GP based regimen) and 83 (26.7%) patients (76 GC and 7 MVAC based regimen), respectively. LND was performed only in 74.9% at RC. However, all 11 UUTR cases underwent LND at RC. According to pathologic stage, organ-confined disease (pT0-2N0, Tis) was found in 161 patients (51.8%), non-organ-confined disease (pT2-4Nx) in 140 (48.2%), including pT2N+ stage in 20 (6.4%), and other positive lymph nodal metastasis in 21 (6.8%) (Table 1). No significant differences in incidence and overall survival in UUTR were observed according different types of urinary diversion ($p = 483$), and the prognosis for survival of Neo was insignificantly better than that of IC (5-year overall survival 78% vs 74%, respectively, $p>0.05$; not shown in tables).

A total of 11 patients (3.5%) from seven Neo and four IC developed UUTR and all patients then underwent NU with only two patients with LND at suspicious peri-hilum and peri-aorta and with only five patients receiving further adjuvant chemotherapy (Table 2). The median time to UUTR after RC was 26 months (not shown in tables). Pathological examination of UUTR patients showed that only two patients had organ-confined disease (pT3aN0) on RC specimens and the remaining nine (81.8%) patients had non-organ-confined disease with five (45.5%) patients with nodal positivity. Local recurrence at the pelvis was observed in six patients, including two urethras, whereas no positive resection margin of ureters and urethra was observed on RC specimens of all 11 patients (Table 2).

In comparison of the 11 patients of the UUTR group with the remaining patients ($n = 300$, non-UUTR group), besides a significantly poorer general condition referred from the ASA score, higher rate of intravesical instillation of agents before RC, and postoperative local recurrence at pelvis, and shorter duration of follow-up in the UUTR group, no significant differences in clinicopathologic, and perioperative parameters were observed between the two groups ($p<0.05$, Table 3). In comparison of median survival between the two groups, the UUTR group had insignificantly poorer survival of approximately nine months than the other group (median survival 65.9 vs. 76.9 months, $p = 0.383$, respectively; Table 3). In assessment of previously known clinicopathological factors from other studies and our significant univariate parameters in prediction of the predictive risk factors of UUTR after RC, the presence of local recurrence at the pelvis (HR 7286.1, CI 3.50-122760.70) and number of positive lymph nodes (HR 9.03, CI 1.22-66.79) were independently significant ($p<0.05$, Table 4).

Discussion

For decades, the schedule and methods for surveillance of UUT after RC have been discussed because of its characteristics of low prevalence (0.7–7.4%) [3,7,8,12,20–22], late diagnosis after postoperative 25–40 months [6,7,23], poor prognosis with a median survival of 10–20 months from diagnosis [6,23], difficulty in detection of abnormal UUT findings in the changed abdomino-pelvic anatomy with diverted intestinal urinary tract of urinary diversions, and contaminated urine specimen from UUT with many degenerating desquamated intestinal epithelial cells to decrease the sensitivity of urine cytology. Many previous studies have attempted to identify several predictive risk factors of UUTR, however, their predictive values varied from those reported in other studies to remain controversial due to different characteristics of the enrolled patients [3,24]. For these limitations, the UUTR was often diagnosed late in a symptomatically advanced state of approximately 30–64%, resulting in poor prognosis [6]. Therefore, an international consensus regarding BC recommended the UUT follow-up regimen with close and thorough examination every six and 12 months with great suspicion [5,9,13,21]. Similar to previous studies, this study included 11 (3.5%) UUTRs diagnosed at median postoperative 26 months after RC, with a median survival of 13 months and 1- and 2- year UUTR-specific survival of 45.5% and 9.1%. In this study, four (36.4%) UUTR patients were diagnosed after symptoms had developed; two cases of gross hematuria, two cases of fever with flank pain. In another case (9.1%), an asymptomatic patient was diagnosed with UUTR after hydronephrosis on a routine CT work-up, and two other (18.2%) patients on abnormal urine cytology.

According to the urothelial characteristics, BC is known as an urothelial cancer affecting the entire urothelium with the risk for development of recurrence from the renal pelvis to the urethra during monitorization [6,12,25]. UUTR is considered to be secondary change to the multifocal metachronous nature of these tumors caused

by both panurothelial field damage by carcinogen to independently transform the epithelial cells at different sites from the renal pelvis to the urethra covered with urothelium, and intraluminal seeding and implantation of tumor cells derived from an initial clone [26,27]. Up to 57% of patients who undergo RC have unsuspected involvement of cancer at the ureter [28,29] and other sites at RC, despite a localized disease state of BC, because BC not only invades directly to adjacent organs through the muscle layer of the bladder, but also spreads to farther organs via vascular and lymphatic systems [30]. Therefore, the incidence of UUTR was not related to either the type of urinary diversion or to the quality of surgery, including operative skills, but to the efforts of experienced clinicians in detection of UUTR [3,8,24]. Some reports have explained the diverse different rates of UUTR from different institutions in that the size of the hospital, the experiences of clinicians, and the thorough and close monitoring schedule after RC were important in detection of UUTR [8].

To overcome the low early detection rate of recurrence in BC and UUTR with current diagnostic modalities, some recent studies have shown the clinical efficacy of some new molecular and epigenetic biomarkers, and immunohistochemical markers in urine and tissue samples from bladder and UUT. The current imaging modalities of UUT monitorization, such as CT, had a burden of cost and radiologic exposure. [3,6,31]. In particular, urine cytology has been known as a potent cost effective tool for screening of BC with a sensitivity of 75–84.6% and specificity of 78–100% for detection of recurrence. However, its results varied

Table 1. Patients' characteristics (n = 311).

	N	%
Median age	64	(46–86)
Male/Female (n,%)	276/35	88.7/11.3
Hypertension/diabetes (n,%)	89/37	28.6/11.9
American society of Anestheology Score (n,%)		
Grade 1	157	50.4
Grade 2	143	46.1
Grade 3	11	3.5
Radical Cystectomy with Orthotopic neobladder (n,%)	168	54.0
with Non-orthotopic ileal conduit	143	46.0
Intravesical chemotherapy (n,%)	45	14.5
Neoadjuvant chemotherapy (n,%)	64	20.5
Extent of LN dissection None (n,%)	78	25.1
Limited	68	21.9
Standard	158	50.7
Extended	7	2.3
Resection margin positivity (n,%)	19	6.1
Ureter/Urethra	6/13	31.6/68.4
No. patients according to pathological tumor stage (n,%)		
pT0, Ta	46	14.8
pTis	29	9.3
pT1	51	16.4
pT2	65	20.9
pT3	84	27.0
pT4	36	11.6
No. patients according to pathological nodal positive (n,%)	41	13.2
Nuclear grade (n,%) Low	34	10.9
Moderate	171	54.9
High	106	34.2
Perineural invasion (n,%)	40	12.9
Lymphovascular invasion (n,%)	87	28.0
Adjuvant chemotherapy (n,%)	84	27.0
Local recurrence (n,%)	39	12.5
Distant metastasis (n,%)	79	25.4
Median follow-up period	53	(13–207)
Survival (n,%)	184	59.2
Median survival time (mo)	46.0	(2–208)

based on intrpretation, which is dependent to some extent on the experience and ability of cytopathologists and on the proportion of the primary detection rate lower than 27% in all UUTR after RC [31]. Another study showed that the different types of urinary diversion also affected the low detection rate of recurrence (12.3% of UUTR in IC and 10.5% in Neo) [31]. In our series, only two (18.2%) IC patients were diagnosed with UUTR after abnormalities in urine cytology. Therefore, the molecular biomarkers, such as Ki-67, p53, and Rb; epigenetic markers; and urine markers such as NMP22, might be new breakthroughs in better detection of tumor recurrence of UUT after RC in combination with current diagnostic modalities [6,32].

In general, incidence of UUTR showed close correlation with the time of follow-up after RC. Most cases of UUTR developed within 25–40 months after RC, with an overall cumulative incidence of 4% at the third year and 7% at the fifth year [6,7], and some cases developed much later, until 10–15 years [12,13,21]. In this study, the median follow-up period was 53 months (13–207 months), which was not quite a long enough period of time for follow-up of UUTR in reference to 10–15 years. However, it might be cautiously said that this study may be representative for RC with an acceptable time of follow-up of UUT, because most of our RC patients (approximately 80%) had completed their follow-up with more than postoperative 36–44 months, and most previous reports also showed a median time of follow-up period of between 30–50 months [3,6,8,23]. Therefore, with our median follow-up period, it was worth discussing the natural histories of 11 UUTRs, although conduct of further studies

Table 2. The demographics of 11 patients with UUTR.

Age (yrs)	Diversion type	Pathology	Neoadj and IV CTx	UUTR (mo)	Recur site	Local recur site	Treatment For UUTR	Pathology of UUTR	UUTR surgery to last F/U	Status
51	Neo	TCC, G2, pT3bN1	None	72	Distal ureter		Surgery and Adjuvant CTx	TCC, pT2N1	13	DOD
58	Neo	TCC, G2, pT3bN2	IV CTx	19	Distal ureter		Surgery and Adjuvant CTx	TCC, pT1Nx	4	DOD
58	IC	Papil, G1, pT3bN0	IV CTx	29	Distal ureter	Rectum	Surgery	Pap, T2N1	5	DOD
64	IC	TCC,G3, pT2N2	None	42	Renal Pelvis	Pelvis	Surgery and Adjuvant CTx	CIS, pT1Nx	31	LWD
65	Neo	Pap, G3, pT3bN0	IV CTx	29	Proximal ureter	Pelvis	Surgery	TCC, TisNx	10	DOD
66	Neo	TCC, G3, pT3bN0	Neoadj CTx	19	Proximal ureter	Common iliac LN	Surgery and Adjuvant CTx	TCC, T1Nx	2	DOD
67	Neo	TCC, G3, pT3aN0	None	45	Proximal ureter		Surgery and Adjuvant CTx	TCC, pT1Nx	4	LWD
68	Neo	TCC, G3, pT3bN0	None	14	Distal ureter		Surgery and Adjuvant CTx	TCC, pT2N0	17	LWD
71	Neo	Pap, G1, pT1N2	IV CTx	18	Renal pelvis	Urethra	Surgery and Adjuvant CTx	Pap, pT2Nx	23	LWD
75	IC	TCC, G3, pT4bN2	IV CTx	26	Distal ureter	Urethra	Surgery	Pap, TaNx	6	DOD
83	IC	TCC, G3, pT3aN0	None	17	Distal ureter		Surgery	TCC, pT1Nx	5	LWD

IV, intravescial chemotherapy; CTx, chemotherapy; F/U; follow-up, Neo, neobladder; IC, ileal conduit; DOD, died of the disease; LWD, lived with the disease; TCC, transitional cell carcinoma; Papil, papillary TCC;

Table 3. Comparison between UUTR and no-UUTR.

	UUTR (n = 11)	No-UUTR (n = 300)	p-value
Gender Male/Female (n,%)	10 (90.9)/1 (9.1)	266 (88.7)/34 (11.3)	0.605
Age (yr)	65.8±8.5	62.7±10.3	0.314
BMI (kg/m^2)	24.9±3.8	23.8±3.2	0.283
Hypertension/Diabetes (n,%)	3 (27.3)/1 (9.1)	86 (28.9)/36 (12.1)	>0.500
IV CTx instillation (n,%)	5 (45.5)	40 (13.3)	0.002
Neoadjuvant CTx. (n,%)	1 (9.1)	63 (21.0)	0.730
Adjuvant CTx (n,%)	7 (63.6)	77 (25.7)	0.015
ASA Grade 1 (n,%)	6 (54.5)	151 (50.3)	0.039
Grade 2	3 (27.3)	140 (46.7)	
Grade 3	2 (18.2)	9 (3.0)	
Hospital stay (day)	21.4±11.4	21.4±15.9	0.998
Total operative time (min)	402.7±159.9	379.6±105.6	0.486
Neobladder/ Ileal conduit (n,%)	7/4 (63.6/36.4)	161/139 (53.7/46.3)	0.120
Pathologic T0 or Ta or Tis (n,%)	0	75 (25.0)	0.282
T1	1 (9.1)	49 (16.3)	
T2	1 (9.1)	64 (21.4)	
T3	8 (72.7)	77 (25.6)	
T4	1 (9.1)	35 (11.7)	
Pathologic node positivity (n,%)	5 (45.5)	38 (12.7)	0.182
Nuclear grade low (n,%)	2 (18.2)	32 (10.7)	0.354
moderate	2 (18.2)	169 (56.3)	
high	7 (63.6)	99 (33.0)	
Resection margin positivity (n,%)	0	19 (6.3)	<0.001
Perineural invasion (n,%)	4 (36.4)	36 (12.0)	0.130
Lymphovascular invasion (n,%)	3 (27.3)	84 (28.0)	0.753
Extent of LN dissection (n,%)			0.320
None	0	78 (26.0)	
Limited	1 (9.1)	67 (22.3)	
Standard	9 (81.8)	149 (49.7)	
Extended	1 (9.1)	6 (2.0)	
Local recurrence (n,%)	6 (65.6)	33 (3.7)	<0.001
Distant metastasis (n,%)	2 (18.2)	77 (25.7)	0.734
Follow-up duration (mo)	50.8±19.6	63.8±42.9	0.049
Survival (n,%)	5 (45.5)	179 (59.7)	0.026
Median survival time (mo)	65.9	76.9	0.383

BMI, body mass index; ASA, American Society of Anesthesiologists; IV, intravesical; CTx, chemotherapy; Tis, T stage with carcinoma in situ; Significant as p<0.05.

with large numbers of subjects with further long-term follow-ups would be necessary in order to obtain more clinical significance for comparison with other studies.

In this series, 25.1% of patients did not undergo pelvic LN dissection at RC to be criticized for their representation of RC patients. The reason for not performing pelvic LND for these patients was first that most of them were early staged BC (To, Ta, and T1) with a superficial low-graded papillary tumor without muscle invasiveness confirmed by transurethral resection. Those patients were clear in LN on imaging studies and intraoperatively without palpable LN enlargement. Papillary tumor was a morphological characteristic of BC limited to the mucosa with a benign nature of growing intravesically, different from a solid mass [32]. However, for the papillary tumor, it was necessary to first confirm its muscle invasiveness transurethrally, because some of them had a pathogenically invasive nature. Second, the superficial noninvasive BC (T0 and Ta, n = 46, 11.8%) almost filled in the entire bladder lumen, which meant an indirect parameter for tumors too largely broad and/or too multifocal to be managed transurethrally. This frequently recurrent multifocal superficial tumorigenic nature refractory to repeat transurethral resection has been suggested as one of the recommended indications for RC [10,24]. And, among patients with these tumors, those with old age greater than 70 years who had multiple underlying comorbidities might have suffered from postoperative morbidity after aggressive LND during RC operations of long duration and their recovery may have been delayed. Therefore, in these cases, the patients did not undergo LND at RC. However, despite the

Table 4. Predictive risk factor of UUTR in Poisson regression analysis.

	Hazard ratio	p-value	95% Confidence Interval
Hospital stay	1.00	0.99	0.81–1.23
ASA score	0.97	0.06	0.94–1.00
Type of Urinary diversion (Neo vs IC)	0.00	0.07	0.00–1.79
Positive resection margin	5.62	0.48	0.05–688.53
Lymph nodal dissection	0.42	0.64	0.01–16.17
Positive lymph node	9.03	0.03	1.22–66.79
Adjuvant chemotherapy	5.07	0.46	0.07–372.36
Pelvic local recurrence	7286.08	0.02	3.50–122760.70
Distant metastasis	18.19	0.16	0.33–1012.56
Pathologic T stage	2.20	0.29	0.51–9.55
Pathologic N stage	0.07	0.38	0.00–27.46

numbers of patients, this study included significantly representative numbers of RC and their UUTRs to be discussed.

This study included a large proportion of RC patients with advanced stage (n = 72, 23.2%) (T3 27.0%, T4 11.6%, and N (+) 13.2%). Especially considering the 11 UUTRs, all Neo patients had pathological stage III. This high proportion of enrolled patients with advanced stage might be attributed one of the ethnic and geographic characteristics of Asian patients with BC. Previous international studies have also shown the existence of disparities among ethnicities and geographic locations, including delays in presentation/diagnosis, inherent biological behavior of the tumor, socioeconomic status, lack of adequate health care access, and differences in exposure to environmental risk factors such as smoking [33–35]. The study showed a high prevalence of non-organ confined and high grade disease in Japanese and Taiwanese people and poorer cancer specific and recurrence free survivals were noted [34,36], similar to our study. Therefore, this study was clinically significant in showing the disease characteristics of BC and UUTR in Korean patients in relation to their ethnic differences from Western peoples, because few Korean studies have reported on UUTR after RC [30,37].

Among the enrolled patients, four patients received carboplatin-based neoadjuvant chemotherapy. Four patients were suspicious for advanced state with single or multiple small positive pelvic LNs at preoperative imaging evaluation. The cisplatin-based combination regimen has been recommended for its clinical efficacy as both neoadjuvant and adjuvant chemotherapy for invasive or advanced BC, and carboplatin proved less effective with deceased efficacy [38,39]. However, in our series, carboplatin based chemotherapy was used because of cisplatin-induced nephrotoxicity, coverage of national insurance, and the anti-tumor efficacy of carboplatin is not inferior to that of cisplatin-based chemotherapy. First, as one patient had baseline chronic kidney disease, the less nephrotoxic carboplatin was used. Second, the guideline of Korean National Insurance covered cisplatin only once, in either neoadjuvant or adjuvant chemotherapies, so that two patients who were suspicious for locally advanced state of BC might need adjuvant chemotherapy after RC. The final reason was that carboplatin based regimen preserved a tumor effect identical to that of the cisplatin based regimen, such as MVAC and GP, and that the maximum response might be obtained immediately after the second course because of the short antitumor effect of carboplatin to facilitate the shorter interval between diagnosis and RC [40,41].

This study did not require a discussion of the quality of surgery, including interpersonal differences of operative skills and distorted proportions of urinary diversion due to its equivalent proportion of Neo and IC (46.0% of IC vs. 54.0% of Neo) compared with other studies [3,7,8,12,13]. Despite the known dis-relationship of UUTR with the quality of surgery, the resection margin of ureter, urethra, and perivesical tissues and pelvic local recurrence closely related to the UUTR were mostly affected by the operator's skills during the complex, and time consuming RC procedure, especially in Neo formation [11,30,42,43]. In this study, despite the clear resection margin on frozen section, the final pathologies turned positive margins in 6.1% of cases, similar to other previous reports (false positive and negative 2–6%) [44,45]. All 11 UUTRs had clear resection margins on final pathology, although six patients later developed UUTR at the distal ureter. This distal UUTR might be explained by a panurothelial field effect in urothelial carcinoma. According to another explanation from Lee et al, intraoperative frozen resection was not an accurate enough analysis to believe the clear UUT after resection of the ureter at RC, because the final pathology indicated that the distal ureter was positive for intramural or juxtavesical ureter involvement and incidence of UUTR development was higher for these conditions [30].

This study analyzed the predictive risk factors for UUTR with most of the previously suggested risk factors from other studies [3,7,8,12,13], such as a positive ureteral/urethral/perivesical margin, presence of CIS, pathological stage, nuclear grade, local recurrence, lymph nodal positivity and recurrent tumors within urinary diversion, including uretroenteric anastomosis (Table 2) [7,8,12,15]. Local recurrence at the pelvis (HR 7286.08, CI 3.5-122760.7, p = 0.02) and positive LN (HR 9.03, CI 1.22-66.79, p = 0.03) were significant risk factors in this study, which have already been proven in other studies. Other well known risk factors, including stage, ureteral and urethral margin involvement, CIS, and grades, did not reach statistical significance and differed from those of other studies [6,20,46] because of small numbers of UUTR cases, which decreased the statistical power. However, our results were similar to those of Balaji et al [22] in that only locally advanced stage was a significant factor without the significance of margins, type of urinary diversion, gender, CIS, and nuclear grade. In this study, 12.5% of local recurrence occurred at a mean time of less than 16.7 (±20.5) months, in accordance with results of previous studies [7,8,12,15]. Three out of five living patients had T3 staged with nodal negative and without local recurrence at the pelvis. The other two patients had staged T1 and T2 despite being nodal positive on the RC specimen and only one local recurrence at the pelvis was noted. Clinically, results of this study indicated that risk of development of UUTR was higher with advanced staged tumors when local recurrence at the pelvis was found during the follow-up period and an increase in the number of positive LN was observed on the final pathology (Table 2). Therefore, urologists should perform a much more careful examination of the UUT with suspicion in these high risk patients.

The type of urinary diversion did not influence the incidence of UUTR. The two different types of urinary diversion were compared in this study under the assumption that incidence of UUTR might be higher with Neo, with poorer prognosis than for IC because Neo has a longer time of mucosal contact from malignant cells in urine and a higher rate of reflux to the upper urinary tract than IC [6,8,12,13,23]. A study by Yang et al reported a long-term effect of UUT change in both functional deterioration and anatomical distortion because of the refluxing and infection related problem [47]. However, this study showed no significant differences of UUTR, similar to other reports [3,22]. This might be suggested that the refluxing urine and longer urinary stasis in the Neo do not increase the risk of UUTR. The frequently timed urinary excretion, peristaltic movement of urine from the UUT, and functional anti-refluxing mechanism of Neo prevent from postoperative reflux of urine resulting in no differences in prevalence of UUTR compared to IC [48]. In addition, the prognosis was opposite to our assumption that IC had insignificantly poorer survival because their preoperative baseline performance states and clinical stages were worse not to qualify for Neo ($p>0.05$, not shown in tables).

The current study has some limitations. A prospective long-term multicenter study with a large number of patients should be conducted in the future for evaluation of suggested risk factors and longitudinal risk assessment of UUTR for evaluation of the potential implications for long-term surveillance. Second, due to its retrospective nature, this study did not include data on biomarkers, therefore, future study would consider the number of risk factors [8], and biomolecular and immunohistochemical markers [5,49,50] with the rate of UUTR. Third, because not all patients underwent LN dissection, this study had a limitation of representation for RC. Finally, the number of UUTR was too small, which weakened the statistical power of other well known risk factors. Despite these limitations, we believe that the current results are clinically informative and will be helpful in strategizing the follow-up plan for patients at risk for UUTR after RC.

In conclusion, this study reports on clinical prognosis and incidence of UUTR after RC with its significant risk factors that the incidence of UUTR was 3.5%, and that the presence of local recurrence at the pelvis and positive LNs were important independent risk factors requiring more careful consideration during follow-ups.

Author Contributions

Conceived and designed the experiments: SHK ESL. Performed the experiments: ESL SHK. Analyzed the data: SHK HKY. Contributed reagents/materials/analysis tools: ESL JHL. Wrote the paper: SHK.

References

1. Quek ML, Stein JP, Clark PE, Daneshmand S, Miranda G, Cai J, et al (2003) Natural history of surgically treated bladder carcinoma with extravesical tumor extension. Cancer 1;98 (5):955–61.
2. Tilki D, Reich O, Svatek RS, Karakiewicz PI, Kassouf W, et al (2010) Characteristics and outcomes of patients with clinical carcinoma in situ only treated with radical cystectomy: an international study of 243 patients. J Urol 183 (5):1757–63.
3. Picozzi S, Ricci C, Gaeta M, Ratti D, Macchi A, et al (2012) Upper Urinary Tract Recurrence Following Radical Cystectomy for Bladder Cancer: A Meta-Analysis on 13,185 Patients. J Urol 183 (5):1757–63.
4. Sanderson KM, Cai J, Miranda G, Skinner DG, Stein JP (2007) Upper tract urothelial recurrence following radical cystectomy for transitional cell carcinoma of the bladder: an analysis of 1,069 patients with 10-year followup. J Urol 177 (6):2088–94.
5. Soukup V, Babjuk M, Bellmunt J, Dalbagni G, Giannarini G, et al (2012) Follow-up after surgical treatment of bladder cancer: a critical analysis of the literature. Eur Urol 62 (2):290–302.
6. Takayanagi A, Masumori N, Takahashi A, Takagi Y, Tsukamoto T (2012) Upper urinary tract recurrence after radical cystectomy for bladder cancer: incidence and risk factors. Int J Urol 19 (3):229–33.
7. Tran W, Serio AM, Raj GV, Dalbagni G, Vickers AJ, et al (2008) Longitudinal risk of upper tract recurrence following radical cystectomy for urothelial cancer and the potential implications for long-term surveillance. J Urol 179 (1):96–100.
8. Volkmer BG, Schnoeller T, Kuefer R, Gust K, Finter F, et al (2009) Upper urinary tract recurrence after radical cystectomy for bladder cancer—who is at risk? J Urol 182 (6):2632–7.
9. Ubrig B, Kories C, Roth S (2013) Follow-up after surgical replacement of the urinary bladder (urinary diversion). Aktuelle Urol 44 (1):55–67.
10. Hautmann RE, Abol-Enein H, Davidsson T, Gudjonsson S, Hautmann SH, et al (2013) ICUD-EAU International Consultation on Bladder Cancer 2012: Urinary diversion. Eur Urol 63 (1):67–80.
11. Tollefson MK, Blute ML, Farmer SA, Frank I (2010) Significance of distal ureteral margin at radical cystectomy for urothelial carcinoma. J Urol 183 (1):81–6.
12. Sanderson KM, Roupret M (2007) Upper urinary tract tumour after radical cystectomy for transitional cell carcinoma of the bladder: an update on the risk factors, surveillance regimens and treatments. BJU Int 100 (1):11–6.
13. Perlis N, Turker P, Bostrom PJ, Kuk C, Mirtti T, et al (2013) Upper urinary tract and urethral recurrences following radical cystectomy: review of risk factors and outcomes between centres with different follow-up protocols. World J Urol 31 (1):161–7.
14. Huang GJ, Kim PH, Skinner DG, Stein JP (2009). Outcomes of patients with clinical CIS-only disease treated with radical cystectomy. World J Urol 27 (1):21–5.
15. Stein JP, Lieskovsky G, Cote R, Groshen S, Feng AC, et al (2001). Radical cystectomy in the treatment of invasive bladder cancer: long-term results in 1,054 patients. J Clin Oncol 1;19 (3):666–75.
16. Theresa M.K, Bernard H.B (2005) Bladder cancer staging. In: Nicholas J.V, Peter T.S,William U,S, Frans M.J.D, W. Marston Linehan, editors. Comprehensive textbook of genitourinary oncology. Philadelphia: Lippincott Williams & Wilkins. pp411–415.
17. Robert H.Y, Grace T.M (2005) Cytology and pathology of carcinomas of the urinary tract. In: Nicholas J.V, Peter T.S, William U,S, Frans M.J.D, W. Marston Linehan, editors. Comprehensive textbook of genitourinary oncology. Philadelphia: Lippincott Williams & Wilkins. pp365–384.
18. Zehnder P, Studer UE, Skinner EC, Dorin RP, Cai J, et al (2011) Super extended versus extended pelvic lymph node dissection in patients undergoing radical cystectomy for bladder cancer: a comparative study. J Urol 186 (4):1261–8.
19. Dhar NB, Klein EA, Reuther AM, Thalmann GN, Madersbacher S, et al (2008) Outcome after radical cystectomy with limited or extended pelvic lymph node dissection. J Urol 179 (3):873–8
20. Kenworthy P, Tanguay S, Dinney CP. The risk of upper tract recurrence following cystectomy in patients with transitional cell carcinoma involving the distal ureter. J Urol 1996 Feb;155 (2):501–3.
21. Huguet J (2013) Follow-up after radical cystectomy based on patterns of tumour recurrence and its risk factors. Actas Urol Esp 37 (6):376–82.
22. Balaji KC, McGuire M, Grotas J, Grimaldi G, Russo P (1999) Upper tract recurrences following radical cystectomy: an analysis of prognostic factors, recurrence pattern and stage at presentation. J Urol 162 (5):1603–6.
23. Furukawa J, Miyake H, Hara I, Takenaka A, Fujisawa M (2007) Upper urinary tract recurrence following radical cystectomy for bladder cancer. Int J Urol 14 (6):496–9.
24. World Health Organization Consensus Conference on Bladder C, Hautmann RE, Abol-Enein H, Hafez K, Haro I, et al (2007) Urinary diversion. Urology. 69 (1 Suppl):17–49.
25. Rabbani F, Perrotti M, Russo P, Herr HW (2001) Upper-tract tumors after an initial diagnosis of bladder cancer: argument for long-term surveillance. J Clin Oncol 1;19 (1):94–100.
26. Sidransky D, Frost P, Von Eschenbach A, Oyasu R, Preisinger AC,et al (1992) Clonal origin bladder cancer. NEJM 12;326 (11):737–40.
27. Kakizoe T (2006) Development and progression of urothelial carcinoma. Cancer science. 97 (9):821–8.

28. Charbit L, Gendreau MC, Mee S, Cukier J (1991) Tumors of the upper urinary tract: 10 years of experience. J Urol 146 (5):1243–6.
29. Sakamoto N, Naito S, Kotoh S, Nakashima M, Nakamura M, Ueda T, et al (1991) Recurrence of bladder tumors following surgery for transitional cell carcinoma of the upper urinary tract. Eur Urol 20 (2):136–9.
30. Lee SE, Byun SS, Hong SK, Chang IH, Kim YJ, et al (2006). Significance of cancer involvement at the ureteral margin detected on routine frozen section analysis during radical cystectomy. Urol Int 77 (1):13–7.
31. Yoshimine S, Kikuchi E, Matsumoto K, Ide H, Miyajima A, et al (2010). The clinical significance of urine cytology after a radical cystectomy for urothelial cancer. Int J Urol 17 (6):527–32.
32. Pasin E, Josephson DY, Mitra AP, Cote RJ, Stein JP (2008) Superficial bladder cancer: an update on etiology, molecular development, classification, and natural history. Rev Urol 10 (1):31–43.
33. Hosain GM, Khan MM, Amiel GE, Lerner SP, Latini DM, et al (2012) Racial/ ethnic differences in upper-tract urothelial cancer. Ethn Dis 22 (3):295–301.
34. Matsumoto K, Novara G, Gupta A, Margulis V, Walton TJ, et al (2011) Racial differences in the outcome of patients with urothelial carcinoma of the upper urinary tract: an international study. BJU Int 108 (8 Pt 2):E304–9.
35. Yee DS, Ishill NM, Lowrance WT, Herr HW, Elkin EB (2011) Ethnic differences in bladder cancer survival. Urology 78 (3):544–9.
36. Li CC, Chang TH, Wu WJ, Ke HL, Huang SP, et al (2003) Significant predictive factors for prognosis of primary upper urinary tract cancer after radical nephroureterectomy in Taiwanese patients. Eur Urol 54 (5):1127–34.
37. Kim B, Choi HJ, Kim MH, Cho KS (2012) Recurrence patterns of bladder transitional cell carcinoma after radical cystectomy. Acta Radiol 1;53 (8):943–9.
38. Apolo AB, Grossman HB, Bajorin D, Steinberg G, Kamat AM (2012) Practical use of perioperative chemotherapy for muscle-invasive bladder cancer: summary of session at the Society of Urologic Oncology annual meeting. Urol Oncol 30 (6):772–80.
39. Sternberg CN, Bellmunt J, Sonpavde G, Siefker-Radtke AO, Stadler WM, et al (2013) ICUD-EAU International Consultation on Bladder Cancer 2012: Chemotherapy for urothelial carcinoma-neoadjuvant and adjuvant settings. Eur Urol 63 (1):58–66.
40. Iwasaki K, Obara W, Kato Y, Takata R, Tanji S, et al (2013) Neoadjuvant gemcitabine plus carboplatin for locally advanced bladder cancer. Jpn J Clin Oncol 43 (2):193–9.
41. Ohyama C, Hatakeyama S, Yoneyama T, Koie T (2014) Neoadjuvant chemotherapy with gemcitabine plus carboplatin followed by immediate radical cystectomy for muscle-invasive bladder cancer. Int J Urol 21 (1):3–4.
42. Fukuta F, Honma I, Muto M, Masumori N, Tsukamoto T (2009) Prognosis of local recurrence after radical cystectomy for bladder cancer. Hinyokika Kiyo 55 (8):469–73.
43. Pejcic T, Hadzi-Djokic J, Acimovic M, Markovic B, Maksimovic H, et al (2007) Local recurrence of bladder cancer after cystectomy with orthotopic bladder substitution and ileal conduit. Acta Chir Iugosl 54 (4):63–7.
44. Raj GV, Tal R, Vickers A, Bochner BH, Serio A, et al (2006) Significance of intraoperative ureteral evaluation at radical cystectomy for urothelial cancer. Cancer 1;107 (9):2167–72.
45. Schoenberg MP, Carter HB, Epstein JI (1996) Ureteral frozen section analysis during cystectomy: a reassessment. J Urol 155 (4):1218–20.
46. Malkowicz SB, Skinner DG (1990) Development of upper tract carcinoma after cystectomy for bladder carcinoma. Urology. 36 (1):20–2.
47. Yang WJ, Cho KS, Rha KH, Lee HY, Chung BH, et al (2006) Long-term effects of ileal conduit urinary diversion on upper urinary tract in bladder cancer. Urology 68 (2):324–7.
48. Eila C. Skinner DGS, John P. Stein.CAMPBELL-WALSH Urology 10th ed. Orthotopic Urinary Diversion. 10th, International edition ed. Louis R. Kavoussi ACN, Alan W. Stein W. Partin, Craig A. Peters, editor. 1600 John F. Kennedy Blvd. Ste 1800 Philadelphia, PA 19103-2899: Saunders, Elsevier Inc.; 2012.
49. Fernandez MI, Parikh S, Grossman HB, Katz R, Matin SF, et al (2012) The role of FISH and cytology in upper urinary tract surveillance after radical cystectomy for bladder cancer. Urol Oncol 30 (6):821–4.
50. Kim WJ, Bae SC (2008) Molecular biomarkers in urothelial bladder cancer. Cancer Sci 99 (4):646–52.

5

BNP Predicts Chemotherapy-Related Cardiotoxicity and Death: Comparison with Gated Equilibrium Radionuclide Ventriculography

Dorthe Skovgaard[1,2]*, Philip Hasbak[2], Andreas Kjaer[1,2]

1 Cluster for Molecular Imaging, University of Copenhagen, Copenhagen, Denmark, **2** Department of Clinical Physiology, Nuclear Medicine and PET, Rigshospitalet and University Hospital of Copenhagen, Copenhagen, Denmark

Abstract

Cardiotoxicity is a dose-limiting side-effect of cancer chemotherapeutics such as anthracyclines. The drug-induced cardiac toxicity is currently monitored with repeated assessments of the left ventricular ejection fraction (LVEF) using multigated equilibrium radionuclide ventriculography (MUGA) or echocardiography. However, the plasma cardiac biomarker B-type natriuretic peptide (BNP) has been suggested for early identification of cardiac dysfunction. The aim of the study was to compare LVEF obtained by MUGA and plasma BNP as predictors of developing congestive heart failure (CHF) or death in a population of anthracycline-treated cancer patients.

Methods: We prospectively followed 333 cancer patients referred to our department for routine monitoring of LVEF with MUGA and measurement of BNP, January-December 2004. Study end points were hospitalization for CHF and death during follow-up 2004-2010. Data were obtained from the Danish National Patient Registry.

Results: During follow-up (mean 1,360 days), 21 of the patients were admitted to hospital with a diagnosis of CHF and 194 of the patients died. BNP levels were significantly higher and LVEF lower in the group of patients that developed CHF. Using cut-off points of BNP>100 pg/ml (HR 5.5; CI 1.8–17.2; p = 0.003) and LVEF <50% (HR 7.9; CI 3.0–21.4; p<0.001) both significantly predicted CHF. Using the same cut-off points only BNP (HR 1.9; CI 1.3-2.9; p = 0.002) and not LVEF (HR 1.1; CI 0.7–1.8; p = 0.58) was predictive of overall death. In multivariate Cox analysis both BNP and LVEF were independent predictors of CHF while age remained the only independent predictor of overall death.

Conclusion: In cancer patients treated with cardiotoxic chemotherapy both BNP and LVEF can significantly predict subsequent hospitalization with CHF. In addition, BNP and not LVEF has a prognostic value in detecting overall death. This prospective study based on the hitherto largest study population supports BNP as a clinical relevant method for monitoring chemotherapy-related cardiac failure and death.

Editor: Claudio Moretti, S.G.Battista Hospital, Italy

Funding: This work was supported by the John and Birthe Meyer Foundation, the A.P. MÅller Foundation, the Danish Medical Research Council, the Danish Heart Foundation, the Research Council of Rigshospitalet and the Research Foundation of the Capital Region. The funders had no role in study design, data collection and analysis, decision to publish, or preparation of the manuscript.

Competing Interests: The authors have declared that no competing interests exist.

* E-mail: dskovgaard@dadlnet.dk

Introduction

Cardiotoxicity associated with intensive chemotherapy affects life quality and overall survival of cancer patients. According to estimates cancer survivors in the US and Europe have a higher risk of cardiovascular death than the actual risk of tumor recurrence [1]. The most common way to prevent the immediate chemotherapy-induced cardiotoxicity from leading to irreversible congestive heart failure (CHF) is to monitor cardiac function during and following treatment by estimating left ventricular ejection fraction (LVEF) using radionuclide ventriculography or echocardiography and then if cardiac impairment is detected, treatment dose are lowered or cardioprotectants are added. International oncology guidelines define cardiotoxicity as a decrease in LVEF greater than 10% or an absolute LVEF value below 50% [2]. However, assessment of LVEF is limited by an inability to detect early changes that can predict late declines in cardiac function and therefore there has been a growing interest in identifying circulating biomarkers as reproducible, sensitive and cost effective ways to identify patients in the risk of developing chemotherapy-related cardiomyopathy [2–4].

B-type natriuretic peptide (BNP) is one of the suggested biomarkers with well-recognized diagnostic and independent prognostic implications in heart failure patients. BNP is secreted by the ventricles in response to end-diastolic pressure and volume [5–7]. Several studies have demonstrated increased plasma BNP levels during cancer therapy with anthracyclines, a group of widely prescribed chemotherpeutic agents with well-known cardiovascular toxicity [6,7]. However, studies have been conflicting with respect to the correlation between BNP concentration and the standard methods of estimating LVEF [8–14]. However, the value of BNP is not to predict LVEF levels but its prognostic and predictive value of developing CHF.

So far, only a few studies have investigated the value of BNP in prediction of clinically endpoints such as manifest cardiac dysfunction following cardiotoxic chemotherapy [6,7,13,15,16].

Therefore, the aim of the study was to evaluate BNP concentration and LVEF obtained by multigated acquisition equilibrium radionuclide ventriculography (MUGA) as predictors of hospital admission for congestive heart failure (CHF) and mortality (death of any cause) in a population of anthracycline-treated cancer patients.

Materials and Methods

The study was designed as a prospective study of 333 cancer patients treated with cardiotoxic chemotherapy with the aim of comparing the predictive value of plasma BNP concentration and LVEF assessed by MUGA for detection of cardiotoxicity and death following cancer treatment. We have previously published data from the same cohort comparing baseline BNP and LVEF as determined by MUGA obtained during chemotherapeutic treatment [8]. Now, we present the long-term follow up data. The study population included all patients consecutively referred to the Department of Clinical Physiology, Nuclear Medicine and PET, Rigshospitalet for routine monitoring of LVEF in relation to treatment with cardiotoxic chemotherapy including anthracyclines in the period January-December 2004. All patients underwent MUGA, routinely performed when half of the cumulative dose of anthracyclines has been given, with estimation of LVEF and a blood sample drawn for BNP measurement as described below.

Data concerning hospital admissions of the patients were obtained from the Danish National Patient Register (2004–2010, mean follow up 1,360 days). The Danish National Patient Register (DNPR) is a nationwide register covering all hospital admissions in Denmark. Every Danish citizen has a personal identification number assigned at birth or immigration which is used by public authorities including DNPR. Each hospital admission is routinely reported to DNPR using the international classification of diseases codes for diagnoses and surgical procedure (ICD-10) [17]. Furthermore, data on the causes of death were obtained from the Danish National register of causes of death [18] but in this study only the dates of death and not the specific causes of death were included in analyzes. The study end points were 1) CHF: hospitalization for congestive heart failure (defined as the ICD-10 codes: DI427 and DI50-DI509) and 2) death: all-cause mortality.

LVEF

LVEF was obtained by multigated acquisition radionuclide ventriculography according to the routine procedure of the department as described in details previously [8]. In brief: a small field-of-view gamma camera (GE starcam) was positioned in a left anterior oblique 30° view with a caudal tilt of 5°–10° adjusted for optimal separation of the ventricles. A bolus of 700–900 MBq of ^{99m}Tc-labelled human serum albumin was injected. LVEF were calculated with GE software programs (ENTEGRA version 1.5; General Electric, Milwaukee, WI, USA). A subgroup of 73 patients had more than one examination (MUGA and BNP).

BNP

Blood was drawn following 20 minutes of rest on the scanner bed prior to the administration of tracer and the BNP concentration was measured in plasma using an ADVIA Centaur two-side sandwich immunoassay technique based on chemiluminescence (Bayer, Leverkusen, Germany) [8,19–21]. BNP cut-off value of 100 pg/mL is routinely used for diagnosing chronic heart failure in the general population [22] and has also been suggested for chemotherapy-related cardiotoxicity [7].

Statistical analyzes

Differences in age, LVEF and BNP according to development of cardiac failure and all-cause mortality were analyzed using unpaired-sample t test. The plasma concentration of BNP were log-transformed before analyzes to ensure normal distribution. The chi-squared test was used for categorical data with dichotomized values for BNP and LVEF. Receiver operating characteristic (ROC) curves were drawn for plasma BNP concentration and LVEF to predict an adverse outcome (CHF or death, respectively) and area under the curves (AUC) were calculated. The prognostic value of BNP and LVEF for predicting either CHF or mortality was studied using Kaplan Meier method and significance was tested using the log rank test. Only (time to) the *first* hospitalization for CHF were included in analyzes. Univariate and multivariate analyses were carried out using Cox proportional hazards regression with age, BNP and LVEF included as covariates. BNP and LVEF were analyzed both as continuous and dichotomized values. Statistical analyses were performed with the use of IBM SPSS (version 20.0).

Results

In total 333 patients (mean age 49, range 11–85 years) were included in the study. The mean follow up was 1,360 days (range 1–2,534 days). Tumor types were breast cancer (24%), various hematological malignancies (35%), uterine/ovarian cancer (10%). The remaining had a wide variety of miscellaneous types of tumors (30%).

During the follow up period 21 patients were admitted to hospital due to a diagnosis of congestive heart failure (CHF) and 239 patients died. Values of age, BNP and LVEF are listed for patients divided in groups according to CHF and all-cause mortality in table 1. BNP levels were significantly increased and LVEF were significantly lower in the group of patients that were subsequently admitted to hospital for CHF. No significant differences were observed (besides age) between survivors and patients that died during the follow up.

Figure 1 shows the receiver operation characteristic curve for BNP for the diagnosis of CHF. The area under the ROC curve was 0.77 (95% CI 0.65–0.90, p<0.001). BNP at the routinely used cut-off value 100 pg/ml showed a sensitivity of 38% and a

Table 1. BNP concentration and left ventricular ejection fraction (LVEF) in patients grouped according to the major end points; hospitalization for congestive heart failure (CHF) and death.

	BNP (pg/ml)	LVEF (%)	Age (years)
CHF (n = 21)	267,8 (107)	51,4 (3)	55 (4)
No CHF (n = 312)	41,3 (4)	61,1 (1)	49 (1)
p value	*0,000*	*0,000*	*0,139*
Dead (n = 194)	65,4 (13)	42,1 (8)	58 (1)
Survivors (n = 139)	61,6 (1)	59,1 (1)	41 (2)
p value	*0,158*	*0,743*	*0,000*

Results are given as mean ± standard deviation (SD).

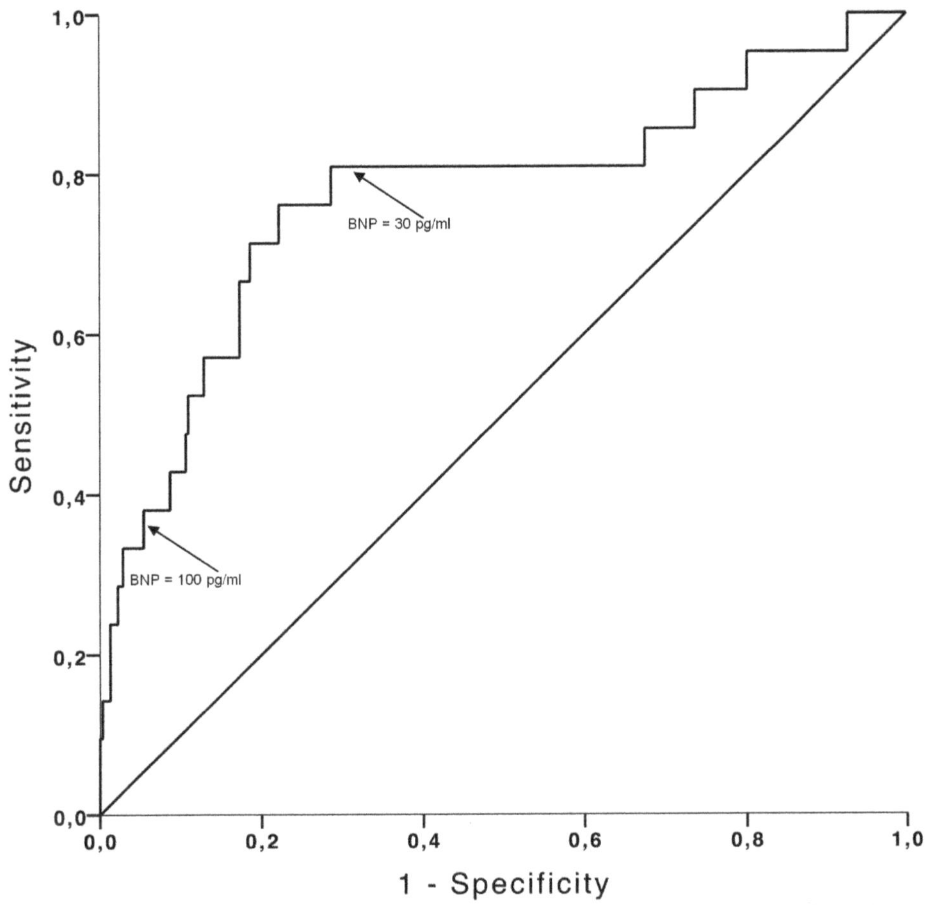

Figure 1. Received operating characteristic (ROC) curve for detection of CHF by BNP in patients treated with cardiotoxic chemotherapy. Area under the curve is 0.77 (95% CI 0.65–0.90, p<0.001). The arrows indicate selected cut-off concentrations of BNP. BNP concentration of 100 pg/ml correspond to a sensitivity 38% of and a specificity of 92% and BNP concentration of 30 pg/ml corresponds to a sensitivity 81% of and a specificity of 62%.

specificity of 92% for detecting CHF (table 2). Decreasing the BNP cut-off level to 30 pg/ml increased the sensitivity (81%) and decreased the specificity (62%) (table 2). When LVEF was used for detection of CHF (figure 2) the area under the ROC curve was 0.67 (CI 0.53–0.81, p = 0.008). A cut-off value of 50% of LVEF corresponding to the currently recommended cut-off value for detection of cardiotoxicity related to chemotherapy [2] resulted in a sensitivity of 48% and specificity of 91% (table 2). A cut-off value of LVEF at 45% resulted in a lower sensitivity (38%) and a high specificity (97%) in discriminating between patients with and without subsequent CHF (table 2), while increasing the cut-off value of LVEF to 55% resulted in a sensitivity of 48% and a lower specificity of 78% (CI: 0.27–0.69 and 0.77-0.80, respectively; p = 0.0130) (table 2). The ability of both BNP and LVEF to detect overall death assessed by ROC curve analysis revealed a low accuracy with AUC<0.6. BNP: AUC 0.58 (CI 0.52–0.64, p = 0.013) and LVEF: AUC 0.56 (CI 0.53–0.66, p = 0.002) (ROC curves according to overall death are not displayed).

Table 2 and table 3 give the sensitivity, specificity, positive and negative predictive values of selected cut-off values of BNP and

Table 2. Prognostic performances of BNP and LVEF in predicting hospitalization for congestive heart failure during follow up.

CHF				
	BNP>100 pg/ml	BNP>30 pg/ml	LVEF<50%	LVEF<45%
Sensitivitet	**38** (20–59)	**81** (58–94)	**48** (27–68)	**29** (13–72)
Specificitet	**92** (91–93)	**62** (61–63)	**91** (90–93)	**98** (97–99)
PPV	**24** (13–38)	**13** (09–15)	**27** (16–39)	**46** (21–72)
NPV	**96** (94–97)	**98** (96–99)	**96** (95–98)	**95** (94–96)
p value	*0.000*	*0.000*	*0.000*	*0.000*

Values in ( ) are 95% confidence interval.

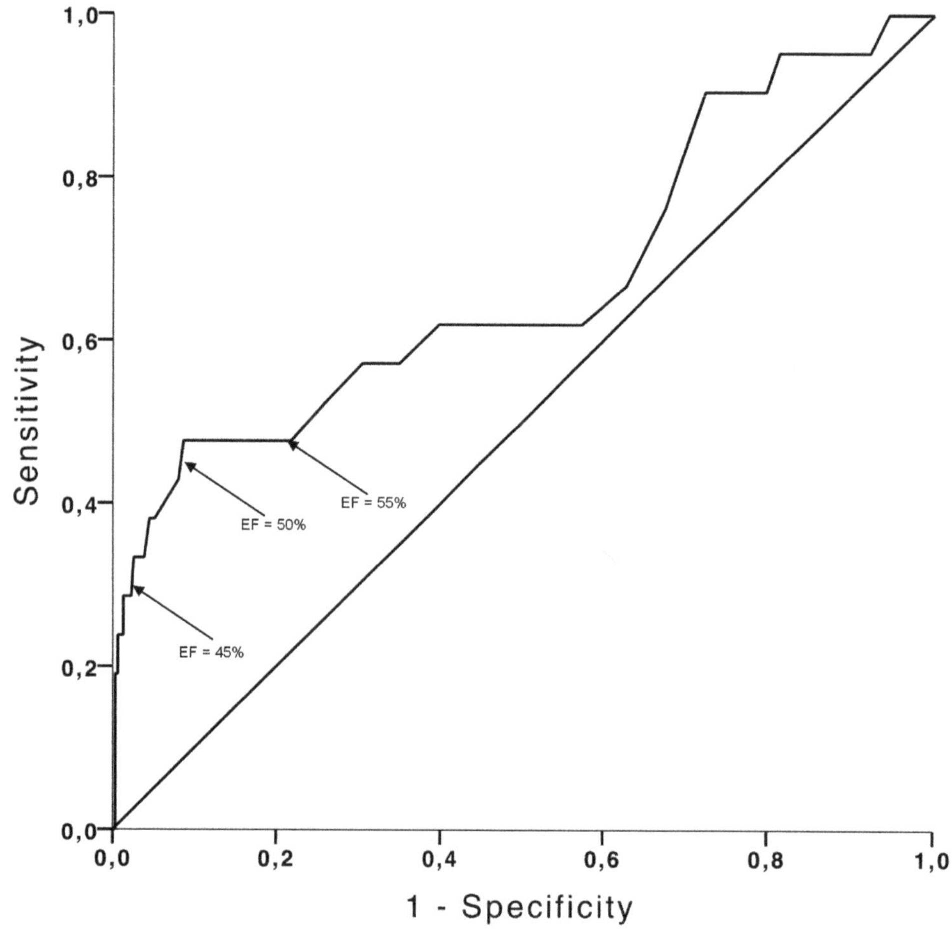

Figure 2. Received operating characteristic (ROC) curve for detection of CHF by LVEF in patients treated with cardiotoxic chemotherapy. Area under the curve is 0.67 (CI 0.53–0.81, p = 0.008). The arrows indicate selected cut-off concentrations for LVEF. A LVEF of 50% correspond to a sensitivity of 48% and a specificity of 91%. The diagnostic performance of LVEF at 45% and 55% showed a sensitivity of 38% and 45% and specificity of 97% and 78%, respectively.

LVEF for the detection of clinical manifest congestive heart failure and overall mortality. Irrespectively of the chosen cut-off values the negative predictive value of both BNP and LVEF were high (> 95%) in selecting patients developing congestive heart failure, while the sensitivity and positive predictive value was moderate. The diagnostic performance of BNP for detection of overall death at the cut-off level of 100 pg/ml showed a low sensitivity (13%) and a high specificity (94%) and lowering cut-off level to 30 pg/ml (a cut-off level also included in our initial analyzes of the baseline data [8]) resulted in higher sensitivity (81%) concurrently with a lower specificity (62%). Regardless of the cut-off values (45%, 50%, 55%) LVEF was non-significant for prediction of overall death by Fischers exact test.

Kaplan-Meier analyses were carried out for the major end points (time to the *first* hospitalization for CHF and time to death) stratified by the selected cut-off values as described above. The Kaplan-Meier curves for cut-off values of BNP>100 pg/ml and LVEF<50% are shown in figures 3–6. Patients with a concen-

Table 3. Prognostic performances of BNP and LVEF in predicting death during follow up.

Death				
	BNP>100 pg/ml	**BNP>30 pg/ml**	**EF<50%**	**EF<45%**
Sensitivitet	**13** (10–15)	**48** (43–52)	**11** (08–14)	**05** (03–06)
Specificitet	**94** (90–97)	**69** (63–75)	**89** (85–93)	**97** (94–99)
PPV	**76** (58–88)	**68** (61–75)	**59** (43–74)	**69** (39–90)
NPV	**44** (42–46)	**49** (44–53)	**42** (40–44)	**42** (41–43)
p value	*0.032*	*0.002*	*0.87*	*0.569*

Values in ( ) are 95% confidence interval.

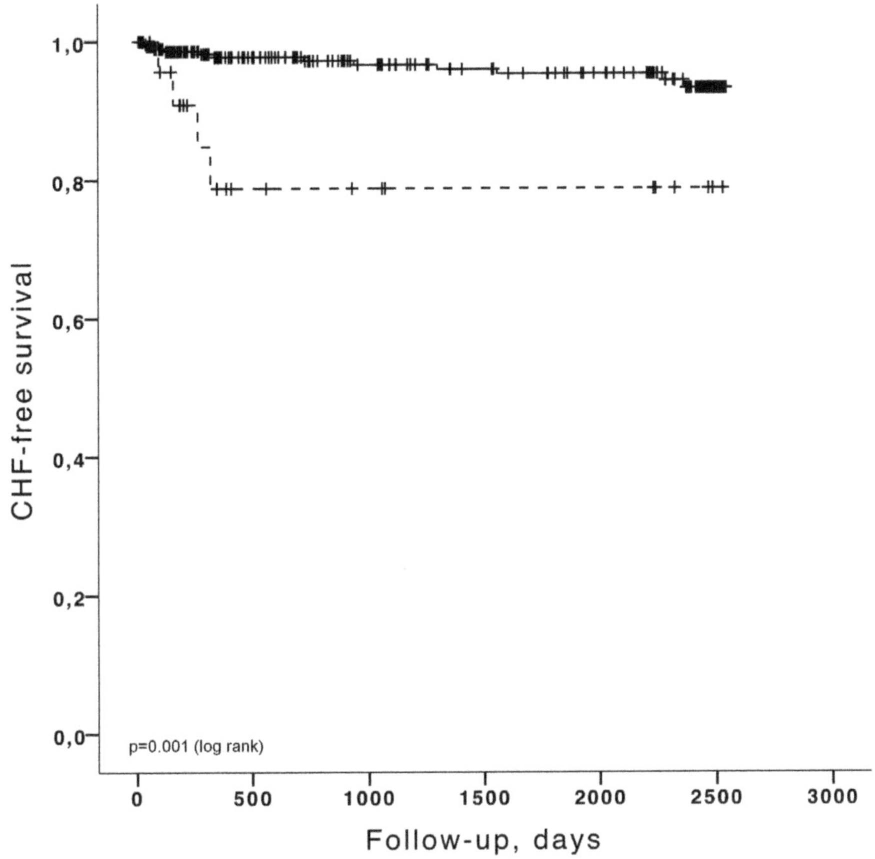

Figure 3. Kaplan-Meier analysis for the probability of CHF hospitalization-free survival according to BNP levels below (black, solid) or above the cut-off level of 100 pg/ml (black, dashed).

tration of BNP>100 pg/ml had a higher risk of developing CHF (figure 3) (log rank p<0.001) and BNP >100 pg/ml was also predictive of overall death (figure 5) (log rank p = 0.003). LVEF< 50% was significantly linked to CHF by Kaplan Meier analysis (figure 4) (log rank p<0.001) but LVEF<50% was not predictive of overall death (figure 6) (log rank p = 0.584). Patients with BNP values above 30 pg/ml had a higher risk of CHF (log rank p< 0.001) and a higher mortality rate (log rank p<0.001). If the cut-off value for LVEF was selected to <45%, LVEF could predict CHF (log rank p = 0.000) but was still not able to differentiate survivors from non survivors (log rank p = 0.351). The unadjusted hazard ratios for the selected cut-off values for prediction of CHF and overall mortality based on univariate Cox regression analysis for age, BNP and LVEF are given in table 4 and table 5.

In a multivariate Cox proportional regression analysis, with age, LVEF and BNP as continuous and dichotomized variables, both LVEF<50% and BNP were statistically significant independent predictors of CHF (LVEF:<50% HR 4.89; CI 1.49–13.53, p = 0.008 and BNP: HR 4.16, CI 1.63–10.42, p = 0.002). When only dichotomized values of BNP and LVEF were entered in the model BNP>30 pg/ml and LVEF<50% remained statistically significant for detection of CHF (BNP>30 pg/ml: HR 4.87, CI 1.55–15.36, p = 0.007 and LVEF<50%: HR 6.13, CI 2.25–16.68, p = 0.000). In a multivariate analysis of BNP and LVEF as dichotomized values according to overall death, age was the only significant independent predictor of overall death (HR 1.04, CI 1.03–1.05, p = 0.000). In addition BNP>100 pg/ml showed a borderline significant value of 0.077 as an independent predictor of overall death (HR 1.47, CI0.96–2.24).

Of the 73 patients with more than one examination no changes in BNP concentration (46.6±9.0 vs. 43.4±7.3 pg/ml, p = 0.544) and no changes in LVEF (0.58±0.01 to 0.58±0.01, p = 0.37) were found from the first to the last examination. In this subgroup, 5 patients were subsequently hospitalized with CHF. Only one of these 5 patients had a significant increase in BNP from below to above the cut-off of 100 pg/ml and in none of the patients, LVEF fell >10% point from the first to the last examination. For the whole group of multi-examined 73 patients, neither an increase in BNP (n = 36) nor a decrease in LVEF of more than 0.10%-point from the first to the last examination or a final LVEF determination of less than 0.50 (n = 10), predicted CHF (BNP: HR 0.63, CI 0.11–3.78, p = 0.61 and LVEF: HR 0.04 CI 0.0–2561, p = 0.57).

Discussion

The present study prospectively investigated BNP concentration and LVEF as predictors of two distinct clinical endpoints (hospitalization for manifest congestive heart failure and overall death) in 333 anthracycline-treated cancer patients. The most important finding was that both BNP and LVEF independently predicted congestive heart failure. However, only BNP and not LVEF was associated with overall mortality. Although the level of BNP can be influenced by e.g. adipositas, pulmonary and renal disease and drugs such as angiontensin converting enzyme

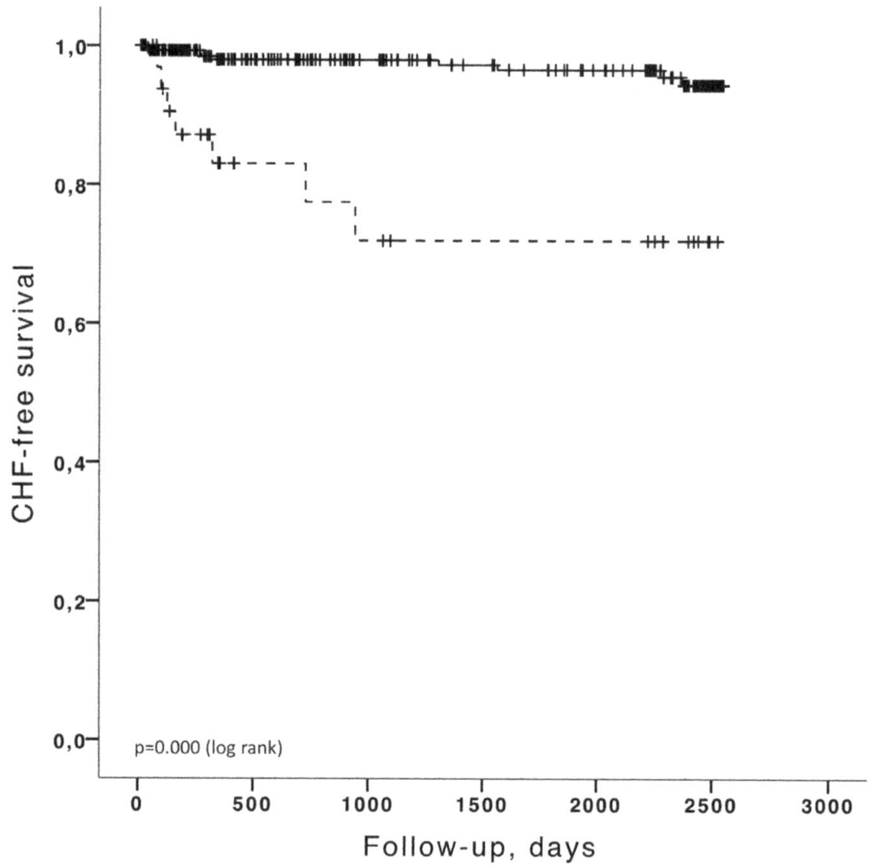

Figure 4. Kaplan-Meier analysis for the probability of CHF hospitalization-free survival according to LVEF above (black, solid) or below 50% (black, solid).

inhibitors, BNP can predict over-all mortality in a wide range of other patient categories such as hypertension, stroke and diabetes [23]

In the literature the reported incidence of cardiovascular toxicity from anticancer treatment is highly variable and depends on the type of drug being used. The patients in the study cohort were treated with anthracycline-containing chemotherapy regimens. Anthracyclines are widely used and have well-known cardiotoxic effects with a reported incidence of 0.9–26% [4]. The cumulated incidence of clinical manifest congestive heart failure in the current study was 6.3% for the entire ~4 year follow up. The relatively high mortality rate (58% died) during the follow-up period most likely reflects aggressive/disseminated malignant disease in the study population.

In this cohort of cancer patients, 21 of the 333 patients were admitted to hospital for congestive heart failure during the follow-up period. If the current recommendations for surveillance of cardiotoxicity in relation to chemotherapy are followed where cardiotoxicity is defined by LVEF<50% (determined by a single examination), only 48% (10 patients) were correctly identified of developing CHF and accordingly 52% of the patients (11 patients) with subsequent cardiac failure were overlooked. Increasing the threshold of LVEF to <55% did not change the number of heart failure patients that would have been identified (10 patients with cardiac failure had LVEF<55%). In comparison a BNP>30 pg/ml could identify 79% (17 patients) of these patients overlooking 21% (4 patients). This emphasizes that the current method based on LVEF is suboptimal in detection of subtle alterations in left ventricular function and that even small increases in BNP (below the recommended routinely used cut-off value) might be applicable in identifying patients at risk of developing cardiac dysfunction. At the routinely used cut-off value of BNP (>100 pg/ml) a substantial part of the patients with subsequent heart failure were not identified (13 patients corresponding to 62%) suggesting that the cut-off value should be decreased if measurements of BNP is applied in the monitoring of cardiotoxicity. However, a major challenge is that 135 patients had BNP levels above 30 pg/ml, resulting in a substantial number of "false positives". This probably reflects a moderate transient increase in BNP during treatment due to acute/subacute cardiotoxicity that only in some patients are irreversible [7]. It was speculated if BNP could serve as a "gatekeeper" implicating that only patients with BNP>30 pg/ml were referred to the more expensive and laborious estimation of LVEF by MUGA. If the 135 patients with BNP >30 pg/ml were subjected to MUGA and LVEF<50% again was considered reference value, then only 8 of the 21 heart failure patients would have been identified. Another possibility could be to use BNP as an additive measure together with LVEF-measurement in the surveillance of cardiotoxic cancer treatment. If these two values (patients having either LVEF<50% *or* BNP>30 pg/ml) were combined 18 of the 21 patients with CHF were identified suggesting that BNP possess meaningful and additive information to the current surveillance based on MUGA. However, by combining BNP and MUGA only 1 more patient was identified compared to BNP>30 pg/ml alone and 150 patients had either

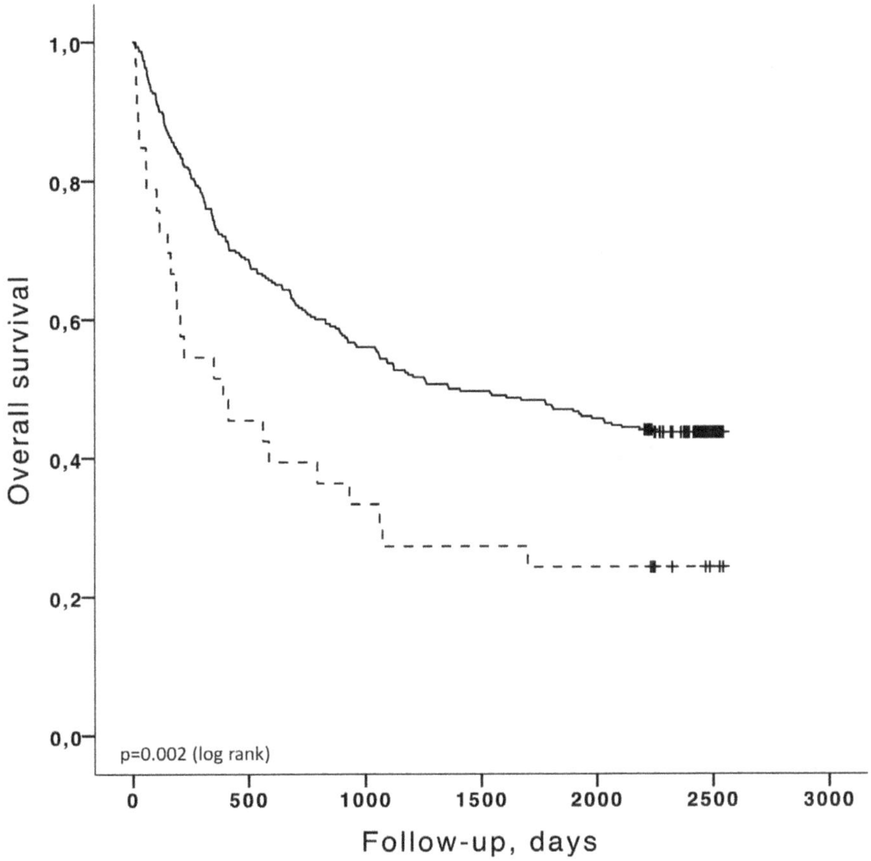

Figure 5. Kaplan-Meier analysis for the probability of over-all survival according to BNP levels below (black, solid) or above the cut-off level of 100 pg/ml (black, dashed).

BNP>30 pg/ml or EF<50, increasing the number of "false positives" compared to BNP>30 pg/ml as the only measure.

It was also speculated if serial measurements of BNP could have improved the diagnostic performance of chemotherapy-induced CHF, since it is well known that repeated measurements in patients with chronic heart failure provide incrementally unique information [22]. Unfortunately, this was only done in 73 of the patients, of whom 5 patients developed congestive heart failure, making the material too small for meaningful statistical analyses.

Several published studies have investigated the role of BNP in diagnosing and risk stratification of chemotherapy-associated cardiotoxicity, however most studies have simply compared BNP levels with LVEF measured by MUGA or echocardiography at baseline or during/after treatment with antracyclines as we did also in our previous publication [8]. Results have shown either no association [10–12] or a correlation between impaired ejection fraction and increased levels of BNP [9,13,24].

There are multiple reasons for these conflicting results including inadequate sample size (most studies include <100 patients), heterogeneity of the studied population with regards to cancer diagnosis, age (adults vs. children), chemotherapeutic agent and treatment regime/cumulative dose. Furthermore, the timing of blood samples drawn for BNP measurements, the laboratory methods and cut off values contributes to the inconsistency of the results. In this study BNP was measured at same the session where MUGA was performed which typically is when half of the cumulative dose of anthracyclines has been given.

Only a few published studies have investigating the use of BNP as predictor of a true clinical end-point such as manifest congestive heart failure. In a study by Pichon et al [7], BNP was correlated to clinical heart failure (as classified by NYHA) in 67 breast cancer patients followed for 62 days (1-984 days) after chemotherapy (anthracyclines with/without trastuzumab) and cut-off level 100 pg/ml was suggested for prediction of CHF. Lee et al [16] studied 86 patients with hematologic malignancies for 2 years and found a correlation between increased BNP concentration and CHF (as diagnosed by Framingham criteria) following antracycline treatment and also Feola et al [6] found that BNP predicted cardiac events (based on reported symptoms or decrease in LVEF>10% at two year follow-up) in 53 breast cancer patients. Other studies focusing on clinical end points have been small including <20 patients [13,25].

Several studies have used NT-ProBNP which despite a longer half-life are considered comparable to BNP [22]. Due to differences in conclusion, study design and importantly the majority of the studies are based on <50 patients it is difficult to draw definite conclusions [26–31].

In addition, a limited number of studies have investigated the possibility of using BNP and other biomarkers in the early detection of anthracycline-induced cardiotoxicity in children/ long-term survivors of childhood cancer with the majority of studies supporting BNP as a useful biomarker of myocardial dysfunction [32–36].

Importantly, the current results presented here, based on the hitherto largest cohorts of patients (333 patients) investigating BNP

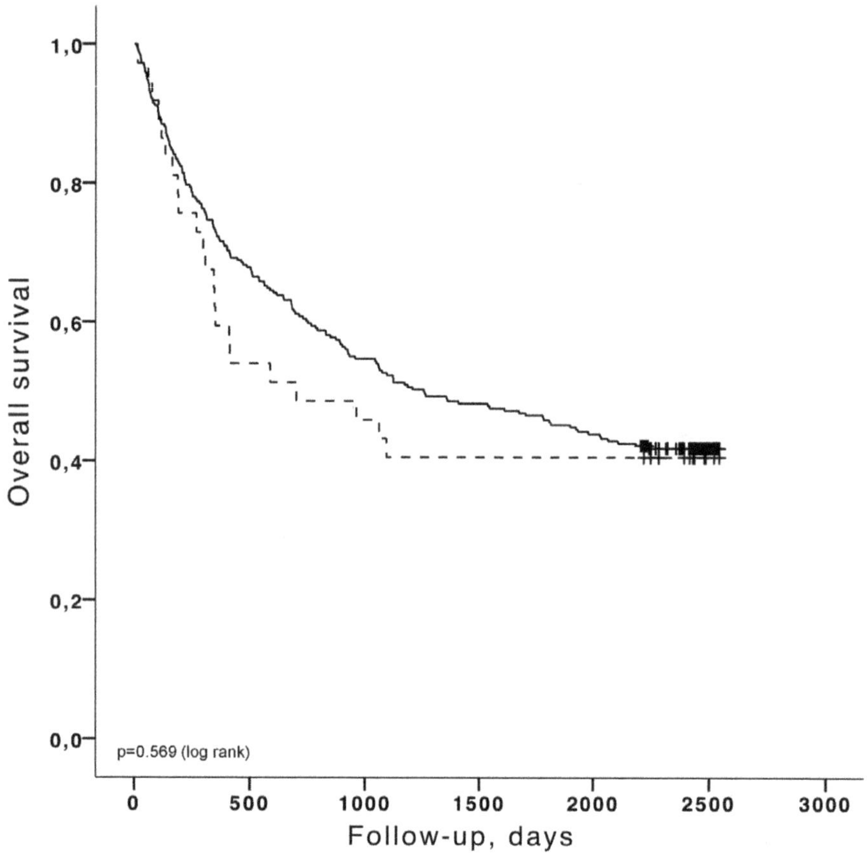

Figure 6. Kaplan-Meier analysis for the probability of over-all survival according to LVEF above (black, solid) or below 50% (black, dashed).

as a predictor of clinical manifest congestive heart failure, clearly show that BNP has an important predictive value comparable or even superior to the currently recommended more time-consuming, radiation exposure involving and expensive MUGA.

There are some important limitations to the study; the incidence of congestive heart failure in the present study might be a conservative estimate since only clinical manifest congestive heart failure treated in hospital and outpatient clinics are recorded. It is possible that we have overlooked patients with subclinical cardiac impairment or patients with only vague clinical symptoms, which would not be categorized as CHF (DI1427 or DI50-509) in the Danish national patient registry.

Furthermore, we have no detailed information on the chemotherapeutic regime, including the cumulative dose of anthracyclines and/or addition of thoracic radiotherapy. This is notable since the cumulative dose of anthracyclines and the addition of other cardiotoxic chemotherapeutics including trastuzumab and also thoracic radiotherapy are established risc factors for developing chemotherapy-related CHF [1]. No baseline medical history with respect to cardiovascular risk factors or concurrent

Table 4. Univariate Cox regression analysis for predicting hospitalization for congestive heart failure in relation to selected cut-off values of BNP concentration and LVEF.

CHF			
	HR	**95% CI**	***p value***
BNP	6.94	2.92–16.50	*0.000*
LVEF	0.000	0.00–0.032	*0.000*
BNP>100 pg/ml	5.51	1.76–17.22	*0.003*
BNP>30 pg/ml	6.02	1.94–18.74	*0.002*
LVEF<50%	7.95	2.95–21.41	*0.001*
LVEF<45%	11.11	2.98–41.44	*0.000*
Age	1.03	1.00–1.07	*0.053*

Table 5. Univariate Cox regression analysis for predicting overall death in relation to selected cut-off values of BNP concentration and LVEF.

Death	HR	95% CI	*p value*
BNP	1.68	1.26–2.34	*0.000*
LVEF	1.76	0.32–9.68	*0.519*
BNP>100 pg/ml	1.94	1.72–2.96	*0.002*
BNP>30 pg/ml	1.70	1.28–2.25	*0.000*
LVEF<50%	1.14	0.73–1.78	*0.569*
LVEF<45%	1.08	0.53–2.25	*0.823*
Age	1.04	1.03–1.05	*0.000*

administration of cardiovascular drugs was obtained. Recently, several studies have shown that adding cardioprotectans such as ACE-1 or Beta-blockers can prevent LVEF reductions in patients undergoing intensive chemotherapy [37]. Lastly, other specific cardiac biomarkers that are reported to detect subclinical chemotherapy-associated cardiac damage (e.g. the troponins, with a high sensitivity for detecting small amounts of myocardial necrosis) were not measured in the current study.

Conclusion

In conclusion, this is the largest patient data set (333 patients) reported till date investigating both plasma BNP concentration and LVEF as predictors of chemotherapy-related cardiotoxicity using distinct clinical end points: hospitalization with a diagnosis of congestive heart failure and overall death. This prospective study shows that for cancer patients treated with cardiotoxic chemotherapy both BNP and LVEF significantly predicted congestive heart failure. Only BNP and not LVEF had diagnostic implications in predicting overall mortality supporting BNP as a clinical relevant factor for monitoring chemotherapy-related cardiac toxicity and death.

A future prospective clinical trial should focus on standardization of the use of BNP concentration for diagnosing patients with irreversible cardiac damage, including determining optimal cut-off level and timing of BNP requiring several samples. In addition, a future focus should be on therapeutic-decision making (e.g. dose adjustment/addition of cardioprotective medical therapy) based on BNP concentration compared to the current approach with assessment of LVEF ideally in a randomized study.

Acknowledgments

We thank the staff at the Department of Clinical Physiology, Nuclear Medicine and PET, Rigshospitalet, Copenhagen for performing the MUGA scans and blood sampling.

Author Contributions

Conceived and designed the experiments: DS PH AK. Performed the experiments: DS. Analyzed the data: DS AK. Wrote the paper: DS PH AK.

References

1. Cardinale D, Cipolla CM (2011) Assessment of cardiotoxicity with cardiac biomarkers in cancer patients. Herz 36: 325–332. 10.1007/s00059-011-3453-4 [doi].
2. Cardinale D, Colombo A, Cipolla CM (2008) Prevention and treatment of cardiomyopathy and heart failure in patients receiving cancer chemotherapy. Curr Treat Options Cardiovasc Med 10: 486–495.
3. Ky B, Carver JR (2011) Biomarker approach to the detection and cardioprotective strategies during anthracycline chemotherapy. Heart Fail Clin 7: 323–331. S1551-7136(11)00022-5 [pii];10.1016/j.hfc.2011.03.002 [doi].
4. Yeh ET, Tong AT, Lenihan DJ, Yusuf SW, Swafford J, et al. (2004) Cardiovascular complications of cancer therapy: diagnosis, pathogenesis, and management. Circulation 109: 3122–3131. 10.1161/01.CIR.0000133187.74800.B9 [doi];109/25/3122 [pii].
5. Doust JA, Glasziou PP, Pietrzak E, Dobson AJ (2004) A systematic review of the diagnostic accuracy of natriuretic peptides for heart failure. Arch Intern Med 164: 1978–1984. 164/18/1978 [pii];10.1001/archinte.164.18.1978 [doi].
6. Feola M, Garrone O, Occelli M, Francini A, Biggi A, et al. (2011) Cardiotoxicity after anthracycline chemotherapy in breast carcinoma: effects on left ventricular ejection fraction, troponin I and brain natriuretic peptide. Int J Cardiol 148: 194–198. S0167-5273(09)01575-7 [pii];10.1016/j.ijcard.2009.09.564 [doi].
7. Pichon MF, Cvitkovic F, Hacene K, Delaunay J, Lokiec F, et al. (2005) Drug-induced cardiotoxicity studied by longitudinal B-type natriuretic peptide assays and radionuclide ventriculography. In Vivo 19: 567–576.
8. Vogelsang TW, Jensen RJ, Hesse B, Kjaer A (2008) BNP cannot replace gated equilibrium radionuclide ventriculography in monitoring of anthracycline-induced cardiotoxity. Int J Cardiol 124: 193–197. S0167-5273(07)00472-X [pii];10.1016/j.ijcard.2007.02.003 [doi].
9. Daugaard G, Lassen U, Bie P, Pedersen EB, Jensen KT, et al. (2005) Natriuretic peptides in the monitoring of anthracycline induced reduction in left ventricular ejection fraction. Eur J Heart Fail 7: 87–93. S1388984204001059 [pii];10.1016/j.ejheart.2004.03.009 [doi].
10. Meinardi MT, van Veldhuisen DJ, Gietema JA, Dolsma WV, Boomsma F, et al. (2001) Prospective evaluation of early cardiac damage induced by epirubicin-containing adjuvant chemotherapy and locoregional radiotherapy in breast cancer patients. J Clin Oncol 19: 2746–2753.
11. Nousiainen T, Jantunen E, Vanninen E, Remes J, Vuolteenaho O, et al. (1999) Natriuretic peptides as markers of cardiotoxicity during doxorubicin treatment for non-Hodgkin's lymphoma. Eur J Haematol 62: 135–141.
12. Nousiainen T, Vanninen E, Jantunen E, Puustinen J, Remes J, et al. (2002) Natriuretic peptides during the development of doxorubicin-induced left ventricular diastolic dysfunction. J Intern Med 251: 228–234. 951 [pii].
13. Okumura H, Iuchi K, Yoshida T, Nakamura S, Takeshima M, et al. (2000) Brain natriuretic peptide is a predictor of anthracycline-induced cardiotoxicity. Acta Haematol 104: 158–163. 46508 [pii];46508 [doi].
14. Garrone O, Crosetto N, Lo NC, Catzeddu T, Vivenza D, et al. (2011) Prediction of Anthracycline Cardiotoxicity after Chemotherapy by Biomarkers Kinetic Analysis. Cardiovasc Toxicol. 10.1007/s12012-011-9149-4 [doi].
15. Dolci A, Dominici R, Cardinale D, Sandri MT, Panteghini M (2008) Biochemical markers for prediction of chemotherapy-induced cardiotoxicity: systematic review of the literature and recommendations for use. Am J Clin Pathol 130: 688–695. B72890MQ9X2W15P5 [pii];10.1309/AJCPB66LRIIVMQDR [doi].
16. Lee HS, Son CB, Shin SH, Kim YS (2008) Clinical correlation between brain natriutetic peptide and anthracyclin-induced cardiac toxicity. Cancer Res Treat 40: 121–126. 10.4143/crt.2008.40.3.121 [doi].
17. Lynge E, Sandegaard JL, Rebolj M (2011) The Danish National Patient Register. Scand J Public Health 39: 30–33. 39/7_suppl/30 [pii];10.1177/1403494811401482 [doi].

18. Helweg-Larsen K (2011) The Danish Register of Causes of Death. Scand J Public Health 39: 26–29. 39/7_suppl/26 [pii];10.1177/1403494811399958 [doi].
19. Gutte H, Mortensen J, Jensen CV, von der Recke P, Petersen CL, et al. (2010) ANP, BNP and D-dimer predict right ventricular dysfunction in patients with acute pulmonary embolism. Clin Physiol Funct Imaging 30: 466–472. CPF967 [pii];10.1111/j.1475-097X.2010.00967.x [doi].
20. Kristoffersen US, Lebech AM, Gerstoft J, Hesse B, Petersen CL, et al. (2008) Right and left cardiac function in HIV-infected patients investigated using radionuclide ventriculography and brain natriuretic peptide: a 5-year follow-up study. HIV Med 9: 180–186. HIV531 [pii];10.1111/j.1468-1293.2007.00531.x [doi].
21. Kjaer A, Hildebrandt P, Appel J, Petersen CL (2005) Neurohormones as markers of right- and left-sided cardiac dimensions and function in patients with untreated chronic heart failure. Int J Cardiol 99: 301–306. S0167527304002633 [pii];10.1016/j.ijcard.2004.02.003 [doi].
22. Januzzi JL Jr. (2012) The role of natriuretic peptide testing in guiding chronic heart failure management: review of available data and recommendations for use. Arch Cardiovasc Dis 105: 40–50. S1875-2136(11)00356-1 [pii];10.1016/j.acvd.2011.10.007 [doi].
23. Hildebrandt P (2009) Natriuretic peptides: prediction of cardiovascular disease in the general population and high risk populations. Dis Markers 26: 227–233. H4034226X421V36T [pii];10.3233/DMA-2009-0632 [doi].
24. Elbl L, Vasova I, Navratil M, Vorlicek J, Malaskova L, et al. (2006) [Comparison of plasmatic levels of B-natriuretic peptide with echocardiographic indicators of left ventricle function after doxorubicin therapy]. Vnitr Lek 52: 563–570.
25. Snowden JA, Hill GR, Hunt P, Carnoutsos S, Spearing RL, et al. (2000) Assessment of cardiotoxicity during haemopoietic stem cell transplantation with plasma brain natriuretic peptide. Bone Marrow Transplant 26: 309–313. 10.1038/sj.bmt.1702507 [doi].
26. Sandri MT, Salvatici M, Cardinale D, Zorzino L, Passerini R, et al. (2005) N-terminal pro-B-type natriuretic peptide after high-dose chemotherapy: a marker predictive of cardiac dysfunction? Clin Chem 51: 1405–1410. clinchem.2005.050153 [pii];10.1373/clinchem.2005.050153 [doi].
27. Romano S, Fratini S, Ricevuto E, Procaccini V, Stifano G, et al. (2011) Serial measurements of NT-proBNP are predictive of not-high-dose anthracycline cardiotoxicity in breast cancer patients. Br J Cancer 105: 1663–1668. bjc2011439 [pii];10.1038/bjc.2011.439 [doi].
28. Kouloubinis A, Kaklamanis L, Ziras N, Sofroniadou S, Makaritsis K, et al. (2007) ProANP and NT-proBNP levels to prospectively assess cardiac function in breast cancer patients treated with cardiotoxic chemotherapy. Int J Cardiol 122: 195–201. S0167-5273(07)00007-1 [pii];10.1016/j.ijcard.2006.11.076 [doi].
29. Sawaya H, Sebag IA, Plana JC, Januzzi JL, Ky B, et al. (2011) Early detection and prediction of cardiotoxicity in chemotherapy-treated patients. Am J Cardiol 107: 1375–1380. S0002-9149(11)00141-X [pii];10.1016/j.amjcard.2011.01.006 [doi].
30. Dodos F, Halbsguth T, Erdmann E, Hoppe UC (2008) Usefulness of myocardial performance index and biochemical markers for early detection of anthracycline-induced cardiotoxicity in adults. Clin Res Cardiol 97: 318–326. 10.1007/s00392-007-0633-6 [doi].
31. Geiger S, Stemmler HJ, Suhl P, Stieber P, Lange V, et al. (2012) Anthracycline-induced cardiotoxicity: cardiac monitoring by continuous wave-Doppler ultrasound cardiac output monitoring and correlation to echocardiography. Onkologie 35: 241–246. 000338335 [pii];10.1159/000338335 [doi].
32. Lipshultz SE, Miller TL, Scully RE, Lipsitz SR, Rifai N, et al. (2012) Changes in cardiac biomarkers during doxorubicin treatment of pediatric patients with high-risk acute lymphoblastic leukemia: associations with long-term echocardiographic outcomes. J Clin Oncol 30: 1042–1049. JCO.2010.30.3404 [pii];10.1200/JCO.2010.30.3404 [doi].
33. Mavinkurve-Groothuis AM, Kapusta L, Nir A, Groot-Loonen J (2008) The role of biomarkers in the early detection of anthracycline-induced cardiotoxicity in children: a review of the literature. Pediatr Hematol Oncol 25: 655–664. 903558793 [pii];10.1080/08880010802244001 [doi].
34. Soker M, Kervancioglu M (2005) Plasma concentrations of NT-pro-BNP and cardiac troponin-I in relation to doxorubicin-induced cardiomyopathy and cardiac function in childhood malignancy. Saudi Med J 26: 1197–1202. 20050218' [pii].
35. Mavinkurve-Groothuis AM, Groot-Loonen J, Bellersen L, Pourier MS, Feuth T, et al. (2009) Abnormal NT-pro-BNP levels in asymptomatic long-term survivors of childhood cancer treated with anthracyclines. Pediatr Blood Cancer 52: 631–636. 10.1002/pbc.21913 [doi].
36. Poutanen T, Tikanoja T, Riikonen P, Silvast A, Perkkio M (2003) Long-term prospective follow-up study of cardiac function after cardiotoxic therapy for malignancy in children. J Clin Oncol 21: 2349–2356. 10.1200/JCO.2003.08.050 [doi];JCO.2003.08.050 [pii].
37. Bosch X, Rovira M, Sitges M, Domenech A, Ortiz-Perez JT, et al. (2013) Enalapril and carvedilol for preventing chemotherapy-induced left ventricular systolic dysfunction in patients with malignant hemopathies: the OVERCOME trial (preventiOn of left Ventricular dysfunction with Enalapril and caRvedilol in patients submitted to intensive ChemOtherapy for the treatment of Malignant hEmopathies). J Am Coll Cardiol 61: 2355–2362. S0735-1097(13)01398-3 [pii];10.1016/j.jacc.2013.02.072 [doi].

6

Associations of Polymorphisms in DNA Repair Genes and MDR1 Gene with Chemotherapy Response and Survival of Non-Small Cell Lung Cancer

Yan Du[1]◑, Tong Su[1]◑, Lijun Zhao[2]◑, Xiaojie Tan[1], Wenjun Chang[1], Hongwei Zhang[1], Guangwen Cao[1]*

1 Department of Epidemiology, Second Military Medical University, Shanghai, China, **2** Department of Pulmonary Medicine, Changhai Hospital, Second Military Medical University, Shanghai, China

Abstract

Objectives: We aimed to determine the associations of genetic polymorphisms of excision repair cross-complementation group 1 (*ERCC1*) rs11615, xeroderma pigmentosum group D (*XPD/ERCC2)* rs13181, X-ray repair cross complementing group 1 (*XRCC1*) rs25487, *XRCC3* rs1799794, and breast cancer susceptibility gene 1 (*BRCA1*) rs1799966 from the DNA repair pathway and multiple drug resistance 1 (*MDR1/ABCB1*) rs1045642 with response to chemotherapy and survival of non-small cell lung cancer (NSCLC) in a Chinese population.

Materials and Methods: A total of 352 NSCLC patients were enrolled to evaluate the associations of the six SNPs with response to chemotherapy and overall survival. Logistic regressions were applied to test the associations of genetic polymorphisms with response to chemotherapy in 161 advanced NSCLC patients. Overall survival was analyzed in 161 advanced and 156 early stage NSCLC patients using the Kaplan-Meier method with log-rank test, respectively. Multivariate Cox proportional hazards model was performed to determine the factors independently associated with NSCLC prognosis.

Results: *BRCA1* rs1799966 minor allele C (TC+CC *vs.* TT, OR = 0.402, 95%CI = 0.204−0.794, p = 0.008) and *MDR1/ABCB1* rs1045642 minor allele A (GA +AA *vs.* GG, OR = 0.478, 95%CI = 0.244−0.934, p = 0.030) were associated with a better response to chemotherapy in advanced NSCLC patients. Survival analyses indicated that *BRCA1* rs1799966 TC+CC genotypes were associated with a decreased risk of death (HR = 0.617, 95% CI = 0.402−0.948, p = 0.028) in advanced NSCLC patients, and the association was still significant after the adjustment for covariates. Multivariate Cox regression analysis showed that *ERCC1* rs11615 AA genotype (*P* = 0.020) and smoking (p = 0.037) were associated with increased risks of death in early stage NSCLC patients after surgery.

Conclusions: Polymorphisms of genes in DNA repair pathway and *MDR1* could contribute to chemotherapy response and survival of patients with NSCLC.

Editor: Xiaoping Miao, MOE Key Laboratory of Environment and Health, School of Public Health, Tongji Medical College, Huazhong University of Science and Technology, China

Funding: This study was supported by Key Project of Shanghai Science and Technology Committee grant (06DZ19503 to G. Cao) and National Natural Science Foundation of China (81025015 to G. Cao). The funding agencies had no role in study design, data collection and analysis, decision to publish, or preparation of the manuscript.

Competing Interests: The authors have declared that no competing interests exist.

* Email: gcao@smmu.edu.cn

◑ These authors contributed equally to this work.

Introduction

Lung cancer is one of the leading causes of cancer deaths worldwide [1]. Non-small-cell lung cancer (NSCLC) is the most common subtype and accounts for 85% of all lung cancer. Most NSCLC patients are at developed advanced tumor stage upon diagnosis and lose the opportunity of surgical resection [2]. Platinum-based combined chemotherapy is a standard treatment for advanced NSCLC. However, the outcome and survival of advanced NSCLC are generally poor, with a 5-year survival rate of only about 15%. In addition, the survival rate of advanced NSCLC varies greatly in different populations with diverse genetic background [3,4]. Furthermore, the therapeutic efficacy of platinum-based regimens was affected by drug resistance. Possible mechanisms of chemoresistance include alterations in drug efflux or influx, DNA repair capacity, and other cellular pathways required for response to DNA damage. For patients with early stage NSCLC that can be surgically excised, the long-term prognosis is not satisfactory and the 5-year survival rate after surgery is less than 50% [5]. The outcome of early stage NSCLC patients receiving surgical treatment is also closely related to individual genetic characteristics, since variation and expression levels of certain genes can affect the survival and adjuvant chemotherapy response [6,7]. Genetic variation analysis in candidate pathways has shown that an individual's genetic background plays an important role in disease development, treatment response, and survival. For example, patients with completely resected NSCLC and negative expression of excision repair cross-complementation group 1 (ERCC1) protein in tumors benefit more from adjuvant cisplatin-based chemotherapy than those with ERCC1 positive expression [8]. Previous studies have shown that tumor-node-metastasis (TNM) staging system, age, performance status and weight loss are associated with NSCLC prognosis; however, the predictive powers of these factors are not optimal. Therefore, it is crucial to identify new biomarkers that can improve prognostic and predictive assessment accuracy to help developing personalized cancer treatment and patient-tailored chemotherapy, and eventually achieving better outcomes for NSCLC patients.

DNA repair capacity (DRC) is a double-edged sword in cancer etiology and treatment. Defects in DNA repair system drastically increase cancer risk [9]. On the other hand, DNA repair mechanism may reduce the therapeutic efficacy of chemotherapy by allowing cancer cells to fix DNA damages caused by these agents [10]. DNA repair involves coordination of many genes in four major DNA repair pathways, which are nucleotide excision repair (NER), base excision repair (BER), double-strand break repair (DSBR), and mismatch repair (MMR) pathways. Single nucleotide polymorphisms (SNPs) in DNA repair genes may modulate DNA repair capacity via influencing protein expression or activities, and therefore affecting lung cancer risk [11–13]. DNA repair gene polymorphisms may be associated with the risk and prognosis of NSCLC. Xeroderma pigmentosum group D (*XPD/ERCC2)* polymorphism can alter the secondary structure of mRNA [14]; and SNP in the X-ray repair cross complementing group 1 (*XRCC1*) gene 5′ untranslated region (UTR) greatly enhance trans-activator Sp1 binding element, therefore decreasing promoter activity and decreasing protein expression [15]. Furthermore, polymorphisms in these genes may also be potential prognostic markers for both chemotherapy response and overall survival of NSCLC patients [16–19].

Multiple drug resistance 1 (*MDR1*, also known as *ABCB1*) gene encodes P-glycoprotein (P-gp), a transmembrane transporter belonging to the ATP-binding cassette family, which can pump out intracellular chemotherapeutics and induce multiple drug resistance. *MDR1/ABCB1* C3435T (rs1045642) polymorphism is associated with expression level and function of MDR1 [20], thus may affect the responses to anticancer drug treatment.

In this study, we selected six previously studied SNPs, located either on the protein coding regions or in regulatory regions of the genes, including *ERCC1* rs11615, *XPD/ERCC2* rs13181 and breast cancer susceptibility gene 1 (*BRCA1*) rs1799966 from the NER pathway; *XRCC1* rs25487 from the BER pathway, *XRCC3* rs1799794 from the DSBR pathway, as well as *MDR1/ABCB1* rs1045642 (Table S1). We first investigated the associations between these SNPs and chemotherapy response in advanced NSCLC patients, then evaluated their relationships with the survival of NSCLC patients who received surgical treatment or chemotherapy.

Materials and Methods

Study population

The participants were recruited at Changhai Hospital of the Second Military Medical University. A total of 352 primary NSCLC patients diagnosed from July 1997 to October 2008 were enrolled (Dataset S1). All patients were histopathologically confirmed as NSCLC. Clinical and histopathologic data of patients were extracted from their medical records. All patients were of ethnic Han Chinese origin. The study protocol conformed to the ethical guidelines of the Declaration of Helsinki (2000), and was approved by the Institutional Review Board of this university. All participants provided written informed consent.

Data collection and follow-up

Of the 352 NSCLC patients, 161 (45.7%) advanced NSCLC patients received evaluable platinum-based chemotherapy. Besides cisplatin (DDP) or carboplatin (CBP), chemotherapy regimens also included gemcitabine (GEM), paclitaxel (TAX), docetaxel (DOC), vinorelbine (NVB), or pemetrexed disodium (PEM). Drug dosages were: DDP 75 mg/m^2 on day 1; CBP area under curve (AUC) $=5-6$ g on day 1; GEM 1250 mg/m^2 on days 1 and 8; TAX 135~175 mg/m^2 on day 1 over 3 hours; DOC 75 mg/m^2 on day 1 over 1 hour; NVB 25 mg/m^2 on days 1 and 8; PEM 500 mg/m^2 on day 1. All drugs were administrated by intravenous infusion every 3–4 weeks for a treatment cycle. Tumor response was assessed after 2 treatment cycles according to the Response Evaluation Criteria in Solid Tumors [21]. Responses were classified into complete response (CR), partial response (PR), stable disease (SD) or progressive disease (PD). Patients with CR, PR or SD were defined as "patients with clinical benefit", and patients with PD were defined as "patients without clinical benefit" [22].

Follow-up was started 2 months after the definite diagnosis. Follow-up was performed by telephone or in-person interview at the outpatient department at an interval of 3 months according to our standard epidemiological procedure. Median follow-up period was 20.8 months (range: 1.0 to 178.6 months).

Genotyping

Genomic DNA was extracted from peripheral blood using QIAmp DNA extraction kits (QIAGEN, Hilden, Germany). SNPs were genotyped using fluorescent-probe real-time quantitative PCR (qPCR) in a LightCycler^{TM}480 (Roche, Basel, Switzerland). Primers and probes (Taqman or Minor Groove Binder [MGB]) were designed and synthesized by GeneCore BioTechnologies (Shanghai, China). The sequences of primers and probes are available in Table S1. Each reaction mixture contained 0.2 μmol/L of primers, 0.2 μmol/L of probes, 0.1 μg–0.5 μg purified templates in Premix Ex Taq reaction system (Takara, Dalian, China). The reactions were programmed at 95°C for 10 s and followed by 40 cycles of 95°C for 10 s and 60°C for 30 s. All samples were successfully genotyped (Dataset S1). For quality control, 5% samples were randomly selected and directly sequenced, and 100% identical results were obtained.

Statistical analysis

Logistic regression analysis was performed to obtain odds ratios (ORs) and their 95% confidence intervals (95% CIs) for the relationships of genetic polymorphisms with chemotherapy response in 161 advanced NSCLC patients. Overall survival (OS) was analyzed using the Kaplan-Meier method in 161 advanced and 156 early stage NSCLC patients separately. Log-rank test was used to compare the survival curves. Forward stepwise multivariate Cox proportional hazards model ($P_{entry}=0.05$, $P_{removal}=0.10$) was performed to determine the factors contributing independently to NSCLC prognosis and estimate the hazard ratios (HRs) and their 95% CIs. Further subgroup analyses stratifying by histology, smoking status, Eastern Cooperative Oncology Group (ECOG) performance status, and stage were

Table 1. Demographic and clinical characteristics of the NSCLC patients.

	Total (n = 352)	Classified according to treatment and follow-up results				
		Early stage patients with surgery (n = 156)	Advanced patients with chemotherapy (n = 161)	Patients without treatment (n = 10)	Patients lost to follow up (n = 25)	P*
Age (year)						0.78
Range	26–90	26–84	30–90	56–76	35–78	
Mean ± SD	59.5±10.6	59.2±9.9	58.9±11.3	66.7±7.8	62.5±9.6	
Sex, n (%)						0.59
Male	246(69.9)	109(69.9)	108(67.1)	8(80.0)	21(84.0)	
Female	106(30.1)	47(30.1)	53(32.9)	2(20.0)	4(16.0)	
Histology, n (%)						0.70
Squamous cell carcinoma	118(33.5)	54(34.6)	52 (32.3)	4(40.0)	8(32.0)	
Adenocarcinoma	181(51.4)	81(51.9)	82(50.9)	3(30.0)	15(60.0)	
Other	53(15.1)	21(13.4)	27(16.8)	3(30.0)	2(8.0)	
Stage, n (%)						-
I	53(15.1)	47(30.1)	(0.0)	0 (0.0)	6(24.0)	
II	77(21.9)	73(46.8)	(0.0)	2(20.0)	2(8.0)	
IIIA	48(13.6)	36(23.1)	8(5.0)	1(10.0)	3(12.0)	
IIIB	54(15.3)	(0.0)	47(29.2)	5(10.0)	2(8.0)	
IV	120(34.1)	(0.0)	106(65.8)	2(10.0)	12(48.0)	
ECOG performance status						0.28
0–1	343(97.4)	154(98.7)	155(96.2)	9(90.0)	24(96.0)	
≥2	9(2.6)	2(1.3)	6(3.7)	1(10.0)	1(4.0)	
Smoking status						0.29†
Never smokers	170(48.3)	80(51.3)	73(45.3)	4(40.0)	13(52.0)	
Ever smokers	182(51.7)	76(48.7)	88(54.7)	6(60.0)	12(48.0)	
<25 pack-years	54(15.3)	27(17.3)	23(14.3)	1(10.0)	3(12.0)	
25–50 pack-years	94(26.7)	37(23.7)	46(28.6)	5(50.0)	6(24.0)	
>50 pack-years	34(9.7)	12(7.7)	19(11.8)	0 (0.0)	3(12.0)	
Radiation therapy						<0.0001
Never received	246(69.9)	124(79.5)	90(55.9)	-	22(88.0)	
Ever received	106(30.1)	32(20.5)	71(44.1)	-	3(12.0)	

Abbreviations: ECOG, Eastern Cooperative Oncology Group; SD, stand deviation.
*P values refer to the comparison between early stage patients with surgery and advanced patients with chemotherapy. Student's t-test was used to compare age as a continuous variable; chi-square test was used to compare categorical variables, except for ECOG performance status, where Fisher's exact test was used.
†Comparisons between never smokers and ever smokers.

also performed. Covariates were adjusted to obtain HRs and corresponding 95% CIs in subgroup analyses. All statistical tests were two-sided and conducted using Statistical Program for Social Sciences (SPSS 16.0 for Windows, SPSS, Chicago, IL). $P<0.05$ was considered as statistically significant.

Results

Patient characteristics

The demographic and clinical characteristics of the patients are shown in Table 1. Of the 352 NSCLC cases, 156 (44.3%) were early stage patients who underwent surgical treatment, 161 (45.7%) were advanced patients at an inoperable stage and received platinum-based chemotherapy, 10 (2.8%) patients refused any treatment for personal reasons, and 25 (7.1%) patients lost to follow up after the first treatment at Changhai Hospital. Most (120/156, 76.9%) early stage NSCLC patients who underwent surgery received preoperative or postoperative adjuvant chemotherapy. Advanced NSCLC patients were more likely to receive radiation therapy compared to early stage patients (44.1% *vs.* 20.5%, p<0.0001). Other demographic and clinical characteristics were similar between early stage and advanced NSCLC patients (p>0.05 for all). Table S2 presented the genotype distributions of these six SNPs in different categories of the NSCLC patients.

Associations of SNPs with chemotherapy response

Of the 161 advanced NSCLC patients that received evaluable platinum-based chemotherapy, the number of patients with CR, PR, SD or PD was 0, 44, 65 and 52, respectively. The overall clinical benefit (CR+PR+SD) rate was 67.7% (109/161). *BRCA1* rs1799966, *MDR1/ABCB1* rs1045642 and clinical stage were

Table 2. Associations of genotype and clinical stage with clinical benefit of chemotherapy among advanced NSCLC patients (N = 161).

	CR+PR+SD, n (%)	PD, n (%)	*P*	OR (95% CI)	Adjusted *P**	Adjusted OR* (95% CI)
BRCA1 rs1799966						
TT	33 (55.0)	27 (45.0)		1.00		1.00
TC+CC	76 (75.2)	25 (24.8)	**0.008**	**0.402 (0.204–0.794)**	**0.013**	**0.410 (0.203–0.831)**
MDR1/ABCB1 rs1045642						
GG	39 (58.2)	28 (41.8)		1.00		1.00
GA +AA	70 (74.5)	24 (25.5)	**0.030**	**0.478 (0.244–0.934)**	**0.045**	**0.488 (0.242–0.984)**
Clinical stage						
III	44 (80.0)	11 (20.0)		1.00		1.00
IV	65 (61.3)	41 (38.7)	**0.016**	**2.523 (1.171–5.437)**	**0.015**	**2.698 (1.214–5.996)**
ERCC1 rs11615						
GG	58 (63.7)	33 (36.3)		1.00		
GA+AA	51 (72.9)	19 (27.1)	0.220	0.655 (0.332–1.290)		
XPD/ERCC2 rs13181						
TT	87 (68.0)	41 (32.0)		1.00		
TG+GG	22 (66.7)	11 (33.3)	0.887	1.061 (0.470–2.393)		
XRCC1 rs25487						
CC	70 (68.6)	32 (31.4)		1.00		
CT+TT	39 (66.1)	20 (33.9)	0.741	1.122 (0.567–2.219)		
XRCC3 rs1799794						
CC	39 (63.9)	22 (36.1)		1.00		
CT+TT	70 (70.0)	30 (30.0)	0.425	0.760 (0.387–1.493)		

Abbreviations: CR, complete response; OR, odds ratio; PD, progressive disease; PR, partial response; SD, stable disease.
*Adjusted for *BRCA1* rs1799966, *MDR1/ABCB1* rs1045642 and clinical stage, adjusted ORs and P values were obtained from multivariate logistic regression analysis by forward stepwise method.

significantly associated with clinical benefit (Table 2). The patients carrying *BRCA1* minor allele C (TC+CC) had significantly more chances of achieving clinical benefit than the patients carrying rs1799966 TT genotype (75.2% *vs.* 55.0%, OR = 0.402, 95%CI = 0.204−0.794, p = 0.008). Similarly, patients carrying *MDR1/ABCB1* rs1045642 minor allele A (GA +AA) had more clinical benefit than patients carrying rs1045642 GG genotype (74.5% *vs.* 58.2%, OR = 0.478, 95%CI = 0.244−0.934, p = 0.030). In addition, the patients with clinical stage IV had significantly less chances of achieving clinical benefit than those with clinical stage III (61.3% *vs.* 80.0%, OR = 2.523, 95%CI = 1.171−5.437, p = 0.016). Furthermore, the associations continued to be significant in multivariate logistic regression analysis, which suggested that *BRCA1* rs1799966 (TC+CC *vs.* TT), *MDR1/ABCB1* rs1045642 (GA+AA *vs.* GG) and clinical stage (IV *vs.* III) were independent factors affecting response to chemotherapy (*BRCA1* rs1799966: adjusted OR = 0.410, 95% CI = 0.203−0.831, adjusted p = 0.013; *MDR1/ABCB1* rs1045642: adjusted OR = 0.488, 95% CI = 0.242−0.984, adjusted p = 0.045; clinical stage: adjusted OR = 2.698, 95% CI = 1.214−5.996, adjusted p = 0.015). No significant associations were observed between the other four SNPs (*ERCC1* rs11615, *XPD/ERCC2* rs13181, *XRCC1* rs25487, *XRCC3* rs1799794) or other characteristics (age, sex, histology, chemotherapy regimens, performance status, smoking status, and radiation therapy) and clinical benefit (p>0.05 for all).

Associations of SNPs with OS of patients with advanced NSCLC

Univariate analyses using Kaplan-Meier curves and log-rank tests indicated that *BRCA1* rs1799966 (TC+CC *vs.* TT genotypes), radiation therapy (ever *vs.* never), and smoking status (never *vs.* ever) were significantly associated with an increased OS of advanced NSCLC patients with log-rank values of p = 0.042, 0.049, and 0.042, respectively (Fig. 1). The stepwise multivariate Cox analysis showed that *BRCA1* rs1799966 (TC+CC *vs.* TT: HR = 0.617, 95% CI = 0.402−0.948, p = 0.028), radiation therapy (ever *vs.* never: HR = 0.611, 95% CI = 0.396−0.944, p = 0.027), and smoking (never *vs.* ever: HR = 0.574, 95% CI = 0.373−0.882, p = 0.011) independently predicted favorable survival of the advanced NSCLC patients. No significant associations were observed between the other SNPs or other characteristics and OS (log-rank p>0.05 for all).

We further examined the association of *BRCA1* rs1799966 with survival in subgroup analyses by categorizing the patients according to histology, smoking status, ECOG performance status, and stage. In with squamous cell carcinoma, those ever smoked, those with ECOG performance status of 1, or those at stage III, *BRCA1* rs1799966 TC+CC genotypes predicted a longer OS than the TT genotype (log-rank p<0.05 for all) (Fig. 2). After adjusting for age, sex, histology, stage, ECOG performance status, smoking status, and radiation therapy in the Cox model, *BRCA1* rs1799966 TC+CC genotypes were associated with a lower risk of death in patients with squamous cell carcinoma (HR = 0.324, 95% CI = 0.137−0.765, p = 0.010), patients ever smoked

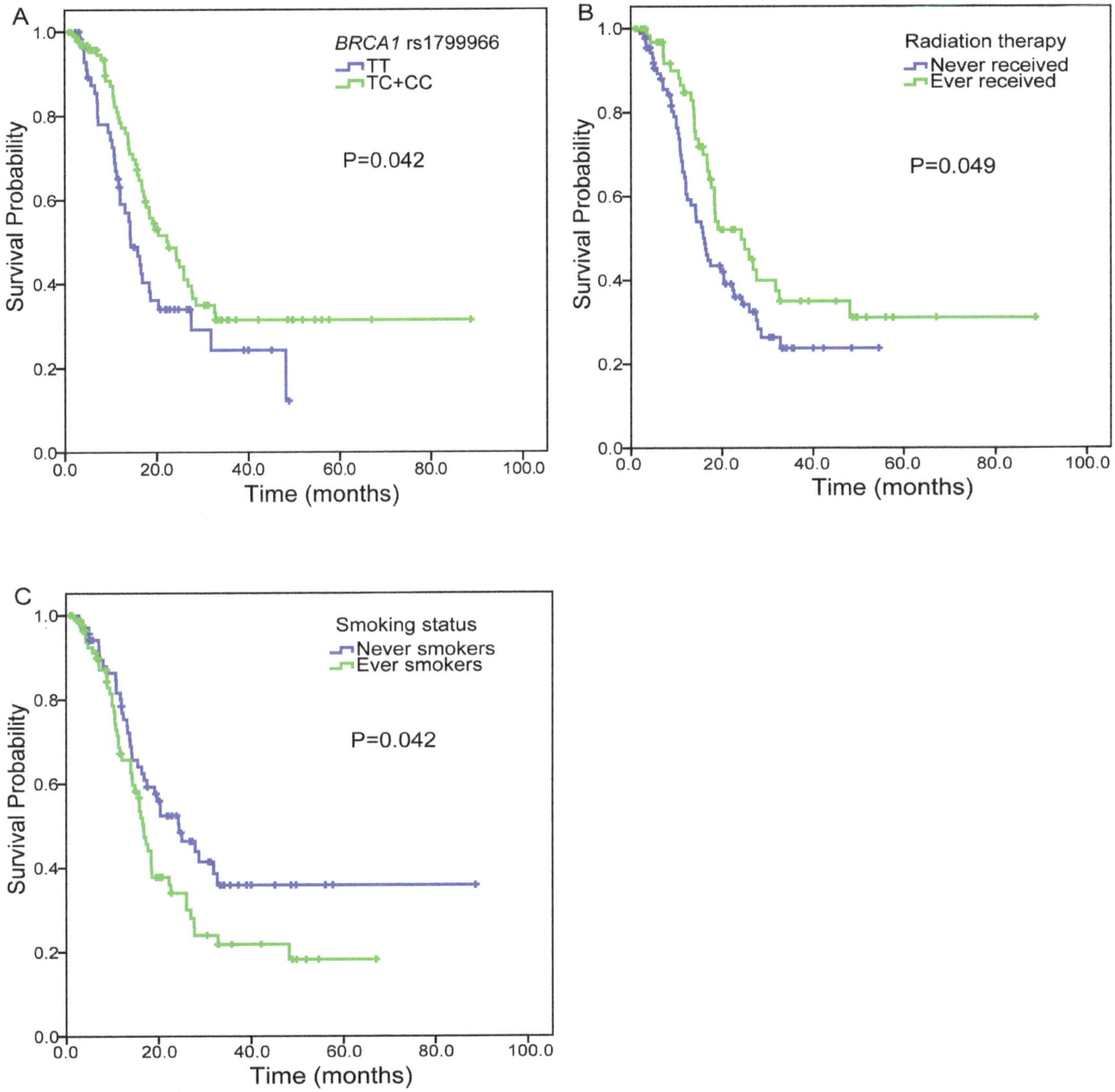

Figure 1. Factors associated with overall survival of advanced NSCLC patients. (A) *BRCA1* rs1799966, (B) radiation therapy, (C) smoking status.

(HR = 0.406, 95% CI = 0.221−0.743, p = 0.004), or those with ECOG performance status of 1 (HR = 0.563, 95% CI = 0.353−0.898, p = 0.016).

Associations of SNPs with postoperative OS of patients with early stage NSCLC

ERCC1 rs11615 and smoking status were statistically significantly associated with OS of early stage NSCLC patients (log-rank p = 0.009 and 0.013, respectively) (Fig. 3). In the stepwise multivariate Cox analysis, patients with *ERCC1* rs11615 AA genotype had an increased risk of death (deaths/cases: 5/9 for AA *vs.* 44/147 for GG+GA, HR = 3.087, 95% CI = 1.197−7.961, p = 0.020,). Smoking was also associated with worse survival (deaths/cases: 30/76 for ever smokers *vs.* 19/80 for never smokers, HR = 1.896, 95% CI = 1.040−3.455, p = 0.037). We did not observe any significant associations of the other SNPs or other characteristics with OS (log-rank p>0.05 for all).

Further stratification analyses in early stage NSCLC patients indicated that *ERCC1* rs11615 AA genotype predicted a significant poorer OS than GG+GA genotypes in patients with squamous cell carcinoma (log-rank p = 0.004), those ever smoked (log-rank p = 0.018), those with ECOG performance status of 1 (log-rank p = 0.007), or those never receiving radiation therapy (log-rank p< 0.001) (Fig. 4). After adjusting for age, sex, histology, stage, ECOG

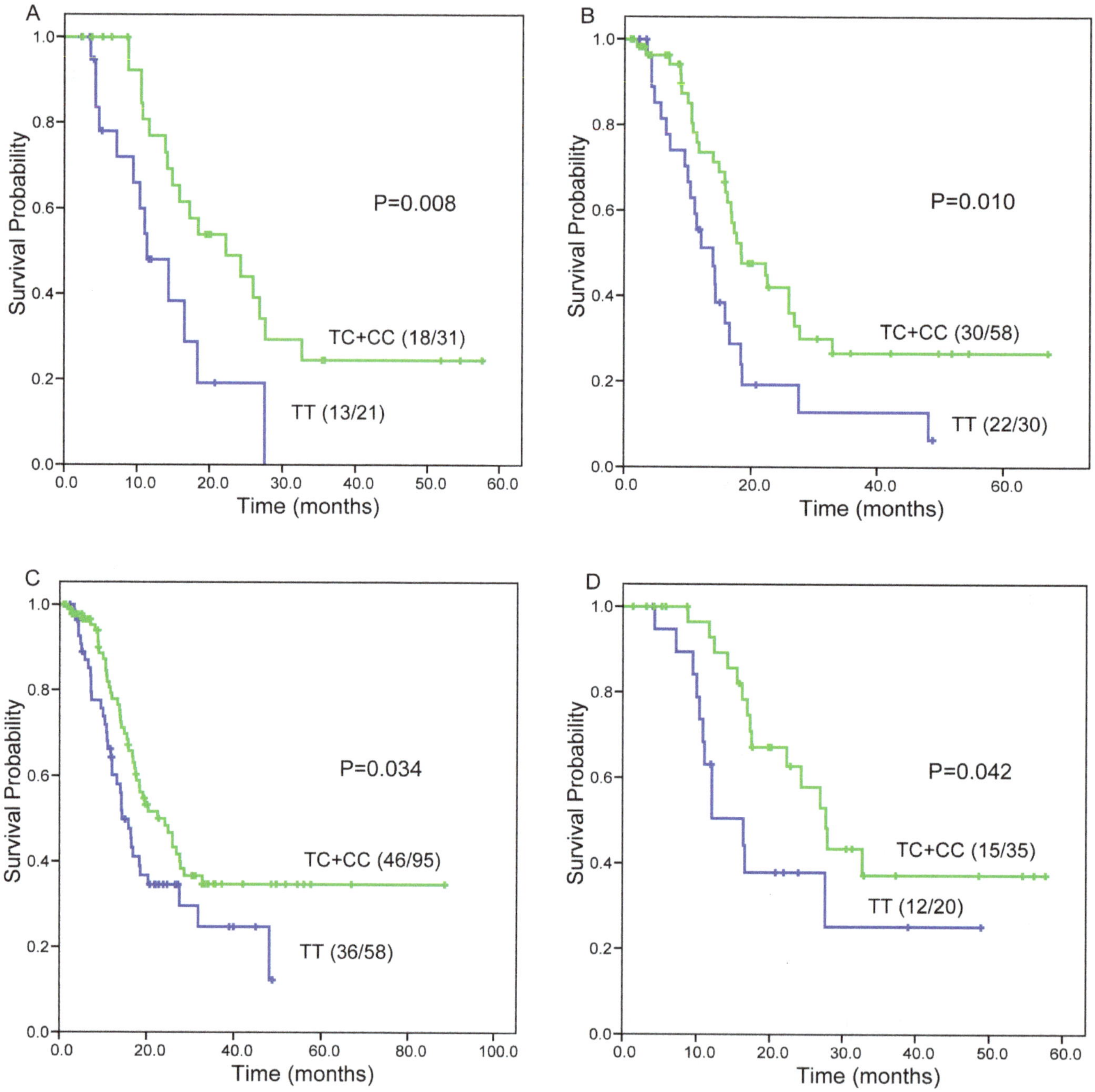

Figure 2. Subgroup analysis results of overall survival in advanced NSCLC patients according to *BRCA1* rs1799966 genotypes (TT *vs.* TC+CC). (A) Squamous cell carcinoma group, (B) ever smokers group, (C) ECOG performance status = 1 group, (D) stage III group. Number in parenthesis, number of deaths/number of cases.

performance status, smoking status, radiation therapy, and adjuvant chemotherapy in the Cox model, *ERCC1* rs11615 AA genotype predicted a higher risk of death in early stage patients with squamous cell carcinoma (HR = 6.633, 95% CI = 1.184−37.164, p = 0.031), those ever smoked (HR = 3.324, 95% CI = 1.040−10.627, p = 0.043), those with ECOG performance status of 1 (HR = 2.835, 95% CI = 1.063−7.560, p = 0.037), or those never receiving radiation therapy (HR = 5.381, 95% CI = 1.857−15.593, p = 0.002).

Discussion

In this study, we evaluated relationships between six SNPs with chemotherapy response and survival of NSCLC in a Han Chinese population. We observed that the minor allele C of *BRCA1* rs1799966 from the DSBR pathway was associated with a better treatment response and a longer survival in advanced NSCLC patients underwent platinum-based chemotherapy. In addition, minor allele A of *MDR1/ABCB1* rs1045642 was significantly associated with clinical benefit of chemotherapy in advanced

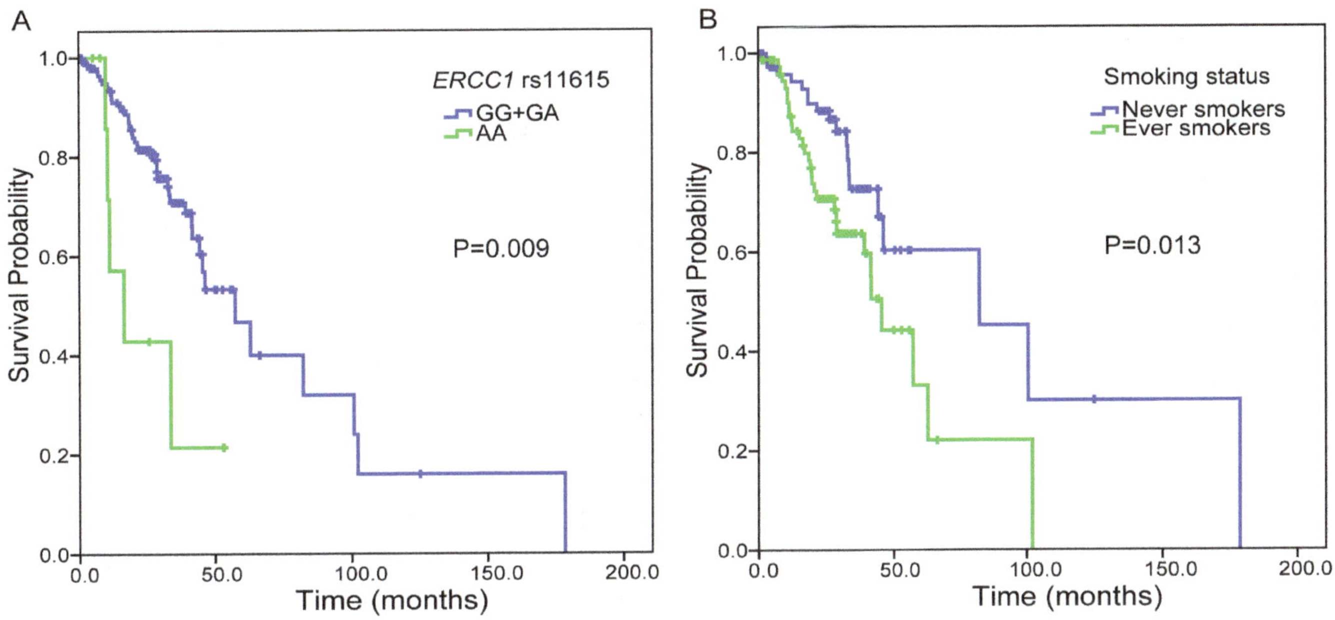

Figure 3. Factors associated with overall survival of early stage NSCLC patients. (A) *ERCC1* rs11615, (B) smoking status.

NSCLC patients. For early NSCLC patients, carriers of *ERCC1* rs11615 AA genotype had an increased risk of death.

BRCA1 gene belongs to the NER system [23], which is the major repair system that reduces platinum-induced DNA damage. *BRCA1* involves in many activities including homologous recombination, nonhomologous end joining, and mismatch repair [24]. BRCA1 protein is a nuclear phosphoprotein with multiple roles not only in DNA damage repair but also in cell cycle checkpoint or cell death machinery [24,25]. *In vitro* studies have reported that BRCA1 can regulate chemotherapy agent sensitivity; for example, the absence of BRCA1 causes high sensitivity to cisplatin [24]. BRCA1 expression is a reliable indicator of chemoresistance in NSCLC patients receiving treatment by DNA-damaging agents such as platinum [26–28]. Patients with lower BRCA1 expression have better survival in platinum-based neoadjuvant chemotherapy [26–28], which is further confirmed by a recent meta-analysis [29]. Genetic polymorphisms may affect the protein expression, structure, and/or function; however, previous studies have rarely investigated the associations between *BRCA1* polymorphisms with NSCLC survival. One study in a Korean population reported no association between *BRCA1* rs1799966 and NSCLC survival; however, they did find *BRCA1* haplotype AACC (rs1799966-rs8176199-rs8067269-rs2070833) predicted shorter survival among advanced NSCLC patients receiving platinum-based chemotherapy [18]. In our analysis, we observed *BRCA1* rs1799966 minor allele C was significantly associated with better chemotherapy response and longer survival in advanced NSCLC patients. rs1799966 is a nonsynonymous SNP in the coding region of the COOH-terminal domain, termed as BRCT, which is essential for homologous recombination in repairing DNA double-stranded breaks [30]. The amino acid change from proline to leucine at position 871 of rs799917 leads to a non-conservative change of the unique structural properties of the BRCA1 protein. In addition, this SNP is in linkage disequilibrium with rs799917, which lies in the middle of a strongly conserved region of the *BRCA1* gene [31].

ERCC1 is another important enzyme in the NER pathway of DNA repair, and is responsible for the 5′ incision of damaged DNA [32]. Previous studies have demonstrated that ERCC1 expression is related to clinical benefit of platinum-based chemotherapy [5,8,33,34], and could be used as a biomarker for NSCLC treatment. The variant genotype in *ERCC1* polymorphisms may destroy or alter the repair functions possibly through changing the expression levels. rs11615 is a synonymous SNP located in codon 118 of the *ERCC1* gene, which encodes the amino acid asparagines. The variant allele of rs11615 may results in altered mRNA level [35]. Studies conducted in different populations showed that the GG genotype of *ERCC1* rs11615 was associated with a better survival in advanced NSCLC patient [36,37]. In contrary, a study conducted in Japan did not find significant associations between *ERCC1* rs11615 and survival [38]. Furthermore, a meta-analysis including 17 studies could not confirm the association of *ERCC1* rs11615 with survival, neither in the overall nor ethnic stratified analyses [39]. The inconsistent results of previous studies may be due to ethnic differences, the stage of the disease, and/or therapeutic variations. Few studies ever investigated the association between rs11615 and survival of early stage NSCLC. In the present study, we detected that the AA genotype of rs11615 was associated with poorer OS in early stage NSCLC patients. One important meta-analysis concluded that high ERCC1 was associated with significantly worse OS in platinum-treated NSCLC patients [40]. These evidences indicate that the variant allele genotype (AA) of rs11615 is related to high expression of ERCC1. However, the effects of radiation therapy are complex. A fraction of our early stage NSCLC patients (32/156, 20.5%) received radiation therapy, thus we cannot rule out the possible influence of radiation therapy on the association of *ERCC1* rs11615 with survival.

One reason of treatment failure in cancer patients is drug resistance, which can be influenced by factors affecting the efflux and influx of chemotherapeutics across the cell membrane. MDR1/ABCB1 is responsible for the efflux of many chemotherapeutics through the cell membrane by hydrolysis of ATP [41]. rs1045642 has a G>A change at cDNA position 3435 in exon 26 and plays a role in the P-gp function [20]. However, results from studies of *MDR1/ABCB1* rs1045642 and platinum-based chemo-

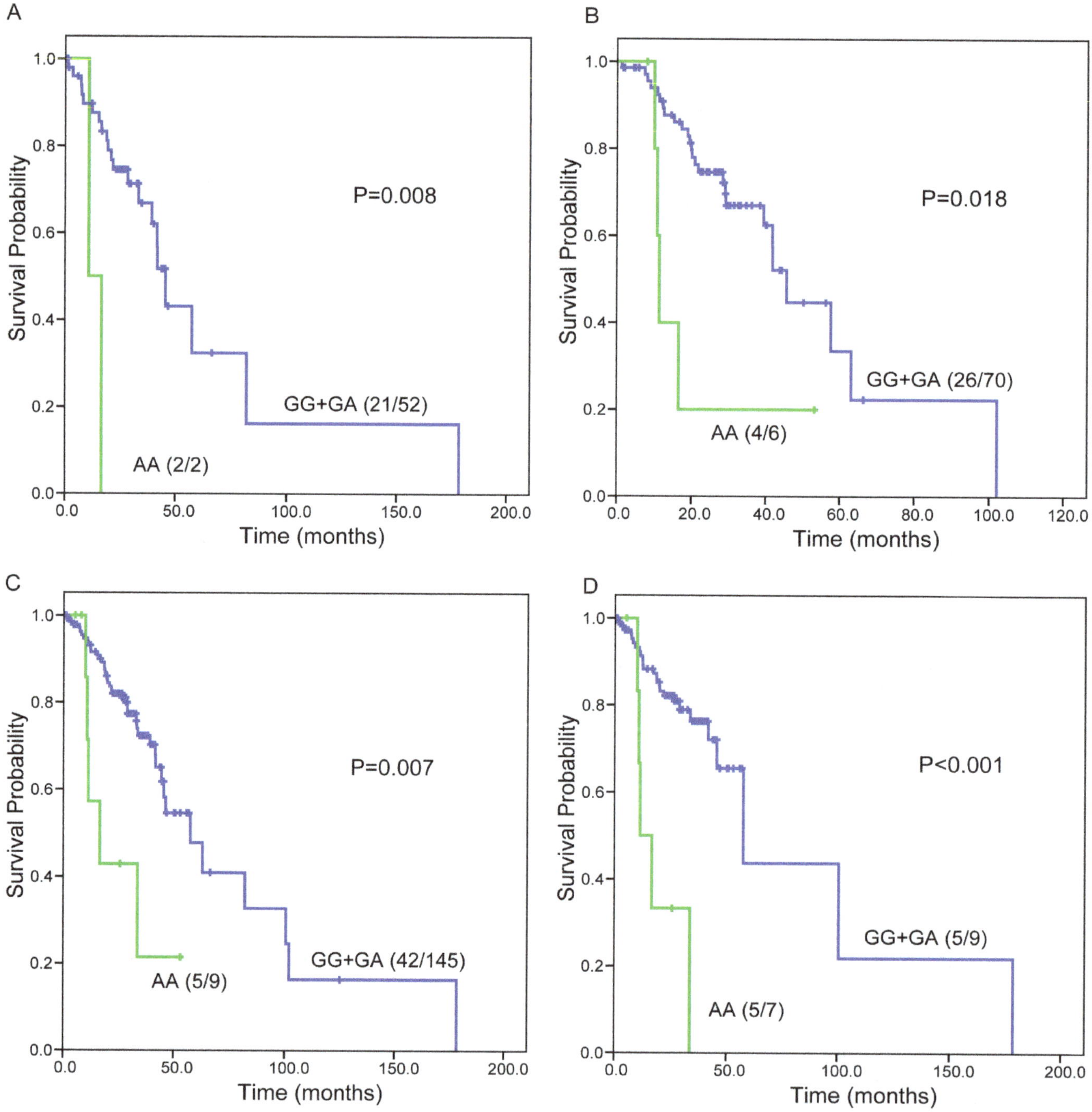

Figure 4. Subgroup analysis results of overall survival in early stage NSCLC patients according to *ERCC1* genotypes (GG+GA vs. AA). (A) Squamous cell carcinoma group, (B) ever smokers group, (C) ECOG performance status = 1 group, (D) never receiving radiation therapy group. Number in parenthesis, number of deaths/number of cases.

therapy response of NSCLC are inconsistent in different populations [36,42]. Recent meta-analyses confirmed this SNP was associated with chemotherapy response in overall and Asian populations [39,43]. However, we obtained opposite results from the meta-analysis findings, showing *MDR1/ABCB1* variant allele carriers had more clinical benefits of chemotherapy. The discrepancy may possibly be explained by potential confounders such as radiation therapy.

Not surprisingly, smoking was associated with NSCLC prognosis in both early and advanced stage patients. Smoking causes impaired lung function, and is the well established risk factor of NSCLC occurrence and poor prognosis. Smoking can cause DNA damages such as DNA adducts and double-strand DNA break lesions [44]. It can also interfere with DNA repair function, thus greatly affecting patient outcomes.

The current study has several limitations. First are the relatively small sample size and a short follow-up period, especially in subgroup analyses, therefore raising the issue of false positive findings. Our results did not reach statistical significance after correcting for multiple comparisons, and these findings need to be further validated. Second, we collected OS data instead of disease-specific survival since it is difficult to confirm the real cause of death in some patients. Third, we only selected limited number of SNPs based on their functions, while other polymorphisms in these genes may affect NSCLC chemotherapy response and prognosis. Last, NSCLC is a heterogeneous group of neoplasm, and multiple mechanisms may determine the response and prognosis, we were unable to account all factors in the current analysis.

To conclude, our study provided further evidences that polymorphisms in DNA repair pathway genes and *MDR1* gene could influence treatment response and survival of NSCLC patients. The mechanisms of how the differences in SNP nucleotide sequences or tandem repeats can affect gene transcription remain largely unclear. Further large-scale studies are needed to elucidate the functions and mechanisms that may help in improving the outcomes of NSCLC patients.

Supporting Information

Table S1 Polymorphism information, primers and probes for genotyping.

Table S2 Genotype distributions of SNPs in NSCLC patients.

Dataset S1.

Author Contributions

Conceived and designed the experiments: GC. Performed the experiments: XT WC HZ. Analyzed the data: YD TS. Contributed reagents/materials/analysis tools: LZ. Contributed to the writing of the manuscript: YD TS GC.

References

1. Jemal A, Bray F, Center MM, Ferlay J, Ward E, et al. (2011) Global cancer statistics. CA Cancer J Clin 61: 69–90.
2. Wu L, Chang W, Zhao J, Yu Y, Tan X, et al. (2010) Development of autoantibody signatures as novel diagnostic biomarkers of non-small cell lung cancer. Clin Cancer Res 16: 3760–3768.
3. Sekine I, Yamamoto N, Nishio K, Saijo N (2008) Emerging ethnic differences in lung cancer therapy. Br J Cancer 99: 1757–1762.
4. Siegel R, Naishadham D, Jemal A (2012) Cancer statistics, 2012. CA Cancer J Clin 62: 10–29.
5. Arriagada R, Bergman B, Dunant A, Le Chevalier T, Pignon JP, et al. (2004) Cisplatin-based adjuvant chemotherapy in patients with completely resected non-small-cell lung cancer. N Engl J Med 350: 351–360.
6. Yoo SS, Choi JE, Lee WK, Choi YY, Kam S, et al. (2009) Polymorphisms in the CASPASE genes and survival in patients with early-stage non-small-cell lung cancer. J Clin Oncol 27: 5823–5829.
7. Park JY, Lee WK, Jung DK, Choi JE, Park TI, et al. (2009) Polymorphisms in the FAS and FASL genes and survival of early stage non-small cell lung cancer. Clin Cancer Res 15: 1794–1800.
8. Olaussen KA, Dunant A, Fouret P, Brambilla E, Andre F, et al. (2006) DNA repair by ERCC1 in non-small-cell lung cancer and cisplatin-based adjuvant chemotherapy. N Engl J Med 355: 983–991.
9. Wei Q, Frazier ML, Levin B (2000) DNA repair: a double-edged sword. J Natl Cancer Inst 92: 440–441.
10. Rosell R, Lord RV, Taron M, Reguart N (2002) DNA repair and cisplatin resistance in non-small-cell lung cancer. Lung Cancer 38: 217–227.
11. Tanaka Y, Maniwa Y, Bermudez VP, Doi T, Nishio W, et al. (2010) Nonsynonymous single nucleotide polymorphisms in DNA damage repair pathways and lung cancer risk. Cancer 116: 896–902.
12. Zienolddiny S, Campa D, Lind H, Ryberg D, Skaug V, et al. (2006) Polymorphisms of DNA repair genes and risk of non-small cell lung cancer. Carcinogenesis 27: 560–567.
13. Zhang X, Miao X, Liang G, Hao B, Wang Y, et al. (2005) Polymorphisms in DNA base excision repair genes ADPRT and XRCC1 and risk of lung cancer. Cancer Res 65: 722–726.
14. Wolfe KJ, Wickliffe JK, Hill CE, Paolini M, Ammenheuser MM, et al. (2007) Single nucleotide polymorphisms of the DNA repair gene XPD/ERCC2 alter mRNA expression. Pharmacogenet Genomics 17: 897–905.
15. Hao B, Wang H, Zhou K, Li Y, Chen X, et al. (2004) Identification of genetic variants in base excision repair pathway and their associations with risk of esophageal squamous cell carcinoma. Cancer Res 64: 4378–4384.
16. Joerger M, Burgers SA, Baas P, Smit EF, Haitjema TJ, et al. (2011) Germline polymorphisms in patients with advanced nonsmall cell lung cancer receiving first-line platinum-gemcitabine chemotherapy: A prospective clinical study. Cancer.
17. Shiraishi K, Kohno T, Tanai C, Goto Y, Kuchiba A, et al. (2010) Association of DNA repair gene polymorphisms with response to platinum-based doublet chemotherapy in patients with non-small-cell lung cancer. J Clin Oncol 28: 4945–4952.
18. Kim HT, Lee JE, Shin ES, Yoo YK, Cho JH, et al. (2008) Effect of BRCA1 haplotype on survival of non-small-cell lung cancer patients treated with platinum-based chemotherapy. J Clin Oncol 26: 5972–5979.
19. Kim M, Kang HG, Lee SY, Lee HC, Lee EB, et al. (2010) Comprehensive analysis of DNA repair gene polymorphisms and survival in patients with early stage non-small-cell lung cancer. Cancer Sci 101: 2436–2442.
20. Hoffmeyer S, Burk O, von Richter O, Arnold HP, Brockmoller J, et al. (2000) Functional polymorphisms of the human multidrug-resistance gene: multiple sequence variations and correlation of one allele with P-glycoprotein expression and activity in vivo. Proc Natl Acad Sci U S A 97: 3473–3478.
21. Therasse P, Arbuck SG, Eisenhauer EA, Wanders J, Kaplan RS, et al. (2000) New guidelines to evaluate the response to treatment in solid tumors. European Organization for Research and Treatment of Cancer, National Cancer Institute of the United States, National Cancer Institute of Canada. J Natl Cancer Inst 92: 205–216.
22. Tibaldi C, Giovannetti E, Vasile E, Mey V, Laan AC, et al. (2008) Correlation of CDA, ERCC1, and XPD polymorphisms with response and survival in gemcitabine/cisplatin-treated advanced non-small cell lung cancer patients. Clin Cancer Res 14: 1797–1803.
23. Yarden RI, Papa MZ (2006) BRCA1 at the crossroad of multiple cellular pathways: approaches for therapeutic interventions. Mol Cancer Ther 5: 1396–1404.
24. Quinn JE, Kennedy RD, Mullan PB, Gilmore PM, Carty M, et al. (2003) BRCA1 functions as a differential modulator of chemotherapy-induced apoptosis. Cancer Res 63: 6221–6228.
25. Lafarge S, Sylvain V, Ferrara M, Bignon YJ (2001) Inhibition of BRCA1 leads to increased chemoresistance to microtubule-interfering agents, an effect that involves the JNK pathway. Oncogene 20: 6597–6606.
26. Taron M, Rosell R, Felip E, Mendez P, Souglakos J, et al. (2004) BRCA1 mRNA expression levels as an indicator of chemoresistance in lung cancer. Hum Mol Genet 13: 2443–2449.
27. Rosell R, Skrzypski M, Jassem E, Taron M, Bartolucci R, et al. (2007) BRCA1: a novel prognostic factor in resected non-small-cell lung cancer. PLoS One 2: e1129.
28. Bonanno L, Costa C, Majem M, Favaretto A, Rugge M, et al. (2013) The predictive value of BRCA1 and RAP80 mRNA expression in advanced non-small-cell lung cancer patients treated with platinum-based chemotherapy. Ann Oncol 24: 1130–1132.
29. Yang Y, Xie Y, Xian L (2013) Breast cancer susceptibility gene 1 (BRCA1) predict clinical outcome in platinum- and toxal-based chemotherapy in non-small-cell lung cancer (NSCLC) patients: a system review and meta-analysis. J Exp Clin Cancer Res 32: 15.
30. Lee KM, Nizza S, Hayes T, Bass KL, Irmisch A, et al. (2007) Brc1-mediated rescue of Smc5/6 deficiency: requirement for multiple nucleases and a novel Rad18 function. Genetics 175: 1585–1595.
31. Chang JS, Yeh RF, Wiencke JK, Wiemels JL, Smirnov I, et al. (2008) Pathway analysis of single-nucleotide polymorphisms potentially associated with glioblastoma multiforme susceptibility using random forests. Cancer Epidemiol Biomarkers Prev 17: 1368–1373.
32. He J, Xu Y, Qiu LX, Li J, Zhou XY, et al. (2012) Polymorphisms in ERCC1 and XPF genes and risk of gastric cancer in an eastern Chinese population. PLoS One, 7:e49308.
33. Lord RV, Brabender J, Gandara D, Alberola V, Camps C, et al. (2002) Low ERCC1 expression correlates with prolonged survival after cisplatin plus gemcitabine chemotherapy in non-small cell lung cancer. Clin Cancer Res 8: 2286–2291.
34. Cobo M, Isla D, Massuti B, Montes A, Sanchez JM, et al. (2007) Customizing cisplatin based on quantitative excision repair cross-complementing 1 mRNA expression: a phase III trial in non-small-cell lung cancer. J Clin Oncol 25: 2747–2754.
35. Yu JJ, Lee KB, Mu C, Li Q, Abernathy TV, et al. (2000) Comparison of two human ovarian carcinoma cell lines (A2780/CP70 and MCAS) that are equally resistant to platinum, but differ at codon 118 of the ERCC1 gene. Int J Oncol 16: 555–560.
36. Isla D, Sarries C, Rosell R, Alonso G, Domine M, et al. (2004) Single nucleotide polymorphisms and outcome in docetaxel-cisplatin-treated advanced non-small-cell lung cancer. Ann Oncol 15: 1194–1203.
37. Dong J, Hu Z, Shu Y, Pan S, Chen W, et al. (2012) Potentially functional polymorphisms in DNA repair genes and non-small-cell lung cancer survival: a pathway-based analysis. Mol Carcinog 51: 546–552.
38. Takenaka T, Yano T, Kiyohara C, Miura N, Kouso H, et al. (2010) Effects of excision repair cross-complementation group 1 (ERCC1) single nucleotide

polymorphisms on the prognosis of non-small cell lung cancer patients. Lung Cancer 67: 101–107.

39. Wei HB, Lu XS, Shang LH, Xu G, Hu J, et al. (2011) Polymorphisms of ERCC1 C118T/C8092A and MDR1 C3435T predict outcome of platinum-based chemotherapies in advanced non-small cell lung cancer: a meta-analysis. Arch Med Res 42: 412–420.
40. Hubner RA, Riley RD, Billingham LJ, Popat S (2011) Excision repair cross-complementation group 1 (ERCC1) status and lung cancer outcomes: a meta-analysis of published studies and recommendations. PLoS One 6:e25164.
41. Campa D, Sainz J, Pardini B, Vodickova L, Naccarati A, et al. (2012) A comprehensive investigation on common polymorphisms in the MDR1/ABCB1 transporter gene and susceptibility to colorectal cancer. PLoS One 7: e32784.
42. Vinolas N, Provencio M, Reguart N, Cardenal F, Alberola V, et al. (2011) Single nucleotide polymorphisms in MDR1 gen correlates with outcome in advanced non-small-cell lung cancer patients treated with cisplatin plus vinorelbine. Lung Cancer 71: 191–198.
43. Yin JY, Huang Q, Zhao YC, Zhou HH, Liu ZQ (2012) Meta-analysis on pharmacogenetics of platinum-based chemotherapy in non small cell lung cancer (NSCLC) patients. PLoS One 7:e38150.
44. Albino AP, Jorgensen ED, Rainey P, Gillman G, Clark TJ, et al. (2009) gammaH2AX: A potential DNA damage response biomarker for assessing toxicological risk of tobacco products. Mutat Res 678: 43–52.

7

Application of a Combination of a Knowledge-Based Algorithm and 2-Stage Screening to Hypothesis-Free Genomic Data on Irinotecan-Treated Patients for Identification of a Candidate Single Nucleotide Polymorphism Related to an Adverse Effect

Hiro Takahashi[1,2,3]*, Kimie Sai[4], Yoshiro Saito[4], Nahoko Kaniwa[4], Yasuhiro Matsumura[5], Tetsuya Hamaguchi[6], Yasuhiro Shimada[6], Atsushi Ohtsu[7], Takayuki Yoshino[7], Toshihiko Doi[7], Haruhiro Okuda[4], Risa Ichinohe[3,8], Anna Takahashi[2], Ayano Doi[3,8], Yoko Odaka[3], Misuzu Okuyama[3], Nagahiro Saijo[9¤a], Jun-ichi Sawada[10¤b], Hiromi Sakamoto[3], Teruhiko Yoshida[3]

1 Graduate School of Horticulture, Chiba University, Matsudo, Chiba, Japan, **2** Plant Biology Research Center, Chubu University, Kasugai, Aichi, Japan, **3** Division of Genetics, National Cancer Center Research Institute, Tokyo, Japan, **4** Division of Medicinal Safety Science, National Institute of Health Sciences, Tokyo, Japan, **5** Division of Developmental Therapeutics, Research Center for Innovative Oncology, National Cancer Center Hospital East, Kashiwa, Chiba, Japan, **6** Gastrointestinal Medical Oncology Division, National Cancer Center Hospital, Tokyo, Japan, **7** Department of Gastrointestinal Oncology, National Cancer Center Hospital East, Kashiwa, Chiba, Japan, **8** Faculty of Horticulture, Chiba University, Matsudo, Chiba, Japan, **9** National Cancer Center Hospital East, Kashiwa, Chiba, Japan, **10** Division of Functional Biochemistry and Genomics, National Institute of Health Sciences, Tokyo, Japan

Abstract

Interindividual variation in a drug response among patients is known to cause serious problems in medicine. Genomic information has been proposed as the basis for "personalized" health care. The genome-wide association study (GWAS) is a powerful technique for examining single nucleotide polymorphisms (SNPs) and their relationship with drug response variation; however, when using only GWAS, it often happens that no useful SNPs are identified due to multiple testing problems. Therefore, in a previous study, we proposed a combined method consisting of a knowledge-based algorithm, 2 stages of screening, and a permutation test for identifying SNPs. In the present study, we applied this method to a pharmacogenomics study where 109,365 SNPs were genotyped using Illumina Human-1 BeadChip in 168 cancer patients treated with irinotecan chemotherapy. We identified the SNP rs9351963 in potassium voltage-gated channel subfamily KQT member 5 (*KCNQ5*) as a candidate factor related to incidence of irinotecan-induced diarrhea. The *p* value for rs9351963 was 3.31×10^{-5} in Fisher's exact test and 0.0289 in the permutation test (when multiple testing problems were corrected). Additionally, rs9351963 was clearly superior to the clinical parameters and the model involving rs9351963 showed sensitivity of 77.8% and specificity of 57.6% in the evaluation by means of logistic regression. Recent studies showed that *KCNQ4* and *KCNQ5* genes encode members of the M channel expressed in gastrointestinal smooth muscle and suggested that these genes are associated with irritable bowel syndrome and similar peristalsis diseases. These results suggest that rs9351963 in *KCNQ5* is a possible predictive factor of incidence of diarrhea in cancer patients treated with irinotecan chemotherapy and for selecting chemotherapy regimens, such as irinotecan alone or a combination of irinotecan with a KCNQ5 opener. Nonetheless, clinical importance of rs9351963 should be further elucidated.

Editor: Olga Y. Gorlova, Geisel School of Medicine at Dartmouth College, United States of America

Funding: This work was supported in part by the Ministry of Education, Culture, Sports, Science, and Technology of Japan (MEXT): Grants-in-Aid for Scientific Research for Young Scientists (B) (nos. 21710211 and 24710222 to H.T.) and Grant-in-Aid for Scientific Research on Innovative Areas (no. 26114703 to H.T.). This work was also supported by the Advanced Research for Medical Products Mining Program of the National Institute of Biomedical Innovation (NIBIO ID10-41), the Futaba Electronics Memorial Foundation, the Research Foundation for the Electrotechnology of Chubu, and the Nakajima Foundation. The funders had no role in study design, data collection and analysis, decision to publish, or preparation of the manuscript.

Competing Interests: The authors have declared that no competing interests exist.

* Email: hiro.takahashi@chiba-u.jp

¤a Current address: Japanese Society of Medical Oncology, Tokyo, Japan
¤b Current address: Pharmaceutical and Medical Devices Agency, Tokyo, Japan

Introduction

Genomic information has been proposed to be utilized as the basis for "personalized" health care. Interindividual variation in a drug response among patients has been well documented to cause serious problems in pharmacotherapy. This variation may be due to multiple factors such as disease phenotypes, genetic and clinical parameters (or environmental factors), and variability in the drug target or allergic response; all of these factors may affect both main and side effects [1,2]. Although some biomarkers [3–9] have been proposed, it is still difficult to determine which group of patients will respond positively, which patients are nonresponders, and which may experience adverse reactions in cases where patients are administered the same medication dose. For effectiveness of personalized medicine in cancer chemotherapy, it is critically important to observe interindividual differences in a drug response and the role of genetic polymorphisms relevant to the drug metabolic pathways and drug response biology in pharmacogenomics [10].

Irinotecan (CPT-11), an anticancer prodrug, is widely used for the treatment of a broad range of carcinomas, such as colorectal, lung, ovarian, and cervical cancers. Unexpected severe diarrhea and neutropenia are prominent adverse effects of irinotecan treatment. The active metabolite SN-38 (7-ethyl-10-hydroxycamptothecin), a topoisomerase I inhibitor, is generated via hydrolysis of the parent compound by carboxylesterases [11], and is subsequently glucuronidated by uridine diphosphate glucuronosyltransferases (UGTs), such as UGT1A1, UGT1A7, or UGT1A9, to form an inactive metabolite, SN-38 glucuronide (SN-38G) [12–14]. Irinotecan is also inactivated by CYP3A4 to produce 7-ethyl-10- [4-N-(5-aminopentanoic acid)-1-piperidino] carbonyloxy-camptothecin (APC; a major CYP3A4 product) and 7-ethyl-10-(4-amino-1-piperidino) carbonyloxycamptothecin (NPC; a minor product) [15,16]. Irinotecan and its metabolites are excreted into the bile and urine via the action of ATP-binding cassette (ABC) transporters, such as P-glycoprotein (P-gp/ABCB1), multiple resistance-associated protein 2 (MRP2/ABCC2), and breast cancer resistance protein (BCRP/ABCG2) [17]. Transport of SN-38 from the plasma into the liver is mediated by the organic anion transporting polypeptide C (OATP-C/SLCO1B1) [18]. Most of the previous pharmacogenetic studies of irinotecan have been focused on *UGT1A1* polymorphisms and have shown clinical relevance of *UGT1A1*28*, a repeat polymorphism in the TATA box [-54_-39A(TA)$_6$TAA>A(TA)$_7$TAA or -40_-39ins TA], to severe adverse effects [3,19,20]. Based on these findings, in 2005, the Food and Drug Administration (FDA) of the United States approved an amendment for the formulation called Camptosar (irinotecan-HCl) (NDA 20-571/S-024/S-027/S-028) and for clinical use of a genetic diagnostic kit for the **28* allele. In parallel with this advance in the USA, clinical relevance to severe neutropenia of *UGT1A1*6* [211G>A(G71R)], another low-activity allele detected specifically in East Asians, as well as **28*, was demonstrated in several studies on Asian patients [5,21–23]. Accordingly, in June 2008, the Ministry of Health, Labor, and Welfare of Japan approved changes to irinotecan formulations (Campto and Topotecin) by adding a warning about the risk of severe adverse effects in patients either homozygous or compound-heterozygous for *UGT1A1*28* and **6* (**28/*28*, **6/*6*, **28/*6*) and also approved clinical use of a diagnostic kit for *UGT1A1*28* and **6*. Severe adverse effects, however, are reported in patients without the genetic variations **6/*6*, **28/*28*, and **28/*6*; therefore, several clinical studies have suggested that polymorphisms of the drug transporter genes, such as *ABCB1*, *ABCC2*, *ABCG2*, and *SLCO1B1*, might affect irinotecan pharmacokinetics (PK)/pharmacodynamics (PD) in Caucasian and Asian patients [22,24–35], as shown in Fig. 1. Nonetheless, the almost all reported results deal with PK in patients and neutropenia induced by irinotecan as an adverse reaction not but with diarrhea. Therefore, other factors responsible for other irinotecan adverse effects, such as diarrhea should be identified.

Diarrhea induced by irinotecan is classified into early- and delayed-onset diarrhea, occurring within 24 hr or ≤24 hr after irinotecan administration, respectively [36]. Irinotecan induces early-onset diarrhea as one of adverse cholinergic effects (acetylcholinelike effects) by inhibiting acetylcholinesterase (AChE) and binding to muscarinic acetylcholine receptors (mAChR) [37,38]. These inhibitory actions are induced by irinotecan, which has an amino group at the C-10 position [37]. Other than that, irinotecan induces delayed-onset diarrhea via rapid deconjugation of SN38G and adsorption of released free SN-38 by β-glucuronidase of intestinal flora [39–41], as shown in Fig. 1. In the present study, we focused on polymorphisms of genes with transporter activity to identify predictive factors of diarrhea induced by irinotecan because there are many genes related to transporter activity in both pathways.

A genome-wide association study (GWAS), also known as a whole-genome association study (WGA study, or WGAS), is an examination of many common genetic variants in different individuals to determine whether a particular variant is associated with a trait. GWAS using hypothesis-free genomic data is a powerful technique for identifying interindividual variation among patients. On the other hand, multiple testing problems are a limitation of this approach. To address this issue, we recently proposed a combined method consisting of a knowledge-based algorithm, 2 stages of screening, and a permutation test for identifying single nucleotide polymorphisms (SNPs) [7]. In general, the objective of a statistical or bioinformatic analysis is the enrichment of important information in a large dataset [42–47]. The use of a knowledge-based algorithm is not a novel concept, but is both practical and useful [48–66]. In the previous study, we found that rs2293347 in the gene of human epidermal growth factor receptor (*EGFR*) is a candidate SNP related to the chemotherapeutic response; we achieved this result by applying our combined method to gastric cancer patients who were treated with fluoropyrimidine [7]. However, our combined method was applied to only 1 dataset. Therefore, the usability of our combined method as a novel approach was still unclear.

We used the combined method in an actual genome-wide pharmacogenomics study of antitumor drugs, particularly irinotecan. We found that rs9351963 in the gene of potassium voltage-gated channel subfamily KQT member 5 (*KCNQ5*) is a candidate SNP related to the adverse response. Rs9351963 may be a potential predictive factor of incidence of diarrhea in cancer patients treated with the cancer prodrug irinotecan.

Materials and Methods

Ethics statement

The study was conducted according to the principles expressed in the Declaration of Helsinki, and the ethics committees of the National Cancer Center and National Institute of Health Sciences, Japan, approved the study protocol. All patients provided written informed consent to participate.

Preparation of hypothesis-free genomic data for cancer patients treated with irinotecan

This study was performed within the framework of the Millennium Genome Project in Japan, and 4 antitumor drugs

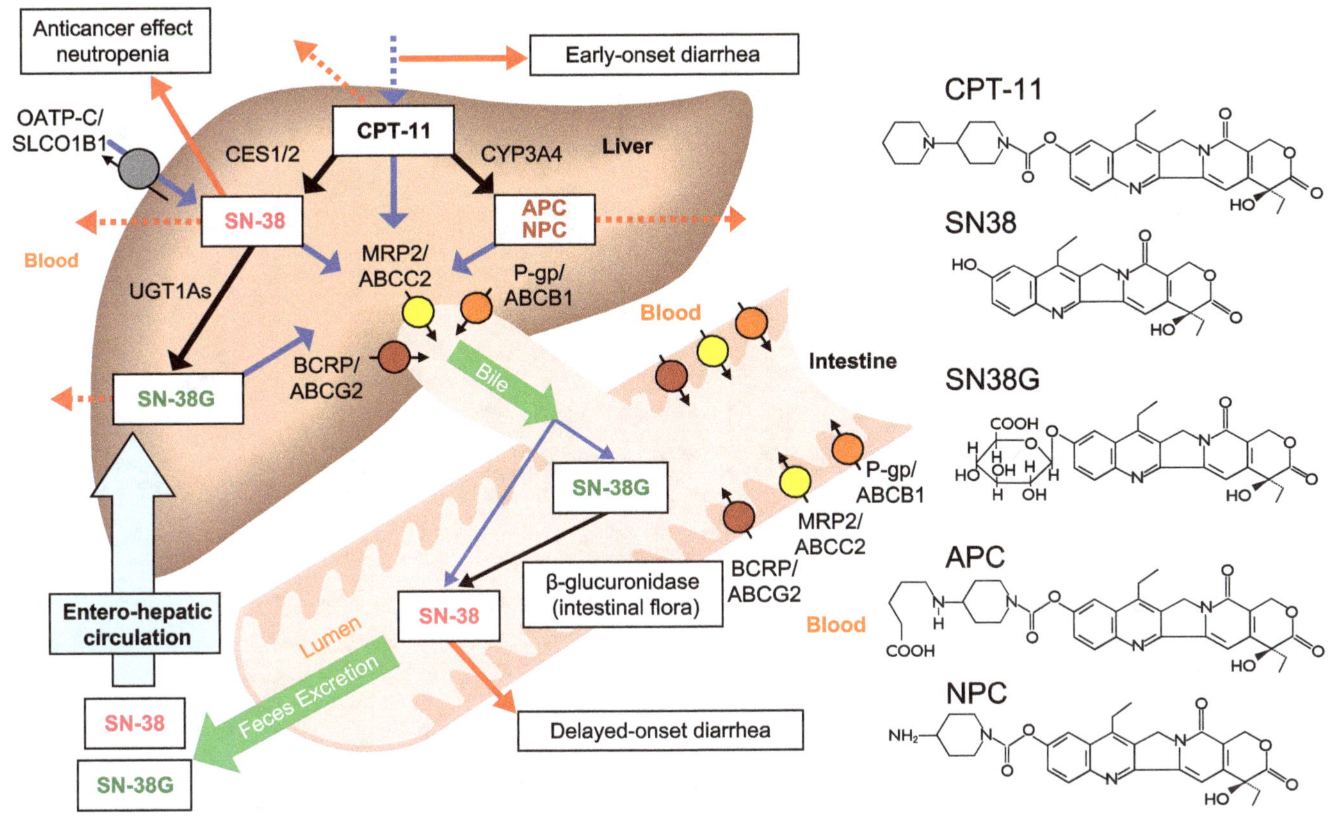

Figure 1. Drug metabolic pathways and the drug response of irinotecan.

were chosen as project targets: gemcitabine, paclitaxel, fluoropyrimidine, and irinotecan. These drugs (alone or in some combination) were administered to approximately 1,000 cancer patients at the National Cancer Center, Japan. Additionally, approximately 1,000 DNA samples were extracted from peripheral blood mononuclear cells and 109,365 SNPs were genotyped using the Illumina Human-1 BeadChip. In this study, we focused on pharmacogenomic properties of irinotecan. Participants included 177 Japanese irinotecan-naïve cancer patients (56 cancer patients treated with irinotecan monotherapy and 121 cancer patients treated with irinotecan combination therapy) at the National Cancer Center Hospital and National Cancer Center Hospital East. A summary of the characteristics of the 176 patients is listed in Table S1. We excluded 1 patient who refused grading of adverse reactions. Furthermore, we excluded 8 patients who did not have genotyping data. Therefore, we analyzed the remaining 168 patients (53 cancer patients treated with irinotecan monotherapy and 115 cancer patients treated with irinotecan combination therapy) in the present study. We defined the 53 patients treated with irinotecan monotherapy as the first dataset and the 168 patients treated with irinotecan chemotherapy (consisting of irinotecan monotherapy and combination therapy) as the second dataset for 2 stages of screening.

Monitoring and adverse effects

A complete medical history and data on physical examination were recorded before the irinotecan therapy. Complete blood cell counts with differentials and platelet counts, as well as blood biochemical variables, were measured once a week during the first 2 months of irinotecan treatment. Adverse events were graded according to the National Cancer Institute - Common Toxicity Criteria (NCI-CTC Version 2.0). Only the highest grade of adverse events was recorded during the first 2 months of irinotecan treatment for each patient and adverse event.

Patient characteristics and clinical parameters

A summary of the patients' characteristics in the two datasets for diarrhea is shown in Table 1. The association of genetic or clinical parameters with incidence of grade ≥2 diarrhea was examined on the basis of Spearman's rank correlation coefficient. "*UGT1A1*6* or **28*" is an effective genetic predictive factor of irinotecan-induced neutropenia and pharmacokinetics in cancer patients [5]. This factor was constructed from 2 polymorphisms: *UGT1A1*6* and **28*.

Fisher's exact test

This statistical test is usually used to determine nonrandom associations between 2 categorical variables [67]. Fisher's exact test is similar to the chi-squared test. If a sample size is large, then the chi-squared test is suitable. Nevertheless, significance values from the chi-squared test are only approximated. Fisher's exact test is used in to analyze contingency tables when the sample sizes are small [67]. We used Fisher's exact test in the present study. The odds ratio (OR) is defined as $a \times d/(b \times c)$, where a is the number of patients that had adverse events with a minor allele, b is the number of patients that did not have adverse events with a minor allele, c is the number of patients that had adverse events with a major allele, and d is the number of patients that did not have adverse events with a major allele. The null hypothesis for Fisher's exact test is OR = 1.

Table 1. Irinotecan-treated cancer patients with SNP information, genetic factor, and clinical parameters for incidence of diarrhea.

Parameters		Diarrhea							
		Irinotecan monotherapy				Irinotecan chemotherapy (including monotherapy)			
		Number of patients		Spearman's rank correlation		Number of patients		Spearman's rank correlation	
		Grade <2	Grade ≥2	ρ	*p* value	Grade <2	Grade ≥2	ρ	*p* value
*UGT1A1**6 or *28	0	15	5	0.056	6.89E−01	64	17	0.009	9.06E−01
	1	21	7			57	16		
	2	3	2			11	3		
Gender	Male	26	11	−0.114	4.15E−01	101	28	−0.012	8.75E−01
	Female	13	3			31	8		
Age		39	14	0.013	9.29E−01	132	36	0.080	3.02E−01
Area		39	14	0.010	9.45E−01	132	36	−0.054	4.88E−01
PS	<2	38	13	0.106	4.50E−01	130	35	0.039	6.15E−01
	≥2	1	1			2	1		
Smoking	0	37	14	−0.119	3.97E−01	111	30	0.008	9.13E−01
	1	2	0			21	6		
Alcohol	0	33	10	0.149	2.88E−01	90	26	−0.036	6.44E−01
	1	6	4			42	10		
Alb	0	18	10	−0.223	1.08E−01	71	24	−0.108	1.62E−01
	1	21	4			60	12		
	2	0	0			1	0		
Hg	0	14	4	0.061	6.65E−01	58	14	0.040	6.05E−01
	1	22	9			67	20		
	2	3	0			6	1		
	3	0	1			0	1		
	4	0	0			1	0		
GOT	0	33	12	−0.014	9.23E−01	108	32	−0.080	3.05E−01
	1	6	2			22	4		
	2	0	0			2	0		
ALP	0	28	8	0.117	4.05E−01	89	23	0.026	7.38E−01
	1	9	6			38	12		
	2	0	0			2	1		
	3	2	0			3	0		
Cr	0	31	13	−0.157	2.62E−01	124	35	−0.060	4.41E−01
	1	8	1			8	1		
C_{max}/dose		39	14	0.049	7.31E−01	132	36	0.019	8.10E−01
AUC ratio		39	14	−0.078	5.81E−01	132	36	−0.109	1.60E−01

Table 1. Cont.

Parameters		Diarrhea								
		Irinotecan monotherapy				Irinotecan chemotherapy (including monotherapy)				
		Number of patients		Spearman's rank correlation		Number of patients		Spearman's rank correlation		
		Grade <2	Grade ≥2	ρ	p value	Grade <2	Grade ≥2	ρ		p value
Concomitant drug - 5-FU	0	39	14	NA	NA	106	28	0.026		7.40E-01
	1	0	0			26	8			
Concomitant drug - CDDP	0	39	14	NA	NA	76	24	−0.076		3.28E-01
	1	0	0			56	12			
Concomitant drug - MMC	0	39	14	NA	NA	121	36	−0.138	†	7.40E-02
	1	0	0			11	0			
Concomitant drug - VP16	0	39	14	NA	NA	129	35	0.014		8.61E-01
	1	0	0			3	1			
Concomitant drug - Amrubicin	0	39	14	NA	NA	132	34	0.210	*	6.25E-03
	1	0	0			0	2			

"*UGT1A1*6* or **28*" is a genetic factor constructed from 2 polymorphisms (UGT1A1*6* and **28*); "2" indicates **6/*6*, **28/*28* or **6/*28*, "1" indicates **6* or **28*, and "0" indicates "other than 2 and 1." Area: body surface area (m^2), PS: performance status, Cr: grade of creatinine, Hg: grade of hemoglobin, Alb: grade of albumin, ALP: grade of alkaline phosphatase, and GOT: grade of glutamic oxaloacetic transaminase. Each laboratory test value (Alb, Hg, GOT, ALP, and Cr) was recorded before the irinotecan therapy. For each type of clinical tests the grade and aberrant values were defined according to the National Cancer Institute - Common Toxicity Criteria (NCI-CTC, Version 2.0). C_{max}/dose: SN38 C_{max}/dose [$10^{-3} \times m^2/L$]. AUC: area under the concentration-time curve. AUC ratio: Ratio of AUC_{SN38}/AUC_{CPT-11}. 5-FU: 5-fluorouracil, CDDP: cisplatin, MMC: mitomycin C, VP16: etoposide. * and † indicate $p<0.05$ and $0.05 \leq p < 0.10$, respectively. For each concomitant drug, 0 means "not administered," 1 indicates administered.

The permutation test

The permutation test theory evolved from the works of Fisher and Pitman in the 1930s [68]. In this study, p values of multiple-comparison analyses were adjusted by applying the permutation test to 2 stages of screening. The case–control (or phenotype) labels were randomly shuffled for the 2 screening stages, and p values were calculated using Fisher's exact test. The lowest p value was selected for the randomized data. This procedure was repeated 100,000 times. Exact p values for the permutation test were calculated based on the distribution of the lowest p values.

Multiple testing correction

The Bonferroni correction is a method used to address the problem of multiple comparisons (also known as the multiple testing problem). It is considered the simplest and most conservative method for control of the family-wise error rate (FWER). In addition, false discovery rate (FDR) controlling procedures, such as the Benjamini-Hochberg (BH) method [69], are more powerful (i.e., less conservative) than the FWER procedures, such as the Bonferroni correction, at the cost of increasing the likelihood of false positives within the rejected hypothesis. In the present study, the BH method was used to calculate the q value. The q value is defined as an FDR analog of the p value.

The Akaike information criterion (AIC)

The AIC is a measure of the relative goodness of fit of a statistical model [70]. A smaller AIC indicates a better fit when comparing fitted objects. The AIC is defined according to the formula -2 × (log likelihood) + $(2 \times n_{par})$, where n_{par} represents the number of parameters in the fitted model, and the log-likelihood value [71] is obtained from the logistic regression model.

The receiver operating characteristic (ROC)

ROC analysis is a graphical plot that illustrates the performance of a binary classifier system as its discrimination threshold is varied. It is built by plotting sensitivity (the number of true positive results divided by the number of true positive samples) against (1 minus specificity) at various threshold settings. (Specificity is the number of true negative results divided by the number of true negative samples.) The area under the curve (AUC) of a ROC curve is an indicator of expected performance of the test. A higher AUC is more desirable, with a value of 1.00 denoting perfect performance (sensitivity and specificity are both 100%), while a value of 0.50 indicates random performance.

Gene set based on gene ontology GO terms

GO has been developed to provide scientists with a controlled terminology system for labeling gene functions in a precise, reliable, computer-readable manner. Data for annotated genes and associated GO terms were obtained from the GO website (http://www.geneontology.org). We compiled a GO term list to select polymorphisms in genes with transporter activity (GO:0005215) and related activities, as shown in Table S2. The numbers of GO terms obtained was 943. GO data were obtained on July 1, 2010.

Results

Association analysis of adverse affects and clinical parameters (or a genetic factor)

The association between clinical parameters (or a genetic factor) and incidence of grade ≥2 diarrhea was examined on the basis of Spearman's rank correlation coefficient, as shown in Table 1. This table shows that no parameter was associated with the adverse response to chemotherapy (incidence of grade ≥2 diarrhea) in the first dataset (patients treated with irinotecan monotherapy). Nonetheless, Amrubicin ($p = 0.00625$) was significantly associated with the response in the second dataset (patients treated with any irinotecan chemotherapy: a combination or monotherapy). Mitomycin C (MMC; $p = 0.0740$) was weakly associated with the response. These clinical factors should be evaluated when constructing diagnostic models involving multiple factors.

Extraction of candidate SNPs using the combined method consisting of the knowledge-based algorithm, 2 stages of screening, and the permutation test

In this study, we applied the combined method to hypothesis-free genomic data on cancer patients treated with irinotecan chemotherapy as shown in Fig. 2. Figure 2A shows an outline of the knowledge-based algorithm for identifying SNPs (KB-SNP). In the previous study, we extracted rs numbers (SNP IDs) related to cancer using a combination of National Center for Biotechnology Information (NCBI) dbSNP and NCBI PubMed [7]. In the present study, we extracted rs numbers from genes linked to specific GO terms instead of the combination of NCBI dbSNP and PubMed. In this analysis, we defined specific GO terms as the terms related to transporter activity.

A total of 6,506 SNPs related to transporter activity were extracted from 109,365 SNPs using KB-SNP (Fig. 2B). Furthermore, we excluded SNPs with a p value <0.2 in the Hardy-Weinberg equilibrium (HWE) or the minor allele frequency (MAF) <0.05. Then the extracted 5,242 SNPs were used in the association study.

We analyzed 53 patients treated with irinotecan monotherapy as the first dataset for first-stage screening in the association study (Fig. 2C). Each p value was calculated using Fisher's exact test for the allele model. A total of 24 SNPs with $p<0.005$ were extracted. In the second stage of screening, 168 patients treated with irinotecan chemotherapy (including 53 patients treated with irinotecan monotherapy) were analyzed to validate these 24 SNPs. Adjustment of a calculated p value for the second stage of screening was conducted using the permutation test for these 2 stages of screening (Fig. 2D). Only rs9351963 in *KCNQ5* showed a statistically significant p value (0.0289), which was determined using the permutation test. The rs9351963 is a common variant (MAF = 0.328). Furthermore, we conducted Fisher's exact test and used the Benjamini-Hochberg method [69] to calculate p and q values for the second dataset only. Seven SNPs had a q value <1, as shown in Table 2. Six SNPs (rs11022922, rs3918305, rs3813627, rs768172, rs3813628, and rs10815019) had $q = 0.802$ as shown in Table 2. This result indicates that 5 out of 6 SNPs were false positive; however, we assessed performance of only rs9351963 in the process of model construction.

Comparison of models based on rs9351963 in *KCNQ5*

We analyzed not only an allele model but also dominant and recessive models of rs9351963 in *KCNQ5* in relation to the first dataset (irinotecan monotherapy), the second dataset (any irinotecan chemotherapy), and the dataset of irinotecan combination chemotherapy (excluding irinotecan monotherapy), as shown in Figure 3. Figure 3A shows that the p value of the allele model was the lowest ($p = 8.86 \times 10^{-5}$, OR = 6.3), and the p value ($p = 1.29 \times 10^{-4}$, OR = 24) of the dominant model was lower than the p value ($p = 0.0358$, OR = 7.0) of the recessive model in the first dataset. In addition, Figure 3B shows that the p value of the

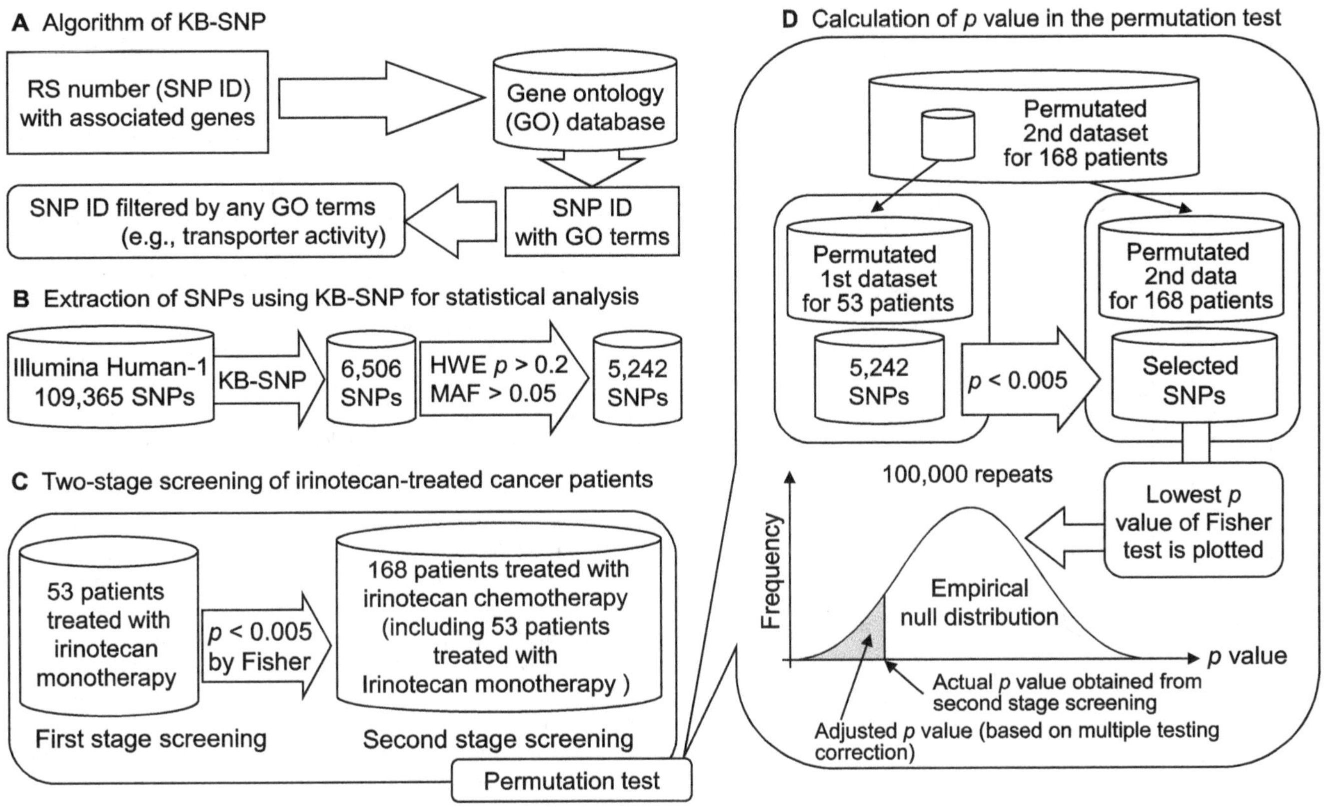

Figure 2. An outline of chemotherapeutic response analysis in irinotecan-treated cancer patients using a combined method consisting of a knowledge-based algorithm for identifying SNPs (KB-SNP), 2 stages of screening, and the permutation test. (A) The KB-SNP algorithm. (B) Extraction of SNPs using KB-SNP for statistical analysis. (C) Two-stage screening of irinotecan-treated cancer patients. (D) Calculation of the *p* value in the permutation test based on the 2 stages of screening. The second dataset (includes first dataset) was permutated. The permutated first dataset was extracted from the permutated second dataset. By using Fisher's exact test, SNPs with $p<0.005$ for the first dataset were selected from among 5,242 SNPs. Among the selected SNPs, those with the lowest *p* value in Fisher's exact test for the second dataset were selected. This procedure was repeated 100,000 times and empirical null distribution was constructed. Using the distribution, the actual *p* value obtained from the second stage of screening was converted to the adjusted *p* value (based on correction of multiple testing problems). At these screening steps, allele models were used for each SNP.

allele model was the lowest ($p = 3.31\times10^{-5}$, OR = 3.1), and the p value ($p = 1.28\times10^{-4}$, OR = 6.7) of the recessive model was lower than the p value ($p = 4.44\times10^{-3}$, OR = 3.3) of the dominant model in the second dataset. Therefore, we evaluated the 3 models using the dataset of irinotecan combination chemotherapy (excluding irinotecan monotherapy; Fig. 3C). Figure 3C shows that the p value ($p = 1.44\times10^{-3}$, OR = 6.9) of the recessive model meant strong statistical significance and the OR was almost equal to OR (= 7.0) in the first dataset, as shown in Figure 3A. Although ORs of the recessive models seemed to have high homogeneity among all 3 datasets, there was no statistical evidence. Therefore, the proportional odds model was used to construct multiple logistic regression models.

Selection of the model of rs9351963 in *KCNQ5* and construction of multiple regression models

We compared the AICs and AUCs using the second dataset in the 8 models: NULL (without parameter), "*UGT1A1*6* or **28*" (an integrated predictive factor based on polymorphisms related to neutropenia), and rs9351963 (genotype of rs9351963 in *KCNQ5*), Amrubicin, MMC, rs9351963+Amrubicin, rs9351963+MMC, and rs9351963+Amrubicin+MMC (Fig. 4A). Figure 4A shows that performance of all models except *UGT1A1 *6* or **28* is better than the performance of the NULL model. Although the Amrubicin+MMC (combination of Amrubicin and MMC) model was better than Amrubicin alone or MMC, the rs9351963 models were clearly better than the Amrubicin+MMC model, as shown in Figures 4A and 4B. Performance of rs9351963+Amrubicin and rs9351963+MMC models was better than performance of the rs9351963 model. Furthermore, performance of the rs9351963+ Amrubicin+MMC model was better than that of rs9351963+ Amrubicin and rs9351963+MMC models. Therefore, we selected the rs9351963+Amrubicin+MMC model as the best one on the basis of AIC. AUC, sensitivity, and specificity of this model were 0.744, 77.8%, and 57.6% in in the ROC curve, respectively, as shown in Figures 4A and 4B.

Discussion

In the present study, we used 2 stages of screening: the method that is based on the concept of joint analysis. Joint analysis is more efficient than replication-based analysis [72]. The first dataset is a part of the second dataset in joint analysis (the latter includes the former). In contrast, the 2 datasets must be independent in a replication-based analysis (which we did not use here). Our 2 stages of screening derived from the joint analysis were used to increase statistical detection power. KB-SNP was performed prior to 2 stages of screening. KB-SNP reduced the number of

Table 2. Extracted 7 SNPs with $q<1$ for the second dataset.

RS number	Allele	MAF	SNP function		Chr	Position[a]	Associated gene symbol	For second dataset		Two stages of screening	
			Type	Location				p_F	q_{BH}		p_{per}
rs9351963	A/C	0.328	cSNP	intron	6	73749861	*KCNQ5*	3.31E-05	0.173	*	0.0289
rs11022922	C/T	0.376	cSNP	intron	14	63472498	*KCNH5*	3.21E-04	0.802		1.0000
rs3918305	A/G	0.402	cSNP	intron	12	109331162	*SVOP*	6.21E-04	0.802		1.0000
rs3813627	G/T	0.435	cSNP	NearGene-5	1	161195148	*TOMM40L*	7.62E-04	0.802		1.0000
rs768172	A/T	0.441	cSNP	intron	7	95805703	*SLC25A13*	7.87E-04	0.802		1.0000
rs3813628	A/C	0.436	cSNP	5'UTR	1	161196166	*TOMM40L*	1.02E-03	0.802		1.0000
rs10815019	A/G	0.222	cSNP	intron	9	4547288	*SLC1A1*	1.20E-03	0.802		1.0000

RS number: reference SNP identification number in dbSNP, MAF: minor allele frequency, Chr: chromosome number, i.e., a position in human genome GRCh37.p10 build 104, p_F indicates a p value calculated using Fisher's exact test, q_{BH} indicates adjusted p_F value by the Benjamini-Hochberg method, p_{per} indicates p values adjusted using a permutation test for multiple testing problems, * indicates $p_{per}<0.05$. NearGene-5 indicates that the SNP is within 2 kb upstream of a gene.

candidate SNPs to 6,506 from 109,365. Approximately 80,000 SNPs can be extracted without knowledge-based reduction of the SNP number. Thus, statistically significant SNPs cannot be extracted from the present data. We could find the statistically significant rs9351963 in *KCNQ5* by applying the combined method to hypothesis-free genomic data.

The KCNQ/K(v)7 potassium channel family consists of 5 members of neural muscarine channel (M channel; from KCNQ1 to KCNQ5) which have a distinct expression pattern and a functional role. Although KCNQ1 is prevalently expressed in the cardiac muscle, KCNQ2, KCNQ3, KCNQ4, and KCNQ5 are expressed in neural tissue [73–75]. On the other hand, a recent study revealed that KCNQ4 and KCNQ5 are the most abundantly expressed KCNQ channels in smooth muscle throughout the gastrointestinal tract [76]. Furthermore, Jepps et al. opined that drugs that selectively block KCNQ4/KCNQ5 might be promising as therapeutics for the treatment of motility disorders such as constipation associated with irritable bowel syndrome [76]. In other words, drugs that selectively open KCNQ4/KCNQ5 might be effective against diarrhea. The KCNQ family gene products assemble as homomeric or heteromeric tetramers to form functional channels that mediate the M-current [77], a current that is suppressed by mAChR activation [78,79]. Irinotecan induces adverse cholinergic effects (acetylcholinelike actions) by inhibiting AChE and binding to mAChR [37,38,80]. Therefore, polymorphisms of *KCNQ5* genes possibly effect incidence of diarrhea as interindividual variation in the drug response among cancer patients treated with irinotecan chemotherapy.

In the present study, only the highest grade of adverse events is recorded during the first 2 months of irinotecan treatment for each patient and each adverse effect. Therefore, incidence of grade ≥2 diarrhea possibly includes cases caused partially by enterohepatic circulation of APC and NPC, but genotype of rs9351963 in *KCNQ5* correlates with the start date of treatment with antidiarrheal agents (Spearman's rank correlation coefficient $\rho=-0.198$, $p=0.00995$). In other words, genotype of rs9351963 may correlates with the diagnosis (or presentiment) of irinotecan induced early-onset diarrhea (diagnosis is made by trained chemotherapists).

The rs9351963 A>C polymorphism is located in an intron, which does not change the amino acid sequence of the protein and may not influence the biological function of the protein itself. Nonetheless, some intronic polymorphisms are effective markers: For example, rs2237892 in intron 15 of *KCNQ1* is associated with susceptibility to type 2 diabetes mellitus in Japanese individuals [81], and the CA simple sequence repeat in intron 1 (CA-SSR1) of the gene of epidermal growth factor receptor (*EGFR*) is associated with the clinical outcome in gefitinib-treated Japanese patients with non-small cell lung cancer [82]. Furthermore, variations related to intronic or synonymous SNPs possibly affect mRNA stability, translational kinetics, and splicing, resulting in alterations at the protein level, e.g., changes of structure or function [83–89]. Although rs9351963 does not have a known function, this SNP is a possible predictive factor of adverse effects of irinotecan-based chemotherapy and is possibly linked to some functional polymorphisms in *KCNQ5*. Their clinical importance needs to be further elucidated.

In the present study, we extracted rs9351963, which showed a p value (0.0289) obtained using a combination of 2 stages of screening and a permutation test from SNPs selected by KB-SNP. In the second dataset, the p value of Fisher's exact test was 3.31×10^{-5}, and the q value was 0.173 calculated by correction of Benjamini-Hochberg method, as shown in Table 2. This value is

A Irinotecan monotherapy

Allele model

rs9351963	Diarrhea Grade < 2	Diarrhea Grade ≥ 2
A	63	11
C	15	17

OR (95%CI): 6.3 (2.3-19)
$p = 8.86 \times 10^{-5}$

Dominant model

rs9351963	Diarrhea Grade < 2	Diarrhea Grade ≥ 2
AA	26	1
AC+CC	13	13

OR (95%CI): 24 (3.1-1139)
$p = 1.29 \times 10^{-4}$

Recessive model

rs9351963	Diarrhea Grade < 2	Diarrhea Grade ≥ 2
AA+AC	37	10
CC	2	4

OR (95%CI): 7.0 (0.87-89)
$p = 0.0358$

B Any irinotecan chemotherapy (including irinotecan monotherapy)

Allele model

rs9351963	Diarrhea Grade < 2	Diarrhea Grade ≥ 2
A	192	33
C	72	39

OR (95%CI): 3.1 (1.8-5.6)
$p = 3.31 \times 10^{-5}$

Dominant model

rs9351963	Diarrhea Grade < 2	Diarrhea Grade ≥ 2
AA	69	9
AC+CC	63	27

OR (95%CI): 3.3 (1.4-8.5)
$p = 4.44 \times 10^{-3}$

Recessive model

rs9351963	Diarrhea Grade < 2	Diarrhea Grade ≥ 2
AA+AC	123	24
CC	9	12

OR (95%CI): 6.7 (2.3-20)
$p = 1.28 \times 10^{-4}$

C Irinotecan combination chemotherapy (excluding irinotecan monotherapy)

Allele model

rs9351963	Diarrhea Grade < 2	Diarrhea Grade ≥ 2
A	129	22
C	57	22

OR (95%CI): 2.3 (1.1-4.7)
$p = 0.0211$

Dominant model

rs9351963	Diarrhea Grade < 2	Diarrhea Grade ≥ 2
AA	43	8
AC+CC	50	14

OR (95%CI): 1.5 (0.53-4.5)
$p = 0.478$

Recessive model

rs9351963	Diarrhea Grade < 2	Diarrhea Grade ≥ 2
AA+AC	86	14
CC	7	8

OR (95%CI): 6.9 (1.9-26)
$p = 1.44 \times 10^{-3}$

Figure 3. Contingency tables for rs9351963 in *KCNQ5* for each model using each dataset. (A) irinotecan monotherapy (first dataset), (B) any irinotecan chemotherapy (including irinotecan monotherapy; second dataset), and (C) irinotecan combination chemotherapy (excluding irinotecan monotherapy). OR: odds ratio. The *p* values were calculated using Fisher's exact test. CI: confidence interval.

statistically insignificant. Therefore, during the 2 stages of screening, it is statistically sufficient to extract rs9351963.

The calculation of probability of occurrence in Bernoulli trials is suitable to for estimation of validity of the repetition number in the permutation process. In this trial, occurrence probability is defined as ${}_{n}C_{k} \times (p_B)^{k} \times (1 - p_B)^{(n-k)}$, where k is the occurrence number, n is the repetition number, and p_B represents probability. If the repetition number is 100,000 for rs9351963 ($p = 0.02891$ [2891/100000]) and the significance level of the test (α) is 0.05, the occurrence probability is ${}_{100000}C_{2891} \times (0.05)^{2891} \times (1-0.05)^{(100000-2891)} = 4.89 \times 10^{-241}$. In statistics, the 99% (or 95%) confidence interval should be considered. The significance level of $\alpha = 0.05$ does not exist in the 99% confidence interval of the p value for rs9351963, because the occurrence probability 4.89×10^{-241} is clearly lower than 0.01. Similarly, if the repetition number is 10,000, the occurrence probability is 3.41×10^{-26}. This way, the occurrence probability is sufficiently low for 10,000 permutations. Nevertheless, we conducted 100,000 permutations to estimate p values more accurately for the permutation test.

Using our combined method involving KB-SNP, we identified rs9351963 as a potential predictive factor of diarrhea in cancer patients treated with irinotecan chemotherapy; however, the comprehensiveness of KB-SNP was limited. Therefore, statistical information regarding the adverse effects of cancer patients treated with irinotecan chemotherapy is shown in Table S3 for incidence of diarrhea ($p<0.05$) and in Table S4 for incidence of neutropenia ($p<0.05$). The relevant data are also provided on the website Genome Medicine Database of Japan (GeMDBJ) [90] (https://gemdbj.nibio.go.jp/). These data will be useful for replication studies or meta-analyses in the future.

In conclusion, in the present study, we applied the combined method to hypothesis-free genomic data on cancer patients treated with irinotecan chemotherapy. By means of this method, rs9351963 in *KCNQ5* was extracted as a candidate SNP related to the incidence of diarrhea. For example, the association of rs9351963 with irinotecan-related diarrhea (OR of 3.14) showed a p value of 3.31×10^{-5} in Fisher's exact test (allele model). Even if this p value were adjusted by means of the permutation test for the effects of multiple testing problems, the adjusted p value would still indicate statistical significance (adjusted p value of $0.0289<0.05$). Additionally, we evaluated the performance of rs9351963 using multiple regression models. rs9351963 was clearly superior to clinical parameters (or environmental factors) and showed a sensitivity of 77.8% and specificity of 57.6% in the multiple regression model, including rs9351963. Recent studies showed that the *KCNQ4* and *KCNQ5* genes encode components of the M channel expressed in gastrointestinal smooth muscles and suggested that these genes are associated with irritable bowel syndrome and similar peristalsis diseases. These results suggest that rs9351963 may be a predictive factor of diarrhea in cancer patients treated with irinotecan chemotherapy. This SNP may also be useful for selection of chemotherapy regimens, such as irinotecan monotherapy or a combination of irinotecan chemo-

A

Parameter	AIC	AUC	Sens.	Spec.
NULL	177	0.500	50.0	50.0
*UGT1A1*6* or **28*	179	0.506	52.8	48.5
rs9351963	162	0.690	75.0	52.3
MMC	173	0.542	100.0	8.3
Amrubicin	172	0.528	5.6	100.0
MMC+Amrubicin	169	0.567	100.0	8.3
rs9351963 + Amrubicin	156	0.718	38.9	93.2
rs9351963 + MMC	159	0.718	75.0	57.6
rs9351963 + Amrubicin + MMC	153	0.744	77.8	57.6

B

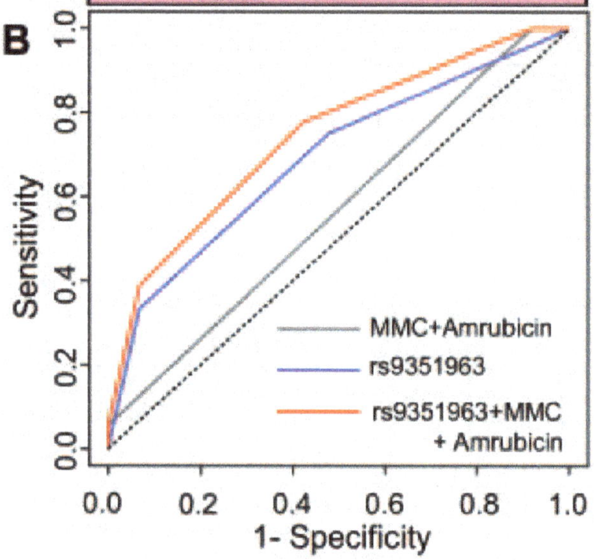

Figure 4. Comparison of AIC, AUC, and ROC curves for logistic regression models. (A) Parameters of each model. (B) The ROC curve of a model consisting of rs9351963+MMC+ Amrubicin. ROC: receiver operating characteristic, AUC: area under the ROC curve, NULL indicates the model without parameters. Each genetic factor conforms to the proportional odds model, AIC: Akaike's information criterion, AUC: area under the ROC curve, Sens.: Sensitivity (%), Spec.: Specificity (%).

therapy with KCNQ5 opener. Furthermore, the result of the present analysis supports usability of our combined method.

Supporting Information

Table S1 Irinotecan-treated cancer patients, genetic factor, and clinical parameters for incidence of diarrhea and neutropenia. "*UGT1A1*6* or **28*" is a genetic factor constructed from 2 polymorphisms (*UGT1A1*6* and **28*); "2" indicates **6/*6*, **28/*28* or **6/*28*, "1" indicates **6* or **28*, and "0" indicates "other than 2 and 1." Area: body surface area (m^2), PS: performance status, Cr: grade of creatinine, Hg: grade of hemoglobin, Alb: grade of albumin, ALP: grade of alkaline phosphatase, and GOT: grade of glutamic oxaloacetic transaminase. Each laboratory test value (Alb, Hg, GOT, ALP, and Cr) was recorded before the irinotecan therapy. For each type of clinical tests the grade and aberrant values were defined according to the National Cancer Institute - Common Toxicity Criteria (NCI-CTC, Version 2.0). C_{max}/dose: SN38 C_{max}/dose [10^{-3}×m^2/L]. AUC: area under the concentration-time curve. AUC ratio: Ratio of AUC_{SN38}/AUC_{CPT-11}. 5-FU: 5-fluorouracil, CDDP: cisplatin, MMC: mitomycin C, VP16: etoposide. * and † indicate $p<0.05$ and $0.05 \leq p<0.10$, respectively. For each concomitant drug, 0 means "not administered," 1 indicates administered.

Table S2 GO term list for transporter activity and the related functions.

Table S3 Statistical information on the chemotherapeutic response (incidence of grade ≥2 diarrhea) of irinotecan-treated cancer patients (*p*<0.05). RS number: reference SNP identification number in dbSNP; *p* values were calculated using Fisher's exact test and *q* values were calculated using the Benjamini-Hochberg (BH) method from *p* values.

Table S4 Statistical information on the chemotherapeutic response (incidence of grade ≥3 neutropenia) of irinotecan-treated cancer patients (*p*<0.05). RS number: reference SNP identification number in dbSNP; *p* values were calculated using Fisher's exact test and *q* values were calculated using the Benjamini-Hochberg (BH) method from *p* values.

Acknowledgments

We thank Ms. Sumiko Ohnami for help with SNP genotyping.

Author Contributions

Conceived and designed the experiments: HT Y. Saito NS JS HS T. Yoshida. Performed the experiments: HT KS NK HO YO MO. Analyzed the data: HT RI AT AD. Contributed reagents/materials/analysis tools: HT YM TH Y. Shimada AO T. Yoshino TD. Contributed to the writing of the manuscript: HT.

References

1. Evans WE, McLeod HL (2003) Pharmacogenomics–drug disposition, drug targets, and side effects. N Engl J Med 348: 538–549.
2. Ingelman-Sundberg M (2008) Pharmacogenomic biomarkers for prediction of severe adverse drug reactions. N Engl J Med 358: 637–639.
3. Ando Y, Saka H, Ando M, Sawa T, Muro K, et al. (2000) Polymorphisms of UDP-glucuronosyltransferase gene and irinotecan toxicity: a pharmacogenetic analysis. Cancer Res 60: 6921–6926.
4. Ma F, Sun T, Shi Y, Yu D, Tan W, et al. (2009) Polymorphisms of *EGFR* predict clinical outcome in advanced non-small-cell lung cancer patients treated with Gefitinib. Lung Cancer 66: 114–119.
5. Minami H, Sai K, Saeki M, Saito Y, Ozawa S, et al. (2007) Irinotecan pharmacokinetics/pharmacodynamics and *UGT1A* genetic polymorphisms in Japanese: roles of *UGT1A1*6* and **28*. Pharmacogenet Genomics 17: 497–504.
6. Sato Y, Laird NM, Nagashima K, Kato R, Hamano T, et al. (2009) A new statistical screening approach for finding pharmacokinetics-related genes in genome-wide studies. Pharmacogenomics J 9: 137–146.
7. Takahashi H, Kaniwa N, Saito Y, Sai K, Hamaguchi T, et al. (2013) Identification of a candidate single-nucleotide polymorphism related to chemotherapeutic response through a combination of knowledge-based algorithm and hypothesis-free genomic data. J Biosci Bioeng 116: 768–773.
8. van Kuilenburg AB, Muller EW, Haasjes J, Meinsma R, Zoetekouw L, et al. (2001) Lethal outcome of a patient with a complete dihydropyrimidine dehydrogenase (DPD) deficiency after administration of 5-fluorouracil: frequency of the common IVS14+1G>A mutation causing DPD deficiency. Clin Cancer Res 7: 1149–1153.
9. Raida M, Schwabe W, Hausler P, Van Kuilenburg AB, Van Gennip AH, et al. (2001) Prevalence of a common point mutation in the dihydropyrimidine dehydrogenase (DPD) gene within the 5′-splice donor site of intron 14 in patients with severe 5-fluorouracil (5-FU)- related toxicity compared with controls. Clin Cancer Res 7: 2832–2839.
10. Efferth T, Volm M (2005) Pharmacogenetics for individualized cancer chemotherapy. Pharmacol Ther 107: 155–176.
11. Slatter JG, Su P, Sams JP, Schaaf LJ, Wienkers LC (1997) Bioactivation of the anticancer agent CPT-11 to SN-38 by human hepatic microsomal carboxylesterases and the in vitro assessment of potential drug interactions. Drug Metab Dispos 25: 1157–1164.

12. Iyer L, King CD, Whitington PF, Green MD, Roy SK, et al. (1998) Genetic predisposition to the metabolism of irinotecan (CPT-11). Role of uridine diphosphate glucuronosyltransferase isoform 1A1 in the glucuronidation of its active metabolite (SN-38) in human liver microsomes. J Clin Invest 101: 847–854.
13. Ciotti M, Basu N, Brangi M, Owens IS (1999) Glucuronidation of 7-ethyl-10-hydroxycamptothecin (SN-38) by the human UDP-glucuronosyltransferases encoded at the *UGT1* locus. Biochem Biophys Res Commun 260: 199–202.
14. Gagne JF, Montminy V, Belanger P, Journault K, Gaucher G, et al. (2002) Common human *UGT1A* polymorphisms and the altered metabolism of irinotecan active metabolite 7-ethyl-10-hydroxycamptothecin (SN-38). Mol Pharmacol 62: 608–617.
15. Haaz MC, Rivory L, Riche C, Vernillet L, Robert J (1998) Metabolism of irinotecan (CPT-11) by human hepatic microsomes: participation of cytochrome P-450 3A and drug interactions. Cancer Res 58: 468–472.
16. Sai K, Saito Y, Fukushima-Uesaka H, Kurose K, Kaniwa N, et al. (2008) Impact of *CYP3A4* haplotypes on irinotecan pharmacokinetics in Japanese cancer patients. Cancer Chemother Pharmacol 62: 529–537.
17. Sparreboom A, Danesi R, Ando Y, Chan J, Figg WD (2003) Pharmacogenomics of ABC transporters and its role in cancer chemotherapy. Drug Resist Updat 6: 71–84.
18. Nozawa T, Minami H, Sugiura S, Tsuji A, Tamai I (2005) Role of organic anion transporter OATP1B1 (OATP-C) in hepatic uptake of irinotecan and its active metabolite, 7-ethyl-10-hydroxycamptothecin: in vitro evidence and effect of single nucleotide polymorphisms. Drug Metab Dispos 33: 434–439.
19. Iyer L, Das S, Janisch L, Wen M, Ramirez J, et al. (2002) UGT1A1*28 polymorphism as a determinant of irinotecan disposition and toxicity. Pharmacogenomics J 2: 43–47.
20. Innocenti F, Undevia SD, Iyer L, Chen PX, Das S, et al. (2004) Genetic variants in the *UDP-glucuronosyltransferase 1A1* gene predict the risk of severe neutropenia of irinotecan. J Clin Oncol 22: 1382–1388.
21. Han JY, Lim HS, Shin ES, Yoo YK, Park YH, et al. (2006) Comprehensive analysis of *UGT1A* polymorphisms predictive for pharmacokinetics and treatment outcome in patients with non-small-cell lung cancer treated with irinotecan and cisplatin. J Clin Oncol 24: 2237–2244.
22. Jada SR, Lim R, Wong CI, Shu X, Lee SC, et al. (2007) Role of *UGT1A1*6*, *UGT1A1*28* and *ABCG2* c.421C>A polymorphisms in irinotecan-induced neutropenia in Asian cancer patients. Cancer Sci 98: 1461–1467.
23. Sai K, Saito Y, Sakamoto H, Shirao K, Kurose K, et al. (2008) Importance of *UDP-glucuronosyltransferase 1A1*6* for irinotecan toxicities in Japanese cancer patients. Cancer Lett 261: 165–171.
24. Sai K, Saito Y, Maekawa K, Kim SR, Kaniwa N, et al. (2010) Additive effects of drug transporter genetic polymorphisms on irinotecan pharmacokinetics/pharmacodynamics in Japanese cancer patients. Cancer Chemother Pharmacol 66: 95–105.
25. Mathijssen RH, Marsh S, Karlsson MO, Xie R, Baker SD, et al. (2003) Irinotecan pathway genotype analysis to predict pharmacokinetics. Clin Cancer Res 9: 3246–3253.
26. Sai K, Kaniwa N, Itoda M, Saito Y, Hasegawa R, et al. (2003) Haplotype analysis of ABCB1/MDR1 blocks in a Japanese population reveals genotype-dependent renal clearance of irinotecan. Pharmacogenetics 13: 741–757.
27. Zhou Q, Sparreboom A, Tan EH, Cheung YB, Lee A, et al. (2005) Pharmacogenetic profiling across the irinotecan pathway in Asian patients with cancer. Br J Clin Pharmacol 59: 415–424.
28. de Jong FA, Marsh S, Mathijssen RH, King C, Verweij J, et al. (2004) ABCG2 pharmacogenetics: ethnic differences in allele frequency and assessment of influence on irinotecan disposition. Clin Cancer Res 10: 5889–5894.
29. de Jong FA, Scott-Horton TJ, Kroetz DL, McLeod HL, Friberg LE, et al. (2007) Irinotecan-induced diarrhea: functional significance of the polymorphic ABCC2 transporter protein. Clin Pharmacol Ther 81: 42–49.
30. Xiang X, Jada SR, Li HH, Fan L, Tham LS, et al. (2006) Pharmacogenetics of SLCO1B1 gene and the impact of *1b and *15 haplotypes on irinotecan disposition in Asian cancer patients. Pharmacogenet Genomics 16: 683–691.
31. Takane H, Miyata M, Burioka N, Kurai J, Fukuoka Y, et al. (2007) Severe toxicities after irinotecan-based chemotherapy in a patient with lung cancer: a homozygote for the SLCO1B1*15 allele. Ther Drug Monit 29: 666–668.
32. Han JY, Lim HS, Shin ES, Yoo YK, Park YH, et al. (2008) Influence of the organic anion-transporting polypeptide 1B1 (*OATP1B1*) polymorphisms on irinotecan-pharmacokinetics and clinical outcome of patients with advanced non-small cell lung cancer. Lung Cancer 59: 69–75.
33. Han JY, Lim HS, Park YH, Lee SY, Lee JS (2009) Integrated pharmacogenetic prediction of irinotecan pharmacokinetics and toxicity in patients with advanced non-small cell lung cancer. Lung Cancer 63: 115–120.
34. Michael M, Thompson M, Hicks RJ, Mitchell PL, Ellis A, et al. (2006) Relationship of hepatic functional imaging to irinotecan pharmacokinetics and genetic parameters of drug elimination. J Clin Oncol 24: 4228–4235.
35. Sai K, Itoda M, Saito Y, Kurose K, Katori N, et al. (2006) Genetic variations and haplotype structures of the *ABCB1* gene in a Japanese population: an expanded haplotype block covering the distal promoter region, and associated ethnic differences. Ann Hum Genet 70: 605–622.
36. Yang X, Hu Z, Chan SY, Chan E, Goh BC, et al. (2005) Novel agents that potentially inhibit irinotecan-induced diarrhea. Curr Med Chem 12: 1343–1358.
37. Kawato Y, Sekiguchi M, Akahane K, Tsutomi Y, Hirota Y, et al. (1993) Inhibitory activity of camptothecin derivatives against acetylcholinesterase in dogs and their binding activity to acetylcholine receptors in rats. J Pharm Pharmacol 45: 444–448.
38. Hyatt JL, Tsurkan L, Morton CL, Yoon KJ, Harel M, et al. (2005) Inhibition of acetylcholinesterase by the anticancer prodrug CPT-11. Chem Biol Interact 157–158: 247–252.
39. Takakura A, Kurita A, Asahara T, Yokoba M, Yamamoto M, et al. (2012) Rapid deconjugation of SN-38 glucuronide and adsorption of released free SN-38 by intestinal microorganisms in rat. Oncol Lett 3: 520–524.
40. Yamamoto M, Kurita A, Asahara T, Takakura A, Katono K, et al. (2008) Metabolism of irinotecan and its active metabolite SN-38 by intestinal microflora in rats. Oncol Rep 20: 727–730.
41. Kuhn JG (1998) Pharmacology of irinotecan. Oncology (Williston Park) 12: 39–42.
42. Takahashi H, Honda H (2006) Modified signal-to-noise: a new simple and practical gene filtering approach based on the concept of projective adaptive resonance theory (PART) filtering method. Bioinformatics 22: 1662–1664.
43. Takahashi H, Kobayashi T, Honda H (2005) Construction of robust prognostic predictors by using projective adaptive resonance theory as a gene filtering method. Bioinformatics 21: 179–186.
44. Takahashi H, Iwakawa H, Nakao S, Ojio T, Morishita R, et al. (2008) Knowledge-based fuzzy adaptive resonance theory and its application to the analysis of gene expression in plants. J Biosci Bioeng 106: 587–593.
45. Takahashi H, Honda H (2006) Prediction of peptide binding to major histocompatibility complex class II molecules through use of boosted fuzzy classifier with SWEEP operator method. J Biosci Bioeng 101: 137–141.
46. Kawamura T, Takahashi H, Honda H (2008) Proposal of new gene filtering method, BagPART, for gene expression analysis with small sample. J Biosci Bioeng 105: 81–84.
47. Takahashi H, Takahashi A, Naito S, Onouchi H (2012) BAIUCAS: a novel BLAST-based algorithm for the identification of upstream open reading frames with conserved amino acid sequences and its application to the *Arabidopsis thaliana* genome. Bioinformatics 28: 2231–2241.
48. Chiba Y, Mineta K, Hirai MY, Suzuki Y, Kanaya S, et al. (2013) Changes in mRNA stability associated with cold stress in Arabidopsis cells. Plant Cell Physiol 54: 180–194.
49. Iwasaki M, Takahashi H, Iwakawa H, Nakagawa A, Ishikawa T, et al. (2013) Dual regulation of *ETTIN* (*ARF3*) gene expression by AS1-AS2, which maintains the DNA methylation level, is involved in stabilization of leaf adaxial-abaxial partitioning in *Arabidopsis*. Development 140: 1958–1969.
50. Kojima S, Iwasaki M, Takahashi H, Imai T, Matsumura Y, et al. (2011) ASYMMETRIC LEAVES2 and Elongator, a histone acetyltransferase complex, mediate the establishment of polarity in leaves of *Arabidopsis thaliana*. Plant Cell Physiol 52: 1259–1273.
51. Kotooka N, Komatsu A, Takahashi H, Nonaka M, Kawaguchi C, et al. (2013) Predictive value of high-molecular weight adiponectin in subjects with a higher risk of the development of metabolic syndrome: From a population based 5-year follow-up data. Int J Cardiol 167: 1068–1070.
52. Matsuo N, Mase H, Makino M, Takahashi H, Banno H (2009) Identification of ENHANCER OF SHOOT REGENERATION 1-upregulated genes during in vitro shoot regeneration. Plant Biotechnol 26: 385–393.
53. Nakagawa A, Takahashi H, Kojima S, Sato N, Ohga K, et al. (2012) Berberine enhances defects in the establishment of leaf polarity in *asymmetric leaves1* and *asymmetric leaves2* of *Arabidopsis thaliana*. Plant Mol Biol 79: 569–581.
54. Nakayama R, Nemoto T, Takahashi H, Ohta T, Kawai A, et al. (2007) Gene expression analysis of soft tissue sarcomas: characterization and reclassification of malignant fibrous histiocytoma. Mod Pathol 20: 749–759.
55. Sano M, Aoyagi K, Takahashi H, Kawamura T, Mabuchi T, et al. (2010) Forkhead box A1 transcriptional pathway in KRT7-expressing esophageal squamous cell carcinomas with extensive lymph node metastasis. Int J Oncol 36: 321–330.
56. Yajima I, Kumasaka MY, Naito Y, Yoshikawa T, Takahashi H, et al. (2012) Reduced GNG2 expression levels in mouse malignant melanomas and human melanoma cell lines. Am J Cancer Res 2: 322–329.
57. Yoshimura K, Mori T, Yokoyama K, Koike Y, Tanabe N, et al. (2011) Identification of alternative splicing events regulated by an Arabidopsis serine/arginine-like protein, atSR45a, in response to high-light stress using a tiling array. Plant Cell Physiol 52: 1786–1805.
58. Takahashi H, Iwakawa H, Ishibashi N, Kojima S, Matsumura Y, et al. (2013) Meta-analyses of microarrays of arabidopsis asymmetric leaves1 (as1), as2 and their modifying mutants reveal a critical role for the ETT pathway in stabilization of adaxial-abaxial patterning and cell division during leaf development. Plant Cell Physiol 54: 418–431.
59. Takahashi H, Murase Y, Kobayashi T, Honda H (2007) New cancer diagnosis modeling using boosting and projective adaptive resonance theory with improved reliable index. Biochem Eng J 33: 100–109.
60. Takahashi H, Nemoto T, Yoshida T, Honda H, Hasegawa T (2006) Cancer diagnosis marker extraction for soft tissue sarcomas based on gene expression profiling data by using projective adaptive resonance theory (PART) filtering method. BMC Bioinformatics 7: 399.
61. Takahashi H, Aoyagi K, Nakanishi Y, Sasaki H, Yoshida T, et al. (2006) Classification of intramural metastases and lymph node metastases of esophageal

cancer from gene expression based on boosting and projective adaptive resonance theory. J Biosci Bioeng 102: 46–52.
62. Takahashi H, Honda H (2006) Lymphoma prognostication from expression profiling using a combination method of boosting and projective adaptive resonance theory. J Chem Eng Jpn 39: 767–771.
63. Takahashi H, Honda H (2005) A new reliable cancer diagnosis method using boosted fuzzy classifier with a SWEEP operator method. J Chem Eng Jpn 38: 763–773.
64. Takahashi H, Masuda K, Ando T, Kobayashi T, Honda H (2004) Prognostic predictor with multiple fuzzy neural models using expression profiles from DNA microarray for metastases of breast cancer. J Biosci Bioeng 98: 193–199.
65. Takahashi H, Tomida S, Kobayashi T, Honda H (2003) Inference of common genetic network using fuzzy adaptive resonance theory associated matrix method. J Biosci Bioeng 96: 154–160.
66. Takahashi H, Nakayama R, Hayashi S, Nemoto T, Murase Y, et al. (2013) Macrophage migration inhibitory factor and stearoyl-CoA desaturase 1: potential prognostic markers for soft tissue sarcomas based on bioinformatics analyses. PLoS One 8: e78250.
67. Fisher RA (1922) On the interpretation of $\chi 2$ from contingency tables, and the calculation of P. J Roy Statistical Society 85: 87–94.
68. Pitman EJG (1938) Significance tests which may be applied to samples from any population. Part III. The analysis of variance test. Biometrika 29: 322–335.
69. Benjamini Y, Hochberg Y (1995) Controlling the false discovery rate: a practical and powerful approach to multiple testing. J R Statist Soc serB 57: 298–300.
70. Akaike H (1974) A new look at the statistical model identification. IEEE T Automat Contr 19: 716–723.
71. Sakamoto Y, Ishiguro M, Kitagawa G (1986) Akaike Information Criterion Statistics. Dordrecht: Reidel Publishing Company.
72. Skol AD, Scott LJ, Abecasis GR, Boehnke M (2006) Joint analysis is more efficient than replication-based analysis for two-stage genome-wide association studies. Nat Genet 38: 209–213.
73. Delmas P, Brown DA (2005) Pathways modulating neural KCNQ/M (Kv7) potassium channels. Nat Rev Neurosci 6: 850–862.
74. Miceli F, Soldovieri MV, Martire M, Taglialatela M (2008) Molecular pharmacology and therapeutic potential of neuronal Kv7-modulating drugs. Curr Opin Pharmacol 8: 65–74.
75. Brown DA, Passmore GM (2009) Neural *KCNQ* (Kv7) channels. Br J Pharmacol 156: 1185–1195.
76. Jepps TA, Greenwood IA, Moffatt JD, Sanders KM, Ohya S (2009) Molecular and functional characterization of Kv7 K+ channel in murine gastrointestinal smooth muscles. Am J Physiol Gastrointest Liver Physiol 297: G107–115.
77. Schwake M, Jentsch TJ, Friedrich T (2003) A carboxy-terminal domain determines the subunit specificity of KCNQ K+ channel assembly. EMBO Rep 4: 76–81.
78. Cavaliere S, Malik BR, Hodge JJ (2013) KCNQ channels regulate age-related memory impairment. PLoS One 8: e62445.
79. Perez C, Vega R, Soto E (2010) Phospholipase C-mediated inhibition of the M-potassium current by muscarinic-receptor activation in the vestibular primary-afferent neurons of the rat. Neurosci Lett 468: 238–242.
80. Blandizzi C, De Paolis B, Colucci R, Lazzeri G, Baschiera F, et al. (2001) Characterization of a novel mechanism accounting for the adverse cholinergic effects of the anticancer drug irinotecan. Br J Pharmacol 132: 73–84.
81. Yasuda K, Miyake K, Horikawa Y, Hara K, Osawa H, et al. (2008) Variants in *KCNQ1* are associated with susceptibility to type 2 diabetes mellitus. Nat Genet 40: 1092–1097.
82. Ichihara S, Toyooka S, Fujiwara Y, Hotta K, Shigematsu H, et al. (2007) The impact of epidermal growth factor receptor gene status on gefitinib-treated Japanese patients with non-small-cell lung cancer. Int J Cancer 120: 1239–1247.
83. Seo S, Takayama K, Uno K, Ohi K, Hashimoto R, et al. (2013) Functional Analysis of Deep Intronic SNP rs13438494 in Intron 24 of *PCLO* Gene. PLoS One 8: e76960.
84. Sauna ZE, Kimchi-Sarfaty C, Ambudkar SV, Gottesman MM (2007) Silent polymorphisms speak: how they affect pharmacogenomics and the treatment of cancer. Cancer Res 67: 9609–9612.
85. Capon F, Allen MH, Ameen M, Burden AD, Tillman D, et al. (2004) A synonymous SNP of the corneodesmosin gene leads to increased mRNA stability and demonstrates association with psoriasis across diverse ethnic groups. Hum Mol Genet 13: 2361–2368.
86. Nackley AG, Shabalina SA, Tchivileva IE, Satterfield K, Korchynskyi O, et al. (2006) Human catechol-*O*-methyltransferase haplotypes modulate protein expression by altering mRNA secondary structure. Science 314: 1930–1933.
87. Nielsen KB, Sorensen S, Cartegni L, Corydon TJ, Doktor TK, et al. (2007) Seemingly neutral polymorphic variants may confer immunity to splicing-inactivating mutations: a synonymous SNP in exon 5 of *MCAD* protects from deleterious mutations in a flanking exonic splicing enhancer. Am J Hum Genet 80: 416–432.
88. Spasovski V, Tosic N, Nikcevic G, Stojiljkovic M, Zukic B, et al. (2013) The influence of novel transcriptional regulatory element in intron 14 on the expression of Janus kinase 2 gene in myeloproliferative neoplasms. J Appl Genet 54: 21–26.
89. Xue G, Aida Y, Onodera T, Sakudo A (2012) The 5′ flanking region and intron1 of the bovine prion protein gene (*PRNP*) are responsible for negative feedback regulation of the prion protein. PLoS One 7: e32870.
90. Yoshida T, Ono H, Kuchiba A, Saeki N, Sakamoto H (2010) Genome-wide germline analyses on cancer susceptibility and GeMDBJ database: Gastric cancer as an example. Cancer Sci 101: 1582–1589.

8

Altered Cerebral Blood Flow One Month after Systemic Chemotherapy for Breast Cancer: A Prospective Study using Pulsed Arterial Spin Labeling MRI Perfusion

Kelly N. H. Nudelman[1,2,3], **Yang Wang**[3,4], **Brenna C. McDonald**[3,4,5], **Susan K. Conroy**[3], **Dori J. Smith**[3], **John D. West**[3,4], **Darren P. O'Neill**[3,4], **Bryan P. Schneider**[1,5,6], **Andrew J. Saykin**[1,3,4,5]*

1 Department of Medical and Molecular Genetics, Indiana University School of Medicine, Indianapolis, Indiana, United States of America, **2** Training in Research for Behavioral Oncology and Cancer Control Program, Indiana University School of Nursing, Indianapolis, Indiana, United States of America, **3** Center for Neuroimaging, Department of Radiology and Imaging Sciences, Indiana University School of Medicine, Indianapolis, Indiana, United States of America, **4** Indiana Alzheimer Disease Center, Indiana University School of Medicine, Indianapolis, Indiana, United States of America, **5** Indiana University Melvin and Bren Simon Cancer Center, Indiana University School of Medicine, Indianapolis, Indiana, United States of America, **6** Department of Medicine, Indiana University School of Medicine, Indianapolis, Indiana, United States of America

Abstract

Cerebral structural and functional alterations have been reported after chemotherapy for non-CNS cancers, yet the causative mechanism behind these changes remains unclear. This study employed a novel, non-invasive, MRI-based neuroimaging measure to provide the first direct longitudinal measurement of resting cerebral perfusion in breast cancer patients, which was tested for association with changes in cognitive function and gray matter density. Perfusion was measured using pulsed arterial spin labeling MRI in women with breast cancer treated with (N = 27) or without (N = 26) chemotherapy and matched healthy controls (N = 26) after surgery before other treatments (baseline), and one month after chemotherapy completion or yoked intervals. Voxel-based analysis was employed to assess perfusion in gray matter; changes were examined in relation to overall neuropsychological test performance and frontal gray matter density changes measured by structural MRI. Baseline perfusion was not significantly different across groups. Unlike control groups, chemotherapy-treated patients demonstrated significantly increased perfusion post-treatment relative to baseline, which was statistically significant relative to controls in the right precentral gyrus. This perfusion increase was negatively correlated with baseline overall neuropsychological performance, but was not associated with frontal gray matter density reduction. However, decreased frontal gray matter density was associated with decreased perfusion in bilateral frontal and parietal lobes in the chemotherapy-treated group. These findings indicate that chemotherapy is associated with alterations in cerebral perfusion which are both related to and independent of gray matter changes. This pattern of results suggests the involvement of multiple mechanisms of chemotherapy-induced cognitive dysfunction. Additionally, lower baseline cognitive function may be a risk factor for treatment-associated perfusion dysregulation. Future research is needed to clarify these mechanisms, identify individual differences in susceptibility to treatment-associated changes, and further examine perfusion change over time in survivors.

Editor: Yu-Feng Zang, Hangzhou Normal University, China

Funding: This study was partially supported by the National Cancer Institute (R01 CA101318, R01 CA087845, P30 CA082709, and R25 CA117865), National Institute on Aging (R01 AG19771, P30 AG10133), and the Indiana CTSI (U54 RR025761, RR027710-01, RR020128), as well as the Indiana Economic Development Corporation (#87884) and an Investigator-Initiated Grant from Siemens Medical Solutions. The funders had no role in study design, data collection and analysis, decision to publish, or preparation of the manuscript.

Competing Interests: Siemens Medical Solutions provided funding in the form of an Investigator-Initiated Grant, for earlier technical research on perfusion imaging. There are no patents, products in development or marketed products to declare.

* E-mail: asaykin@iupui.edu

These authors contributed equally to this work.

Introduction

Breast cancer treatment has made great strides, leading to an overall five-year survival rate of 89% according to SEER [1]. Given this high survival rate, resulting side effects are an area of increasing concern. Cognitive dysfunction in particular has been associated with breast cancer, chemotherapy, radiation, and anti-estrogen treatments, underscoring the need to clarify the mechanisms of disease and treatment effects on cognition [2–15].

Neuroimaging has been used to measure structural and functional effects of cancer and chemotherapy treatment, including treatment-associated frontal gray matter density (GMD) decrease in breast cancer patients [16–18]. However, characterization of the full spectrum of cerebral alterations associated with chemotherapy is far from complete; one novel area of investigation is the effect of chemotherapy on resting cerebral perfusion using pulsed arterial spin labeling (PASL) magnetic resonance imaging (MRI). PASL is a noninvasive advanced technique capable of

Table 1. Sample Demographics.

	Ctx+ (N = 27)	Ctx− (N = 26)	HC (N = 26)	P^a
Age at Baseline (yrs.)	49.9 (7.6), (36–69)	52.0 (8.9), (31–68)	48.4 (10.1), (32–69)	0.350
Education (yrs.)	15.4 (2.8), (10–20)	15.4 (2.5), (11–20)	15.6 (2.1), (12–20)	0.954
Estimated Full Scale IQ (Barona Index) [49]	110.1 (6.7), (89–117)	111.1 (6.2), (98–117)	111.2 (5.2), (99–116)	0.760
Handedness (R,L/Amb)	26,1	24,2	24,2	0.662
White, Non-Hispanic	77.8%	88.5%	80.8%	0.588
CES-D raw score: Baseline	10.9 (9.7), (0–38)	9.0 (8.8), (0–34)	7.2 (7.6), (0–28)	
CES-D raw score: 1 M	14.6 (9.3), (2–33)	9.8 (9.7), (0–40)	6.9 (7.0), (0–25)	0.216
STAI-S raw score: Baseline	35.1 (15.0), (20–78)	28.9 (8.0), (20–47)	30.9 (10.2), (20–55)	
STAI-S raw score: 1 M	35.4 (12.4), (20–62)	32.2 (13.0), (20–64)	32.4 (12.4), (20–62)	0.601
Inter-scan interval (days)	158.7 (68.9), (73–387)	177.2 (72.2), (106–480)	159.6 (28.0), (116–253)	0.465
Cancer stage: 0 (DCIS)	0	6		
Cancer stage: I	11	18		0.000
Cancer stage: II	12	2		
Cancer stage: III	4	0		
Received radiotherapy	2	16		0.000
On anti-estrogen therapy[b]: Baseline	0	1 TAM		
On anti-estrogen therapy: 1 M	1 ANA, 1 TAM, 1 LET	11 TAM, 1 TAM/LEU, LET, 2 ANA, 1 EXE, 1 RAL		
Chemotherapy Regimen[c,d]				
DOX/CYC/paclitaxel	8			
DOC/CYC	8			
DOC/carboplatin	6			
DOC/DOX/CYC	2			
DOC/cisplatin	1			
DOX/CYC	1			
paclitaxel	1			

Values are Mean (Standard Deviation), (Range).
1 M = one month post chemotherapy completion (or yoked intervals).
[a]P value for one-way ANOVA with treatment groups for age, education, IQ, handedness, ethnicity, interscan interval, and radiotherapy; group-by-time analysis with treatment group for CESD and STAI, chi-square with treatment group for cancer stage.
[b]ANA = anastrozole; TAM = tamoxifen, LET = letrozole; EXE = exemestane; RAL = raloxifene; LEU = lueprolide acetate.
[c]Nine Ctx+ patients were also treated with trastuzumab, one was also treated with sunitinib, and one was also treated with bevacizumab.
[d]DOX = doxorubicin, CYC = cyclophosphamide, DOC = docetaxel.

measuring blood flow by using magnetically labeled arterial blood water as an endogenous contrast tracer. This technique can provide quantitative, stable, and physiologically meaningful images [19]. It has been shown to be well-suited to longitudinal studies of cerebral perfusion in healthy and diseased individuals, or as a surrogate marker of metabolism [20]. Based on previous prospective breast cancer studies, observed GMD decrease post-treatment suggests the likelihood of accompanying hypoperfusion; however, patterns of increased and decreased activation observed during cognitive task performance post-treatment might indicate the presence of hyperperfusion as well [16–18,21–22]. To test these competing hypotheses, we conducted the first controlled prospective study of cerebral perfusion in breast cancer patients treated with (Ctx+) and without (Ctx−) standard-dose chemotherapy and healthy controls (HC) using PASL MRI. We predicted that the Ctx+ group would evidence statistically significant changes in brain perfusion compared to the HC and Ctx− control groups post-treatment, in response to or in order to compensate for chemotherapy-induced cellular, vascular, or other tissue damage, and that this change would correlate with cognitive performance. Additionally, we analyzed perfusion changes for associations with previously reported frontal GMD change to investigate the functional independence of these measures and underlying mechanisms [18].

Methods

Ethics Statement

All participants gave written informed consent according to the Declaration of Helsinki under a protocol approved by the Indiana University Institutional Review Board.

Overall Study Design

This manuscript focuses on a subset of data from a prospective, longitudinal investigation of cancer and treatment-related cognitive effects which includes a comprehensive study protocol of neuroimaging, neurocognitive, and behavioral assessments as well as biomarker investigation. Other aspects of this and a related cohort have previously been reported [17,18,21,23]. In brief, study participants include Ctx+ and Ctx− female breast cancer patients and demographically matched HC. For Ctx+ patients, all study measures were acquired at baseline (after surgery but before radiation, chemotherapy, and/or anti-estrogen treatment), approximately one month after chemotherapy treatment completion, and approximately one year later. These time points were chosen to allow examination of both sub-acute and longer-term effects of treatment, with a particular focus on the effects of chemotherapy. Ctx− patients and HC were studied at yoked intervals (see Table 1). In addition to the PASL and T1 sequences examined for this report, the detailed MRI examination included PD/T2 and FLAIR structural sequences, working and episodic memory functional MRI tasks, magnetic resonance spectroscopy, and diffusion tensor imaging. Neurocognitive assessment included a targeted research battery with emphasis on episodic memory and executive functioning, as well as measures briefly assessing other neuropsychological domains (e.g., general intellectual ability, language, attention, processing speed, visuospatial and motor skills, etc.). Self-report measures included demographic and medical information, treatment sequelae, self-perceived cognition, mood and anxiety, and diet and lifestyle factors. Finally, blood samples were acquired for routine labs, genetic analyses, and banked for future investigation of potential biomarkers. Blood work was typically acquired in the early morning, while other study measures were acquired over the course of one or two study visits depending on participant preference. MRI scanning was conducted prior to cognitive assessment whenever possible, though timing of study measures varied depending on scheduling availability.

Participants

The study cohort consisted of 27 Ctx+ patients, 26 Ctx− patients, and 26 HC. Only patients with non-invasive (stage 0) or non-metastatic invasive (stages I, II, or III) disease were included; additional exclusion criteria for all participants included prior cancer, substance abuse, and other medical, neurological, and psychiatric risk factors which might affect cerebral structure or function, as described in McDonald et al., 2013 [18]. Based on these criteria, 213 individuals were determined to be ineligible during phone screening. Another 15 individuals were excluded after enrolling in the study due to subsequent determination of ineligibility (e.g., tissue expanders, claustrophobia, etc.), withdrawal, or loss to follow-up, and 18 more individuals were excluded from this analysis due to lack of relevant data or scan quality, yielding 79 eligible participants with required data.

All Ctx+ patients were treated with common standard-dose chemotherapy regimens. Eight neoadjuvant chemotherapy patients' baseline measures were completed before surgery as well as chemotherapy; these individuals did not differ significantly from the other Ctx+ patients for any demographic factors, depression, or anxiety. Patients were recruited via the Indiana University Melvin and Bren Simon Cancer Center recruitment core and affiliated clinical practices. Demographically matched healthy controls were recruited via community advertisements.

Demographic and treatment characteristics are summarized in Table 1. The Center for Epidemiologic Studies-Depression Scale (CES-D) and the State Trait Anxiety Inventory-State subscale (STAI-S) were used to measure depressive symptoms and anxiety at each visit [24,25]. Self-reported caffeine consumption on scan days was also obtained. Demographic and treatment variables were assessed for statistical significance using SPSS 19 (SPSS Statistics 19, IBM Corporation, Somers, NY), using ANOVA, general linear models, and chi-square analyses as appropriate.

MRI Acquisition

Scans were acquired on a Siemens Tim Trio 3T whole-body MRI scanner using a 12-channel receiver-only head coil. Subjects were scanned in a conscious resting state with closed eyes. Cerebral perfusion measurements were obtained using a previously published scan protocol [19]. Briefly, a Q2TIPS PASL sequence using the PICORE labeling scheme was applied. Utilizing a 10 cm labeling region with 25 mm spacing from the distal edge of the labeled region to the image section, an adiabatic inversion pulse for labeling was followed by optimized inversion time delays $TI_1 = 700$ ms and $TI_2 = 1800$ ms, chosen so as to minimize intravascular signal intensity at 3T. Images were acquired using a gradient-echo single shot EPI readout, with acquisition parameters: TR/TE = 3000/13 ms, FOV = 224 mm, and matrix = 64×64. The imaging region consists of 16 contiguous ascending axial slices of 7 mm thickness. Each perfusion measurement consists of 100 dynamic (50 control and label image pairs) plus one M_0 image (the equilibrium brain tissue magnetization used to normalize the difference perfusion map) with a scan time of approximately 5 minutes. The scanner's built-in 3D online prospective acquisition correction (PACE) was used to minimize head motion artifact during acquisition. A high resolution T1-weighted magnetization prepared rapid gradient echo (MPRAGE) image and a high resolution EPI whole brain scan were acquired for subsequent reference and normalization; T2-weighted and fluid attenuated inversion recovery (FLAIR) sequences were also acquired to examine for incidental pathology.

Image Analysis

PASL scan processing was performed using previously published methods [14]. In brief, labeled images were subtracted from matched control images to create a perfusion-weighted time series; these were used to create quantitative regional perfusion maps for each scan, which were normalized to Montréal Neurological Institute (MNI) space in SPM8 (Wellcome Department of Cognitive Neuroscience, London, UK), resampled to 2 mm^3 voxels, and smoothed with a FWHM kernel of 6×6×8 mm. Image analyses in SPM8 were run with and without age at baseline and scan-day caffeine consumption as covariates given previous findings of perfusion variance [26,27]. However, inclusion of these variables is not shown as groups were balanced and these variables did not significantly alter any results.

A general linear model approach was utilized to conduct statistical parametric mapping on a voxel-by-voxel basis in SPM8. To specifically examine perfusion in gray matter, the Pick Atlas gray matter mask was used as an explicit mask in all analyses [28]. MRI image acquisition and analysis of GMD was performed as described in McDonald et al., 2013 [18].

Baseline analyses using a random effects model were performed to identify voxels with initial perfusion differences between groups. Weighted contrast vectors were entered for each group in the design matrix as described in McDonald et al., 2013 [18]. To test for areas in which cancer patients showed hypoperfusion relative to controls at baseline, −1 was entered in the Ctx+ and Ctx− baseline columns, while 2 was entered in the control baseline column. Alternate directionality and other interactions were similarly tested. The voxel-wise critical significance threshold (P_{crit}) was set to 0.001 uncorrected, with a minimum cluster extent (k) of 100 voxels for this and subsequent tests to reduce noise.

An unbiased F test of overall effects was performed to identify any statistically significant perfusion differences between groups and times. The cluster of voxels with the most significant perfusion difference was used to graph group-by-time contrast estimates and 90% confidence intervals. All groups were tested alone for

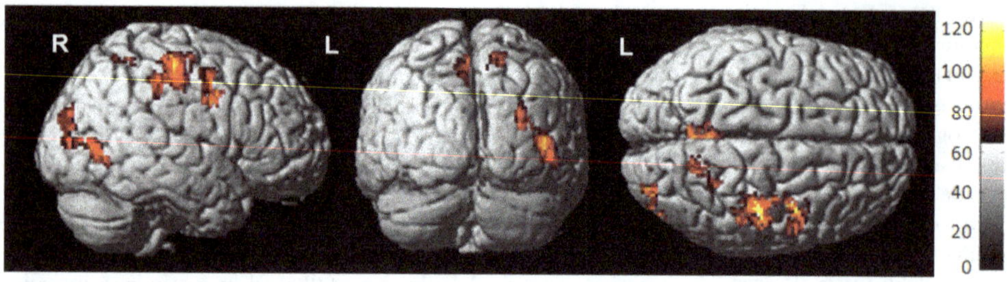

Figure 1. Group-by-time analysis (F test). Surface rendering of perfusion differences from baseline to one month post-treatment for all groups (P_{crit}<0.001 uncorrected, k = 100). Colored areas indicate statistically significant changes between groups and/or times; red to yellow color scale indicates increasing statistical significance, with yellow areas indicating the most significant regions.

perfusion change over time using weighted contrast vectors. Based on these results, the Ctx+ group was analyzed for perfusion increase over time relative to HC in an interaction model, also using weighted contrast vectors.

Perfusion and Cognition Analysis

Due to the small cohort size, we chose to investigate cognition utilizing an overall neuropsychological performance test score (global score), generated by averaging scores for eight neuropsychological domains in a similar fashion as in Conroy et al., 2013 [29] and Ahles et al., 2008 and 2010 [3,4]. To discern whether chemotherapy was associated with a change in cognition, global score change was assessed for association with treatment group in SPSS 19 using a one-way ANOVA. Based on the results, global baseline score was chosen for testing with Ctx+ perfusion change. We extracted baseline and post-treatment cluster scores for the right precentral gyrus (area of significant increase in Ctx+ compared to HC) using MarsBar in SPM8, and subtracted baseline from post-treatment scores to obtain a change score for each Ctx+ individual [30]. Ctx+ perfusion change scores were tested for Pearson correlation with global baseline scores in SPSS.

Perfusion and GMD Change Association Analysis

To test for association of GMD and perfusion, we compared the previously identified frontal GMD change clusters with the more regionally diffuse pattern of change observed for perfusion. Association was only tested in the Ctx+ group, since only this group had statistically significant changes in both measures. To analyze this association, we extracted the two frontal clusters where significant GMD decreases occurred after chemotherapy using MarsBar in SPM8 and averaged them to obtain one GMD measure for each subject at each time point [30]. The measures at baseline were subtracted from the post-treatment measures, yielding a change score for each individual. These GMD change scores were used as the covariate of interest in a multiple regression testing for association with whole brain perfusion change. Perfusion change was measured by subtracting PASL baseline scans from post-treatment scans using the ImCalc utility in SPM8 to create new scans only including regions of change.

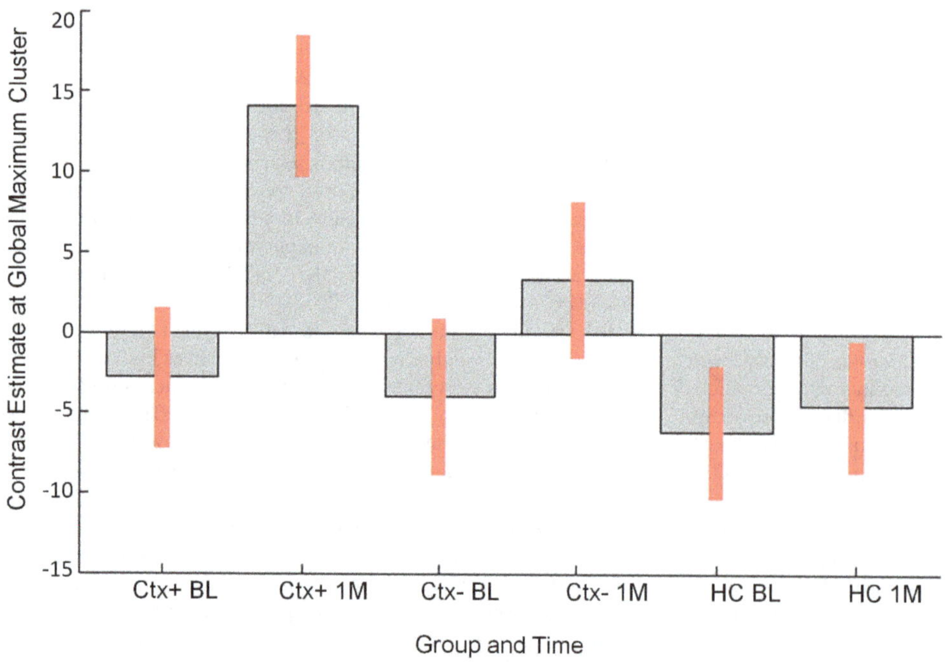

Figure 2. Maximum perfusion change. Right postcentral gyrus perfusion signal from overall F test graphed by group and time (Red bars indicate 90% confidence intervals (C.I.)). Key: BL = baseline, 1 M = one month post-treatment.

Table 2. Regional Perfusion Changes for the Overall F Test, All Groups by Times.

x[a]	y[a]	z[a]	k[b]	T	Z	$P_{FWE-corr}$[c]	Region description (for cluster peak)
44	−24	56	437	8.32	4.87	0.009	R Postcentral G (BA3)
16	−58	54	112	7.91	4.72	0.018	R Precuneus (BA7)
48	−70	2	268	7.78	4.67	0.022	R M Temporal G (BA37)
42	0	48	183	7.74	4.65	0.024	R Precentral G (BA6)
−10	−46	50	264	6.39	4.10	0.217	L Precuneus (BA7)

[a]MNI coordinates.
[b]Cluster extent.
[c]Peak-level p value.
Key: R= Right, L= Left, G= Gyrus, BA= Brodmann Area, I= Inferior, M= Middle, S= Superior.

Table 3. Regional Perfusion Changes for Ctx+ Post-Treatment Increase.

x[a]	y[a]	z[a]	k[b]	T	Z	$P_{FWE-corr}$[c]	Region description (for cluster peak)
46	−22	56	673	5.32	5.09	0.012	R Postcentral G (BA3)
32	−84	24	1464	5.20	4.98	0.000	R S Occipital G (BA19)
66	−24	34	116	5.03	4.83	0.552	R Postcentral G (BA2)
−14	12	−10	119	4.27	4.14	0.540	L Lentiform Nucleus
−6	−86	26	425	4.26	4.14	0.059	L Cuneus (BA19)
−6	−64	56	207	4.22	4.10	0.282	L Precuneus (BA7)
−16	−94	−16	101	4.20	4.08	0.612	L I Occipital G (BA17)
−54	−18	54	128	4.07	3.96	0.507	L Postcentral G (BA3)

[a]MNI coordinates.
[b]Cluster extent.
[c]Cluster-level p value.
Key: R= Right, L= Left, G= Gyrus, BA= Brodmann Area, I= Inferior, M= Middle, S= Superior.

Table 4. Regional Perfusion Changes for Ctx+ Increase Relative to Controls.

x[a]	y[a]	z[a]	k[b]	T	Z	$P_{FWE-corr}$[c]	Region description (for cluster peak)
40	−24	60	151	4.22	4.10	0.429	R Precentral G (BA4)

[a]MNI coordinates.
[b]Cluster extent.
[c]Cluster-level p value.
Key: R = Right, L = Left, G = Gyrus, BA = Brodmann Area, I = Inferior, M = Middle, S = Superior.

After multiple regression association testing of frontal GMD change with whole brain perfusion change in SPM8, again using the Pick Atlas gray matter mask, positive and negative associations were analyzed. Covarying for age did not significantly alter the results and is not reported. To graph GMD and perfusion, statistically significant perfusion change clusters from the positive association were extracted using MarsBar and averaged to one change score per individual; these were plotted against the GMD change measure. One individual's perfusion and GMD scores were more than three standard deviations below the mean. Inclusion/exclusion of this individual's scores did not alter the statistical significance of the findings, so these data points are excluded from the graphical presentation of the results.

Results

Demographic and Baseline Comparisons

Ctx+ patients had significantly higher stage disease than Ctx− patients ($X^2 = 18.82$, df = 3, $P<0.001$), as expected given current treatment protocols, and most had not received either radiotherapy or hormone therapy by one month post-chemotherapy treatment. There were no other statistically significant demographic differences or group-by-time interactions with depression or anxiety symptoms (CES-D, STAI-S, Table 1). The second scan occurred on average six months after the baseline visit; interscan intervals did not differ significantly between groups (Table 1). Eight patients received neoadjuvant treatment; these individuals did not demonstrate statistically significant demographic differences or group-by-time interactions with depression or anxiety symptoms compared to adjuvant Ctx+, Ctx−, or HC groups.

Baseline comparisons indicated no significant between-group differences in perfusion.

Perfusion Change: Chemotherapy Group Hyperperfusion

An F test across all groups and both time points indicated statistically significant perfusion change over time, primarily in the right hemisphere (Figure 1, Table 2). The cluster of maximal change, located in the right postcentral gyrus, is presented for all groups and both time points (Figure 2). In this region, the Ctx+ group showed hyperperfusion at one month post-treatment relative to both comparison groups. For this and subsequent image analyses, results including MNI coordinates, cluster extents, multiple comparison-corrected *P* values, T and Z scores, and regions are presented in Tables 2–5.

To further elucidate group differences in change over time, each group was tested individually. Only the Ctx+ group had statistically significant perfusion change, demonstrating an increase in perfusion from baseline to one month post-treatment, primarily in superior and posterior brain regions (Figure 3, Table 3). To determine how much of this increase was statistically significantly different than controls, we analyzed group-by-time interactions; results indicated that the Ctx+ group perfusion increased relative to HC specifically in the right precentral gyrus after treatment, indicating that these patients had resting state hyperperfusion discernible by MRI compared to controls (Figure 4, Table 4). Table 6 lists mean perfusion for both time points as well as perfusion change for the right precentral gyrus cluster.

The eight neoadjuvant patients were not analyzed separately, as the study design was not powered to detect subgroup effects. However, in the neoadjuvant-treated participants the mean perfusion increase in the right postcentral gyrus was almost identical to that observed for the adjuvant Ctx+ participants and Ctx+ group as a whole. The three Ctx+

Table 5. Regional Perfusion Changes for Ctx+ Perfusion and GMD Positive Association.

x[a]	y[a]	z[a]	k[b]	T	Z	$P_{FWE-corr}$[c]	Region description (for cluster peak)
12	18	−24	578	10.13	6.33	0.006	R Rectal G (BA11)
−50	−60	−22	153	9.71	6.20	0.317	L Fusiform G (BA37)
44	48	−10	136	8.26	5.68	0.377	R M Frontal G (BA11)
−4	50	−24	285	7.61	5.43	0.084	L Rectal G (BA11)
22	44	50	513	7.34	5.31	0.011	R S Frontal G (BA8)
−42	−58	44	248	7.20	5.25	0.120	L I Parietal Lobule (BA40)
34	−40	56	264	6.85	5.09	0.103	R Postcentral G (BA40)
−8	58	40	255	6.71	5.03	0.112	L S Frontal G (BA9)
−38	42	38	189	6.52	4.49	0.219	L S Frontal G (BA9)
−48	−58	44	114	6.10	4.73	0.470	L I Parietal Lobule (BA40)
38	64	12	608	5.92	4.64	0.005	R M Frontal G (BA10)
24	−10	−12	121	5.74	4.54	0.439	R Amygdala
−22	−8	0	159	5.07	4.17	0.298	L Lentiform Nucleus

[a]MNI coordinates.
[b]Cluster extent.
[c]Cluster-level p value.
Key: R= Right, L= Left, G= Gyrus, BA= Brodmann Area, I= Inferior, M= Middle, S= Superior.

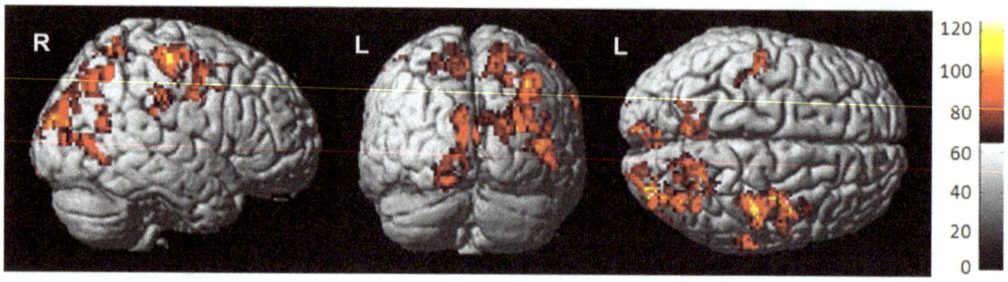

Figure 3. Ctx+ group post-treatment hyperperfusion. Surface rendering of Ctx+ increase from baseline to one month post-treatment indicates that bilateral superior and posterior brain regions demonstrate hyperperfusion post-treatment.

patients who received anti-estrogen treatment in this interval also displayed a post-chemotherapy perfusion increase, though there was insufficient power for a formal assessment of hormonal effects or interactions. Given that only two Ctx+ patients received radiotherapy treatment during this interval, this factor is also unlikely to contribute significantly to the observed variation.

Chemotherapy-Associated Hyperperfusion and Cognition

To clarify the clinical significance of this perfusion increase, we assessed perfusion change for correlation with cognitive performance. Change in the global neuropsychological test score from baseline to post-treatment was not statistically significantly different between groups, although all groups showed an increase over time likely attributable to practice effects (Table 7). In the Ctx+ group, baseline global score was negatively correlated ($r = -0.629$, $P<0.001$) with right precentral gyrus perfusion change from baseline to one month (Figure 5), indicating that individuals with lower baseline cognitive performance showed greater perfusion increase over time.

Perfusion and GMD Association

Because the chemotherapy-associated perfusion increase was not located in the frontal regions where GMD decrease was observed by McDonald et al., 2013 [18], we hypothesized that these effects might be independent. When the frontal GMD decrease was analyzed for association with whole brain perfusion change, we observed that there were statistically significant regions of bilateral frontal and parietal perfusion change positively correlated with GMD change (Figure 6, Table 5), indicating that decreased frontal GMD was associated with lower perfusion in these regions ($r = 0.553$, $P = 0.003$). However, if the frontal GMD decrease was associated with the hyperperfusion observed in Ctx+ patients, we would expect to see significant negative association in the superior and posterior regions. In this analysis there were no statistically significant regions of negative association, supporting our hypothesis that these are independent effects.

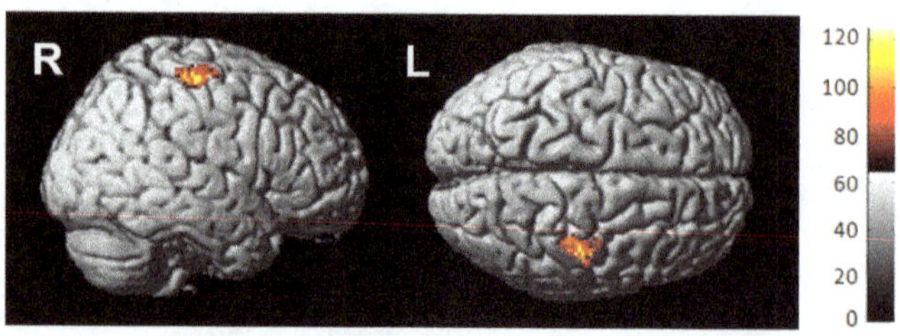

Figure 4. Ctx+ perfusion increase compared to HC. Surface rendering of Ctx+ increase compared to HC over time indicates statistically significant perfusion increase in Ctx+ in the right precentral gyrus post-treatment.

Discussion

This is the first prospective, longitudinal study documenting the effects of chemotherapy on resting cerebral perfusion in breast cancer patients. Given conflicting evidence from other measures of cerebral effects of chemotherapy, we investigated two competing hypotheses, chemotherapy-induced hypo- or hyper-perfusion. Although previous evidence suggests that aspects of the cancer disease process and/or host factors in cancer patient may induce cerebral structural and functional alterations, in the present study there were no statistically significant between-group perfusion differences at baseline [18,21,29–33]. This initial observation suggests that breast cancer itself is not associated with changes in cerebral perfusion. Although requiring replication and possibly specific to the present cohort, the lack of baseline differences suggests that treatment-associated findings are unlikely to be confounded by cancer-induced changes. This is important to note, as it may suggest that perfusion is a more specific indicator of cerebral alterations after chemotherapy, as other functional neuroimaging measures have shown differential alterations both prior to and after chemotherapy.

Although perfusion and metabolism are normally coupled, a previous cerebral resting state metabolic study using fluorodeoxyglucose [^{18}F] positron emission tomography (PET) by Silverman et al., 2007 did not find significant differences between control and adjuvant chemotherapy-treated groups, though they did identify a significant correlation between metabolism and the Rey-Osterrieth Complex Figure delayed recall performance in chemotherapy-treated subjects [22]. They also found differential perfusion in Ctx+ group patients compared to controls during a functional [^{15}O] PET study. Using functional MRI, McDonald and colleagues found differential activation in Ctx+ group patients, further supporting the idea that chemotherapy may alter perfusion and activation [21]. Thus it appears that PET and MRI may be complementary detection methods for perfusion and metabolic changes in response to chemotherapy. This new PASL data adds another perspective to prior findings, indicating that perfusion is altered in the resting state as well as during tasks,

Table 6. Right Precentral Gyrus Perfusion Group Means.

	Ctx+ (N = 27)	Ctx− (N = 26)	HC (N = 26)	P^a
Cluster Perfusion: Baseline	35.0 (10.7), (18.1–53.7)	33.9 (13.3), (2.5–57.5)	35.9 (10.4), (18.1–57.7)	0.821
Cluster Perfusion: 1 M	49.7 (18.9), (21.5–96.6)	38.8 (16.5), (−2.6–81.7)	33.9 (10.6), (12.8–56.8)	0.002
Cluster Perfusion: Change[b]	15.0 (16.7), (−9.6–57.2)	4.9 (14.7), (−22.1–33.9)	−2.0 (9.0), (−20.9–11.5)	0.000

Values are Mean (Standard Deviation), (Range). 1 M = one month post-treatment.
[a]Significance, one way ANOVA with treatment group.
[b]Change = 1 M − Baseline.

and may be related to previously identified metabolic, cognitive, and structural changes in breast cancer patients.

To date, the precise mechanisms underlying chemotherapy-induced cognitive alterations are unknown. In addition to possible direct neurotoxic injury, several pathways that could influence cerebral structure and function have been posited as potentially affected by chemotherapy, including immune response, DNA repair, oxidative stress, and altered hormone levels or signaling, all of which may be genetically modulated [34–36]. Although only small amounts of chemotherapeutic agents have been measured in the brain, this may still be enough to provoke various cellular responses including inflammation and oxidative stress, less effective DNA repair, and possibly cell death, leading to structural and functional alterations and cognitive dysfunction [37–41]. All chemotherapy drugs utilized in this cohort are alkylating agents, anthracyclines, platinating agents, or taxanes; these antineoplastic agents target various aspects of DNA repair and cell cycle division, and cause apoptosis. A systemic response to cell death could include several of the mechanisms listed above, and have widespread indirect cerebral effects, such as hyperperfusion. Interestingly, paclitaxel and docetaxel have been shown to have peripheral anti-angiogenic effects, and doxorubicin and paclitaxel have been associated with vascular toxicity [42–44]. Since all but one patient received paclitaxel or docetaxel, and only one patient in the Ctx+ group was on bevacizumab during the study, we could not draw any conclusions on the effects of anti-angiogenesis on perfusion; however, the individual receiving bevacizumab did experience increased perfusion post-treatment, consistent with other Ctx+ patients. The study was also not powered to examine any specific vascular toxicity related to doxorubicin or paclitaxel; this will be an important factor to consider in future studies. Although chemotherapy-altered estrogen signaling is still a possible causal mechanism, changes were likely not related to anti-estrogen treatments or aromatase inhibitors, since only three individuals out of 27 in the Ctx+ group were taking these types of medications at one month post-treatment [45]. Although this study was not powered to assess these individuals as a separate group, they did display hyperperfusion that was greater than that observed for the Ctx− or HC groups, though not as large as the Ctx+ group increase as a whole. Based on this evidence, we conclude that anti-estrogen or aromatase inhibitors are unlikely to contribute significantly to the observed hyperperfusion. Radiotherapy was similarly different between groups, with nearly all Ctx+ patients receiving this treatment following the one month post-chemotherapy time point, whereas the majority of Ctx− received radiotherapy before this time point. This emphasizes the specificity of the chemotherapy effect on cerebral perfusion, as radiotherapy is unlikely to confound these results. Finally, caffeine consumption is known to influence cerebral blood flow. We only obtained general self-reported caffeine consumption on scan days, and so were not powered to do a detailed analysis of the variance accounted for by this measure; however, basic self-reported caffeine consumption was not significantly different between groups, suggesting that this was not a confounding factor for this analysis.

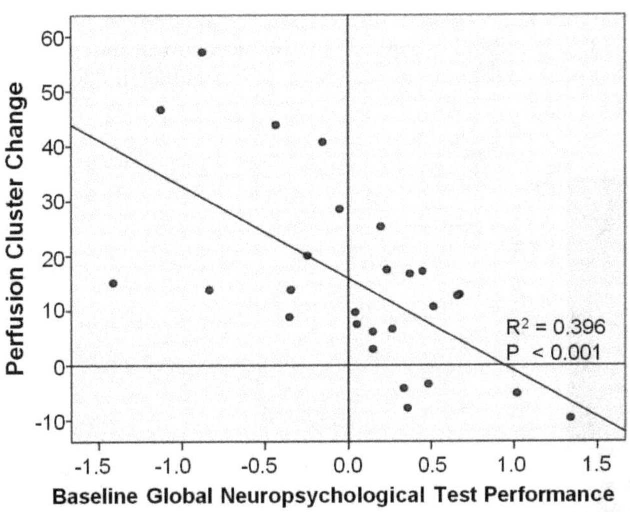

Figure 5. Ctx+ baseline cognitive performance and perfusion change correlation. Individual baseline global neuropsychological test performance (x-axis) graphed with right precentral gyrus perfusion cluster (statistically significant increase in Ctx+ vs. HC from baseline to post-treatment) change from baseline to one month post-treatment, indicating a significant negative correlation of baseline cognition with perfusion change.

Our observation that the statistically significant Ctx+ increase in cerebral perfusion was negatively correlated with baseline neuropsychological test performance suggests that baseline cognitive reserve may indicate an indirect protective mechanism; perhaps the Ctx+ post-treatment perfusion increase is an unsuccessful compensatory mechanism that is most pronounced in individuals with lower cognitive ability [4]. Future research should focus on identifying the biological mechanism driving the potential protective effect of baseline cognitive performance/reserve.

The statistically significant pre- and postcentral gyri regions of chemotherapy-associated cerebral perfusion increase reported here were independent of frontal GMD decreases noted in this cohort. However, bilateral frontal and parietal decreases in perfusion were observed that correlated with GMD decreases. These regional perfusion alterations may be influenced by different mechanisms. This is supported by previous investigations

Table 7. Global Cognitive Performance.

	Ctx+ (N = 27)[a]	Ctx− (N = 25)[a]	HC (N = 26)	p^b
Global score: Baseline	0.1 (0.6), (−1.-1.3)	0.2 (0.6), (−1.6–1.0)	0.0 (0.7), (−1.7–1.0)	0.8
Global score: 1 M	0.2 (0.6), (−1.0–1.4)	0.3 (0.6), (−1.3–1.3)	0.2 (0.7), (−1.8–1.3)	0.8
Global score change[c]	0.1 (0.2), (−0.2–0.9)	0.2 (0.2), (−0.2–0.5)	0.2 (0.2), (−0.1–0.8)	0.6

Values are Mean (Standard Deviation), (Range). 1 M = one month post-treatment.
[a]Due to missing neuropsychological data, a global score could not be calculated for one Ctx+ individual at 1 M (1 M Ctx+ N = 26), as well as one Ctx− individual at either time point.
[b]Significance, one way ANOVA with treatment group.
[c]Change = 1 M − Baseline.

in Alzheimer's disease suggesting that PASL and MRI GMD measures are complementary and have similar sensitivity; consequently if these measures were associated we would likely have detected this in our study [46]. Assuming different mechanisms are involved, one reason for the lack of correlation could be the influence of individual demographic and risk factors on susceptibility; for instance, it may be that some individuals may have genetic polymorphisms impairing drug clearance, leading to toxicity, cell death, and hypoperfusion, while others are physiologically predisposed to inflammation, which might lead to hyperperfusion. The observed lack of association indicates that there are some individuals who experience both hyperperfusion and decreased GMD post-treatment; future studies should examine whether these two measures have additive relationships with cognitive performance or complaints, which may perhaps explain why only a subgroup of breast cancer survivors appear to experience long-term cognitive dysfunction.

Further studies should also examine possible correlations of perfusion with other imaging methods, in order to further clarify the mechanistic basis of chemotherapy-induced cognitive alterations, with the long-term goal of developing preventative measures or treatments targeting these effects. While some cognitive alterations have been observed in survivors of breast cancer years after treatment, other studies show patient improvement by one year post-treatment [4,17,21,47]. If brain changes such as those observed in this study persist, they may be contributing to long-term cognitive sequelae, prioritizing perfusion as a target for therapeutic measures [48]. Future studies should utilize multimodal imaging and long-term prospective designs to clarify the mechanistic basis and persistence of this adverse effect, to help determine the focus of therapeutic efforts and pharmaceutical intervention in this patient population. Additional research could also use animal models to investigate the association of mechanisms such as direct neurotoxicity and immune response with neuroimaging measures; findings from such studies could provide important cues for therapeutic efforts.

This first study of cerebral perfusion in a prospective cohort of breast cancer patients and healthy controls provides evidence that chemotherapy is associated with alterations in cerebral perfusion, independent of cancer effects. We found statistically significant hyperperfusion in superior and posterior regions after chemotherapy, which was not seen in patients who did not receive chemotherapy or controls. While this hyperperfusion was independent of frontal GMD decrease after chemotherapy, regional frontal and parietal hypoperfusion post-treatment did correlate with GMD decreases in these patients. The regional dissociation between hyperperfusion and GMD reduction suggests the involvement of independent functional mechanisms, as well as potential influence of

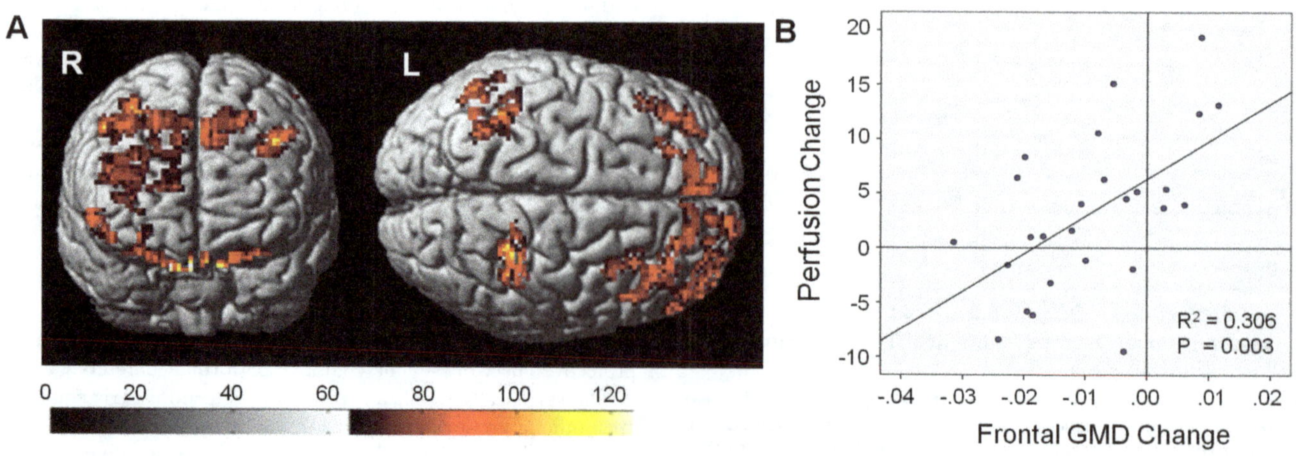

Figure 6. Perfusion and GMD positive association. A) Surface rendering of positive association between frontal GMD decrease and bilateral frontal and parietal perfusion change; association does not overlap with regions of Ctx+ hyperperfusion. B) Frontal GMD decrease (x-axis) graphed with average of all positively associated clusters of perfusion change (y-axis); decreased GMD is associated with decreased primarily frontal perfusion.

individual risk factors, providing important information to guide future investigation towards therapeutic and preventative strategies.

Acknowledgments

The authors thank Kim Wagler-Ziner, PhD, the Indiana University-Melvin and Bren Simon Cancer Center recruitment core, and our oncologist colleagues for their invaluable assistance with patient recruitment. We also thank Michele A. Beal, RT, and Courtney R. Robbins, RT for their assistance with scan acquisition. Finally, we are very grateful to our participants for their time and effort; this research would not have been possible without their willingness to participate during a particularly challenging time in their lives.

Author Contributions

Conceived and designed the experiments: BCM AJS. Performed the experiments: DJS DPO. Analyzed the data: KN YW BCM SKC JDW BPS AJS. Contributed reagents/materials/analysis tools: YW JDW AJS. Wrote the paper: KN YW.

References

1. Howlader N, Noone AM, Krapcho M, Neyman N, Aminou R, et al. (2012) SEER Cancer Statistics Review, 1975–2009 (Vintage 2009 Populations), National Cancer Institute. Available: http://seer.cancer.gov/csr/1975_2009_pops09/.
2. Agrawal K, Onami S, Mortimer JE, Pal SK (2010) Cognitive changes associated with endocrine therapy for breast cancer. Maturitas 67: 209–214.
3. Ahles TA, Saykin AJ, McDonald BC, Furstenberg CT, Cole BF, et al. (2008) Cognitive function in breast cancer patients prior to adjuvant treatment. Breast Cancer Res Treat 110: 143–152.
4. Ahles TA, Saykin AJ, McDonald BC, Li Y, Furstenberg CT, et al. (2010) Longitudinal assessment of cognitive changes associated with adjuvant treatment for breast cancer: impact of age and cognitive reserve. J Clin Oncol 28: 4434–4440.
5. Collins B, Mackenzie J, Stewart A, Bielajew C, Verma S (2009) Cognitive effects of chemotherapy in post-menopausal breast cancer patients 1 year after treatment. Psychooncology 18: 134–143.
6. Falleti MG, Sanfilippo A, Maruff P, Weih L, Phillips KA (2005) The nature and severity of cognitive impairment associated with adjuvant chemotherapy in women with breast cancer: a meta-analysis of the current literature. Brain Cogn 59: 60–70.
7. Fan HG, Houede-Tchen N, Yi QL, Chemerynsky I, Downie FP, et al. (2005) Fatigue, menopausal symptoms, and cognitive function in women after adjuvant chemotherapy for breast cancer: 1- and 2-year follow-up of a prospective controlled study. J Clin Oncol 23: 8025–8032.
8. Holohan KN, Von Ah D, McDonald BC, Saykin AJ (2013) Neuroimaging, cancer, and cognition: state of the knowledge. Semin Oncol Nurs 29: 280–287.
9. Jim HS, Donovan KA, Small BJ, Andrykowski MA, Munster PN, et al. (2009) Cognitive functioning in breast cancer survivors: a controlled comparison. Cancer 115: 1776–1783.
10. Quesnel C, Savard J, Ivers H (2009) Cognitive impairments associated with breast cancer treatments: results from a longitudinal study. Breast Cancer Res Treat 116: 113–123.
11. Wefel JS, Lenzi R, Theriault R, Buzdar AU, Cruickshank S, et al. (2004) 'Chemobrain' in breast carcinoma?: a prologue. Cancer 101: 466–475.
12. Wefel JS, Lenzi R, Theriault RL, Davis RN, Meyers CA (2004) The cognitive sequelae of standard-dose adjuvant chemotherapy in women with breast carcinoma: results of a prospective, randomized, longitudinal trial. Cancer 100: 2292–2299.
13. Bender CM, Sereika SM, Berga SL, Vogel VG, Brufsky AM, et al. (2006) Cognitive impairment associated with adjuvant therapy in breast cancer. Psychooncology 15: 422–430.
14. Schilder CM, Eggens PC, Seynaeve C, Linn SC, Boogerd W, et al. (2009) Neuropsychological functioning in postmenopausal breast cancer patients treated with tamoxifen or exemestane after AC-chemotherapy: cross-sectional findings from the neuropsychological TEAM-side study. Acta Oncol 48: 76–85.
15. Ahles TA, Root JC, Ryan EL (2012) Cancer- and cancer treatment-associated cognitive change: an update on the state of the science. J Clin Oncol 30: 3675–3686.
16. Inagaki M, Yoshikawa E, Matsuoka Y, Sugawara Y, Nakano T, et al. (2007) Smaller regional volumes of brain gray and white matter demonstrated in breast cancer survivors exposed to adjuvant chemotherapy. Cancer 109: 146–156.
17. McDonald BC, Conroy SK, Ahles TA, West JD, Saykin AJ (2010) Gray matter reduction associated with systemic chemotherapy for breast cancer: a prospective MRI study. Breast Cancer Res Treat 123: 819–828.
18. McDonald BC, Conroy SK, Smith DJ, West JD, Saykin AJ (2013) Frontal gray matter reduction after breast cancer chemotherapy and association with executive symptoms: a replication and extension study. Brain Behav Immun 30 Suppl: S117–125.
19. Wang Y, Saykin AJ, Pfeuffer J, Lin C, Mosier KM, et al. (2011) Regional reproducibility of pulsed arterial spin labeling perfusion imaging at 3T. Neuroimage 54: 1188–1195.
20. Detre JA, Wang J, Wang Z, Rao H (2009) Arterial spin-labeled perfusion MRI in basic and clinical neuroscience. Curr Opin Neurol 22: 348–355.
21. McDonald BC, Conroy SK, Ahles TA, West JD, Saykin AJ (2012) Alterations in Brain Activation during Working Memory Processing Associated with Breast Cancer and Treatment: A Prospective Functional MRI Study. J Clin Oncol 30: 2500–2508.
22. Silverman DH, Dy CJ, Castellon SA, Lai J, Pio BS, et al. (2007) Altered frontocortical, cerebellar, and basal ganglia activity in adjuvant-treated breast cancer survivors 5-10 years after chemotherapy. Breast Cancer Res Treat 103: 303–311.
23. Conroy SK, McDonald BC, Ahles TA, West JD, Saykin AJ (2013) Chemotherapy-induced amenorrhea: a prospective study of brain activation changes and neurocognitive correlates. Brain Imaging Behav 7: 491–500.
24. Radloff LS (1977) The CES-D Scale: A self-report depression scale for research in the general population. Appl Psychol Meas 1: 385–401.
25. Spielberger CD (1983) State-Trait Anxiety Inventory. Palo Alto, CA: Consulting Psychologists Press, Inc.
26. Wierenga CE, Clark LR, Dev SI, Shin DD, Jurick SM, et al. (2013) Interaction of age and APOE genotype on cerebral blood flow at rest. J Alzheimers Dis 34: 921–935.
27. Wang DJ, Chen Y, Fernandez-Seara MA, Detre JA (2011) Potentials and challenges for arterial spin labeling in pharmacological magnetic resonance imaging. J Pharmacol Exp Ther 337: 359–366.
28. Maldjian JA, Laurienti PJ, Kraft RA, Burdette JH (2003) An automated method for neuroanatomic and cytoarchitectonic atlas-based interrogation of fMRI data sets. Neuroimage 19: 1233–1239.
29. Conroy SK, McDonald BC, Smith DJ, Moser LR, West JD, et al. (2013) Alterations in brain structure and function in breast cancer survivors: effect of post-chemotherapy interval and relation to oxidative DNA damage. Breast Cancer Res Treat 137: 493–502.
30. Brett M AJ, Valabregue R, Poline JB (2002) Region of interest analysis using an SPM toolbox. 8th International Conference on Functional Mapping of the Human Brain. Sendai, Japan: NeuroImage.
31. Cimprich B, Reuter-Lorenz P, Nelson J, Clark PM, Therrien B, et al. (2010) Prechemotherapy alterations in brain function in women with breast cancer. J Clin Exp Neuropsychol 32: 324-331.
32. Scherling C, Collins B, Mackenzie J, Bielajew C, Smith A (2012) Prechemotherapy differences in response inhibition in breast cancer patients compared to controls: a functional magnetic resonance imaging study. J Clin Exp Neuropsychol 34: 543–560.
33. Scherling C, Collins B, Mackenzie J, Bielajew C, Smith A (2011) Prechemotherapy differences in visuospatial working memory in breast cancer patients compared to controls: an FMRI study. Front Hum Neurosci 5: 122.
34. Ahles TA, Saykin AJ (2007) Candidate mechanisms for chemotherapy-induced cognitive changes. Nat Rev Cancer 7: 192–201.
35. Saykin AJ, Ahles TA, McDonald BC (2003) Mechanisms of chemotherapy-induced cognitive disorders: neuropsychological, pathophysiological, and neuroimaging perspectives. Semin Clin Neuropsychiatry 8: 201–216.
36. Walker CH, Drew BA, Antoon JW, Kalueff AV, Beckman BS (2012) Neurocognitive effects of chemotherapy and endocrine therapies in the treatment of breast cancer: recent perspectives. Cancer Invest 30: 135–148.
37. Dietrich J, Han R, Yang Y, Mayer-Proschel M, Noble M (2006) CNS progenitor cells and oligodendrocytes are targets of chemotherapeutic agents in vitro and in vivo. J Biol 5: 22.
38. Gangloff A, Hsueh WA, Kesner AL, Kiesewetter DO, Pio BS, et al. (2005) Estimation of paclitaxel biodistribution and uptake in human-derived xenografts in vivo with (18)F-fluoropaclitaxel. J Nucl Med 46: 1866–1871.
39. Ginos JZ, Cooper AJ, Dhawan V, Lai JC, Strother SC, et al. (1987) [13N]cisplatin PET to assess pharmacokinetics of intra-arterial versus intravenous chemotherapy for malignant brain tumors. J Nucl Med 28: 1844–1852.
40. Troy L, McFarland K, Littman-Power S, Kelly BJ, Walpole ET, et al. (2000) Cisplatin-based therapy: a neurological and neuropsychological review. Psychooncology 9: 29–39.
41. Verstappen CC, Heimans JJ, Hoekman K, Postma TJ (2003) Neurotoxic complications of chemotherapy in patients with cancer: clinical signs and optimal management. Drugs 63: 1549–1563.
42. Bar-Joseph H, Ben-Aharon I, Tzabari M, Tsarfaty G, Stemmer SM, et al. (2011) In vivo bioimaging as a novel strategy to detect doxorubicin-induced damage to gonadal blood vessels. PLoS One 6:e23492.
43. Vacca A, Ribatti D, Iurlaro M, Merchionne F, Nico B, et al. (2002) Docetaxel versus paclitaxel for antiangiogenesis. J Hematother Stem Cell Res 11: 103–118.

44. Wang J, Lou P, Lesniewski R, Henkin J (2003) Paclitaxel at ultra low concentrations inhibits angiogenesis without affecting cellular microtubule assembly. Anticancer Drugs 14: 13–19.
45. Pachnicki JP, Czeczko NG, Tuon F, Cavalcanti TS, Malafaia AB, et al. (2012) Immunohistochemical evaluation of estrogen and progesterone receptors of pre and post-neoadjuvant chemotherapy for breast cancer. Rev Col Bras Cir 39: 86–92.
46. Dashjamts T, Yoshiura T, Hiwatashi A, Yamashita K, Monji A, et al. (2011) Simultaneous arterial spin labeling cerebral blood flow and morphological assessments for detection of Alzheimer's disease. Acad Radiol 18: 1492–1499.
47. Ahles TA, Saykin AJ, Furstenberg CT, Cole B, Mott LA, et al. (2002) Neuropsychologic impact of standard-dose systemic chemotherapy in long-term survivors of breast cancer and lymphoma. J Clin Oncol 20: 485c493.
48. de Ruiter MB, Reneman L, Boogerd W, Veltman DJ, van Dam FS, et al. (2011) Cerebral hyporesponsiveness and cognitive impairment 10 years after chemotherapy for breast cancer. Hum Brain Mapp 32: 1206–1219.
49. Barona A, Reynolds C, Chastain R (1984) A demographically based index of pre-morbid intelligence for the WAIS-R. J Consult Clin Psych 52: 885–887.

9

Determinants of Long-Term Outcome in Patients Undergoing Simultaneous Resection of Synchronous Colorectal Liver Metastases

Qi Lin[1,9], Qinghai Ye[2,9], Dexiang Zhu[1,9], Ye Wei[1,9], Li Ren[1,9], Lechi Ye[1], Qingyang Feng[1], Pingping Xu[1], Peng Zheng[1], Minzhi Lv[3], Jia Fan[2], Jianmin Xu[1]*

1 Department of General Surgery, Zhongshan Hospital, Fudan University, Shanghai, China, **2** Department of Liver Surgery, Zhongshan Hospital, Fudan University, Shanghai, China, **3** Department of Biostatistics, School of Public Health, Fudan University, Shanghai, China

Abstract

Background: It remains unclear which patients can benefit from simultaneous resection of synchronous colorectal liver metastases (SCRLMs). This study aimed to examine the prognostic value of patient- and tumor-related factors in predicting long-term outcomes of patients undergoing simultaneous resection of SCRLMs and to help patients select a suitable therapeutic regimen and proper surveillance.

Methods: Clinicopathological and outcome data of 154 consecutive SCRLM patients who underwent simultaneous resection between July 2003 and July 2013 were collected from our prospectively established SCRLM data and analyzed with univariate and multivariate methods, and the prognostic index (PI) was formulated based on the regression coefficients (β) of the Cox model. The patients were classified into high- and low-risk groups according to the PI value; the cut-off point was the third quartile.

Results: The 5-year overall survival rate was 46%, and the 5-year disease-free survival rate was 35%. Five factors were found to be independent predictors of poor overall survival (OS) by multivariate analysis: positive lymph node status, vascular invasion, *BRAF* mutation, the distribution of bilobar liver metastases (LMs) and non-R0 resection of LMs. Compared to low PI (≤5.978), high PI (>5.978) was highly predictive of shorter OS. Three factors were found to be independent predictors of poor disease-free survival (DFS) by multivariate analysis: tumor deposits, *BRAF* mutation and bilobar LM distribution. We also determined the PI for DFS. Compared to low PI (≤2.945), high PI (>2.945) was highly predictive of shorter DFS.

Conclusions: Simultaneous resection of SCRLM may lead to various long-term outcomes. Patients with low PI have longer OS and DFS, while those with high PI have shorter OS and DFS. Thus, patients with high PI may receive more aggressive treatment and intensive surveillance, This model needs further validation.

Editor: Beicheng Sun, The First Affiliated Hospital of Nanjing Medical University, China

Funding: This project received financial support from the Key Projects of the Clinical Disciplines, which is administered by the Ministry of Health (Projects from 2010-2012), Shanghai Science and Technology Committee Talent Program (12XD1401900) and Outstanding Academic Leaders Project of Health System in Shanghai (XBR2011031). The funders had no role in study design, data collection and analysis, decision to publish, or preparation of the manuscript.

Competing Interests: The authors have declared that no competing interests exist.

* Email: xujmin@aliyun.com

9 These authors contributed equally to this work.

Introduction

Colorectal cancer (CRC) is the third most commonly diagnosed cancer in males and the second in females, with over 1.2 million new cancer cases and 608,700 deaths estimated to have occurred worldwide in 2008 [1]. Approximately 25% of CRC patients present with synchronous colorectal liver metastases (SCRLMs) at the time of initial diagnosis, and 25~50% of patients subsequently develop metachronous colorectal liver metastases (MCRLMs) at the time of disease recurrence [2]. The median survival is 2.3 to 21.3 months for patients with unresectable liver metastases (LMs) [3]. A subset of patients with either SCRLM or MCRLM benefit from radical surgery and may even achieve a cure; approximately 25~50% of patients with surgically resected colorectal liver metastasis (CRLM) survive 5 or more years [4–7].

Unfortunately, the optimal surgical strategy for patients presenting with SCRLM remains controversial. Traditionally, patients have undergone a two-stage procedure with resection of the primary colorectal tumor followed by chemotherapy and subsequent liver resection. Presently, an increasing number of studies have demonstrated that simultaneous resection is an acceptable and safe option due to advances in the surgical technique of liver resection and enhancements in anesthesia and critical care [3,4,8,9]. This strategy has potential benefits in terms of cost and quality of life, particularly as using contemporary chemotherapy regimens may damage the liver parenchyma and leave patients ineligible for surgical resection [3].

Several previous studies have reported prognostic factors for patients undergoing two-stage resection [5,8–10]; however, few have examined the factors that influence long-term outcome in patients exclusively undergoing simultaneous resection, and the sample size was very small [4,11].

This study aimed to examine the prognostic value of patient- and tumor-related factors in predicting long-term outcomes in a cohort of prospectively collected patients undergoing simultaneous resection of SCRLMs and to help patients to select a suitable therapeutic regimen and proper surveillance.

Patients and Methods

Inclusion Criteria

We reviewed our prospectively collected SCRLM database between July 2003 and July 2013 and identified 154 consecutive patients treated with simultaneous curative surgery for initially resectable SCRLM. The selection criteria for simultaneous surgery have been reported previously: [12] expected radical resection of primary disease and margin-negative resection of liver LMs (R0), no unresectable extrahepatic disease and adequate predicted volume of the post-resection hepatic remnant. All deaths occurred were due to colorectal cancer. Patients who underwent previous hepatic resections or ablations of the CRLM, experienced perioperative death or had incomplete materials were excluded from this study. The study was approved by the institutional review board of Zhongshan Hospital. All of the patients provided written consent.

Data Collection

Clinicopathological data for each patient were collected from our prospectively collected SCRLM database. The tumors were staged using the 7th edition of The International Union Against Cancer (UICC)/American Joint Committee on Cancer (AJCC) Tumor, Node, Metastasis (TNM) classification system [13]. *KRAS* and *BRAF* mutations were detected by pyrosequencing, and the timing of perioperative chemotherapy was recorded. The follow-up regimen included routine computed tomography of the chest, abdomen and pelvis and regular colonoscopic surveillance. Disease recurrence was recorded on the basis of clinical, endoscopic or radiological findings at the time of diagnosis. The date of last follow-up, vital status and recurrence of LM were determined and recorded for all patients. Overall survival (OS) was calculated from the date of diagnosis to the date of death due to CRC or last follow-up. Disease-free survival (DFS) was measured from the date of surgery until the date of documented disease recurrence.

Statistical Analysis

Summary statistics were obtained using established methods and are presented as percentages or median values with standard deviations. Categorical data are summarized as percentages and were analyzed using chi-squared analysis or Fisher's exact test. OS and DFS were analyzed using the Kaplan-Meier method; survival curves were compared using the log-rank test. Univariate and multivariate analyses were performed using the Cox proportional hazards model; significant prognostic factors in univariate analysis were entered into the Cox proportional hazards model using stepwise selection to identify independent predictors. The prognostic index (PI) of patients was calculated based on the regression coefficients (β) of the Cox model: $PI = \beta 1 \times 1 + \beta 2 \times 2 + \ldots + \beta n \times n$. The patients were classified into high- and low-risk groups according to the PI value; the cut-off point was the third quartile [14–16]. All of the statistical analyses were performed using SPSS 16.0 software (SPSS, Chicago, IL, USA). Two-sided P-values were calculated, and $P<0.05$ was considered significant.

Results

Clinicopathological Characteristics of the Patients

From July 2003 to July 2013, a total of 189 patients underwent simultaneous CRC and hepatic resection; 35 patients were excluded because of benign hepatic disease, incomplete material or the presence of other malignant tumors. Detailed clinicopathological data of the 154 patients who underwent simultaneous resection of SCRLMs are shown in Table 1. The majority of patients were male (57.8%) and younger than 60.0 years (66.2%). Most patients presented with a primary colon tumor (69.5%). The average number of metastases was 1.97±1.30 (1.0–8.0). The average size of the largest metastasis was 3.86±2.45 cm (0.5 cm–15 cm).

As shown in Fig. 1, Kaplan-Meier survival analysis revealed that the OS (Fig. 1a) and DFS (Fig. 1b) of CRC patients with bilobar LMs were significantly poorer than those patients with unilobar LMs (P<0.001; P<0.001, respectively), indicating a crucial impact of LMs distribution on clinical outcome in patients.

Operative Details and Perioperative Chemotherapy

A total of 7 patients (4.5%) underwent resection of extrahepatic metastases, and pathologically identified margin involvement was noted in 8 patients (5.2%). A total of 46 patients (29.9%) had 60 complications as follows: ascites (11), subphrenic fluid (9), pleural effusion (8), wound infection and fat liquefaction (6), small bowel obstruction (5), pneumonia and atelectasis (5), intra-abdominal infection (3), hemorrhage/hematoma (3), transient hepatic dysfunction (2), bile leakage (2), intestinal leakage (2) and others (4). All of the complications were successfully treated medically or by percutaneous drainage. Regarding adjuvant treatment, a total of 38 patients (24.7%) received preoperative chemotherapy; all of the patients received adjuvant chemotherapy. The routinely used chemotherapy regiments were FOLFOX, FOLFIRI and XELOX.

Overall Survival Analysis

Follow-up information was obtained for the 154 patients through July 2013. The median OS calculated from the time of diagnosis of the disease was 49 months. The 5-year OS rate was 46%. The median follow-up period was 36 months. At the last follow-up, 49 (31.8%) patients had died; 78 (50.6%) patients experienced tumor recurrence; 52 (35.6%) had recurrence in the liver only, 12 (8.2%) had recurrence in the lung only and 14 (9.6%) had recurrence in other sites. Among the 52 (35.6%) patients with recurrence in the liver only, 13 (25%) underwent a repeat R0 resection, and 39 (75%) received adjuvant chemotherapy. The former had a good prognosis, as determined with the Kaplan-Meier method (P = 0.013) (Fig. 2).

In univariate analyses, the following factors were significantly associated with poor OS: CEA level (>5 ng/ml), positive lymph node status, vascular invasion, nerve invasion and *BRAF* mutation in the primary tumor, number of metastases (≥4), bilobar distribution, and non-R0 resection of LMs. Multivariate analysis indicated that positive lymph node status, vascular invasion, *BRAF* mutation, bilobar LM distribution and non-R0 resection of LMs were significantly associated with poor prognosis. The details of the univariate and multivariate analyses are shown in Table 2.

Table 1. Clinicopathological characteristics of the 154 patients who underwent simultaneous resection of primary and synchronous colorectal liver metastases.

Variable		N (%)
Clinical characteristics		
Age	≤60	102 (66.2)
	>60	52 (33.8)
Gender	Male	89 (57.8)
	Female	65 (42.2)
Primary tumor site	Colon	107 (69.5)
	Rectum	47 (30.5)
Histological type	Adenocarcinoma	130 (84.4)
	Mucinous adenocarcinoma	24 (15.6)
Tumor differentiation	Well, moderate	82 (53.2)
	Poor and others	72 (46.8)
Primary tumor (T) stage	T1	3 (1.9)
	T2	5 (3.2)
	T3	25 (16.2)
	T4	121 (78.7)
Primary nodal (N) stage	N0	58 (37.7)
	N1	68 (44.1)
	N2	28 (18.2)
Tumor deposits	Negative	90 (58.4)
	Positive	64 (41.6)
Vascular invasion	Negative	127 (82.5)
	Positive	27 (17.5)
Nerve invasion	Negative	135 (87.7)
	Positive	19 (12.3)
No. of metastases	≤3	129 (83.8)
	≥4	25 (16.2)
Largest metastasis	<5 cm	111 (72.1)
	≥5 cm	43 (27.9)
Tumor distribution	Unilobar	109 (70.8)
	Bilobar	45 (29.2)
Extrahepatic metastases	No	147 (95.5)
	Yes	7 (4.5)
Resection margin	R0	146 (94.8)
	R1	8 (5.2)
CEA	≤5 ng/ml	87 (56.5)
	>5 ng/ml	67 (43.5)
KRAS status	Wild type	111 (72.1)
	Mutated	43 (27.9)
BRAF status	Wild type	140 (90.9)
	Mutated	14 (9.1)
Primary tumor operation	Right hemicolectomy	58 (37.7)
	Left hemicolectomy	51 (33.1)
	Rectectomy	45 (29.2)
Liver operation	Wedge resection	115 (74.7)
	Hemihepatectomy	28 (18.2)
	Extended hepatectomy	3 (1.9)
	Unknown extent of hepatic resection	8 (5.2)
Treatment	Perioperative chemotherapy	38 (24.7)
	Postoperative chemotherapy	154 (100)

Based on the results of multivariate analyses, the PI for OS was calculated as follows: PI = (1.413×positive lymph nodes) + (1.074×vascular invasion) + (0.928×*BRAF* mutation) + (0.846×bilobar LM distribution) + (1.945×non-R0 LM resection) (β values was shown in Table 2). Kaplan-Meier estimates were calculated according to the PI value, and the cut-off point was the third quartile. A high PI (>5.978) was found to be highly predictive of the short-term outcome (P<0.001) (Fig. 3a). The 5-year OS rate for patients with low PI (≤5.978) was 55%, whereas the 5-year survival rate for patients with high PI (>5.978) was 0%.

Disease-free Survival Analysis

The 5-year DFS of the 154 CRLM patients was 35%. In univariate analyses, tumor deposits, *BRAF* mutation, number of LMs (≥4), bilobar LM distribution and extrahepatic metastases resection were significantly associated with shorter DFS. Multivariate analysis indicated that tumor deposits, *BRAF* mutation and bilobar LM distribution were significantly associated with shorter DFS. The details of the univariate and multivariate analyses are shown in Table 3.

The PI for DFS was calculated as follows: PI = (1.257×*BRAF* mutation) + (0.844×bilobar LM distribution) + (0.730×tumor deposits) (β values was shown in Table 3). Kaplan-Meier estimates were calculated according to the PI value; the cut-off point was the third quartile. A high PI (>2.945) was found to be highly predictive of the short-term outcome (P<0.001) (Fig. 3b). The 5-year DFS rate for patients with a low PI (≤2.945) was 41%, whereas the 3-year survival rate for patients with a high PI (> 2.945) was 5%.

Subgroup Analysis for Colon and Rectal Cancer

In consideration of the heterogeneity between colon and rectal cancer, we performed the categorized analysis according to high and low PI value for colon and rectal cancer patients respectively. Kaplan-Meier estimates were calculated according to high and low PI value. In colon cancer patients, a high PI (>5.978) was found to be highly predictive of the short-term OS (P<0.001) (Fig. 4a) and also high PI (>2.945) was found to be highly predictive of the short-term DFS (P<0.001) (Fig. 4b). In rectal cancer patients, a high PI (>5.978) was found to be highly predictive of the short-term OS (P = 0.001) (Fig. 5a), but high PI (>2.945) was not found to be highly predictive of the short-term DFS (P = 0.145) (Fig. 5b).

Discussion

In recent decades, the strategy of delayed hepatectomy has gained popularity and has been established as the standard surgical practice. Some authors hold the view that simultaneous resections may increase the rate of postoperative complications [17]. Given that the morbidity and mortality associated with hepatectomy have decreased substantially over the past 20 years, the classic paradigm of a staged operation for SCRLMs has been questioned. Specifically, given the improved feasibility and safety of major hepatic resections, some investigators have suggested that the simultaneous approach to SCRLMs may be preferable. Other large studies, including meta-analyses [3,4,8,9], have also shown that simultaneous resections are not associated with increased rates of hepatic or colon complications compared with delayed resection. Finally, as demonstrated by some large studies and meta-analyses examining the timing of hepatectomy for patients

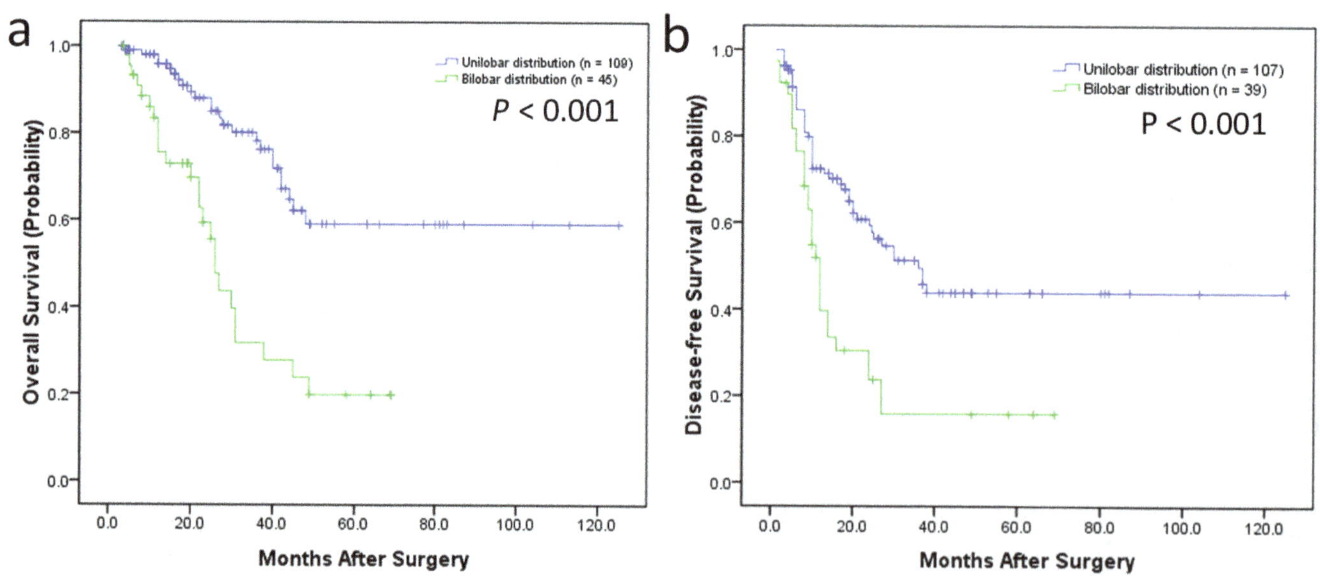

a) No. at risk

	0.0	20.0	40.0	60.0	80.0	100.0	120.0
Unilobar distribution	109	65	35	12	8	3	0
Bilobar distribution	45	23	7	3	0	0	0

b) No. at risk

	0.0	20.0	40.0	60.0	80.0	100.0	120.0
Unilobar distribution	107	47	21	9	6	2	0
Bilobar distribution	39	9	4	2	0	0	0

Figure 1. Kaplan-Meier estimates of the OS and DFS according to the tumor distribution (bilobar or unilobar). a) Kaplan–Meier curves illustrating the OS of bilobar distribution versus unilobar distribution patients. The OS of tumor bilobar distribution patients was significantly shorter than that of tumor unilobar distribution patients (P<0.001). b) Kaplan–Meier curves illustrating the DFS of bilobar distribution versus unilobar distribution patients. The DFS of tumor bilobar distribution patients was significantly shorter than that of tumor unilobar distribution patients (P< 0.001).

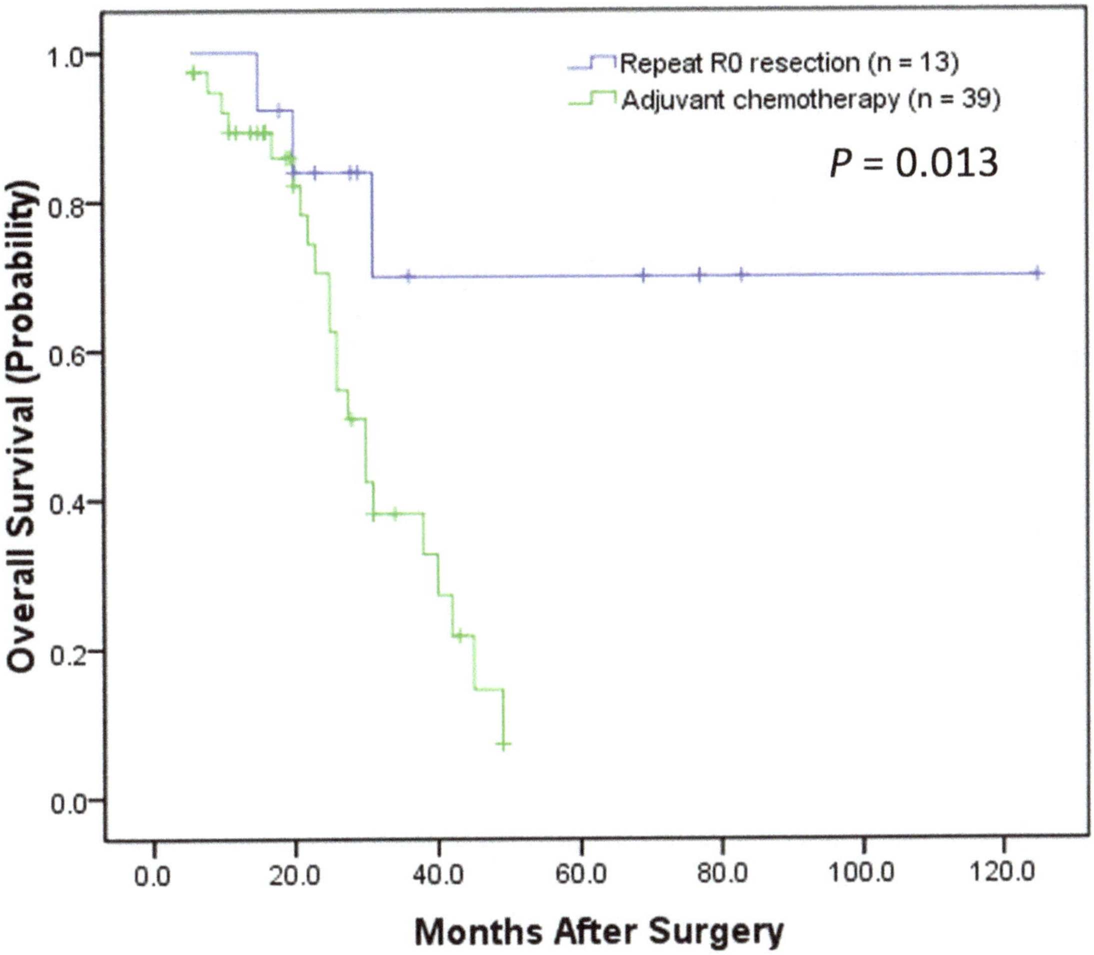

No. at risk							
Reresection	13	11	4	4	2	1	1
Chemotherapy	39	23	6	0	0	0	0

Figure 2. Kaplan-Meier curves illustrating the OS of patients with liver-only recurrence who underwent a repeat R0 resection versus those who underwent adjuvant chemotherapy only. Patients who underwent a repeat R0 resection had a good prognosis compared to those who underwent adjuvant chemotherapy only (P = 0.013).

with SCRLMs, long-term OS and DFS are similar between the simultaneous and delayed resection groups [3,4,18]. In our study, the median overall survival was 49 months, the 5-year OS rate was 46%, and the 5-year DFS was 35%. These findings are in agreement with present studies [3,4,8,9,11,19].

Recently, Abbott AM et al [18] found significant predictors of short outcomes for CRLMs about complications, mortality, and prolonged length of stay including age >70 years, male gender, nonprivate health insurance, and Elixhauser score. However, the most important problem is identifying determinants of the long-term outcome. Few studies have examined factors that are prognostic of OS and DFS following synchronous resection, and the sample sizes were very small [10,19–22]. Most studies have used a Clinical Risk Score (including nodal status of the primary tumor, a disease-free interval from discovery of the primary tumor to discovery of LM<12 months, >1 tumor, a preoperative CEA level >200 ng/ml and size of the largest tumor >5 cm) [20] and the Basingstoke Predictive Index (including >3 hepatic metastases, node-positive primary disease, a poorly differentiated primary tumor, presence of extra-hepatic disease, tumor diameter ≥5 cm, CEA level >60 ng/ml and positive resection margins) for risk-categorizing patients who may benefit from intensive surveillance as well as for the selection of adjuvant therapy and trials [21]. However, there were more MCRLMs in these studies, and the prognostic factor "discovery of liver metastasis of <12 months" is unsuitable for predicting recurrence in SCRLM patients after simultaneous resection, as the OS and DFS of SCRLM patients are shorter than those of MCRLM patients. Furthermore, additional emphasis is now focused on tumor molecular stratification. Thus, the Clinical Risk Score must be updated. In our study, we found significant independent predictors of short OS, including positive lymph node status, vascular invasion, *BRAF*

Table 2. Univariate and multivariate analyses of associations between clinicopathological characteristics and overall survival after curative resection of liver metastases.

Prognostic factor	Univariate analysis			Multivariate analysis			
	HR	95% CI	P	HR	95% CI	P	β
Age (>60:≤60)	0.644	0.346–1.198	0.165				
Sex (Female:Male)	1.378	0.785–2.417	0.264				
Primary tumor site (Rectum:Colon)	1.288	0.720–2.307	0.394				
Histological type (Mucinous adenocarcinoma: Adenocarcinoma)	0.846	0.360–1.990	0.702				
Tumor differentiation (Well, moderate: Poor and others)	1.422	0.801–2.524	0.230				
Primary tumor (T) stage (T3,T4:T1,T2)	1.596	0.387–6.576	0.517				
Primary nodal (N) stage (N1,N2:N0)	3.336	1.617–6.885	0.001	4.108	1.907–8.853	<0.001	1.413
Tumor deposits (Positive:Negative)	1.688	0.962–2.962	0.068				
Vascular invasion (Positive:Negative)	2.358	1.121–4.555	0.011	2.928	1.410–6.080	0.004	1.074
Nerve invasion (Positive:Negative)	2.384	1.055–5.388	0.037				
CEA (>5 ng/ml:≤5 ng/ml)	2.109	1.050–4.238	0.036				
KRAS status (Mutated: Wild type)	1.494	0.835–2.672	0.176				
BRAF status (Mutated: Wild type)	3.232	1.498–6.976	0.003	2.531	1.102–5.811	0.029	0.928
No. of LMs (≥4:≤3)	3.988	2.094–7.595	<0.001				
Tumor distribution (Bilobar:Unilobar)	3.522	2.003–6.193	<0.001	2.331	1.265–4.294	0.007	0.846
Size of LM (≥5 cm:<5 cm)	1.489	0.808–2.744	0.202				
Resection margin (R1:R0)	12.381	4.969–30.847	<0.001	6.992	2.066–23.661	0.002	1.945
Extrahepatic metastases resection (Yes: No)	1.903	0.590–6.136	0.282				
Chemotherapy (Postoperative:Perioperative)	0.959	0.527–1.746	0.891				

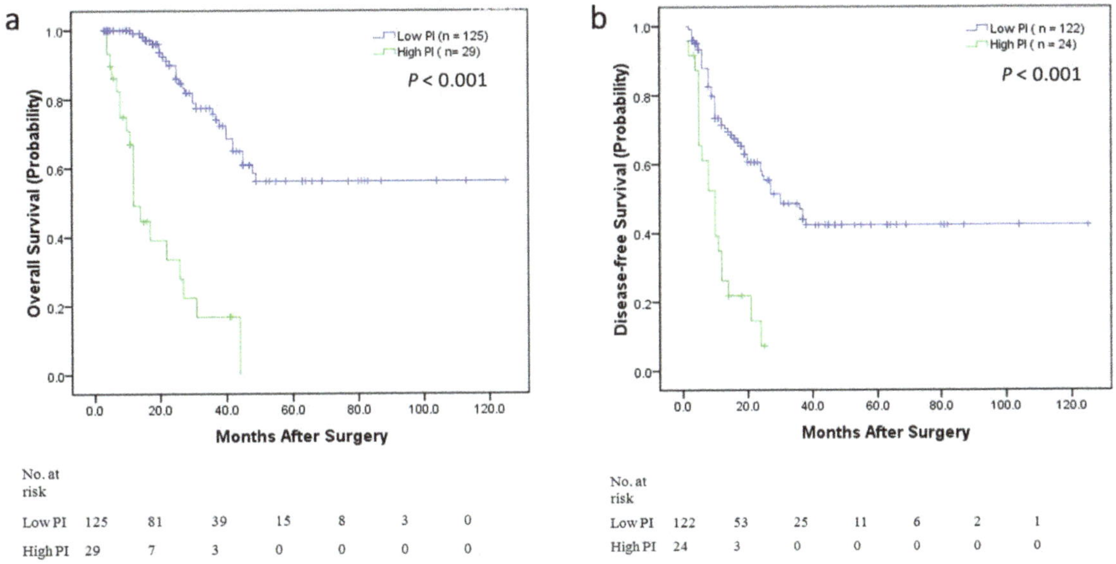

Figure 3. Kaplan-Meier estimates of OS and DFS from categorized analysis. a) OS categorized by high prognostic index (PI) and low PI. Patients with low PI had longer OS, whereas those with high PI had shorter OS (P<0.001). b) DFS categorized by high PI and low PI. Patients with low PI had longer DFS, whereas those with high PI had shorter DFS (P<0.001).

mutation, bilobar LM distribution and non-R0 resection of LMs. We determined the PI using these predictors, and a high PI (> 5.978) was found to be highly predictive of short OS (P<0.001). We also performed categorized analysis using tumor deposits, *BRAF* mutation and bilobar LM distribution for DFS, and we found that a high PI (>2.945) was highly predictive of short-term DFS (P<0.001). We also performed the categorized analysis according to high and low PI value for colon and rectal cancer patients respectively. In colon cancer patients, a high PI was found to be highly predictive of the short-term OS and DFS. In rectal cancer patients, a high PI was found to be highly predictive of the short-term OS, but high PI was not found to be highly predictive of the short-term DFS, because of the small sample of rectal cancer.

In contrast to previous series, the number of LMs [10,20–22] and the size of LMs [20,21] were not independent predictors in our study. We examined different cut-offs for number and size in the univariate analyses, and we found that the hazard ratio of number of LMs (≤3; ≥4) and size of LMs (<5 cm; ≥5 cm) was maximal, in agreement with the above studies [10,20–22]. Therefore, we preliminarily concluded that if R0 resection is achieved, the number and size of LMs do not conclusively influence OS; however, additional evidence is needed. In many studies, a high preoperative CEA has been associated with poor survival, particularly at higher cut-off levels [11,19–21]. However, our study and other studies [10,22] have failed to show that CEA is a significant prognostic factor, which could partially be due to the use of different cut-off values. In fact, we examined different cut-off values in univariate analyses and found that the hazard ratio of CEA >5 ng/ml/<5 ng/ml was maximal.

We first found that bilobar LM distribution and *BRAF* mutation of the primary tumor are independently associated with worse OS and DFS, respectively. Very few studies have explored the predictive role of bilobar distribution. In our study, OS and DFS of CRC patients with bilobar LMs were significantly poorer than those patients with unilobar LMs, indicating a crucial impact of LMs distribution on clinical outcome in patients.

KRAS and *BRAF*, which function downstream of the epidermal growth factor receptor (EGFR) signaling pathway, play important roles in the initiation and progression of CRC. Mutant *KRAS* is a predictor of resistance to EGFR monoclonal antibodies; thus, mutations in this gene are useful markers in clinical practice for patients with metastatic CRC [23]. Other studies have reported that *BRAF* mutations appear to be prognostic rather than predictive, as patients with metastatic CRC who do not receive cetuximab also have markedly reduced survival when their tumors harbor a *BRAF* mutation [24,25]. Therefore, it is essential to include these two genes in studies attempting to identify prognostic predictors for SCRLM. In the current study, we determined that *BRAF* is an independent predictor of both OS and DFS.

Despite the theoretical advantages of neo-adjuvant chemotherapy, including the eradication of microscopic neoplastic foci, practical evidence for its benefit in patients with resectable SCRLM is weak. According to the results of the EORTC 40983 randomized trial, perioperative chemotherapy improves the outcome of resectable CRLM patients [26]; however, the control group in this trial only underwent surgery without adjuvant chemotherapy. Our study and some retrospective series specifically focused on resectable synchronous metastases have failed to demonstrate any survival advantage in patients receiving neoadjuvant treatments compared to adjuvant chemotherapy [27,28]. Reddy SK et al [27] suggested that chemotherapy administered after but not before SCRLM resection is associated with improved DFS and OS. Another study including patients with SCRLMs and MCRLMs demonstrated that the effects of pre- and post-operative chemotherapy are indistinguishable [29] and that chemotherapy administered after but not before resection is associated with a good prognosis [30]. Prospective randomized trials are needed to determine the optimal timing of chemotherapy.

Conclusions

Despite the limitations of the patient data showing a fair amount of early censoring, based on our preliminary data, we can make a conclusion that simultaneous resection of SCRLM may produce

Table 3. Univariate and multivariate analyses of associations between clinicopathological characteristics and disease-free survival after curative resection of liver metastases.

Prognostic factor	Univariate analysis			Multivariate analysis			
	HR	95% CI	P	HR	95% CI	P	β
Age (>60:≤60)	0.671	0.408–1.104	0.116				
Sex (Female:Male)	1.529	0.971–2.409	0.067				
Primary tumor site (Rectum:Colon)	1.313	0.819–2.104	0.258				
Histological type (Mucinous adenocarcinoma: Adenocarcinoma)	0.620	0.298–1.292	0.202				
Tumor differentiation (Well, moderate: Poor and others)	1.423	0.898-2.255	0.133				
Primary tumor (T) stage (T3,T4:T1,T2)	1.539	0.484–4.893	0.465				
Primary nodal (N) stage (N1,N2:N0)	1.611	0.991–2.620	0.054				
Tumor deposits (Positive:Negative)	2.149	1.360–3.396	0.001	2.076	1.304–3.306	0.002	0.730
Vascular invasion (Positive:Negative)	1.482	0.828–2.652	0.485				
Nerve invasion (Positive:Negative)	1.453	0.722–2.926	0.295				
CEA (>5 ng/ml: ≤5 ng/ml)	1.429	0.868–2.352	0.160				
KRAS status (Mutated: Wild type)	1.509	0.941–2.419	0.088				
BRAF status (Mutated: Wild type)	4.400	2.263–8.553	<0.001	3.514	1.791–6.896	0.000	1.257
No. of LMs (≥4:≤3)	2.333	1.251–4.351	0.008				
Tumor distribution (Bilobar:Unilobar)	2.343	1.465–3.749	<0.001	2.325	1.443–3.746	0.001	0.844
Size of LM (≥5 cm:<5 cm)	1.420	0.872–2.312	0.159				
Extrahepatic metastases resection (Yes: No)	2.670	1.068–6.675	0.036				
Chemotherapy (Postoperative:Perioperative)	1.108	0.663–1.852	0.696				

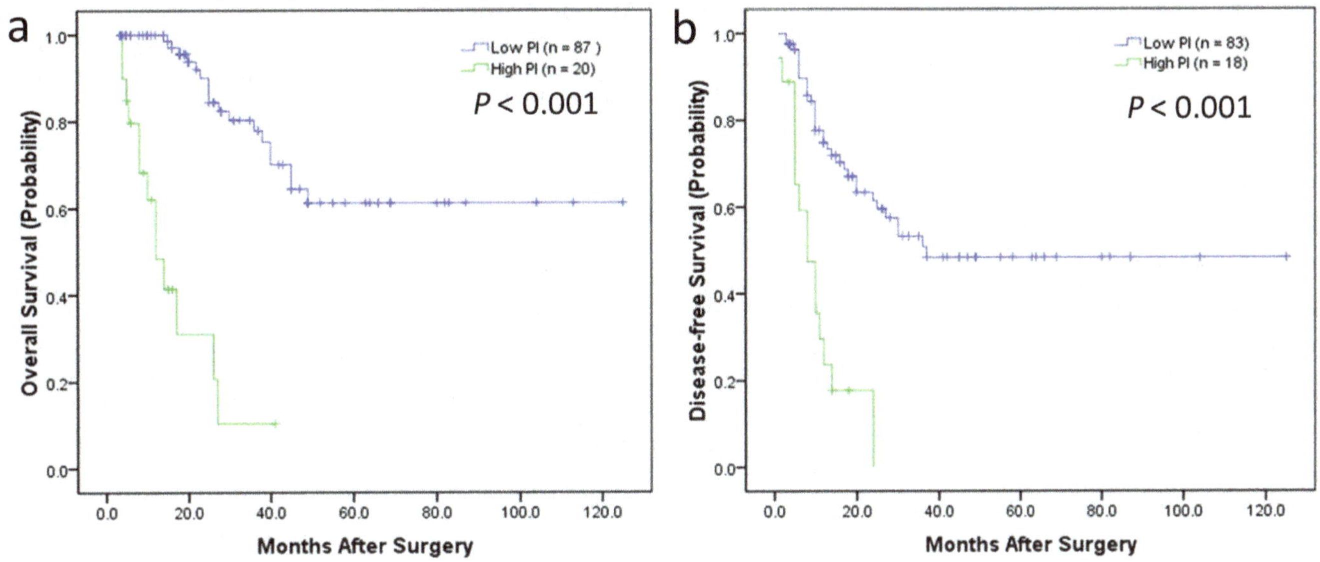

a)

No. at risk							
Low PI	87	55	29	12	7	3	0
High PI	20	3	1	0	0	0	0

b)

No. at risk							
Low PI	83	37	19	9	5	2	0
High PI	18	1	0	0	0	0	0

Figure 4. Kaplan-Meier estimates of OS and DFS from categorized analysis in colon cancer patients. a) OS categorized by high prognostic index (PI) and low PI. Patients with low PI had longer OS, whereas those with high PI had shorter OS (P<0.001). b) DFS categorized by high PI and low PI. Patients with low PI had longer DFS, whereas those with high PI had shorter DFS (P<0.001).

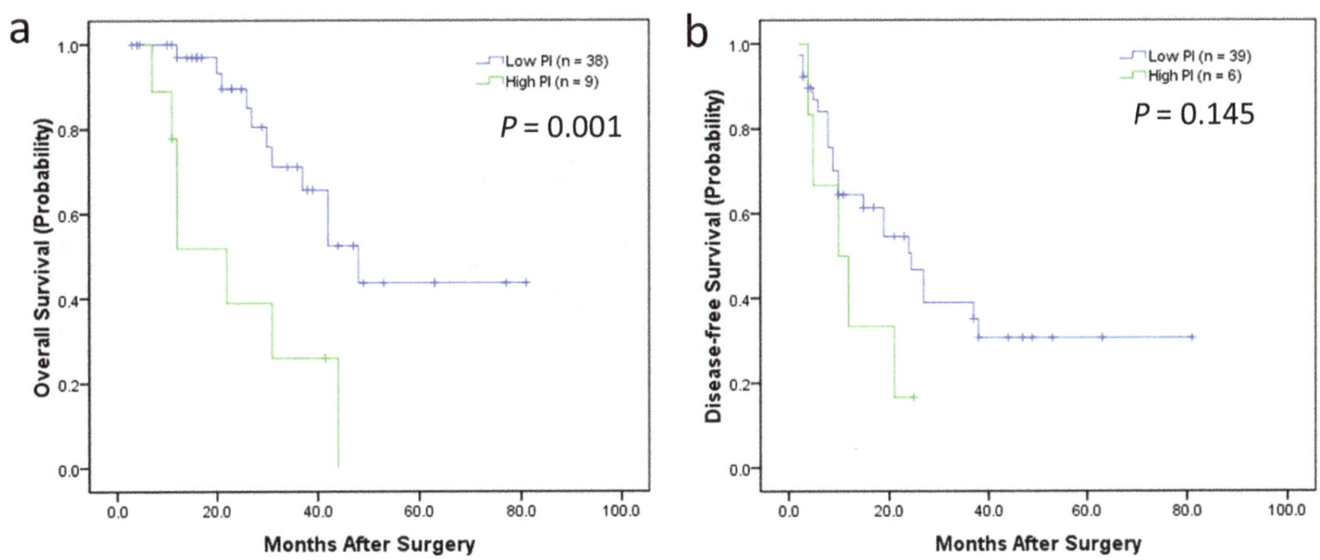

a)

No. at risk						
Low PI	38	26	10	3	1	0
High PI	9	4	2	0	0	0

b)

No. at risk						
Low PI	39	16	6	2	1	0
High PI	6	2	0	0	0	0

Figure 5. Kaplan-Meier estimates of OS and DFS from categorized analysis in rectal cancer patients. a) OS categorized by high prognostic index (PI) and low PI. Patients with low PI had longer OS, whereas those with high PI had shorter OS (P<0.001). b) DFS categorized by high PI and low PI. The OS of high PI patients was not significantly shorter than that of low PI patients (P = 0.145).

good long-term outcomes. Patients with low PI have longer OS and DFS, while those with high PI have shorter OS and DFS. Thus, patients with high PI may be provided more aggressive treatment and intensive surveillance, This model needs further validation.

Author Contributions

Conceived and designed the experiments: QL QY DZ YW LR JX. Performed the experiments: QL QY DZ YW LR LY QF PX PZ JF JX. Analyzed the data: QL QY DZ YW ML JX. Wrote the paper: QL QY DZ.

References

1. Jemal A, Bray F, Center MM, Ferlay J, Ward E, et al. (2011) Global cancer statistics. CA Cancer J Clin 61: 69–90.
2. Van Cutsem E, Rivera F, Berry S, Kretzschmar A, Michael M, et al. (2009) Safety and efficacy of first-line bevacizumab with FOLFOX, XELOX, FOLFIRI and fluoropyrimidines in metastatic colorectal cancer: the BEAT study. Ann Oncol 20: 1842–1847.
3. Yin Z, Liu C, Chen Y, Bai Y, Shang C, et al. (2013) Timing of hepatectomy in resectable synchronous colorectal liver metastases (SCRLM): Simultaneous or delayed? Hepatology 57: 2346–2357.
4. Mayo SC, Pulitano C, Marques H, Lamelas J, Wolfgang CL, et al. (2013) Surgical management of patients with synchronous colorectal liver metastasis: a multicenter international analysis. J Am Coll Surg 216: 707–716; discussion 716–708.
5. Adam R, Delvart V, Pascal G, Valeanu A, Castaing D, et al. (2004) Rescue surgery for unresectable colorectal liver metastases downstaged by chemotherapy: a model to predict long-term survival. Ann Surg 240: 644–657; discussion 657–648.
6. Manfredi S, Lepage C, Hatem C, Coatmeur O, Faivre J, et al. (2006) Epidemiology and management of liver metastases from colorectal cancer. Ann Surg 244: 254–259.
7. Robertson DJ, Stukel TA, Gottlieb DJ, Sutherland JM, Fisher ES (2009) Survival after hepatic resection of colorectal cancer metastases: a national experience. Cancer 115: 752–759.
8. Martin RC 2nd, Augenstein V, Reuter NP, Scoggins CR, McMasters KM (2009) Simultaneous versus staged resection for synchronous colorectal cancer liver metastases. J Am Coll Surg 208: 842–850; discussion 850–842.
9. Slesser AA, Simillis C, Goldin R, Brown G, Mudan S, et al. (2013) A meta-analysis comparing simultaneous versus delayed resections in patients with synchronous colorectal liver metastases. Surg Oncol 22: 36–47.
10. Malik HZ, Prasad KR, Halazun KJ, Aldoori A, Al-Mukhtar A, et al. (2007) Preoperative prognostic score for predicting survival after hepatic resection for colorectal liver metastases. Ann Surg 246: 806–814.
11. de Santibanes E, Fernandez D, Vaccaro C, Quintana GO, Bonadeo F, et al. (2010) Short-term and long-term outcomes after simultaneous resection of colorectal malignancies and synchronous liver metastases. World J Surg 34: 2133–2140.
12. Xu JM, Qin XY, Wang JP, Zhang SZ, Zhong YS, et al. (2011) Chinese guidelines for the diagnosis and comprehensive treatment of hepatic metastasis of colorectal cancer. Journal of Cancer Research and Clinical Oncology 137: 1379–1396.
13. Sobin LH, Gospodarowicz MK, Wittekind C, International Union against Cancer. (2009) TNM classification of malignant tumours. Chichester, West Sussex, UK; Hoboken, NJ: Wiley-Blackwell.
14. Sebastian SO, Gonzalez JM, Paricio PP, Perez JS, Flores DP, et al. (2000) Papillary thyroid carcinoma: prognostic index for survival including the histological variety. Arch Surg 135: 272–277.
15. Teramukai S, Ochiai K, Tada H, Fukushima M, Japan Multinational Trial Organization OC (2007) PIEPOC: a new prognostic index for advanced epithelial ovarian cancer—Japan Multinational Trial Organization OC01-01. J Clin Oncol 25: 3302–3306.
16. Francart J, Vaes E, Henrard S, Legrand C, Baas P, et al. (2009) A prognostic index for progression-free survival in malignant mesothelioma with application to the design of phase II trials: a combined analysis of 10 EORTC trials. Eur J Cancer 45: 2304–2311.
17. Kimura F, Miyazaki M, Suwa T, Kakizaki S, Itoh H, et al. (1996) Reduced hepatic acute-phase response after simultaneous resection for gastrointestinal cancer with synchronous liver metastases. British Journal of Surgery 83: 1002–1006.
18. Abbott AM, Parsons HM, Tuttle TM, Jensen EH (2013) Short-Term Outcomes after Combined Colon and Liver Resection for Synchronous Colon Cancer Liver Metastases: A Population Study. Annals of Surgical Oncology 20: 139–147.
19. John SK, Robinson SM, Rehman S, Harrison B, Vallance A, et al. (2013) Prognostic factors and survival after resection of colorectal liver metastasis in the era of preoperative chemotherapy: an 11-year single-centre study. Dig Surg 30: 293–301.
20. Fong Y, Fortner J, Sun RL, Brennan MF, Blumgart LH (1999) Clinical score for predicting recurrence after hepatic resection for metastatic colorectal cancer: analysis of 1001 consecutive cases. Ann Surg 230: 309–318; discussion 318–321.
21. Rees M, Tekkis PP, Welsh FK, O'Rourke T, John TG (2008) Evaluation of long-term survival after hepatic resection for metastatic colorectal cancer: a multifactorial model of 929 patients. Ann Surg 247: 125–135.
22. Settmacher U, Dittmar Y, Knosel T, Schone U, Heise M, et al. (2011) Predictors of long-term survival in patients with colorectal liver metastases: a single center study and review of the literature. Int J Colorectal Dis 26: 967–981.
23. De Roock W, Claes B, Bernasconi D, De Schutter J, Biesmans B, et al. (2010) Effects of KRAS, BRAF, NRAS, and PIK3CA mutations on the efficacy of cetuximab plus chemotherapy in chemotherapy-refractory metastatic colorectal cancer: a retrospective consortium analysis. Lancet Oncol 11: 753–762.
24. Laurent-Puig P, Cayre A, Manceau G, Buc E, Bachet JB, et al. (2009) Analysis of PTEN, BRAF, and EGFR status in determining benefit from cetuximab therapy in wild-type KRAS metastatic colon cancer. J Clin Oncol 27: 5924–5930.
25. Tol J, Nagtegaal ID, Punt CJ (2009) BRAF mutation in metastatic colorectal cancer. N Engl J Med 361: 98–99.
26. Nordlinger B, Sorbye H, Glimelius B, Poston GJ, Schlag PM, et al. (2008) Perioperative chemotherapy with FOLFOX4 and surgery versus surgery alone for resectable liver metastases from colorectal cancer (EORTC Intergroup trial 40983): a randomised controlled trial. Lancet 371: 1007–1016.
27. Reddy SK, Zorzi D, Lum YW, Barbas AS, Pawlik TM, et al. (2009) Timing of multimodality therapy for resectable synchronous colorectal liver metastases: a retrospective multi-institutional analysis. Ann Surg Oncol 16: 1809–1819.
28. Allen PJ, Kemeny N, Jarnagin W, DeMatteo R, Blumgart L, et al. (2003) Importance of response to neoadjuvant chemotherapy in patients undergoing resection of synchronous colorectal liver metastases. J Gastrointest Surg 7: 109–115; discussion 116–107.
29. Araujo R, Gonen M, Allen P, Blumgart L, DeMatteo R, et al. (2013) Comparison between perioperative and postoperative chemotherapy after potentially curative hepatic resection for metastatic colorectal cancer. Ann Surg Oncol 20: 4312–4321.
30. Nanji S, Cleary S, Ryan P, Guindi M, Selvarajah S, et al. (2013) Up-front hepatic resection for metastatic colorectal cancer results in favorable long-term survival. Ann Surg Oncol 20: 295–304.

10

Novel Secondary Somatic Mutations in Ewing's Sarcoma and Desmoplastic Small Round Cell Tumors

Yunyun Jiang[1]⁹, Vivek Subbiah[1,2]*⁹, Filip Janku[1], Joseph A. Ludwig[3], Aung Naing[1], Robert S. Benjamin[3], Robert E. Brown[4], Pete Anderson[2,5], Razelle Kurzrock[1,6]

1 Department of Investigational Cancer Therapeutics (Phase I Clinical Trials Program), Division of Cancer Medicine, The University of Texas MD Anderson Cancer Center, Houston, Texas, United States of America, **2** Department of Pediatrics, The University of Texas MD Anderson Cancer Center, Houston, Texas, United States of America, **3** Department of Sarcoma Medical Oncology, The University of Texas MD Anderson Cancer Center, Houston, Texas, United States of America, **4** From the Department of Pathology, UT Health-Department of Pathology and Laboratory medicine, Houston, Texas, United States of America, **5** Pediatric Hematology/Oncology/BMT, Levine Children's Hospital/Levine Cancer Institute, Charlotte, North Carolina, United States of America, **6** Center for Personalized Cancer Therapy and Division of Hematology & Oncology, University of California San Diego - Moores Cancer Center, La Jolla, California, United States of America

Abstract

Background: Ewing's sarcoma (ES) and desmoplastic small round cell tumors (DSRCT) are small round blue cell tumors driven by an N-terminal containing EWS translocation. Very few somatic mutations have been reported in ES, and none have been identified in DSRCT. The aim of this study is to explore potential actionable mutations in ES and DSRCT.

Methodology: Twenty eight patients with ES or DSRCT had tumor tissue available that could be analyzed by one of the following methods: 1) Next-generation exome sequencing platform; 2) Multiplex PCR/Mass Spectroscopy; 3) Polymerase chain reaction (PCR)-based single- gene mutation screening; 4) Sanger sequencing; 5) Morphoproteomics.

Principal Findings: Novel somatic mutations were identified in four out of 18 patients with advanced ES and two of 10 patients with advanced DSRCT (six out of 28 (21.4%));*KRAS* (n = 1), *PTPRD* (n = 1), *GRB10* (n = 2), *MET* (n = 2) *and PIK3CA* (n = 1). One patient with both PTPRD and GRB10 mutations and one with a GRB10 mutation achieved a complete remission (CR) on an Insulin like growth factor 1 receptor (IGF1R) inhibitor based treatment. One patient, who achieved a partial remission (PR) with IGF1R inhibitor treatment, but later developed resistance, demonstrated a *KRAS* mutation in the post-treatment resistant tumor, but not in the pre-treatment tumor suggesting that the RAF/RAS/MEK pathway was activated with progression.

Conclusions: We have reported several different mutations in advanced ES and DSRCT that have direct implications for molecularly-directed targeted therapy. Our technology agnostic approach provides an initial mutational roadmap used in the path towards individualized combination therapy.

Editor: Benjamin Edward Rich, Dana-Farber Cancer Institute, United States of America

Funding: The University of Texas MD Anderson Cancer Center is supported by Cancer Center Support Grant no. CA 016672. Vivek Subbiah acknowledges the Bob Howe Research Funds. The funders had no role in study design, data collection and analysis, decision to publish, or preparation of the manuscript.

Competing Interests: The authors have declared that no competing interests exist.

* Email: vsubbiah@mdanderson.org

⁹ These authors contributed equally to this work.

Introduction

Ewing's sarcoma (ES) and desmoplastic small round cell tumor (DSRCT) are small cell sarcomas characterized by the translocation of chromosome 22 to chromosome 11, resulting in fusion of the *EWSR1* gene to the *FLI1* gene (and several rarer fusion partners) [1,2] in the case of ES (*EWSR1-FLI1*), and to the *WT1* gene in the case of DSRCT (*EWSR1-WT1*) [3,4,5]. While both are mediated by the EWS translocated chimera, the clinical presentation, pathologic features, and response to therapy are different. They have been treated with similar chemotherapy regimens using a multi-disciplinary approach but this does not reflect similar biology. Although genotypically and phenotypically different, historically they have been grouped together based on their shared sensitivity to chemotherapies otherwise used for Ewing's sarcoma. For Ewing's sarcoma, in the United States, the current cytotoxic chemotherapy-based standard of care promoted by the Children's Oncology Group has resulted in steadily improved survival rates over the last four decades for the 60% of ES patients fortunate enough to present with radiographically localized disease [6]. Twenty-three percent of patients present with metastatic disease at diagnosis. Unfortunately, despite equivalent response rates among those who present with metastatic disease, the antineoplastic responses are often short-lived and the 5-year survival of this patient population remains stubbornly in the 30% range [1,7]. Early phase studies have demonstrated remarkable responses in patients with advanced ES treated with an insulin-like growth factor-1 receptor (IGF1R) antibody, with or without an mTOR inhibitor, albeit in only a small subset (10–14%) of individuals [1,8,9,10,11,12,13]. To date, no predictive biomarkers of IGF-1R response have been identified and only recently have resistance mechanisms, such as shift from the IGF-1R/IGF-1 axis towards IR-A/IGF-2, been identified [11,14]. For patients with DSRCT, the chemotherapy, radiotherapy, and surgical approaches have not been standardized, given the extreme rarity of the disease. [15,16,17]. The most commonly used cytotoxic regimens employ alkylator and anthracycline chemotherapy similar to those administered in Ewing's sarcoma.

Recent identification of molecular mutations such as *BRAF* V600E in some melanomas as well as ALK rearrangements in non-small cell lung cancer has enabled targeted therapies directed toward such anomalies and significantly altered the therapeutic landscape for afflicted patients [18,19]. While *EWSR1-FLI1* and *EWSR1-WT1* translocations occur in virtually all ES and DSRCT patients, respectively, the resulting fusion proteins have not proved to be druggable targets. Therefore, an alternative approach would be to expand the therapeutic focus to ancillary genetic aberrations infrequently encountered in those tumor types. Toward that end, a recent study using sequence-based genotyping identified mutations in 4% (three of 75 patients or cell lines with ES), including *BRAF*, *CTNNB1*, and *NRAS* [20]. No somatic mutations have been identified in patients (total = 24 samples) with DSRCT [20]. We recently reported germline Protein tyrosine phosphatase delta (PTPRD) mutations in a small pilot study in patients with Ewing's sarcoma [21].

Here we report potential actionable mutations identified in four patients with advanced ES and in two patients with advanced DSRCT. The mutations include *KRAS* (G13N), *PTPRD* (W775D), *GRB10* (Q107stop and V109A), *MET* (T1010I and N375S) and *PIK3CA* (M1040I and G1049S). Correlations with response and resistance to IGF1R inhibitor based regimen in these patients are discussed.

Patients and Methods

We reviewed 62 consecutive patients with advanced metastatic ES or DSRCT who were referred to the Department of Investigational Cancer Therapeutics (A Phase 1 program) and/or the Department of Pediatrics or Department of Sarcoma at The University of Texas MD Anderson Cancer Center (MD Anderson). Of the 62 patients, 28 patients had tumor archival tissue available that could be analyzed by one of the following methods: 1) next-generation sequencing using the Clinical Laboratory Improvement Amendment (CLIA)-approved FoundationOne platform (Foundation Medicine, Cambridge, MA; 182 genes tested); 2) CLIA-approved mutation screening by Multiplex PCR/Mass Spectroscopy (Knight Cancer Institute, Oregon, Ohio; 53 genes tested); 3) CLIA-approved polymerase chain reaction (PCR)-based single- gene mutation screening in the Department of Pathology at MD Anderson (up to 10 genes tested); 4) next-generation whole exome sequencing in the Center of Targeted Therapy CORE at MD Anderson; 5) Sanger sequencing; 6) immunohistochemical and morphoproteomic analyses of tumor samples collected from patient # 1 were performed, as previously described [11,22]. Briefly, for patient # 1, morphoproteomics and immunohistochemical probes were used to detect p-ERK1/2 (Thr202/Tyr204) ([Cell Signaling Technology, Beverly, MA] along with negative controls [11,22]. Testing was done according to tissue availability, test and physicians' choice. This study and all treatments were approved by the MD Anderson Institutional Review Board and conducted in accordance with the MD Anderson Institutional Review Board requirements. The data from this manuscript is based on CLIA certified next generation sequencing from commercially available resources. As such we do not have access to the primary data set. However, data can be made available to researchers upon request. Because this is a retrospective analysis the consent requirements were waived by the MD Anderson Institutional Review Board and informed consents were obtained from patients for collection of samples at the time of screening or enrollment of patients to the clinical trials.

Results

Among the 28 patients tested for molecular aberrations, 18 had ES and 10 had DSRCT. Four ES patients (22.2%) and two DSRCT patients (20%) had secondary mutations, including *GRB10* (n = 2), *PTPRD* (n = 1), *KRAS* (n = 1), *MET* (n = 2) and *PIK3CA* (n = 1) (Table 1). All patients had metastatic disease. The medium age of the 28 patients at diagnosis was 22 years (range 9 to 52 years). Twenty were men and most had been heavily pretreated with chemotherapy with a median of four prior systemic treatments at the time of tissue acquisition (range, 0 to11). The prior therapies consisted of standard front-line alkylator and anthracycline-based chemotherapy as is standard in the USA and Europe: vincristine, adriamycin, cyclophosphamide, ifosfamide and etoposide. In addition, several patients were treated with additional standard second-line and third -line agents like temozolomide/irinotecan, topotecan/cyclophosphamide and gemcitabine/docetaxel.

Of interest, both of the patients with *GRB10* mutations (cases #2 and #3, Table 1) responded to therapy with an IGF1R plus mTOR inhibitor and both achieved a complete remission (CR) [10]. One of the patients (case #2) also attained a prior CR with IGF1R inhibitor alone [8,11,13] (Figure 1). Case # 2 had been selected for an in-depth molecular analyses with the use of next generation exome sequencing and Foundation One (Foundation Medicine) 182 gene panel interrogation because of her excellent response (CR) after IGF1R inhibitor therapy. Because of the finding of *GRB10* mutation in case #2, mutational analysis of *GRB10* was also performed on tumor from case #3 (who also achieved a CR after IGF1R inhibitor therapy) and, remarkably, was also positive by Sanger sequencing.

The Grb10 protein sends a negative feedback signal to IGF1R, hence inhibiting the IGF1R signal; a loss of function *GRB10* mutation may therefore be expected to be associated with activated IGF1-R signaling (Figure 2) [23,24]. Case # 2 also demonstrated a protein tyrosine phosphatase receptor type D (PTPRD) mutation that would truncate this protein (Table 1). The PTPRD protein dephosphorylates STAT3, whereas IGF1R is important in STAT3 phosphorylation [21,25]. A PTPRD mutation would be expected to inhibit STAT3 dephosphorylation, resulting in accumulated phosphorylated STAT3 (Figure 2). Because of the role of IGF1R in enabling STAT3 phosphorylation, inhibiting IGF1R might diminish the up regulation of STAT3 phosphorylation effected by mutated PTPRD. Of interest, increased expression of phospho-STAT3 has been implicated in ES pathogenesis [26].

One patient (Case # 1, Table #1) received IGF1R/mTOR inhibitor therapy and achieved a partial remission (PR) for 6 months, but developed resistance to the therapy. A *KRAS* mutation was identified in the resistant tumor, but not in the pre-treatment tumor. This was c.37_38GG>AA and was reported in the 53 gene sequenom panel (Knight Diagnostics assay). In addition, immunohistochemistry-based morphoproteomics in the tumor specimen showed that the ras/Raf kinase/extracellular signal-regulated kinase (ERK) pathway was constitutively activated with chromogenic signal observed, up to 3+ in nucleus and ± in

Table 1. Ewing's sarcoma and Desmoplastic small round cell tumor (DSRCT) patients whose tumors were analyzed for somatic aberrations.

Pt#	Diagnosis	Mutation	Methods used for molecular analysis
1	Ewing's	KRAS: G13N	Knight Diagnostics 53 gene panel (Sequenome) Foundation One 182 gene panel (Foundation Medicine), MDACC single gene PCR based assay
2	Ewing's	PTPRD:W775stop GRB10:Q107stop	Foundation One 182 gene panel (Foundation Medicine), Next generation sequencing
3	Ewing's	GRB10: V109A	Sanger sequencing
4	Ewing's	MET: T1010I	MDACC single gene PCR based assay
5	Ewing's	none	"
6	Ewing's	none	"
7	Ewing's	none	"
8	Ewing's	none	"
9	Ewing's	none	"
10	Ewing's	none	"
11	Ewing's	none	"
12	Ewing's	none	"
13	Ewing's	none	"
14	Ewing's	none	"
15	Ewing's	none	"
16	Ewing's	none	"
17	Ewing's	none	Foundation One 182 gene panel (Foundation Medicine), Next generation sequencing
18	Ewing's	none	MDACC single gene PCR based assay
19	DSRCT	MET:N375S	"
20	DSRCT	PIK3CA:M1040I&G1049S	"
21	DSRCT	none	"
22	DSRCT	none	"
23	DSRCT	none	"
24	DSRCT	none	"
25	DSRCT	none	"
26	DSRCT	none	"
27	DSRCT	none	"
28	DSRCT	none	"

the cytoplasm, for p-ERK 1/2 (Thr 202/Tyr 204) (Figure 3). A fourth patient (Table 1, Case # 4), whose tumor demonstrated a *MET* mutation did not receive IGF1R inhibitor therapy. The mutation was detected in codon 1010 (ACT to ATT) of the *MET* gene that would change the encoding amino acid from Thr to Ile (p.T1010I) using a screening assay (PCR-based primer extension analysis).

Of the ten DSRCT patients tested, one patient had a *MET* mutation. Mutation was detected in codon 375 (AAC to AGC) of the *MET* gene that would change the encoding amino acid from Asn to Ser (N375S). The other had two mutations in the *PIK3CA* gene (Table # 1, Case #19 and # 20). Mutation was detected in codon 1040 (ATG to ATA) in exon 20 of the *PIK3CA* gene that would change the encoding amino acid from Met to Ile (M1040I). A second mutation detected in codon 1049 (GGT to AGT) of the *PIK3CA* gene that would change the encoding amino acid from Gly to Ser (G1049S).

Discussion

Our study shows that 21.4% of patients (6 of 28) with advanced, heavily pretreated Ewing's sarcoma family of tumors (ES, n = 18; DSRCT, n = 10) had secondary somatic molecular aberrations, including mutations in *KRAS*, *PTPRD*, *GRB10*, *MET* and *PIK3CA*. Interestingly, we recently reported germline PTPRD mutations in three out of eight (37.5%) patients with metastatic Ewing's sarcoma [21]. Previous studies by Shukla et al [17] reported molecular aberrations in 3 of 75 patients with ES (4%) and 0 of 24 patients with DSRCT [20]. The higher incidence of somatic mutations in our current study may be due to evolution of technologies. Shukla et al [17] had used a 29 gene panel sequenom assay while we used a range of evolving technologies, including next generation exome sequencing, a 53-gene panel sequenom (Knight Diagnostics) and a 182 gene panel (Foundation One next generation panel) in selected patients. In addition, our patients all had advanced disease with multiple prior therapies. While the number and type of prior therapies could have an effect on the

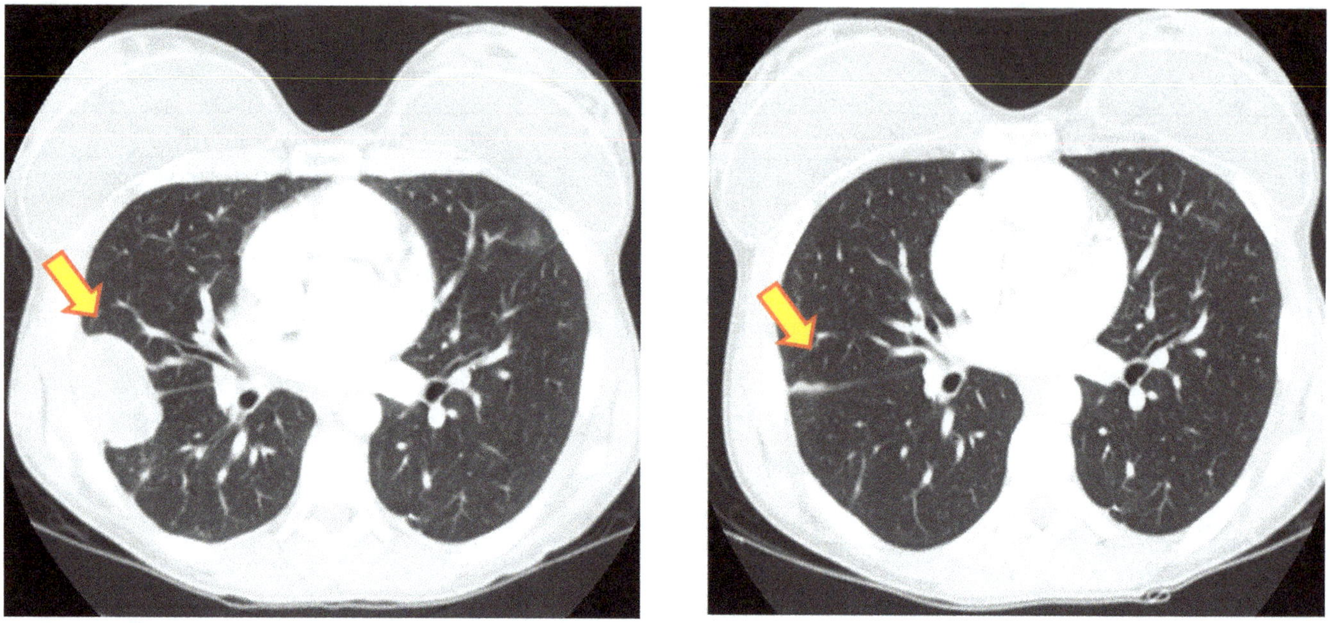

Figure 1. CT of the chest in Case # 2 with Ewing's sarcoma response to single agent IGF1R antibody alone [11]. Left panel shows lung metastases before IGF1R antibody therapy and right panel shows response to therapy after six weeks of treatment [11].

evolution of type and pattern of mutation, our study did not reveal a pattern, though a larger group may be needed for a robust analysis of specific associations. Shukla et al. [17] found *BRAF*, *NRAS* and *CTNNB1* mutations in their ES patients and cell lines, while we found *KRAS*, *PTPRD*,*GRB10* and *MET*. Together, these results suggest that advanced and resistant ES (and DSRCT) may be driven by diverse secondary aberrations.

The specific genetic aberrations and their correlation with response and resistance may be also illuminating. For instance, patient 1 (Table 2) achieved a PR on combined IGF1R and mTOR inhibitor therapy lasting six months. In that patient, tissue was available (both pre- and post-treatment tumors) and only the post-treatment tumor showed a *KRAS* mutation. This result suggests an adaptive mechanism of resistance to IGF1R/mTOR attributable to the RAS/RAF/MEK pathway (Figure 2) and is consistent with those shown previously by morphoproteomic analysis where resistance to IGF1R/mTOR inhibitor was associated with ERK activation [11]. An impact of the *KRAS* mutation was confirmed in this patient's tumor tissue by immunohistochemistry-based morphoproteomics which demonstrated that the Ras/Raf kinase/extracellular signal-regulated kinase (ERK) pathway was constitutively activated with chromogenic signal observed, up to 3+ in nucleus and ± in the cytoplasm, for p-ERK 1/2 (Thr 202/Tyr 204) (Figure 3). Acquired *KRAS* mutations have also been implicated as a mechanism of resistance after anti-EGFR targeted therapy in colorectal cancer. [27,28,29,30]. In addition, it has been shown that the emergence of *KRAS* mutant clones can be detected months before radiographic progression [27,29]. In colorectal cancer, it has been suggested that early initiation of a MEK inhibitor may be a rational strategy for delaying or reversing drug resistance [27,29]. While it was not possible to provide this particular patient with a MEK inhibitor concurrently with combined IGF-1R/mTOR inhibition, due to constraints inherent in clinical trials, joint blockade of the MAPK and PI3K/Akt/mTOR cascades +/− IGF-1R inhibition may be an interesting approach for patients who acquire resistance to IGF-1R/mTOR-based therapies.

Patient 2 (ES) (Table 1) initially received IGF1R antibody treatment and achieved a CR for nearly three years before developing resistance [11]. After subsequent enrollment in a study of combined IGF1R/mTOR inhibition, she achieved a second CR that lasted two years. Two mutations were identified in her tumor sample collected between the two lines of treatment, a *GRB10* Q107stop mutation and a *PTPRD* W775 stop mutation. The latter mutation results in a truncated non-functional protein product incapable of dephosphorylating STAT3 [25]. (Of interest, STAT3 phosphorylation is found in about 50% of Ewing's sarcomas [22].) The loss of PTPRD function would be expected to suppress STAT3 dephosphorylation and lead to accumulated phosphorylated STAT3, especially under conditions of activated p-IGF1R [26,31] (Figure 2). One could reasonably speculate that patient 2 responded to IGF1R therapy, even in the presence of a mutated PTPRD, because p-STAT3 remains critically dependent on intact IGF-1R signaling for downstream effects.

As mentioned, patient 2 (Table 2) also had a *GRB10* mutation. The growth factor receptor-bound protein 10 (Grb10) is reported to be an mTORC1 substrate that acts downstream of IGF1R pathway [23,24]. The mTORC1 protein regulates the phosphorylation of Grb10 at S501 and S503, which indirectly results in the inhibition of PI3K, and thus regulates the IGF1R pathway through a negative feedback [24] (Figure 2). Mutation of Q107 to a stop codon, as found in this patient, would be expected to lead to a truncated Grb10 protein and loss of the phosphorylation sites on Grb10. This, in turn, would be expected to abrogate the negative feedback regulation of Grb10 and result in enhanced IGF1R pathway activity. Among a number of possible mechanisms of acquired resistance, this mutation may therefore have contributed to the eventual development of resistance to the IGF1R inhibitor treatment.

Patient 3 (ES) (table 1) achieved a CR, which lasted for two years in response to a combination regimen using an IGF1R and an mTOR inhibitor. This patient was specifically studied for a GRB10 mutation because of the similarity in his outcome to that of patient #2. A *GRB10* V109A mutation was identified in his

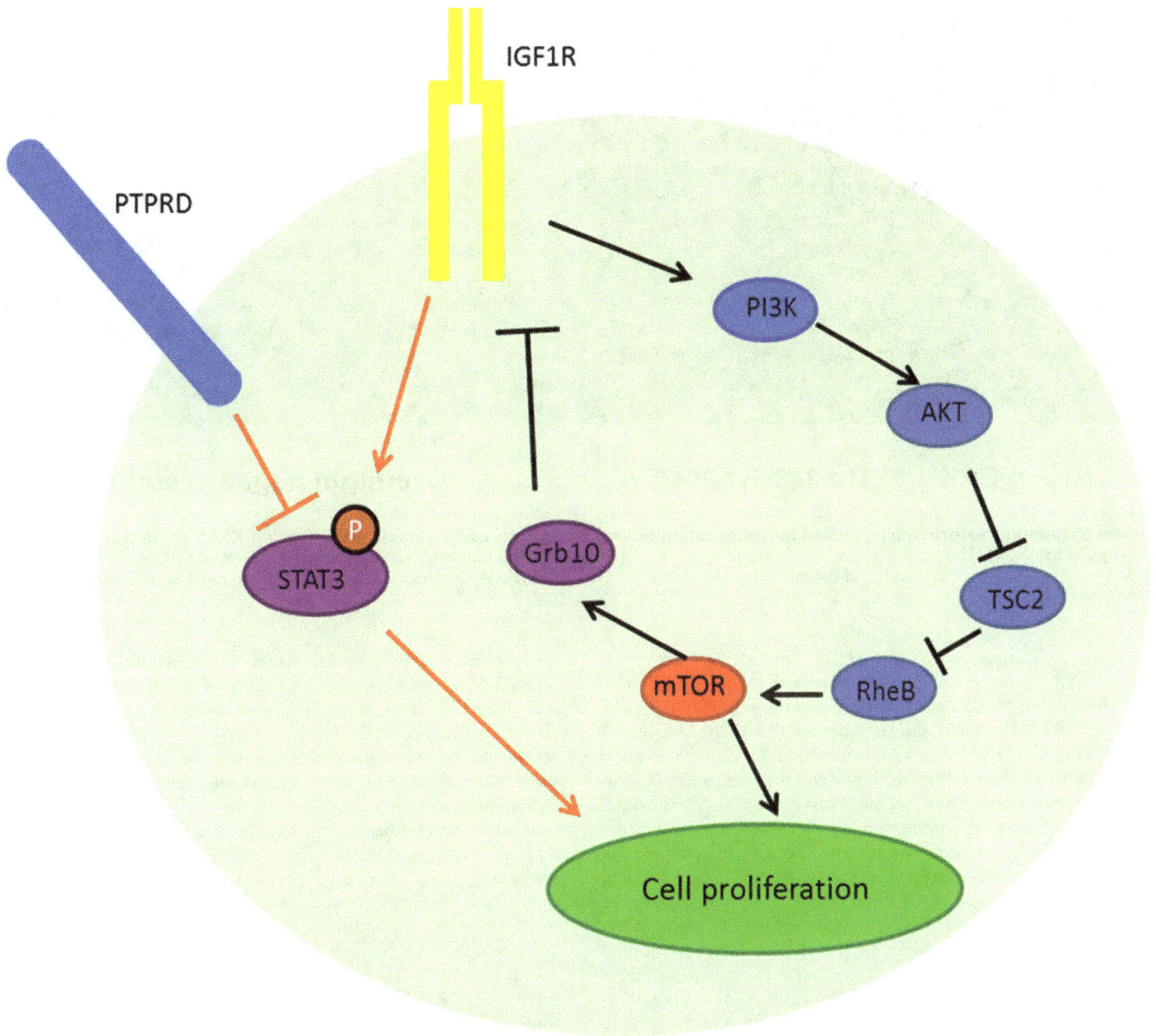

Figure 2. Schematic figure of the IGF1R pathway, regulation of STAT3 phosphorylation and negative feedback of Grb10. IGF1R is one of the regulators for STAT3 phosphorylation while PTPRD dephosphorylates STAT3. STAT3 is recruited to IGF1R for phosphorylation. IGF1R is modulated by several downstream cascades, including PI3K, AKT and mTOR. mTOR phosphorylates Grb10, which in turn inhibits the IGF1R pathway.

tumor tissue, which would not be expected to abrogate GRB10 function as the Q107 stop mutation previously noted in patient 2. However, it is possible that the V109A mutation resulted in a sufficient conformational change of the Grb10 protein to impair the negative feedback to the IGF1R pathway.

In addition to the mutations in *GRB10* and *PTPRD* that can directly affect IGF-1R signaling, an unexpected mutation in MET was identified in patients with ES and DSRCT. Patient 4 (ES, Table 2) demonstrated a *MET* T1010I mutation, which has been reported in lung cancer patients [32] but never in ES. MET belongs to the receptor tyrosine kinase (RTK) family and has been known to stimulate cancer cell growth [33]. The T1010I mutation is located in the juxtamembrane domain, which is essential for catalytic function of receptor tyrosine kinases [34]. The mutation may compromise the negative feedback function of the MET pathway, and thus lead to tumor growth. Patient 19 (DSRCT, Table 2) also demonstrated a *c-MET* N375S mutation in his tumor tissue. This is the most frequent mutation in *MET* and has primarily been reported in patients with lung cancer. However, this is the first time that the mutation has been reported in a patient with DSRCT. The N375S mutation has been previously observed as contributing to the resistance of MET to its inhibitors [35].

Patient 20 (DSRCT, Table 2) demonstrated two *PIK3CA* mutations, M1040I and G1049S, both located in the kinase domain of p110α near the activation loop [36]. The protein product expressed by *PIK3CA* is p110α, which forms a PI3K complex with p85α [37]. The PI3K/AKT/mTOR pathway regulates cell proliferation and tumor growth [38]. The M1040I and G1049S mutations are located in the kinase domain of p110α,

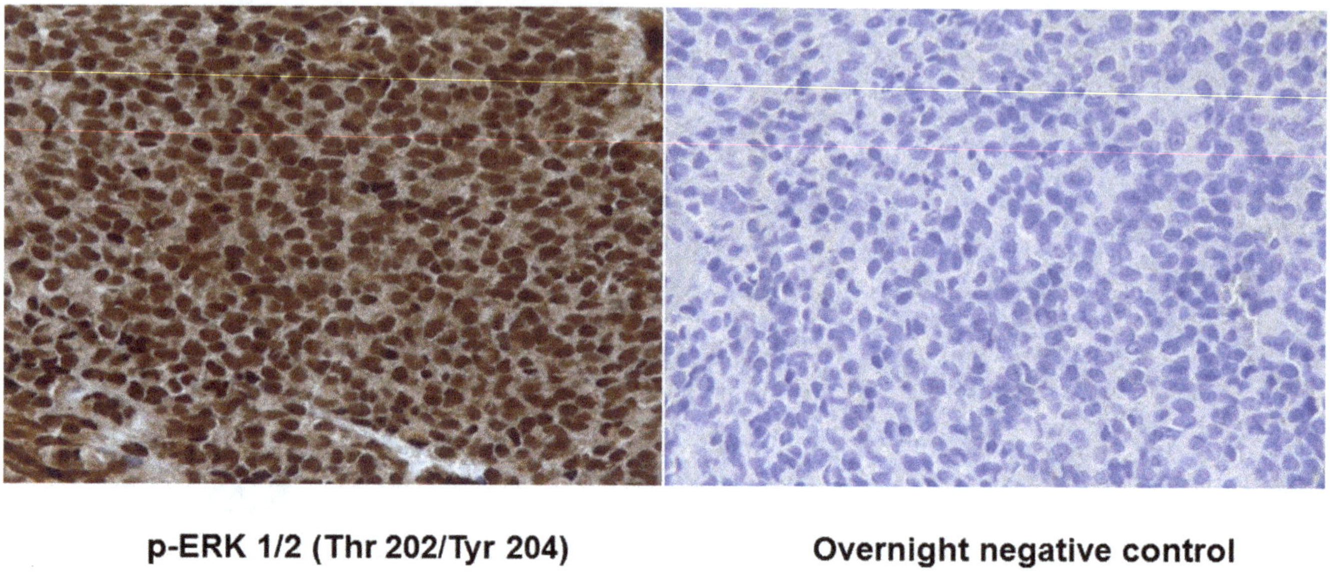

Figure 3. Immunohistochemistry based morphoproteomics of Ewing's sarcoma sample that showed KRAS mutation post IGF1R therapy (Patient 1). The Ras/Raf kinase/extracellular signal-regulated kinase (ERK) pathway was constitutively activated with chromogenic signal observed, up to 3+ in nucleus and ± in the cytoplasm, for p-ERK 1/2 (Thr 202/Tyr 204) (left hand panel) with the overnight negative control (Right hand panel).

near the activation loop [36]. H1047 mutations have been reported to result in enhanced kinase activity [39], one may hypothesize that M1040 and G1049 mutations located in the same helix with H1047 would similarly bolster the kinase activity of p110α by inducing an active conformation of the kinase activation loop. Yet, the precise role of these mutations in ES or DSRCT as well as the effectiveness of PI3K inhibitors remains to be validated.

There are several important limitations to this study. First, it is a descriptive study. Indeed, the analysis was largely retrospective with a variety of different methods used for molecular profiling. Second, the patients selected for in-depth molecular assessment were enriched for those who had responded to biologically-targeted therapy. Third, there was a lack of matched normal tissue, so it is unclear to what extent some of these aberrations might be somatic versus germ-line. Fourth, there were limitations in tissue availability and an evolution in the technologies used to analyze molecular features. As a result, while our research identified the emergence of a number of novel mutations in ES and DSRCT, their frequency and association with response requires additional study. Lastly, a series of controlled experiments are needed to test and validate the functional impact of some of these aberrations. Our findings should therefore be viewed as hypothesis generating.

In summary, we have reported diverse secondary aberrations in advanced ES and DSRCT. Some of these aberrations may be actionable and, therefore, potentially have implications for molecularly-directed targeted therapy. As the technology to assess whole genomes, transcriptomes and more is evolving rapidly, it is likely that these techniques will be increasingly applied, and may reveal even more complex molecular portfolios for patients with metastatic Ewing's sarcoma and desmoplastic small round cell tumor.

Table 2. Characteristics of Ewing's sarcoma and DSRCT patients with somatic mutations.

Patient* #	Age at Dx	Pathology/fusion type	Best Reponse to IGF1R inhibitor	Best Response to IGF1R+mTOR inhibitor	Mutation	Time of tumor sample
1	16	CD99+;EWSR1(22q12)	N/A	**PR**	KRAS G13N (c.37_38GG>AA)	Tumor resistant to IGF1R+ mTOR inhibitor (Pre-treatment sample did not show KRAS mutation)
2	24	CD99+;EWSR1(22q12)	**CR**	**CR**	PTPRD W775stop GRB10 Q107stop	Tumor resistant to IGF1R inhibitor
3	13	CD99+;EWSR1(22q12)	N/A	**CR**	GRB10 V109A	Before treatment with IGF1R inhibitor
4	20	CD99+;EWSR1(22q12)	N/A	N/A	MET T1010I	
19	13	EWSR1-WT1	N/A	N/A	MET N375S	
20	52	EWSR1-WT1	N/A	N/A	PIK3CA M1040I, G1049S	

* Patient numbers according to Table 1.
Abbreviations: CR- Complete remission, PR- Partial remission,N/A-Not applicable.

Author Contributions

Conceived and designed the experiments: YJ VS FJ RK. Performed the experiments: YJ VS REB RK. Analyzed the data: YJ VS FJ JAL AN RSB REB PA RK. Contributed reagents/materials/analysis tools: YJ VS FJ JAL AN REB PA RK. Wrote the paper: YJ VS FJ JAL AN RSB REB PA RK. Provided sarcoma expertise: VS JAL RSB PA. Prepared the figures: YJ VS. Reviewed the final manuscript: YJ VS FJ JAL AN RSB REB PA RK.

References

1. Subbiah V, Anderson P, Lazar AJ, Burdett E, Raymond K, et al. (2009) Ewing's sarcoma: standard and experimental treatment options. Curr Treat Options Oncol 10: 126–140.
2. Delattre O, Zucman J, Plougastel B, Desmaze C, Melot T, et al. (1992) Gene fusion with an ETS DNA-binding domain caused by chromosome translocation in human tumours. Nature 359: 162–165.
3. Sawyer JR, Tryka AF, Lewis JM (1992) A novel reciprocal chromosome translocation t(11;22)(p13;q12) in an intraabdominal desmoplastic small round-cell tumor. Am J Surg Pathol 16: 411–416.
4. Gerald WL, Rosai J, Ladanyi M (1995) Characterization of the genomic breakpoint and chimeric transcripts in the EWS-WT1 gene fusion of desmoplastic small round cell tumor. Proc Natl Acad Sci U S A 92: 1028–1032.
5. Ladanyi M, Gerald WL (1996) Specificity of the EWS/WT1 gene fusion for desmoplastic small round cell tumour. J Pathol 180: 462.
6. Grier HE, Krailo MD, Tarbell NJ, Link MP, Fryer CJ, et al. (2003) Addition of ifosfamide and etoposide to standard chemotherapy for Ewing's sarcoma and primitive neuroectodermal tumor of bone. N Engl J Med 348: 694–701.
7. Miser JS, Krailo MD, Tarbell NJ, Link MP, Fryer CJ, et al. (2004) Treatment of metastatic Ewing's sarcoma or primitive neuroectodermal tumor of bone: evaluation of combination ifosfamide and etoposide–a Children's Cancer Group and Pediatric Oncology Group study. J Clin Oncol 22: 2873–2876.
8. Naing A, Kurzrock R (2010) Chemotherapy resistance and retreatment: a dogma revisited. Clin Colorectal Cancer 9: E1–4.
9. Naing A, Kurzrock R, Burger A, Gupta S, Lei X, et al. (2011) Phase I trial of cixutumumab combined with temsirolimus in patients with advanced cancer. Clin Cancer Res 17: 6052–6060.
10. Naing A, Lorusso P, Fu S, Hong DS, Anderson P, et al. (2012) Insulin Growth Factor-Receptor (IGF-1R) Antibody Cixutumumab Combined with the mTOR Inhibitor Temsirolimus in Patients with Refractory Ewing's Sarcoma Family Tumors. Clin Cancer Res.
11. Subbiah V, Naing A, Brown RE, Chen H, Doyle L, et al. (2011) Targeted morphoproteomic profiling of Ewing's sarcoma treated with insulin-like growth factor 1 receptor (IGF1R) inhibitors: response/resistance signatures. PLoS One 6: e18424.
12. Subbiah V, Kurzrock R (2012) Ewing's sarcoma: overcoming the therapeutic plateau. Discov Med 13: 405–415.
13. Kurzrock R, Patnaik A, Aisner J, Warren T, Leong S, et al. (2010) A phase I study of weekly R1507, a human monoclonal antibody insulin-like growth factor-I receptor antagonist, in patients with advanced solid tumors. Clin Cancer Res 16: 2458–2465.
14. Huang HJ, Angelo LS, Rodon J, Sun M, Kuenkele KP, et al. (2011) R1507, an anti-insulin-like growth factor-1 receptor (IGF-1R) antibody, and EWS/FLI-1 siRNA in Ewing's sarcoma: convergence at the IGF/IGFR/Akt axis. PLoS One 6: e26060.
15. Philippe-Chomette P, Kabbara N, Andre N, Pierron G, Coulomb A, et al. (2012) Desmoplastic small round cell tumors with EWS-WT1 fusion transcript in children and young adults. Pediatr Blood Cancer 58: 891–897.
16. Hayes-Jordan A, Anderson PM (2011) The diagnosis and management of desmoplastic small round cell tumor: a review. Curr Opin Oncol 23: 385–389.
17. Quaglia MP, Brennan MF (2000) The clinical approach to desmoplastic small round cell tumor. Surg Oncol 9: 77–81.
18. Chapman PB, Hauschild A, Robert C, Haanen JB, Ascierto P, et al. (2011) Improved survival with vemurafenib in melanoma with BRAF V600E mutation. N Engl J Med 364: 2507–2516.
19. Kwak EL, Bang YJ, Camidge DR, Shaw AT, Solomon B, et al. (2010) Anaplastic lymphoma kinase inhibition in non-small-cell lung cancer. N Engl J Med 363: 1693–1703.
20. Shukla N, Ameur N, Yilmaz I, Nafa K, Lau CY, et al. (2012) Oncogene mutation profiling of pediatric solid tumors reveals significant subsets of embryonal rhabdomyosarcoma and neuroblastoma with mutated genes in growth signaling pathways. Clin Cancer Res 18: 748–757.
21. Jiang Y, Janku F, Subbiah V, Angelo LS, Naing A, et al. (2013) Germline PTPRD mutations in Ewing sarcoma: biologic and clinical implications. Oncotarget 4: 884–889.
22. Subbiah V, Brown RE, Jiang Y, Buryanek J, Hayes-Jordan A, et al. (2013) Morphoproteomic profiling of the mammalian target of rapamycin (mTOR) signaling pathway in desmoplastic small round cell tumor (EWS/WT1), Ewing's sarcoma (EWS/FLI1) and Wilms' tumor(WT1). PLoS One 8: e68985.
23. Hsu PP, Kang SA, Rameseder J, Zhang Y, Ottina KA, et al. (2011) The mTOR-regulated phosphoproteome reveals a mechanism of mTORC1-mediated inhibition of growth factor signaling. Science 332: 1317–1322.
24. Yu Y, Yoon SO, Poulogiannis G, Yang Q, Ma XM, et al. (2011) Phosphoproteomic analysis identifies Grb10 as an mTORC1 substrate that negatively regulates insulin signaling. Science 332: 1322–1326.
25. Veeriah S, Brennan C, Meng S, Singh B, Fagin JA, et al. (2009) The tyrosine phosphatase PTPRD is a tumor suppressor that is frequently inactivated and mutated in glioblastoma and other human cancers. Proc Natl Acad Sci U S A 106: 9435–9440.
26. Lai R, Navid F, Rodriguez-Galindo C, Liu T, Fuller CE, et al. (2006) STAT3 is activated in a subset of the Ewing sarcoma family of tumours. J Pathol 208: 624–632.
27. Misale S, Yaeger R, Hobor S, Scala E, Janakiraman M, et al. (2012) Emergence of KRAS mutations and acquired resistance to anti-EGFR therapy in colorectal cancer. Nature 486: 532–536.
28. Vilar E, Tabernero J (2012) Cancer: Pinprick diagnostics. Nature 486: 482–483.
29. Diaz LA Jr, Williams RT, Wu J, Kinde I, Hecht JR, et al. (2012) The molecular evolution of acquired resistance to targeted EGFR blockade in colorectal cancers. Nature 486: 537–540.
30. Bouchahda M, Karaboue A, Saffroy R, Innominato P, Gorden L, et al. (2010) Acquired KRAS mutations during progression of colorectal cancer metastases: possible implications for therapy and prognosis. Cancer Chemother Pharmacol 66: 605–609.
31. Zhang W, Zong CS, Hermanto U, Lopez-Bergami P, Ronai Z, et al. (2006) RACK1 recruits STAT3 specifically to insulin and insulin-like growth factor 1 receptors for activation, which is important for regulating anchorage-independent growth. Mol Cell Biol 26: 413–424.
32. Ma PC, Kijima T, Maulik G, Fox EA, Sattler M, et al. (2003) c-MET mutational analysis in small cell lung cancer: novel juxtamembrane domain mutations regulating cytoskeletal functions. Cancer Res 63: 6272–6281.
33. To CT, Tsao MS (1998) The roles of hepatocyte growth factor/scatter factor and met receptor in human cancers (Review). Oncol Rep 5: 1013–1024.
34. Puri N, Ahmed S, Janamanchi V, Tretiakova M, Zumba O, et al. (2007) c-Met is a potentially new therapeutic target for treatment of human melanoma. Clin Cancer Res 13: 2246–2253.
35. Krishnaswamy S, Kanteti R, Duke-Cohan JS, Loganathan S, Liu W, et al. (2009) Ethnic differences and functional analysis of MET mutations in lung cancer. Clin Cancer Res 15: 5714–5723.
36. Huang CH, Mandelker D, Schmidt-Kittler O, Samuels Y, Velculescu VE, et al. (2007) The structure of a human p110alpha/p85alpha complex elucidates the effects of oncogenic PI3Kalpha mutations. Science 318: 1744–1748.
37. Vanhaesebroeck B, Waterfield MD (1999) Signaling by distinct classes of phosphoinositide 3-kinases. Exp Cell Res 253: 239–254.
38. Vivanco I, Sawyers CL (2002) The phosphatidylinositol 3-Kinase AKT pathway in human cancer. Nat Rev Cancer 2: 489–501.
39. Samuels Y, Diaz LA Jr, Schmidt-Kittler O, Cummins JM, Delong L, et al. (2005) Mutant PIK3CA promotes cell growth and invasion of human cancer cells. Cancer Cell 7: 561–573.

11

Low Molecular Weight Procyanidins from Grape Seeds Enhance the Impact of 5-Fluorouracil Chemotherapy on *Caco-2* Human Colon Cancer Cells

Ker Y. Cheah[1,2], Gordon S. Howarth[2,3], Keren A. Bindon[4], James A. Kennedy[4,5], Susan E. P. Bastian[1]*

1 Wine Science and Business Group, School of Agriculture, Food and Wine, Waite Campus, The University of Adelaide, PMB 1, Glen Osmond, Australia, **2** Centre for Paediatric and Adolescent Gastroenterology, Children, Youth and Women's Health Service, North Adelaide, Australia, **3** School of Animal and Veterinary Sciences, Roseworthy Campus, The University of Adelaide, Australia, **4** The Australian Wine Research Institute, Urrbrae, Adelaide, Australia, **5** Department of Viticulture and Enology, California State University, Fresno, California, United States of America

Abstract

Objective: Grape seed procyanidins (PC) are flavan-3-ol oligomers and polymers known for their biological activity in the gut. Grape seed extract (GSE) have been reported to reduce intestinal injury in a rat model of mucositis. We sought to investigate effects of purified PC fractions differing in mean degree of polymerization (mDP) combined with 5-Fluorouracil (5-FU) chemotherapy on the viability of colon cancer cells (Caco-2).

Design: SixPC fractions (F1-F6) were isolated from Cabernet Sauvignon seeds at two ripeness stages: pre-veraison unripe (immature) and ripe (mature), utilizing step gradient, low-pressure chromatography on a Sephadex LH-20 resin. Fractions were tested on Caco-2 cells, alone and in combination with 5-FU. Eluted fractions were characterized by phloroglucinolysis and gel permeation chromatography. Cell viability was determined by the 3-(4,5-Dimethylthiazol-2yl)-2,5-diphenyl-tetrazolium bromide) (MTT) assay.

Results: All isolated fractions significantly reduced Caco-2 cell viability compared to the control (P<0.05), but F2 and F3 (mDP 2–6) were the most active fractions (immature F2 = 32% mDP 2.4, F3 = 35% mDP 5.8 and mature F2 = 13% mDP 3.6 and F3 = 17% mDP 5.9; percentage of viable cells remaining) on Caco-2 cells. When combined with 5-FU, immature fractions F1-F3 enhanced the cell toxicity effects of 5-FU by 27–73% (*P*<0.05). Mature seed PC fractions (F1–F4) significantly enhanced the toxicity of 5-FU by 60–83% against Caco-2 cells (*P*<0.05). Moreover, some fractions alone were more potent at decreasing viability in Caco-2 cells (*P*<0.05; immature fractions = 65–68% and mature fractions = 83–87%) compared to 5-FU alone (37%).

Conclusions: PCs of mDP 2–6 (immature F1-F3 and mature F1 and F4)not only enhanced the impact of 5-FU in killing Caco-2 cells, but also surpassed standard 5-FU chemotherapy as an anti-cancer agent.The bioactivity of PC is therefore attributed primarily to lower molecular weight PCs.

Editor: Rajeev Samant, University of Alabama at Birmingham, United States of America

Funding: Professor Gordon Howarth is supported by a South Australian Health and Medical Research Institute Cancer Council Senior Research Fellowship. The current study was performed under the collaboration between Wine Science and Business Group, The University of Adelaide and Australian Wine Research Institute (AWRI). The funders had no role in study design, data collection and analysis, decision to publish, or preparation of the manuscript.

Competing Interests: The authors have have declared that no competing interests exist.

* E-mail: sue.bastian@adelaide.edu.au

Introduction

Colorectal cancer has the second highest mortality, and is the fourth most frequently diagnosed form of cancer in the United States [1]. The primary treatment for colon cancer involves surgical bowel resection and chemotherapy, most often by 5-Fluorouracil (5-FU) [2]. Unfortunately, chemotherapy cannot discriminate between normal and cancer cells, and it targets areas where cells are replaced at a high rate, such as in the mouth and gut [3]. This leads to the development of mucositis (gastrointestinal toxicity). Current mucositis treatments are largely ineffective as they target only the symptoms, but not the pathogenesis of the condition [3]. Thus, it is important to seek new alternative treatments which not only target mucositis but also enhance chemotherapeutic action without compromising the well-being of patients.

Increasingly, grape seed extracts (GSEs) are being studied due to their reported health benefits for a variety of disorders such as cancer [4],cardiovascular disease[5,6] and ulcerative colitis [7,8]. The beneficial effects of GSEs have been attributed to polyphenolic procyanidins (PCs) [9], comprising flavan-3-ol subunits. The polymer length of PC is described by the degree of polymerization (DP). Due to their polymerized structure, cellular absorption is restricted to oligomers with a lower DP, leaving the larger DP molecules for adsorption in the gut lumen following oral administration [10,11]. A number of studies have reported the polymerization and galloylation of PCs to be responsible for their anti-proliferative effects on transformed cells [9,12,13].

There is increasing evidence suggesting GSEs are effective at reducing the proliferation of cancer cells without being cytotoxic to normal cells [14]. Additionally, GSE has demonstrated partial amelioration of intestinal damage in a rat model of intestinal mucositis and has reduced gastrointestinal cell toxicity following chemotherapy treatment in normal IEC-6 intestinal cells [15]. However, the bioactive components in GSE remain unknown. The primary aim of the current study was to identify the chemical composition of the bioactive PC fractions, and investigate their potential in combination with 5-FU chemotherapy, for their effects on the viability of colon cancer cells. When in combination with 5-FU, certain PC fractions further enhanced toxicity in colon cancer cells.

Materials and Methods

Ethic statements

Cabernet Sauvignon grape samples were obtained from commercial vineyards, Accolade Wines (Orlando) in the Langhorne Creek growing region of South Australia, which has a latitude 35°16′11.56″S and a longitude 139°00′14.47″E, with an elevation approximately 28 m above sea level. No permits were required for the described study, which complied with all relevant regulations.

Grape sampling and preparation

Grape samples were collected at different stages of ripeness: immature (preveraison, green seeds) and mature (25–26° Brix, brown seeds) during the 2009 growing season. Grape berries were prepared according to a previously described method [16] in which grapes were collected and kept frozen at −20°C. While still frozen, seeds were removed from the flesh with a scalpel. Seeds were then wiped clean of flesh with a paper towel and re-frozen at −20°C prior to extraction.

Preparation and extraction of seed procyanidins (PCs)

PC extraction commenced by extracting seeds (100 g) overnight for 18 h in 70% acetone (200 mL, v/v) and ascorbic acid (1 g/L). The extract was concentrated under reduced pressure at 35°C (HeidolphLaborota 4011 rotary evaporator, John Morris Scientific, Adelaide, Australia), and lyophilized to a dry powder (Dynavac FD3 freeze drier, Dynavac Pty Ltd, Sydney, Australia). Yields for each samples were: immature 6.31 g and mature 10.29 g. PC seed powder (5 g) was dissolved in 50 mL of methanol (60%, v/v) containing trifluoroacetic acid (TFA) (0.05%, v/v) and then applied (~18.3 mL/min) to a 300 mm x 21 mm glass column (Michel-Miller, Vineland, NJ, USA) containing Sephadex LH20 chromatography resin (Amersham, Uppsala, Sweden) to an approximate bed volume of 93 mL, and washed off in 250 mL of methanol (60%, v/v) containing TFA (0.05%, v/v) to remove low molecular weight monomers. PC was then recovered in 150 mL of aqueous acetone (70%, v/v) and the extracts was concentrated in a rotary evaporator at 35°C to remove acetone. The aqueous solution was extracted with hexane to remove residual lipophilic material using a separatory funnel. The aqueous extract was freeze-dried into powder and recovered amount for two extracts were; immature, 2.5 g and mature, 0.9 g respectively. Powders were kept under nitrogen and at −20°C prior to fractionation.

For fractionation of PCs, seed PC powder (0.5 g) was dissolved in methanol (60%, v/v) containing TFA (0.05%, v/v) and applied to the same column under identical conditions. PC seed extract was fractionated according to a step-gradient elution method described previously [16] to produce 6 fractions with increasing mean degree of polymerization (mDP) and molecular weights of PCs designated as F1 to F6. The eluted fractions were concentrated under pressure at 35°C to remove organic solvents and further lyophilized into dry powder. The isolated fractions were stored at −20°C prior to analysis. Grape seed extract was a generous gift from Tarac Technologies (GraPex seed tannin; North Adelaide, South Australia) and was included in the study as a control. GSE (1 g) was dissolved in methanol (60%, v/v) containing TFA (0.05%, v/v) and fractionated accordingly.

Acid catalysis of PC in the presence of excess phloroglucinol (Phloroglucinolysis)

Phloroglucinolysis was used to determine subunit composition, mDP and galloylation of PC. Pholoroglucinolysis was performed according to a previously described method [16]. Seed fractions were dissolved in methanol (10 mg/mL, v/v) and equal volumes (25 μL) of extract and phloroglucinol solution (0.2 N HCL and 100 g/L phloroglucinol and 20 g/L ascorbic acid) to give a final PC concentration of 5 g/L. The phloroglucinolysis reaction was carried out at 50°C for 25 min and analysed by RP-HPLC using (−)-epicatechin (Sigma Aldrich, St. Louis, MO) as the quantitative standard.

Gel Permeation Chromatography (GPC)

Gel permeation chromatography was performed based on a previously described method [16]. The GPC technique characterises information on the size distribution of PC for each fraction. Fractionated samples (10 mg/mL) were dissolved in methanol and further diluted with 4 volumes of HPLC mobile phase (*N,N*-dimethylformamide containing glacial acetic acid (1%, v/v), water (5%, v/v) and 0.15 M lithium chloride). The flow-rate was maintained at 1 ml/min with a column temperature of 60°C and elution was monitored at 280 nm. The maximum amount of PC injected onto the column was 40 μg. PC seed fractions from a previous study[17] were used as standards for calibration. Calibration curves of fractionated PCs with their cumulative mass distribution were plotted and the mean molecular mass of the fractions was predicted at 50%.

Ferric reducing antioxidant power (FRAP) assay

This assay was carried out following a modified protocol [18]. Briefly, FRAP reagent was prepared (300 mM acetate buffer, pH 3.6, 10 mM 2,4,6-tri[2-pyridyl]-s-triazine (TPTZ) solution in 40 mM HCL, 20 mM ferrous chloride; in 10:1:1 v/v) and kept in the dark at 37°C prior to analysis. Fractions were dissolved in dimethylsulfoxide (DMSO) (0.1 mg/mL) and 15 μL were added to 96-well plates. 15 μL of FRAP reagent was added to the wells containing the fractions and the plate was read at 593 nm after 4 min (Multiskan Spectrum, Therma Electron Corporation, Vantaa, Finland) using Skanit software 2.2. Ferrous sulphate (0.1–1 mM) was used to construct a standard curve and FRAP values of test compounds were expressed as mMFe(II)/g of sample. Each treatment was tested in triplicate and the whole experiment was repeated three times. The data are expressed as mean ± SEM of 3 independent experiments.

Cell preparation and experimental treatment

The human colon cancer cell line, Caco-2 was obtained from American Type Culture Collection (ATCC, Manassas, USA). Cells were maintained in Dulbecco Modified Eagle Medium (DMEM) at 37°C and in a 5% CO_2 incubator. Media were replaced twice in each week. PC fractions were dissolved in DMSO and kept at −20°C prior to analysis. Caco-2 cells were seeded at 1000 cells/well in 96-well tissue culture plates (Grenier Bio-one, Victoria, Australia) and incubated at 37°C in 5% CO_2 for 48 h to allow attachment. After 48 h of incubation, the media were replaced with different concentrations of seed fractions dissolved in DMEM (μg/mL) containing <0.025% (v/v) of DMSO and 5-FU (100 μM) (DBL, Mayne Pharma Pty. Ltd., Victoria, Australia). Cells were further incubated at 37°C, 5% CO_2 for 24, 48 and 72 hrs.

MTT assay

The (3-(4,5-Dimethylthiazol-2yl)-2,5-diphenyl-tetrazolium bromide) (MTT) assay was performed based on a previously described method, with slight modification [19]. After exposure to the treatments (seed extracts and 5-FU), 50 μL of MTT (1 mg/mL in Dulbecco's Phosphate Buffered Saline) was added to each well and further incubated at 37°C, 5% CO_2 for 4 h. After 4 h, the medium was aspirated and 100 μL of DMSO added to dissolve the formazan product. Plates were placed on a shaking incubator for 15 min and read at 570 nm by a UV spectrophotometer. Each treatment was tested in triplicate and the whole experiment was repeated three times. The data are expressed as mean ± SEM of 3 independent experiments. Data were expressed as number of viable cells compared with the percentage of control cells treated with serum free DMEM. Control cells represent either cell treated with serum free DMEM only or cell treated with 100 μM 5-FU.

Statistical analysis

Each cell-based experiment was performed at least 3 times. Statistical analyses were performed using XLSTAT version 12.0 for Windows or PASW statistic version 18. Statistical analysis was determined by two-way ANOVA with Tukey's*post-hoc* test.

A Pearson's correlation coefficient was calculated to determine the relationship between cell viabilities, PC composition and antioxidant value. Statistical significance was considered at $P<0.05$.

Chemicals

Acetone, ascorbic acid, methanol, trifluoroacetic acid (TFA), phloroglucinol, (−)-epicatechin, N,N-dimethylformamide, lithium chloride, sodium acetate (CH3COONa), 2,4,6-tri[2-pyridyl]-s-triazine (TPTZ), ferrous chloride and methanol were purchased from Sigma Chemical Co. Ltd, St Louis, MO. Hydrochloric acid (HCL), glacial acetic acid, Folin-ciocalteau reagent and ferrous sulphate were purchased from AnalaR, BDH, MERCK, Pty. Ltd., Australia. Tissue culture solutions include Dulbecco's Modified Eagle's Minimum Essential Medium (DMEM), Dulbecco's Phosphate Buffered Saline, dimethyl sulfoxide (DMSO) and 3-(4,5-Dimethylthiazol-2yl)-2,5-diphenyl-tetrazolium bromide) (MTT) were purchased from Gibco BRL, Life Tehnologies Pty Ltd, Australia.Pty. Ltd.

Instrumentation

An Agilent model 1100 HPLC (Agilent Technologies Australia Pty Ltd., Melbourne, Australia) was used with Chemstation software for chromatographic analyses.

Results

Characterization of PC fractions

GSE was included in the current study as a control. The PC composition of GSE is illustrated in Table 1. Compared to Cabernet Sauvignon seed extracts, GSE had low mass conversion (23.8% w/w) and also a lower molecular mass, as measured by phloroglucinolysis and GPC. The PC terminal subunits in GSE were mostly dominated by (−)-epicatechin-3-*O*-gallate. Due to the apparently low contribution of PCs in GSE, we isolated PCs from fresh Cabernet Sauvignon seed harvested at different stages as previous reports showed a high mass conversion in unprocessed grape seeds [16].

Comparing purified PC from both seed samples, the immature seed had higher mass conversion (87%) compared to mature seeds (71%) (Table 2). The purified PCs were further fractionated into 6 fractions with increasing mDP or molecular mass. The mass conversion yield for conversion of PC into known PC was >49%, except for the highest mDP F6 (approximately 37%). The major differences between immature and mature seed fractions were that mature fractions had a higher proportion of (−)-epicatechin terminal subunits (9-30%) compared to the immature fractions (2-11%). Both mature and immature seed fractions showed a similar pattern of decreasing (−)-epicatechin terminal subunits with increasing mDP. Interestingly, the increases in polymerisation or molecular weight were mainly controlled by (−)-epicatechin-3-*O*-gallate extension subunits. The galloylation of immature fractions ranged from 15-35% and mature fractions range from 9–24%. Immature F2 had the highest galloylation (35%), mainly driven by a high proportion of (−)-epicatechin-3-*O*-gallate (88%).

Antioxidant capacity of seed fractions

The antioxidant capacity of seed fractions was measured by the FRAP assay (Figure 1). GSE, which contained a mixture of oligomers and polymers of PCs, was included as a positive control to determine the antioxidant activity of the seed fractions. Compared to GSE (5 mM/g), all the fractions had higher FRAP values, ranging from 5.4–8.8 mM/g. The antioxidant capacity of the fractions decreased in the more polymerized PC fractions. The FRAP values were negatively correlated with mDP ($r^2 = -0.81$, $P<0.05$).

Effects of seed fractions on the viability of Caco-2 cells

The cytotoxic effects of seed fractions on Caco-2 cells were determined by the MTT assay (Figure 2). Caco-2 cells were exposed to seed fractions for 72 hr and the data expressed as IC_{50}, defined as the dose of each compound that inhibited cell viability to 50%, representing the mean value of three independent experiments. All fractions showed a degree of toxicity as indicated by decreased absorbance values. The IC_{50}value (mean of the three independent experiments) for immature seed fractions (F1-F6) ranged from 17.7–70.2 μg/mL (Figure 2A). The number of viable cells was positively correlated with the mDP of immature seed fractions ($r^2 = 0.48$, $P<0.05$) i.e., the fractions with highest mDP (F5 and F6) were less toxic to Caco-2 cells. Similar trends in terms of cytotoxic effects were also observed for the application of mature seed fractions (Figure 2B), where the number of viable cells was similarly correlated with the mDP of the fractions ($r^2 = 0.50$, $P<0.05$). Mature seed fractions exhibited stronger cytotoxicity compared to immature seed fractions (Figure 2A and 2B).

The combined effect of isolated seed fractions and 5-FU on the viability of Caco-2 cells

The combined effect of seed fractions and 5-FU on Caco-2 cells was investigated (Figure 3). For immature seed fractions, the viability of Caco-2 cells was significantly inhibited by all seed fractions (Figure 3A). Compared to GSE (67%), F2 and F3 of immature seed extracts were more toxic to Caco-2 cells (F2, 32% and F3, 35% of control value, $P<0.05$). However, when seed

Table 1. The chemical profiles of commercial grape seed extracts (GSE) and its isolated fractions characterized by phloroglucinolysis and gel permeation chromatography (GPC).

Procynidin	MC[a]	mDP[b]	galloylation	MM[c]	MM[d]	Mass[e]	Terminal subunits[f]			Extension subunits[f]		
Fraction	(%)		(%)	(subunit)	(GPC 50%)	(%)	C	E	ECG	C-P	E-P	ECG-P
GSE Control[g]	23.8	5.9	19	1871	1400	100	20.1	14.0	65.9	8.9	53.0	38.1
F1	37.1	2.0	6	593	974	7	43.7	40.3	16.0	19.1	63.4	17.5
F2	34.8	3.0	18	961	1870	8	22.3	16.9	60.8	11.6	59.8	28.6
F3	30.7	4.4	22	1423	3330	9	19.6	12.3	68.1	7.5	52.6	39.9
F4	14.4	6.5	23	2108	4490	11	19.6	10.3	70.2	7.6	47.3	45.1
F5	19.2	7.5	21	2432	4490	5	21.8	11.4	66.8	7.0	48.2	44.8
F6	28.7	9.1	21	2928	4400	5	22.4	10.6	67.1	6.3	48.9	44.8

[a]Mass conversion based on % recovery of procyanidin by phloroglucinolysis based on the gravimetric mass. [b]Mean degree of polymerization in epicatechin units. [c]Molecular mass as determined by phloroglucinolysis. [d]Molecular mass as determined by GPC at 50% procyanidin elution. [e]Percent composition of procyanidin fractions by gravimetric recovery. [f]Percent composition of subunits (in moles) with the following subunit abbreviations: (-P), phloroglucinol adduct of extension subunit; C, (+)-catechin; EC, (−)-epicatechin; ECG, (−)-epicatechin-3-O-gallate. [g]Crude grape seed extract of which 55% w/w eluted in F0 and 45% w/w was recovered as procyanidin for further fractionation.

fractions were present with 5-FU (100 uM), the growth inhibitory effects of 5-FU were significantly enhanced ($P<0.05$) (Figure 3A). 5-FU significantly reduced cell viability to 62% of control values ($P<0.05$). F1-F3 significantly enhanced the growth inhibitory activity of 5-FU (27%, 73% and 56% respectively compared to 5-FU control; $P<0.05$). F2 could therefore be considered a more potent chemotherapy agent than unfractionated commercially available GSE, which only enhanced the growth inhibitory effect of 5-FU by 55% ($P<0.05$; compared to 5-FU control). Moreover, we also found that immature F2 (32%) and F3 (35%) were more potent than 5-FU (62% of control value; $P<0.05$) at reducing Caco-2 viability.

Mature seed fractions behaved in a similar manner to immature seed fractions (Figure 3B). Mature seed fractions significantly reduced cell viability ($P<0.05$). F2 and F3 were more cytotoxic to Caco-2 cells (13% and 17% respectively, $P<0.05$) than GSE (47%) (Figure 3B). When cells were exposed to seed fractions and 5-FU, all seed fractions enhanced the capacity of 5-FU to reduce cell viability. GSE significantly enhanced the growth inhibition of 5-FU by 49%. However, F1-F4 significantly enhanced the growth inhibitory effect of 5-FU (62%, 83%, 80% and 60% respectively compared to 5-FU control; $P<0.05$). Moreover, the F2 (13%), F3 (17%) and F4 (50%) fractions were more potent than 5-FU alone (65% of control value; $P<0.05$) (Figure 3B).

Discussion

Grape seed PCs have been reported to exert health-promoting properties, particularly in the gut [14,15,20,21]. In addition to its anti-cancer efficacy, GSE has been demonstrated to reduce gastrointestinal toxicity following chemotherapy treatment in healthy animals and in normal intestinal cells [15]. Although there is growing evidence to support the chemotherapeutic properties of GSE in colon cancer, identification of the bioactive components responsible remains undefined.

In the current study, PC fractions isolated from commercially available GSE showed different mDPs and molecular sizes. However, these fractions had very low conversion yields (< 37%), indicating that less than 40% of the fractions were characterised using the selected analysis techniques, which was unacceptable for this study. The explanation for the low conversion yield in PC fractionsmay have been due to oxidation occurring during generation of GSEs from the winemaking process. Thus, it was decided to isolate PC fractions from fresh grapes collected at different maturities: immature (pre-veraison) and mature (ripe). This decision was based on the observation that immature seeds have a higher conversion yield than mature seeds [22], substantiated by the current study. Moreover, future studies utilizing mass spectrometry are warranted to further define the purity of PCs isolated from grape seeds.

The cytotoxic effects of PC fractions on cancer cells have been reported previously [9,12,13]. However, whether these effects occurred through extracellular signalling or following uptake of PCs was not attempted. The present study showed that the most active fractions affecting the viability of Caco-2 cells contained smaller oligomers: F2 and F3. The more potent cytotoxic effects observed in Cabernet Sauvignon seed fractions compared to GSE may have reflected a lower PC yield in GSE (~24%) compared to PC isolated from fresh grapes (~60%).

Absorption of PC across cell membranes was greatly dependent upon their mDPs [23,24]. Only certain lower mDP PCs are absorbed during transit in the gut, leaving the larger mDP PCs (mDP >7) deposited in the gut lumen. This result supports the current data whereby F2 and F3 (mDP 2–6) and likely to be

Table 2. The chemical profile of immature and mature fractions characterized by phloroglucinolysis and gel permeation chromatography (GPC).

Procynidin	MC[a]	mDP[b]	galloylation	MM[c]	MM[d]	Mass[e]	Terminal subunits[f]			Extension subunits[f]		
Fraction	(%)		(%)	(subunit)	(GPC 50%)	(%)	C	E	ECG	C-P	E-P	ECG-P
Immature[g]	86.5	4.9	24	1593	3334	100	19.6	9.5	70.9	6.6	47.6	45.8
F1	48.7	2.0	15	619	882	7.7	35.8	11.0	53.1	22.7	65.0	12.3
F2	64.0	2.4	35	818	1280	12.9	9.6	2.2	88.3	12.4	61.1	26.0
F3	65.1	5.8	22	1893	5670	17.9	17.4	3.3	79.3	7.0	53.4	39.6
F4	62.7	10.0	23	3262	7600	24.4	17.5	4.1	78.4	5.8	47.9	46.3
F5	52.7	16.3	23	5313	7810	28.4	20.1	5.0	75.0	5.5	46.0	48.5
F6	37.7	18.8	22	6063	7940	8.8	24.4	4.6	71.0	5.4	47.3	47.3
Mature[g]	71.2	4.4	20	1404	2863	100	27	20.7	52.6	7.7	48.1	44.3
F1	64.0	2.3	9	706	896	10.9	36.8	30.2	32.9	20.0	62.1	17.9
F2	64.2	3.6	20	1150	1550	14.2	21.3	12.2	66.5	10.3	56.6	33.1
F3	66.0	5.9	23	1927	3620	21.3	19.5	9.3	71.1	6.7	49.0	44.4
F4	68.0	8.7	24	2840	6620	27.4	19.5	9.1	71.5	5.8	45.4	48.8
F5	54.1	12.0	23	3906	7190	17.6	21.1	9.3	69.6	5.9	45.9	48.2
F6	36.5	15.1	21	4886	7400	8.7	22.3	10.2	67.4	5.8	47.5	46.6

[a]Mass conversion based on % recovery of procyanidin by phloroglucinolysis based on the gravimetric mass. [b]Mean degree of polymerization in epicatechin units. [c]Molecular mass as determined by phloroglucinolysis. [d]Molecular mass as determined by GPC at 50% procyanidin elution. [e]Percent composition of procyanidin fractions by gravimetric recovery. [f]Percent composition of subunits (in moles) with the following subunit abbreviations: (-P), phloroglucinol adduct of extension subunit; C, (+)-catechin; EC, (−)-epicatechin; ECG, (−)-epicatechin-3-*O*-gallate. [g]Purifiedprocyanidin from immature (preveraison) and mature (ripe) Cabernet Sauvignon seeds prior to fractionation.

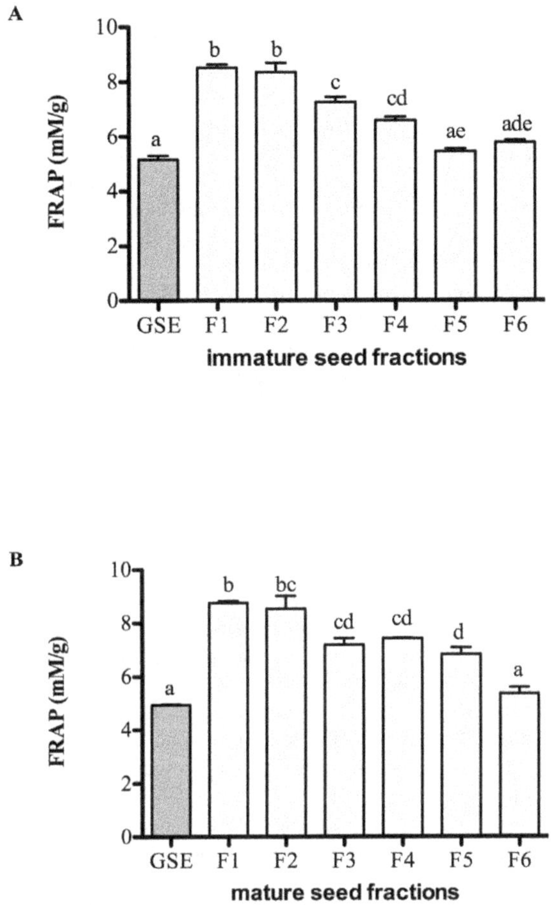

Figure 1. Antioxidant activity of the fractions from immature (A) and mature (B) seed extracts measured by Ferric reducing antioxidant power (FRAP) assay. Results are expressed as mean ± SEM of 3 independent experiments. Statistical analysis was determined by one-way ANOVA with Tukey's*post-hoc* test. Values with different letters (a,b,c) in each column are statistically different at $P<0.05$.

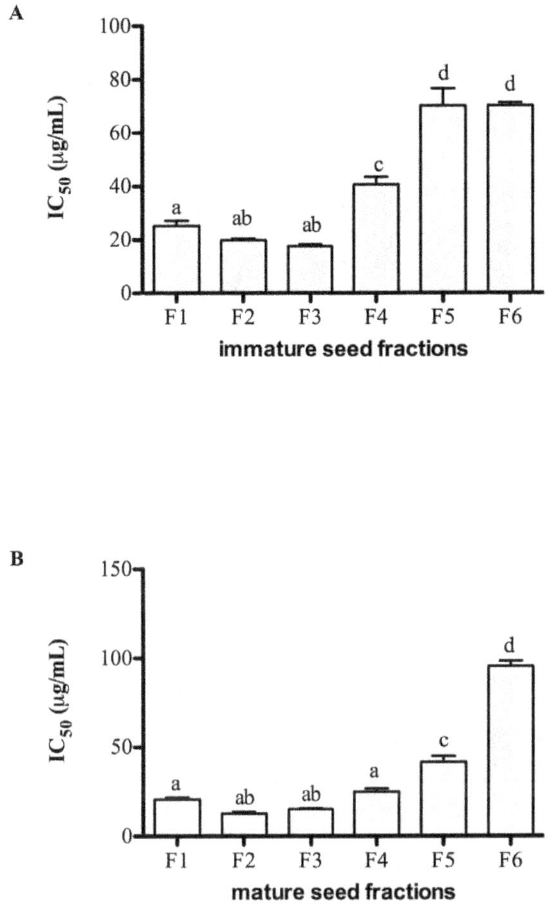

Figure 2. Viability of Caco-2 cells after exposure to fractions from immature (A) and mature (B) seed extracts for 72 hr measured by 3-(4,5-Dimethylthiazol-2yl)-2,5-diphenyl-tetrazolium bromide (MTT) assay. Data are expressed as IC_{50} or dose (μg/mL) inhibiting cell viability to 50% (mean ± SEM) of 3 independent experiments. Statistical analysis was determined by one-way ANOVA with Tukey's*post-hoc* test. Values with different letters (a,b,c) in each column were statistically different at $P<0.05$.

absorbed across the cell membranes were more potent than fractions with a higher mDP, which exert a surface effect only. However, F2 and F3 were more bioactive than F1, possibly due to their higher percentage of galloylation and proportion of epicatechin-3-*O*-gallate as terminal subunits, compared to F1. This result is in agreement with other studies in which PC fractions with higher galloylation were more cytotoxic than PC fractions with lower galloylation when tested on colon cancer cells [9,25]. However, the actual mechanism of PCs on cell growth remains unknown. Absorbed PC may play a vital role in interfering with cell signalling pathways. PCs have been reported to be inhibitors of androgen receptors in prostate cancer cells[26,27] and epidermal growth factor receptors on colon cancer cells [28]. In addition, PCs are known to attenuate the PI3-kinase (serine/threonine protein kinase) pathway [14] which could lead to induction of cell cycle arrest at G1 phase [20] and activation of the apoptosis-inducing pathway [29]. Future studies investigating the endpoints of cell growth and apoptosis including PI uptake, caspase 3 activity and sub-G1 DNA content are warranted.

Previous findings have demonstrated that the cytotoxic effects of PCs are dependent on their mDP [9,13]. Nevertheless, the current study showed that fractions with higher mDP (7–16) failed to exert cytotoxic effects on colon cancer cells. However, the current study used a different solvent system to isolate PC fractions compared to other studies [9,30]. This solvent system isolates PC fractions with a wider range of molecular mass (619–6063 g/mol) and mDP (2–9) compared to other methods (molecular mass of 552–1232 g/mol, mDP 1–4); implying that the previous studies only measured limited PC fractions (<1200 g/mol) for their biological activities.

The antioxidant capacity of PCs is greatly dependent upon their degree of polymerization and galloylation [9]. The reduction of metal ions, as measured by the FRAP assay, is believed to be positively correlated with the number of hydroxyl groups present in the molecules, and that the points of attachment to transition metal ions in the flavonoid molecules are at the *o*-catechol group of ring B [31]. However, this was not the case in the current study. PC fractions with higher mDP were weaker antioxidants, which is in agreement with previous studies [32,33]. Fractions with larger subunits tend to self-aggregate and cause stereochemical hindrance [33,34], thereby exposing fewer hydroxyl groups for radical scavenging activities. Future studies should be performed to address the antioxidant properties of grape seed PCs including the impact on cellular antioxidant status.

The current study was performed based on the basis of a previous study of GSE and chemotherapy on the viability of colon

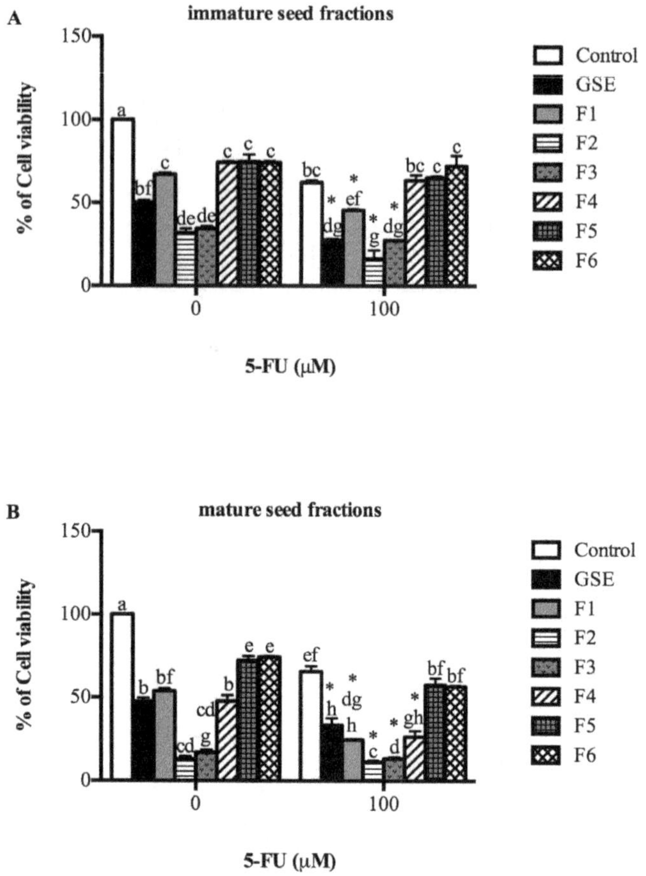

Figure 3. Combined effects of immature (A) and mature (B) fractions and 5-FU on Caco-2 cells for 72 hr measured by 3-(4,5-Dimethylthiazol-2yl)-2,5-diphenyl-tetrazolium bromide (MTT) assay. Data are presented as percentage of cell viability relative to viability of control cells. Data are expressed as mean ± SEM of 3 independent experiments. Statistical analysis was determined by two-way ANOVA with Tukey's*post-hoc* test. Values with different letters (a,b,c) in each column were statistically different at $P<0.05$. * indicates significant difference in 5-FU treated group when compared to 5-FU control.

cancer cells [35]. The doses of grape seed fractions in the current study were selected based on the basis of this previous study. 5-FU is an anti-metabolite drugs which block DNA synthesis via inhibition of thymidylate synthase [3].When seed extract fractions were combined with 5-FU, they not only enhanced the impact of 5-FU in killing Caco-2 cells, but also surpassed 5-FU as an anti-cancer agent. In the current study, the effects of PC fractions and 5-FU on Caco-2 cell viability were examined over 24–72 hr. 5-FU (100 uM) significantly reduced cancer cells viability to 60–80%, gastrointestinal toxicity in cancer patients. Exposure of PC fraction and 5-FU to cells for 24–48 hr did show a trend towards a synergistic effect but was not significant (data not shown). Moreover, greater time exposure (72 hr) to PC fractions and 5-FU resulted in greatest reduction of cell viability. The current study also revealed that mature seed fractions were superior to immature seed fractions as chemotherapeutic agents against colon cancer *in vitro*. The chemical profile of the mature seed fractions showed that these effects could be driven by their higher proportion of (−)-epicatechin as terminal subunits compared to the immature seed extract. Another possible explanation could have been the distribution within each fraction of a higher proportion of low molecular weight material in the mature seeds than immature seeds.

The current study showed that the most active fractions affecting the viability of Caco-2 were F2 and F3. However, whether these effects occurred through extracellular signalling or following uptake of PCs is not known. Further studies are warranted to determine the intestinal absorption of PC fractions in normal intestinal cell lines. TheMTT assay is an indirect measure of cell viability based on metabolic activity. The reduction of cell viability observed in the current study could be attributed to an effect on cell cycle or cell proliferation. Hence, additional studies investigating cell cycle, cell proliferation and cell death activities (Annexin V/PI staining, LDL release assay, caspase-3 and Bcl-2 quantification) could provide evidence of the impact of specific sizes of PCs oncell signalling. Testing PC fractions in other colon cell lines (normal and neoplastic) might exclude general toxicity and provide further evidence of PC potential.

In conclusion, further studies are warranted to determine the molecular mechanism of F2 and F3 on cellular pathways associated with colonic neoplasia. Mature seed PC extracts not only have potential uses in human health, but alsoin turn value-add to the wine producing industry, as the mature grape seeds are the major by-products of winemaking. Our data provides compelling evidence that combining PC fractions and 5-FU may be a potential chemopreventative agent in colon cancer treatment regimens; however, further confirmatory *in vitro* studies are required with different classes of chemotherapy drugs followed by *in vivo* cancer model trials to better define the potential role of grape seed PCs against colon cancer.

Author Contributions

Conceived and designed the experiments: KYC GSH JAK SEPB. Performed the experiments: KYC KAB. Analyzed the data: KYC GSH KAB JAK SEPB. Contributed reagents/materials/analysis tools: GSH SEPB. Wrote the paper: KYC GSH KAB JAK SEPB.

References

1. Jemal A, Siegel R, Xu J, Ward E (2010) Cancer statistics, 2010. CA Cancer J Clin 60: 277–300.
2. Van Cutsem EJ, Kataja VV, Force EGT (2005) ESMO Minimum Clinical Recommendations for diagnosis, adjuvant treatment and follow-up of colon cancer. Ann Oncol 16 Suppl 1: i16–17.
3. Keefe DM, Sonis ST, Bowen JM (2008) Emerging drugs for chemotherapy-induced mucositis. Expert Opin Emerg Drugs 13: 511–522.
4. Huang S, Yang N, Liu Y, Gao J, Huang T, et al. (2012) Grape seed proanthocyanidins inhibit colon cancer-induced angiogenesis through suppressing the expression of VEGF and Ang1. Int J Mol Med 30: 1410–1416.
5. Du Y, Guo H, Lou H (2007) Grape seed polyphenols protect cardiac cells from apoptosis via induction of endogenous antioxidant enzymes. J Agric Food Chem 55: 1695–1701.
6. Huang S, Yang N, Liu Y, Hu L, Zhao J, et al. (2012) Grape seed proanthocyanidins inhibit angiogenesis via the downregulation of both vascular endothelial growth factor and angiopoietin signaling. Nutr Res 32: 530–536.
7. Wang YH, Ge B, Yang XL, Zhai J, Yang LN, et al. (2011) Proanthocyanidins from grape seeds modulates the nuclear factor-kappa B signal transduction pathways in rats with TNBS-induced recurrent ulcerative colitis. Int Immunopharmacol 11: 1620–1627.
8. Cheah KY, Bastian SE, Acott TM, Abimosleh SM, Lymn KA, et al. (2013) Grape seed extract reduces the severity of selected disease markers in the proximal colon of dextran sulphate sodium-induced colitis in rats. Dig Dis Sci 58: 970–977.
9. Ugartondo V, Mitjans M, Tourino S, Torres JL, Vinardell MP (2007) Comparative antioxidant and cytotoxic effect of procyanidin fractions from grape and pine. Chem Res Toxicol 20: 1543–1548.

10. Scalbert A, Morand C, Manach C, Remesy C (2002) Absorption and metabolism of polyphenols in the gut and impact on health. Biomed Pharmacother 56: 276–282.
11. Choy YY, Jaggers GK, Oteiza PI, Waterhouse AL (2013) Bioavailability of intact proanthocyanidins in the rat colon after ingestion of grape seed extract. J Agric Food Chem 61: 121–127.
12. Pierini R, Kroon PA, Guyot S, Ivory K, Johnson IT, et al. (2008) Procyanidin effects on oesophageal adenocarcinoma cells strongly depend on flavan-3-ol degree of polymerization. Mol Nutr Food Res 52: 1399–1407.
13. Lizarraga D, Lozano C, Briede JJ, van Delft JH, Tourino S, et al. (2007) The importance of polymerization and galloylation for the antiproliferative properties of procyanidin-rich natural extracts. FEBS J 274: 4802–4811.
14. Engelbrecht AM, Mattheyse M., Ellis B., Thomas M., Smith R., Peters S., Smith C., Myburgh K. (2007) Proanthocyanidin from grape seeds inactivates the PI3-kinase/PKB pathway and induces apoptosis in a colon cancer cell line. Cancer Letters 258: 144–153.
15. Cheah KY, Howarth GS, Yazbeck R, Wright TH, Whitford EJ, et al. (2009) Grape seed extract protects IEC-6 cells from chemotherapy-induced cytotoxicity and improves parameters of small intestinal mucositis in rats with experimentally-induced mucositis. Cancer Biol Ther 8: 382–390.
16. Bindon KA, Kennedy JA (2011) Ripening-induced changes in grape skin proanthocyanidins modify their interaction with cell walls. J Agric Food Chem 59: 2696–2707.
17. Bindon KA, Smith PA, Kennedy JA (2010) Interaction between grape-derived proanthocyanidins and cell wall material. 1. Effect on proanthocyanidin composition and molecular mass. J Agric Food Chem 58: 2520–2528.
18. Benzie IF, Szeto YT (1999) Total antioxidant capacity of teas by the ferric reducing/antioxidant power assay. J Agric Food Chem 47: 633–636.
19. Huynh-Delerme C, Huet H, Noël L, Frigieri A, Kolf-Clauw M (2005) Increased functional expression of P-glycoprotein in Caco-2 TC7 cells exposed long-term to cadmium. Toxicology in Vitro 19: 439–447.
20. Kaur M, Agarwal R., Agarwal C. (2008) Grape seed extract induced cell cycle arrest and apoptosis in human colon carcinoma cells. Nutrition Cancer 60: 2–11.
21. Dinicola S, Cucina A, Pasqualato A, D'Anselmi F, Proietti S, et al. (2012) Antiproliferative and Apoptotic Effects Triggered by Grape Seed Extract (GSE) versus Epigallocatechin and Procyanidins on Colon Cancer Cell Lines. Int J Mol Sci 13: 651–664.
22. Kennedy JA, Taylor AW (2003) Analysis of proanthocyanidins by high-performance gel permeation chromatography. J Chromatogr A 995: 99–107.
23. Spencer JP, Schroeter H, Shenoy B, Srai SK, Debnam ES, et al. (2001) Epicatechin is the primary bioavailable form of the procyanidin dimers B2 and B5 after transfer across the small intestine. Biochem Biophys Res Commun 285: 588–593.
24. Deprez S, Mila I, Huneau JF, Tome D, Scalbert A (2001) Transport of proanthocyanidin dimer, trimer, and polymer across monolayers of human intestinal epithelial Caco-2 cells. Antioxid Redox Signal 3: 957–967.
25. Actis-Goretta L, Romanczyk LJ, Rodriguez CA, Kwik-Uribe C, Keen CL (2008) Cytotoxic effects of digalloyl dimer procyanidins in human cancer cell lines. J Nutr Biochem 19: 797–808.
26. Choi KC, Park S, Lim BJ, Seong AR, Lee YH, et al. (2010) Procyanidin B3, an inhibitor of histone acetyltransferase, enhances the action of antagonist for prostate cancer cells via inhibition of p300-dependent acetylation of androgen receptor. Biochem J 433: 235–244.
27. Park SY, Lee YH, Choi KC, Seong AR, Choi HK, et al. (2011) Grape seed extract regulates androgen receptor-mediated transcription in prostate cancer cells through potent anti-histone acetyltransferase activity. J Med Food 14: 9–16.
28. Kern M, Tjaden Z, Ngiewih Y, Puppel N, Will F, et al. (2005) Inhibitors of the epidermal growth factor receptor in apple juice extract. Mol Nutr Food Res 49: 317–328.
29. Dinicola S, Cucina A, Pasqualato A, Proietti S, D'Anselmi F, et al. (2010) Apoptosis-inducing factor and caspase-dependent apoptotic pathways triggered by different grape seed extracts on human colon cancer cell line Caco-2. Br J Nutr 104: 824–832.
30. Torres JL, Varela B, Garcia MT, Carilla J, Matito C, et al. (2002) Valorization of grape (Vitis vinifera) byproducts. Antioxidant and biological properties of polyphenolic fractions differing in procyanidin composition and flavonol content. J Agric Food Chem 50: 7548–7555.
31. Rice-Evans CA, Miller NJ, Paganga G (1996) Structure-antioxidant activity relationships of flavonoids and phenolic acids. Free Radic Biol Med 20: 933–956.
32. Nomoto H, Iigo M, Hamada H, Kojima S, Tsuda H (2004) Chemoprevention of colorectal cancer by grape seed proanthocyanidin is accompanied by a decrease in proliferation and increase in apoptosis. Nutr Cancer 49: 81–88.
33. Faria A, Calhau C, de Freitas V, Mateus N (2006) Procyanidins as Antioxidants and Tumor Cell Growth Modulators. Journal of Agricultural and Food Chemistry 54: 2392–2397.
34. Poncet-Legrand C, Cartalade D, Putaux J-L, Cheynier V, Vernhet A (2003) Flavan-3-ol Aggregation in Model Ethanolic Solutions: Incidence of Polyphenol Structure, Concentration, Ethanol Content, and Ionic Strength. Langmuir 19: 10563–10572.
35. Cheah KY, Howarth GS, Bastian SE (2014) Grape seed extract dose-responsively decreases disease severity in a rat model of mucositis; concomitantly enhancing chemotherapeutic effectiveness in colon cancer cells. PLoS One 9: e85184.

12

Prospective Study of the Evolution of Blood Lymphoid Immune Parameters during Dacarbazine Chemotherapy in Metastatic and Locally Advanced Melanoma Patients

Grégoire Mignot[1,2¶], Alice Hervieu[1,2,3¶], Pierre Vabres[2,3], Sophie Dalac[3], Geraldine Jeudy[3], Blandine Bel[3], Lionel Apetoh[1,2,4], François Ghiringhelli[1,2,4*]

1 INSERM, UMR866, Dijon, France, **2** Faculté de Médecine, Université de Bourgogne, Dijon, France, **3** Service de Dermatologie, Centre Hospitalier Universitaire le Bocage, Dijon, France, **4** Oncologie médicale, Centre Georges François Leclerc, Dijon, France

Abstract

Background: The importance of immune responses in the control of melanoma growth is well known. However, the implication of these antitumor immune responses in the efficacy of dacarbazine, a cytotoxic drug classically used in the treatment of melanoma, remains poorly understood in humans.

Methods: In this prospective observational study, we performed an immunomonitoring of eleven metastatic or locally advanced patients treated with dacarbazine as a first line of treatment. We assessed by flow cytometry lymphoid populations and their activation state; we also isolated NK cells to perform in vitro cytotoxicity tests.

Results: We found that chemotherapy induces lymphopenia and that a significantly higher numbers of naïve $CD4^+$ T cells and lower proportion of Treg before chemotherapy are associated with disease control after dacarbazine treatment. Interestingly, NK cell cytotoxicity against dacarbazine-pretreated melanoma cells is only observed in NK cells from patients who achieved disease control.

Conclusion: Together, our data pinpoint that some immune factors could help to predict the response of melanoma patients to dacarbazine. Future larger scale studies are warranted to test their validity as prediction markers.

Editor: Nikolas K. Haass, University of Queensland Diamantina Institute, Australia

Funding: This work was supported by ligue nationale contre le cancer (équipe labellisée), Institut National du Cancer and by a French Government grant managed by the French National Research Agency under the program "Investissements d'Avenir" with reference ANR-11-LABX-0021 (Lipstic Labex). G. M. was supported by a grant from the Fondation pour la Recherche Médicale. The funders had no role in study design, data collection and analysis, decision to publish, or preparation of the manuscript.

Competing Interests: The authors have declared that no competing interests exist.

* Email: fghiringhelli@cgfl.fr

¶ GM and AH are first senior authors on this work.

Introduction

In the last few years, there have been many considerable changes in the treatment of metastatic melanoma, with the development of BRAF and MEK tyrosine kinase inhibitors and monoclonal antibody immunotherapies, such as anti CTLA-4 and anti PD-1, which have proved efficacy both in term of clinical response and overall survival. However, in metastatic melanoma patients who presented side effects, no indications or failure of targeted therapies or immunotherapy, "classical" cytotoxic chemotherapy is still used, namely dacarbazine (DTIC).

It has been shown that some cytotoxic drugs could affect the immune system and the antitumor immune response. The first mechanism is directly related to the cytotoxic property of these agents on cancer cells. The seminal discovery was that cancer death induced by some chemotherapies could prime $CD8^+$ T cell antitumor immune response. This phenomenon is an essential contributor to the antitumor effect of some major anticancer drugs such as anthracyclines and oxaliplatin both in mice and humans [1–4]. The second phenomenon involves the capacity of some anticancer agents to selectively kill or affect the biology of some immune cells. Anticancer drugs can eliminate immunosuppressive cells and enhance antitumor immune responses [5–7] or mitigate cytotoxic antitumor immunity by inducing some immunosuppressive mechanisms [8]. In a recent work, using a mouse melanoma model B16F10, we identified DTIC immunological effect. While DTIC did not directly affect immune cells in this mouse model, we observed that DTIC triggered the expression of NKG2D ligands on tumor cells that led to activation of natural killer (NK) cells, interferon (IFN)γ secretion, then activation of cytotoxic T cells [9,10]. We also observed that *in vitro* DTIC treatment enhanced NKG2D ligand expression on human melanoma cell lines. We thus formulated the hypothesis that for some patients, DTIC may also enhance NK cell toxicity toward melanoma cells and that this could be related to the clinical response to DTIC.

To address this question, we performed immunomonitoring of lymphoid subpopulations of patients with metastatic melanoma before and after a first cycle of DTIC treatment.

Material & Methods

Patients

To monitor immune markers that could potentially be implicated in melanoma as prognosis and/or prediction for treatment response, we immunomonitored patients from the university Hospital of Dijon (France), bearing unresectable or metastatic melanoma. All patients gave their written informed consent and were treated with the cytotoxic chemotherapy DTIC at 1 g/m^2 every four weeks. The response rate was evaluated one month after the third cycle of treatment by CT scan, according to RECIST criteria 1.1. This trial received approbation of the ethics committee of the Hospital of Dijon under the number 2010/55 eudract n: 2010-02358-34 and was conducted following the Declaration of Helsinki's protocol. Patient whose death was related to cancer are counted as "dead", the others are censored after their last sign-of-life.

Blood sample preparation

Blood samples were obtained from patients before the first and second cycle of chemotherapy. Blood was collected in vacutainer tubes, with EDTA for determination of total leukocytes, lymphocytes and granulocytes concentration or with citrate for immunomonitoring. Citrated samples were diluted 1:1 with RPMI1640 (Lonza) and centrifugated on a cushion of lymphocyte separation medium (Eurobio). Peripheral blood mononuclear cells (PBMC) were collected and washed once with phosphate buffered saline (PBS) 5% bovine serumalbumin (BSA). 5% of the pellet was taken for further polymerase chain reaction (PCR) analysis, 10% for flow cytometry analysis and the remaining cells underwent NK cell separation with an NK cell isolation kit (Miltenyi Biotech), followed by separation on AutoMACS (Miltenyi).

Cytotoxicity assay

The MelC human melanoma cell line was a kind gift from Dr Anne Caignard. MelC cells, previously treated with PBS or DTIC (0.4 g/L) were incubated overnight either alone or with freshly purified NK cells from patients. Tumor cells were harvested and death was assayed using DAPI (4′,6′-diamidino-2-phénylindole) staining (Sigma Aldrich) by flow cytometry. Tumor cells were identified by their characteristic size and granularity, and cells positives for DAPI staining were considered dead.

PCR analysis

Total RNA from PBMC was extracted using TRIZOL (Invitrogen) as recommended by the manufacturer. The RNAs were rehydrated and measured with a NanoDrop 1000 (Thermo-Scientific). Reverse transcription was performed using the kit "M-MLV Reverse Transcriptase" (Invitrogen) as recommended by the manufacturer using a Biometra thermocycler. The quantitative PCR reaction was performed using the kit "SYBR Green PCR Master Mix" (Applied Biosystems) according to manufacturer's recommendations, on an Applied 7500 device (Applied Biosystems). Relative mRNA levels were determined using the difference in cycle threshold (ΔCt) method. Values were expressed relative to *ACTB*. We detected *ACTB* (with primers GATCATTGCTCC-TCCTGAGC and TGCGCAAGTTAGGTTTTGTC), *EOMES* (CAGCACCACCTCTACGAACA and CGCCACCAAACTGA-GTGAT), *TBX21* (AACATCCTGTAGTGGCTGGTG and C-CACCTGTTGTGGTCCAAGT) and *RORC* (AAGCAGGAG-CAATGGAAGTG and GCAATCTCATCCTCGGAAAA).

Flow cytometry

Blood counts (leukocytes, granulocytes, lymphocytes and monocyte counts) were performed on the Xn2000 (Sysmex) device, which is the device used for clinical blood count in Dijon's hospital routine care. Fluorescent data were produced using a LSRII cytometer (BD Pharmingen). PBMC were stained in PBS/5%BSA with antibodies indicated in Table 1. All antibodies were purchased from Biolegend (Ozyme) and used according to the manufacturer's protocol. Analyses were done with FlowJo software (Tristar). Events were considered positive if their fluoresence was higher than matched- isotype control staining peak fluorescence. The gating strategy is summarized in Fig. S1 & S2.

Statistical analysis

We used Mann-Whitney's test for nonparametric means comparison. Student's t test was used when variance were tested comparable by Fisher-Snedecor's test. Paired tests were used when applicable. Linear correlations were assessed using the Pearson correlation coefficient. All tests were performed and graphed with GraphPad Prism 6 software. All p values were two-tailed. A p value inferior to 0.05 was considered statistically significant for all experiments and is indicated with *.

Results

Patients

Eleven patients were included in this prospective observational trial. Patients' clinical characteristics are described in Table 2. In our cohort, one patient exhibited partial response, two showed disease stabilization and eight had progressive disease following DTIC treatment. Patients that showed partial response or disease stabilization after DTIC were grouped as "disease control". So, in our cohort, there were 3 (27%) patients with disease control and 8 (73%) with progressive disease, which is consistent with the published response rates to DTIC in the literature [11,12]. Survival analysis (Fig. S3) underscores that patients with progressive disease have a shorter survival than those with disease control (median survival 7 vs 19.5 months, respectively, Mantel-Cox'test $p = 0.0379$).

Blood count

A total blood count was performed before the first and second cycle of chemotherapy. One injection of DTIC induced no change in the total number of leucocytes (Fig. 1A). When looking at leukocyte types, we observed a drop in total lymphocyte count (Fig. 1B, $p = 0.0439$), whereas no significant modifications were observed for monocyte (Fig. 1C) or granulocyte counts (Fig. 1D). Neither lymphocyte nor monocyte counts before or after chemotherapy were associated with disease control (not shown). Surprisingly, patients with disease control showed a tendency of higher granulocyte counts after treatment compared to the progressive disease group (Fig. 1E).

T cells

We did not observe differences in total number of CD4$^+$ or CD8$^+$ T cells before and after chemotherapy (Fig. 2A), although a tendency could be observed for both, accounting for the diminution of total lymphocyte count (Fig. 1B). When looking at memory and naïve subpopulations, we observed that chemotherapy did not significantly affect the number of naïve CD4$^+$ T cells

Table 1. Antibodies for flow cytometry analysis.

Antigen	Clone	Panel 1	Panel 2	Panel 3
CD3	UCHT1	PE	PE/Cy7	PE
CD4	RPA-T4	PerCP		PerCP
CD8	HIT8a	PE/Cy7		
CD16	3G8		Alexa fluor 700	
CD45RA	HI100	Brillant Violet 570		
CD56	MEM-188		PE	
CD69	FN50	Alexa Fluor 647	Alexa Fluor 488	
FOXP3	206D			Alexa Fluor 647

PerCP: Peridinin chlorophyll; PE: Phycoerythrin; Cy7: Cyanine-7.

(Fig. 2B) or naïve CD8$^+$ T cells (not shown). However, high numbers of naïve (CD45RA$^+$) CD4$^+$ T cells before chemotherapy are seen in patients with controlled disease (Fig. 2C). Neither the numbers of CD4$^+$ or CD8$^+$ T cells after one cycle of chemotherapy, nor naïve CD8$^+$ T cell number are correlated with clinical outcome (Not shown).

T cell polarization

The polarization state of T cells was determined using the monitoring of master controller transcription factors using RT-qPCR. There was a strong correlation between expression of *EOMES*, coding for eomesodermin, before and after treatment and survival (Fig. 3A), thus suggesting that CD8$^+$ or NK cells anti-tumor cytotoxic responses would be associated with longer survival. We did not find any correlation between the expression of *TBX21*, a gene coding for T-bet, before and after chemotherapy and overall survival (Fig. 3B). Conversely, after chemotherapy, the Th17 transcription factor, *RORC*, was associated with longer survival (Fig. 3C).

Regulatory T cells

We evaluated the proportion of FOXP3 positive cells amongst the CD3$^+$CD4$^+$ double-positive lymphocyte cells. There was a tendency for the proportion of FOXP3 expression to positively correlate with tumor stage (Fig. 4A). We noted that chemotherapy did not significantly affect FOXP3$^+$ cell numbers (Fig. 4B). However, we observed that, before chemotherapy, patients with disease control had fewer FOXP3$^+$ than those with progressive disease (Fig. 4C).

NK

Treatment had no significant effect on total number of either CD56^{hi} or CD56^{dim}CD16$^+$NK cell subsets (Fig. 5A). We also did not detect significant modifications of the activation state of NK cell subsets after chemotherapy using CD69 labeling (Fig. S4). Furthermore, we did not see any association between CD56^{dim}CD16$^+$ NK cell activation and response. However, we observed a higher activation of CD56^{hi} NK cells in patients with disease control after chemotherapy (Fig. 5B) thus suggesting that DTIC may help activation of CD56^{hi} NK cells in these patients.

We previously demonstrated that, in a mouse model, DTIC induces the expression of NK cell activating ligands on the surface of melanoma cells. This causes a better detection and lysis of DTIC-treated targets by NK cells [10]. To validate this observation in a human context, we tested in this cohort the cytotoxic properties of purified NK cells from patients before chemotherapy, against a human melanoma cell line *ex vivo* pretreated with DTIC at a dosage that triggers expression of NKG2D ligand [10]. We observed that NK purified from patients with progressive disease are unable to lyse either DTIC-treated targets or PBS-treated targets [13] (Fig. 5C, left panel), with a cytotoxicity -if any- comparable to the background mortality, i.e. the death of target cells cultured without NK cells, that is 6+/−1% (IC95[3.7–8.2]) and 5+/−1% (IC95[2.1–8.2]) for PBS- and DTIC-treated MelC cell, respectively. In contrast, NK cells from patients with disease control seem to have better capacity to kill pretreated DTIC target cells (Fig. 5C, right panel).

Discussion

To our knowledge, this study is the first that performs a systematic study of the effect of alkylating chemotherapy on all blood lymphoid cell subsets in melanoma patients. We observed that chemotherapy modestly but significantly affects the total number of lymphocytes, which is reduced after chemotherapy. This observation could be linked to the toxicity of this anticancer drug. However chemotherapy did not affect the number of CD8$^+$ or CD4$^+$ T cells or Treg or NK cells thus underscoring that such treatment is not a major immunosuppressive treatment.

High expression of *EOMES* gene, encoding eomesodermin is also correlated with longer survival. Eomesodermin has been described as a master regulator of cytotoxic CD8$^+$ T cells [14], and can also be expressed by NK cells in mice [15]. This suggest that the intrinsic presence of a cytotoxic cellular response could be important for DTIC efficacy, thus corroborating our previous mouse findings that DTIC antitumor effects are dependent on CD8 T cells and NK cells [10].

After treatment, high expression of *RORC*, coding for RORγt, a transcription factor responsible for CD4$^+$ Th17 differentiation, correlates with better survival. Th17 cell induction has already been described with various melanoma treatments, such as vaccination [16], anti-PD-1 [17], anti-CTLA4 [18], as well as other anticancer drugs such as cyclophosphamide [19]. Furthermore, it has been described that Th17 cells can drive antigen-dependent tumor shrinkage [20,21]. We hypothesize that Th17 cell induction after treatment could be a surrogate marker of efficacy. This event could be related to the association of high granulocyte counts in responder patients after treatment, because Th17 cells are well known to be important in the activation and recruitment of neutrophils.

CD4$^+$ T cell subsets seem to be associated with clinical outcome. In particular, the presence of higher number of naïve CD4$^+$ T cells at baseline is associated with better response to DTIC. In patients

Table 2. Patients' clinical characteristics.

Patient n°	Age	Sex	Histological type	Breslow score (mm)	Stade	Metastasis	Response	Survival (month)
1	85	Female	Desmoplastic	4	IIIC	Skin, lymph node	PR	18†
2	87	Female	Mucosal	N/A	II (*)		PD	6†
3	88	Female	Lentigo maligna	3,1	IV M1b	Lung, Lymph node	SD	21 No treatment
4	77	Male	Lentigo maligna	11	IV M1b	Lung, skin	PD	13†
5	66	Female	N/A	2,6	IIIC	Skin, lymph node	PD	1 Ipilimumab
6	95	Male	Superficial-spreading	3,5	IV M1b	Lung, skin, lymph node	PD	3†
7	62	Male	Superficial-spreading	1,1	IV M1c	Lung, lymph node, liver, bone, thyroide	PD	8†
8	69	Male	N/A	3,5	IV M1b	Lung	PD	12 Ipilimumab
9	44	Female	Superficial-spreading	1,6	IV M1c	Lung, lymph node, liver, brain	PD	3†
10	74	Female	Acral-lentiginous	2,4	IIIC	Skin	SD	9 No treatment
11	72	Female	Superficial-spreading	1,31	IV M1a	Skin, lymph node	PD	9†

PD: progressive disease.
PR: partial response.
SD: stable disease.
†: dead.
(*): Patient n°2 was inoperable, due to initial extension of its nasal tumor.

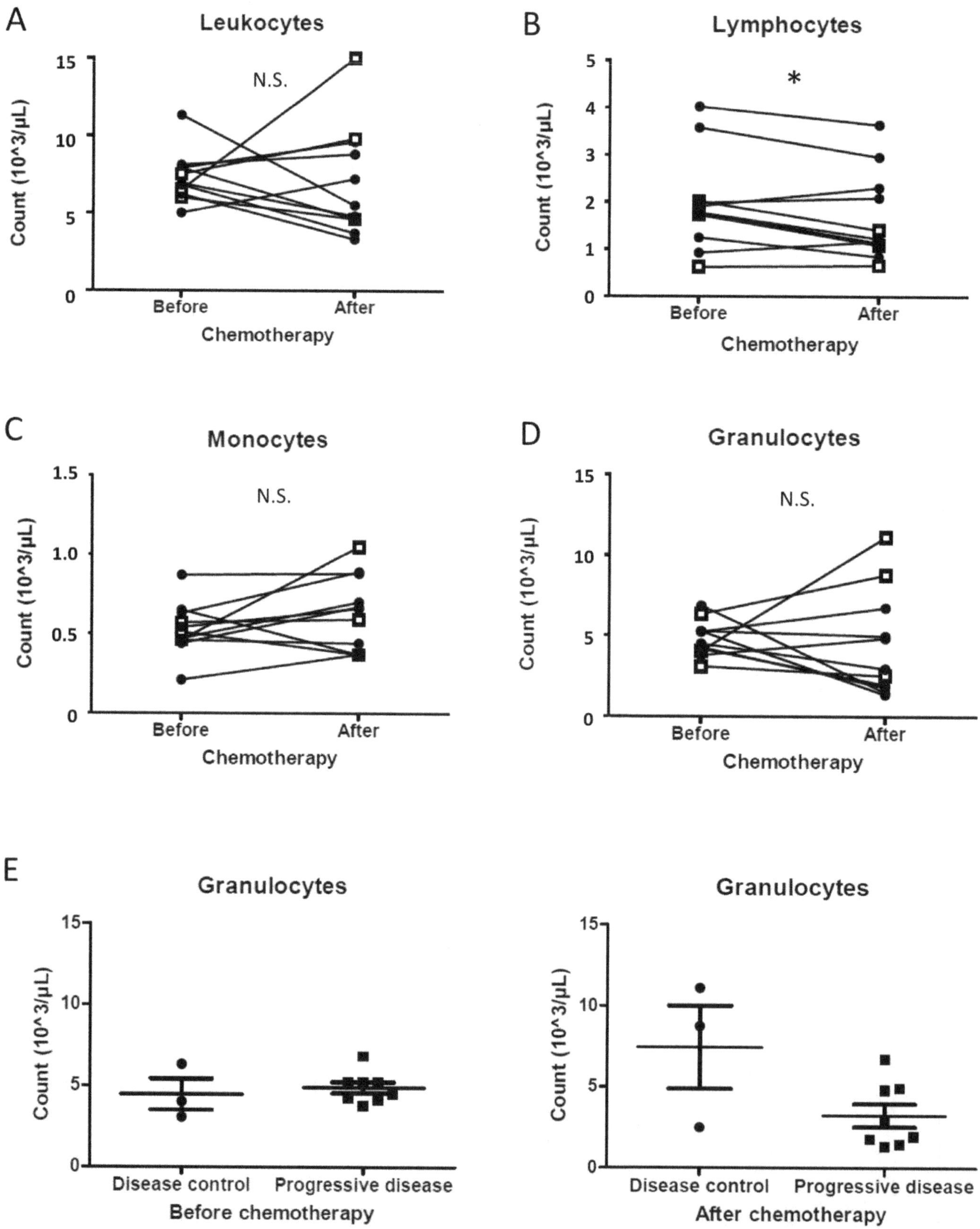

Figure 1. Chemotherapy causes changes in blood cells. We retrieved clinical data about leukocytes (A), lymphocytes (B), monocytes (C) and granulocytes (D) before the first ("Before") and second ("After") DTIC treatment. Black filled diamonds represent data from patients with progressive disease and white squares represent data from patients with disease control. For panel E, we compared granulocytes counts between patient groups before the first and second treatment (left and right panel, respectively).

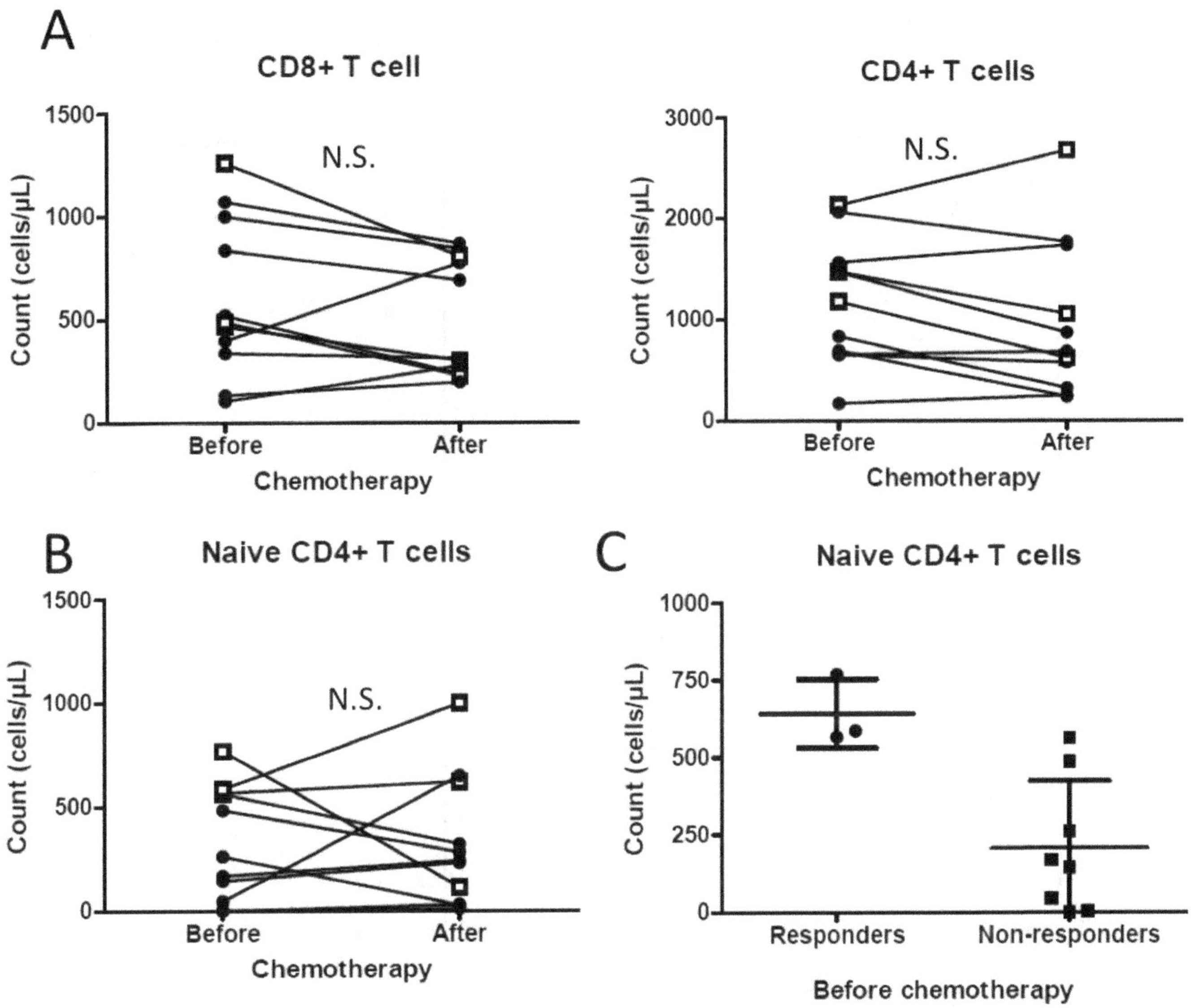

Figure 2. Treatment impacts T cell sub-populations. Panel A shows $CD8^+$ (left panel) and $CD4^+$ (right panel) T cell counts before and after chemotherapy. B and C: Naïve $CD4^+$ T cell counts before and after chemotherapy (B) and between patient groups (C). Black filled diamonds represent data from patients with progressive disease and white squares represent data from patients with disease control.

with low numbers of naïve $CD4^+$ T cells, we suspect that there is an increase in the number of memory and exhausted lymphocytes. Indeed, in chronic inflammatory situations such as cancer, the presence of chronic antigen stimulation leads to an exhausted or senescent memory phenotype of $CD4^+$ T cells. These cells are known to dampen anti-tumor immune response efficacy [22]. Such cells are known to accumulate in peripheral blood of cancer patients [23]. It is possible that the high number of exhausted lymphocytes could impair chemotherapy associated antitumor immune response, thus rendering such drug less effective. In addition, our study corroborates the previous finding that higher Treg rate is associated with advanced clinical stage [24]. Moreover, higher Treg number at baseline is associated with absence of response to DTIC. Such data suggest that high tumor burden and/or immunosuppressive state could impair antitumor efficacy of DTIC probably by inhibiting drug related antitumor immune response.

The major finding of this study is the relationship between NK cell activity and response to DTIC. We analyzed the two subsets of peripheral blood NK cells, that are described as functionnaly different[25]: $CD56^{hi}$ NK cells can secrete high amounts of cytokines [26], and $CD56^{lo}CD16^+$ are perceived as cytotoxic [27]. Our results show that, while DTIC did not affect the total number of NK cells, $CD56^{hi}$ NK cells from patients with disease control have a higher activation status than the patients with progressive disease. We previously showed that DTIC can enhance NKG2D ligand expression by melanoma cells [10]. In a mouse model, we showed that this causes IFNγ secretion by NK cells, followed by major histocompatibility complex expression by tumor cells, hence better recognition by T cells. We selected here a melanoma cell line in which DTIC *ex vivo* treatment induced up regulation of NKG2D ligands. We and others already described how these cells are killed by NK cells thanks to NKG2D-recognition [9,10,28]. Using this setting, we could see here that NK cells from responder patients seem to have a stronger capacity to kill DTIC- pretreated

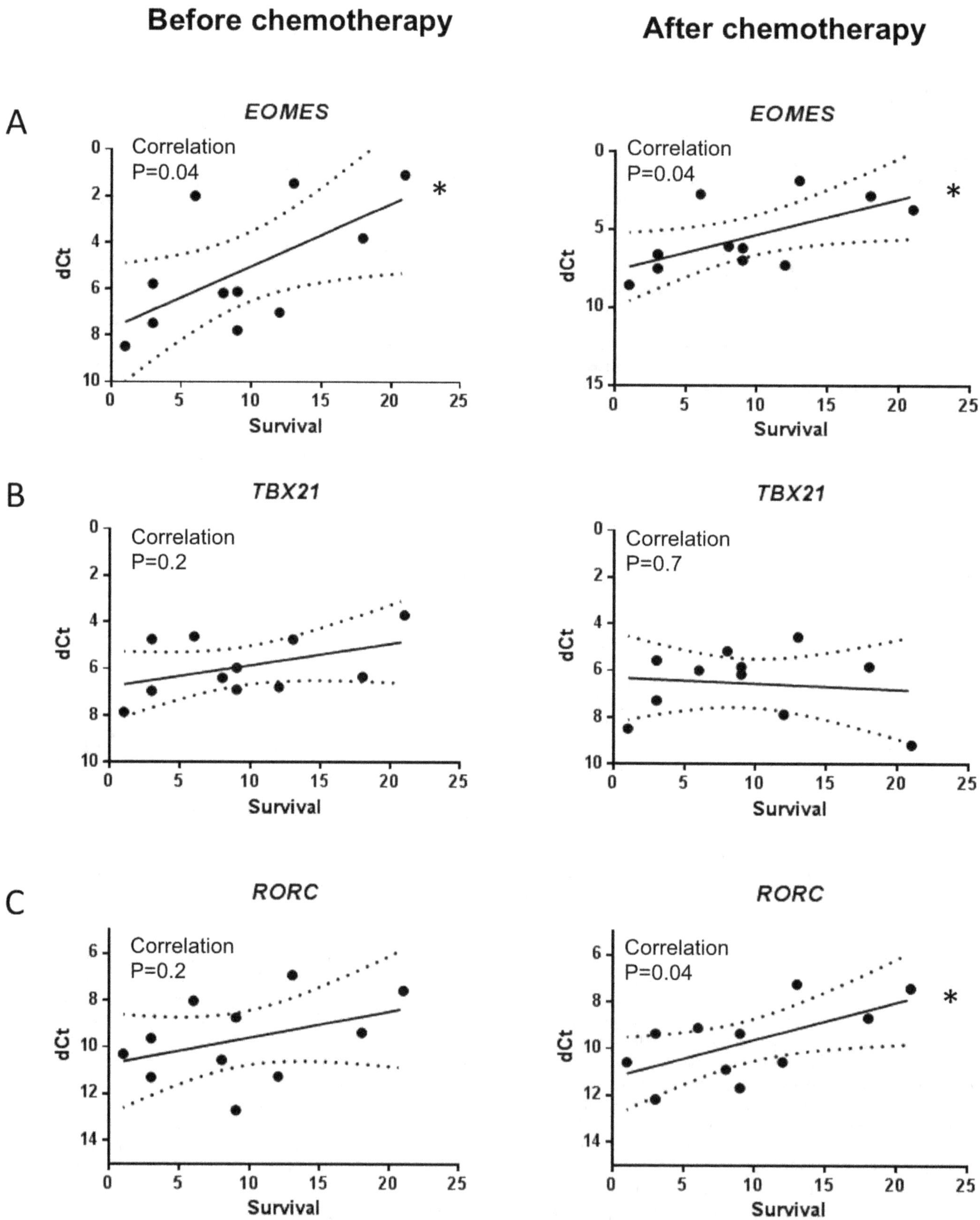

Figure 3. Correlation between T cell transcription factors and survival. We performed RT-qPCR on RNA from PBMC. Figure depicts relation between survival (in months) and expression level of indicated genes: *EOMES* (A), *TBX21* (B), *RORC* (C).

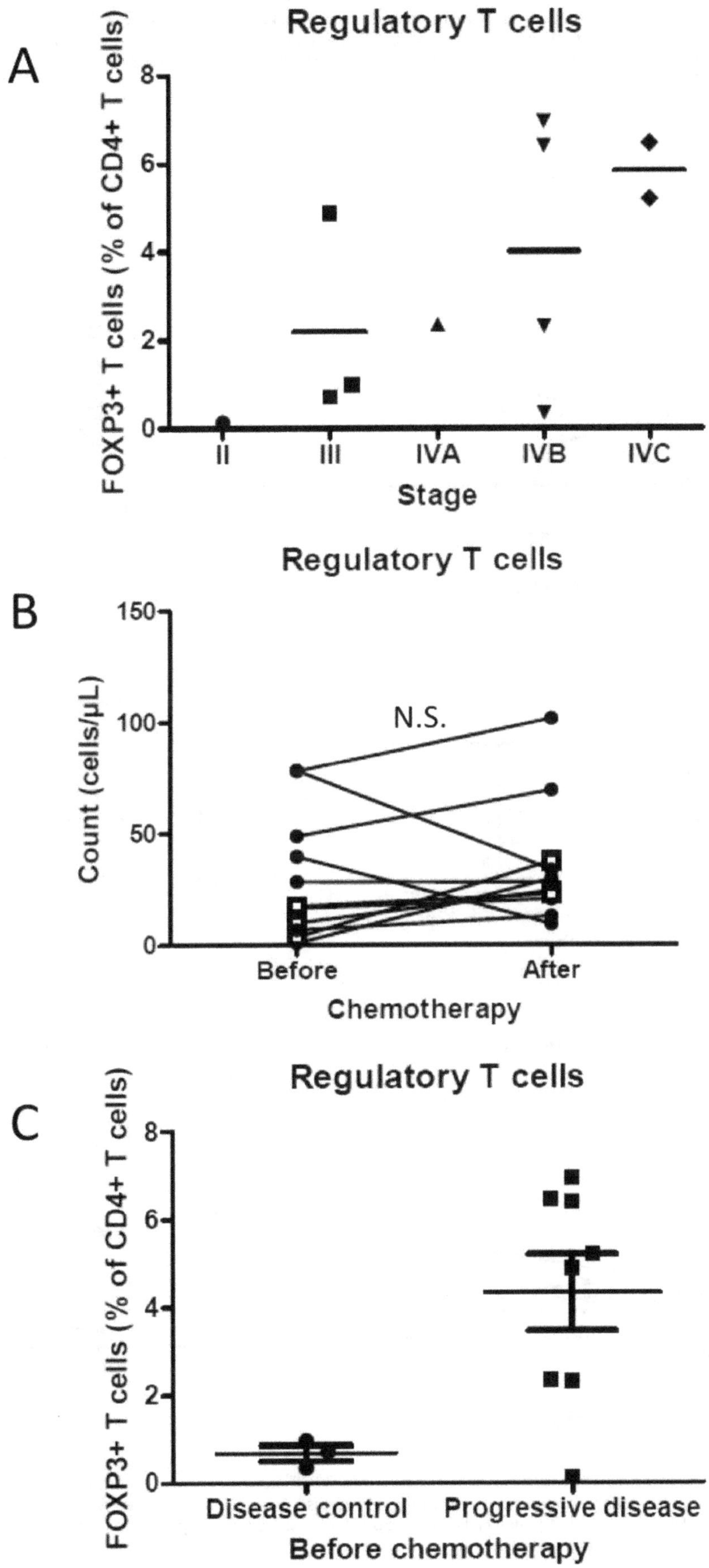
A
Regulatory T cells
FOXP3+ T cells (% of CD4+ T cells)
8
6
4
2
0
II
III
IVA
IVB
IVC
Stage
B
Regulatory T cells
Count (cells/µL)
150
100
50
0
N.S.
Before
After
Chemotherapy
C
Regulatory T cells
FOXP3+ T cells (% of CD4+ T cells)
8
6
4
2
0
Disease control
Progressive disease
Before chemotherapy

Figure 4. Regulatory T cells are associated with tumor grade and response to chemotherapy. A: The proportion of $FOXP3^+$ amongst $CD4^+$ T cells (Treg) is depicted in function of tumor grade of the corresponding patient. B: Treg numbers are depicted before and after treatment with DTIC. Black filled diamonds represent data from patients with progressive disease and white squares represent data from patients with disease control. C: Proportion of Treg amongst $CD4^+$ T cells.

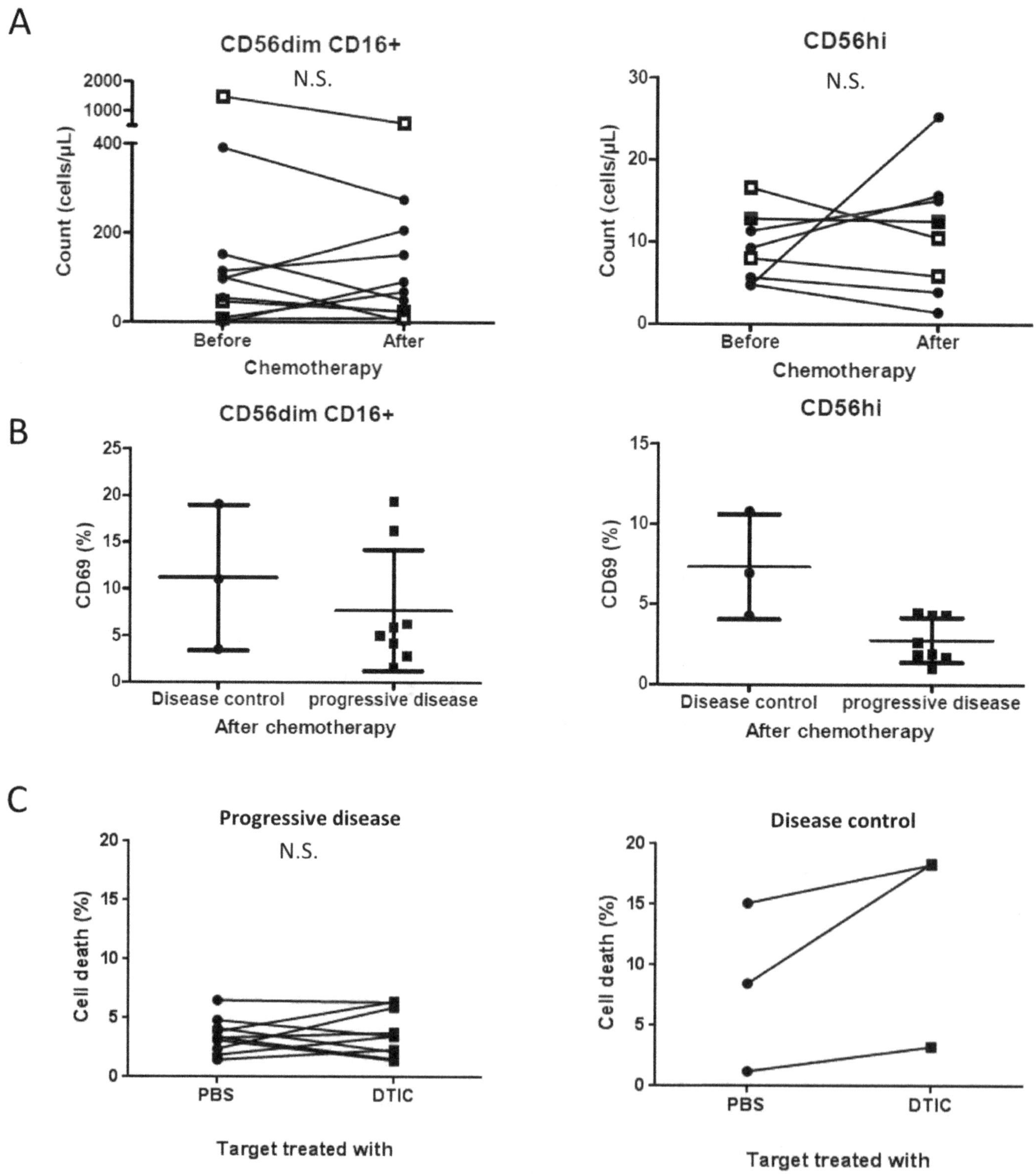

Figure 5. NK cell activity is related to chemotherapy response. A: $CD56^{dim}CD16^+$ (left panel) cells and $CD56^{hi}CD16^-$ (right panel) NK cells counts. Black filled diamonds represent data from patients with progressive disease and white squares represent data from patients with disease control. B: CD69 expression by $CD56^{dim}CD16^+$ (left panel) cells and $CD56^{hi}CD16^-$ NK cells (right panel). C: Death of MelC cells pretreated with PBS or DTIC, and cocultured with NK cells isolated from patients.

cancer cells than NK cells from patients with progressive disease. This is coherent with the published literature, as Anne Caignard's group described how NK cell phenotypes and functions vary according to tumor stage and treatment [28,29]. Indeed, they showed that NK cell receptor NKP46 expression by NK cells seems diminished in patient bearing metastatic melanoma, and that chemotherapy could increase expression of NKP46 by NK cells, but IFNγ secretion and degranulation are decreased after chemotherapy in ex-vivo assays, due to up-regulation of inhibiting factor NKG2A [28,29]. They also showed no variation of NKG2D expression by NK cells after chemotherapy or according to tumor stage. Our data support that alkylating chemotherapy such as DTIC is only effective in patients with functional NK cells and support that either some patients have intrinsic more proficient NK cells or that the tumor drives an immunosuppressive state, which blunts NK cell function. The second hypothesis is more probable because we described that pretreatment of melanoma cell line with DTIC enhanced the cytotoxicity of NK cells from healthy volunteers [10] and that high number of Treg before chemotherapy is associated with absence of response to DTIC.

Taken together, our study underscores some immune properties of DTIC and gives some preliminary data to isolate predictive factors of response. We believe that the two most promising factors are the importance of naïve CD4 T cell number and NK cell activity to predict response to chemotherapy. First, our results show that high Treg number and low number of naïve $CD4^+$ T cells are associated with disease progression after chemotherapy. These patients are presumably those with exhausted memory cells and may greatly benefit from immune-based treatments, such as anti-CTLA4 or anti-PD1 antibody, because these two treatments aim to reverse immune inhibition and exhaustion. Furthermore, patients having highly cytotoxic NK cells could be better candidates to DTIC-based treatment, as they may benefit the most from its immune effects, enhancing NK- and $CD8^+$T cell based cytotoxicity. Larger studies are warranted to validate these results.

Supporting Information

Figure S1 Flow cytometry strategy. We present here the gating strategy for flow fluorocytometry analysis. We present two examples of NK cell CD69 labelling.

Figure S2 Flow cytometry strategy for FOXP3 analysis. We present gating strategy for FOXP3+ analysis by flow fluorocytometry. We show two examples of FOXP3 labelling.

Figure S3 Survival curves. Comparison of survival curves of patient with progressive disease or disease control.

Figure S4 Activation of NK cells is not related to chemotherapy. We compared NK cell activation before and after chemotherapy. We used CD69 labelling by flow cytometry to assess activation of $CD56^{hi}$ (A) and $CD56^{dim}CD16^+$ NK cells (B).

Acknowledgments

We thank Anne Caignard (Hopital Cochin, Paris, France) for providing us the MelC melanoma cell line [28].

Author Contributions

Conceived and designed the experiments: FG GM. Performed the experiments: GM AH PV SD GJ BB. Analyzed the data: GM FG. Contributed reagents/materials/analysis tools: GM FG. Contributed to the writing of the manuscript: GM FG LA AH.

References

1. Tesniere A, Schlemmer F, Boige V, Kepp O, Martins I, et al. (2010) Immunogenic death of colon cancer cells treated with oxaliplatin. Oncogene 29: 482-491.
2. Apetoh L, Ghiringhelli F, Tesniere A, Obeid M, Ortiz C, et al. (2007) Toll-like receptor 4-dependent contribution of the immune system to anticancer chemotherapy and radiotherapy. Nat Med 13: 1050–1059.
3. Ghiringhelli F, Apetoh L, Tesniere A, Aymeric L, Ma Y, et al. (2009) Activation of the NLRP3 inflammasome in dendritic cells induces IL-1beta-dependent adaptive immunity against tumors. Nat Med 15: 1170–1178.
4. Obeid M, Tesniere A, Ghiringhelli F, Fimia GM, Apetoh L, et al. (2007) Calreticulin exposure dictates the immunogenicity of cancer cell death. Nat Med 13: 54–61.
5. Chalmin F, Ladoire S, Mignot G, Vincent J, Bruchard M, et al. (2010) Membrane-associated Hsp72 from tumor-derived exosomes mediates STAT3-dependent immunosuppressive function of mouse and human myeloid-derived suppressor cells. J Clin Invest 120: 457–471.
6. Mignot G, Ullrich E, Bonmort M, Menard C, Apetoh L, et al. (2008) The critical role of IL-15 in the antitumor effects mediated by the combination therapy imatinib and IL-2. J Immunol 180: 6477–6483.
7. Vincent J, Mignot G, Chalmin F, Ladoire S, Bruchard M, et al. (2010) 5-Fluorouracil selectively kills tumor-associated myeloid-derived suppressor cells resulting in enhanced T cell-dependent antitumor immunity. Cancer Res 70: 3052–3061.
8. Bruchard M, Mignot G, Derangere V, Chalmin F, Chevriaux A, et al. (2013) Chemotherapy-triggered cathepsin B release in myeloid-derived suppressor cells activates the Nlrp3 inflammasome and promotes tumor growth. Nat Med 19: 57–64.
9. Hervieu A, Mignot G, Ghiringhelli F (2013) Dacarbazine mediate antimelanoma effects via NK cells. Oncoimmunology 2: e23714.
10. Hervieu A, Rebe C, Vegran F, Chalmin F, Bruchard M, et al. (2013) Dacarbazine-mediated upregulation of NKG2D ligands on tumor cells activates NK and CD8 T cells and restrains melanoma growth. J Invest Dermatol 133: 499–508.
11. Bhatia S, Tykodi SS, Thompson JA (2009) Treatment of metastatic melanoma: an overview. Oncology (Williston Park) 23: 488–496.
12. Rosenberg SA (2011) Cell transfer immunotherapy for metastatic solid cancer-what clinicians need to know. Nat Rev Clin Oncol 8: 577–585.
13. Jacobs JF, Nierkens S, Figdor CG, de Vries IJ, Adema GJ (2012) Regulatory T cells in melanoma: the final hurdle towards effective immunotherapy? Lancet Oncol 13: e32–42.
14. Pearce EL, Mullen AC, Martins GA, Krawczyk CM, Hutchins AS, et al. (2003) Control of effector CD8+ T cell function by the transcription factor Eomesodermin. Science 302: 1041–1043.
15. Gordon SM, Chaix J, Rupp LJ, Wu J, Madera S, et al. (2012) The transcription factors T-bet and Eomes control key checkpoints of natural killer cell maturation. Immunity 36: 55–67.
16. Duran-Aniotz C, Segal G, Salazar L, Pereda C, Falcon C, et al. (2013) The immunological response and post-treatment survival of DC-vaccinated melanoma patients are associated with increased Th1/Th17 and reduced Th3 cytokine responses. Cancer Immunol Immunother 62: 761–772.
17. Dulos J, Carven GJ, van Boxtel SJ, Evers S, Driessen-Engels LJ, et al. (2012) PD-1 blockade augments Th1 and Th17 and suppresses Th2 responses in peripheral blood from patients with prostate and advanced melanoma cancer. J Immunother 35: 169–178.
18. von Euw E, Chodon T, Attar N, Jalil J, Koya RC, et al. (2009) CTLA4 blockade increases Th17 cells in patients with metastatic melanoma. J Transl Med 7: 35.
19. Viaud S, Flament C, Zoubir M, Pautier P, LeCesne A, et al. (2011) Cyclophosphamide induces differentiation of Th17 cells in cancer patients. Cancer Res 71: 661–665.
20. Muranski P, Boni A, Antony PA, Cassard L, Irvine KR, et al. (2008) Tumor-specific Th17-polarized cells eradicate large established melanoma. Blood 112: 362–373.
21. Martin-Orozco N, Muranski P, Chung Y, Yang XO, Yamazaki T, et al. (2009) T helper 17 cells promote cytotoxic T cell activation in tumor immunity. Immunity 31: 787–798.
22. Goding SR, Wilson KA, Xie Y, Harris KM, Baxi A, et al. (2013) Restoring immune function of tumor-specific CD4+ T cells during recurrence of melanoma. J Immunol 190: 4899–4909.
23. Montes CL, Chapoval AI, Nelson J, Orhue V, Zhang X, et al. (2008) Tumor-induced senescent T cells with suppressor function: a potential form of tumor immune evasion. Cancer Res 68: 870–879.

24. De Panfilis G, Campanini N, Santini M, Mori G, Tognetti E, et al. (2008) Phase- and stage-related proportions of T cells bearing the transcription factor FOXP3 infiltrate primary melanoma. J Invest Dermatol 128: 676–684.
25. Moretta A, Marcenaro E, Parolini S, Ferlazzo G, Moretta L (2008) NK cells at the interface between innate and adaptive immunity. Cell Death Differ 15: 226–233.
26. Poli A, Michel T, Thérésine M, Andrès E, Hentges F, et al. (2009) CD56bright natural killer (NK) cells: an important NK cell subset. Immunology 126: 458–465.
27. Messaoudene M, Fregni G, Fourmentraux-Neves E, Chanal J, Maubec E, et al. (2014) Mature cytotoxic CD56(bright)/CD16(+) natural killer cells can infiltrate lymph nodes adjacent to metastatic melanoma. Cancer Res 74: 81–92.
28. Fregni G, Perier A, Pittari G, Jacobelli S, Sastre X, et al. (2011) Unique functional status of natural killer cells in metastatic stage IV melanoma patients and its modulation by chemotherapy. Clin Cancer Res 17: 2628–2637.
29. Fregni G, Messaoudene M, Fourmentraux-Neves E, Mazouz-Dorval S, Chanal J, et al. (2013) Phenotypic and functional characteristics of blood natural killer cells from melanoma patients at different clinical stages. PLoS One 8: e76928.

13

Progesterone Receptor Status and Ki-67 Index may Predict Early Relapse in Luminal B/HER2 Negative Breast Cancer Patients

Yu Zong[1], Li Zhu[1]*, Jiayi Wu[1], Xiaosong Chen[1], Ou Huang[1], Xiaochun Fei[2], Jianrong He[1], Weiguo Chen[1], Yafen Li[1], Kunwei Shen[1]*

1 Comprehensive Breast Health Center, Shanghai Ruijin Hospital affiliated to Medical School of Shanghai Jiaotong University, Shanghai, China, **2** Pathology Department, Shanghai Ruijin Hospital affiliated to Medical School of Shanghai Jiaotong University, Shanghai, China

Abstract

Purpose: Few studies has documented early relapse in luminal B/HER2-negative breast cancer. We examined prognostic factors for early relapse among these patients to improve treatment decision-making.

Patients and Methods: A total 398 patients with luminal B/HER2-negative breast cancer were included. Kaplan-Meier curves were applied to estimate disease-free survival and Cox regression to identify prognostic factors.

Results: Progesterone receptor (PR) negative expression was associated with higher tumor grade ($p<.001$) and higher Ki-67 index ($p=.010$). PR-negative patients received more chemotherapy than the PR-positive group ($p=.009$). After a median follow-up of 28 months, 17 patients (4.3%) had early relapses and 8 patients (2.0%) died of breast cancer. The 2-year disease-free survival was 97.7% in the PR-positive and 90.4% in the PR-negative groups (Log-rank $p=.002$). Also, patients with a high Ki-67 index (defined as >30%) had a reduced disease-free survival (DFS) when compared with low Ki-67 index group (≤ 30%) (98.0% vs 92.4%, respectively, Log-rank $p=.013$). In multivariate analysis, PR negativity was significantly associated with a reduced DFS (HR = 3.91, 95% CI 1.29–11.88, $p=.016$).

Conclusion: In this study, PR negativity was a prognostic factor for early relapse in luminal B/HER2-negative breast cancer, while a high Ki-67 index suggested a higher risk of early relapse.

Editor: Anthony W. I. Lo, The Chinese University of Hong Kong, Hong Kong

Funding: This study was supported by Shanghai Natural Science Foundation 11ZR1422900, National Natural Science Foundation of China (Young Investigators) 81102017 and Wu Jieping Medical Foundation 320.6750.12285. The funders had no role in study design, data collection and analysis, decision to publish, or preparation of the manuscript.

Competing Interests: The authors have declared that no competing interests exist.

* Email: zhuli8@hotmail.com (LZ); kwshen@medmail.com.cn (KS)

Introduction

The most commonly diagnosed cancer among Chinese women in 2009 was of the breast, with an incidence of $42.55/10^5$, accounting for 16.8% of all new cancer cases among women [1]. Recent gene expression studies have confirmed that breast cancer is no longer a single disease with variable morphology, but with high molecular heterogeneity [2]. Breast cancer is now identified as at least 4 subtypes: Luminal A, Luminal B, HER2-enriched and basal-like by gene profiles [3,4]. Since certain immunohistochemical (IHC) markers can provide prognosis and predictive treatment information and also have easy clinical accessibility [5,6], these have been used in an attempt to determine intrinsic subtypes. A simplified IHC classification including estrogen receptor (ER), progesterone receptor (PR), HER2, and Ki-67 index is now considered a surrogate for establishing breast cancer subtype [7] and could be equivalent to intrinsic subtypes by gene profiling [8–10].

Luminal B breast cancer is classified as higher nuclear grade [2], lower expression of ER-related genes [11,12], and higher expression of proliferative genes [13,14] compared to luminal A, thus representing a heterogeneous disease. IHC classification defines Luminal B tumors as ER- and/or PR-positive, HER2-negative, and Ki-67 labeling index (Ki-67 index) ≥14%, or as ER- and/or PR-positive, HER2 over-expressed or amplified, any and Ki-67 index [7], although this is still a heterogeneous group. It has been reported that Luminal B had a 1.86 times greater risk of early relapse, but not late relapse, compared to luminal A [15]. Also, Luminal B cancers were relatively insensitive to endocrine therapy compared with Luminal A types [8] and to chemotherapy when compared with HER2-enriched and basal-like breast cancers [16–20]. In this study, we emphasized Luminal B/HER2-negative breast cancers since they lack the use of anti-HER2 treatment [15].

PR is an ER-regulated gene which mediates the effect of progesterone on the development of both the normal mammary gland and breast cancer [21]. The predictive value of PR status of the benefit of adjuvant tamoxifen in ER-positive breast cancer remains controversial [22–25]. It has recently been reported that

PR loss is a prognosis factor in Luminal B breast cancers regardless of HER2 status [26].

Ki-67 index is a proliferation-related factor which associated with poor prognosis in breast cancer [27,28]. Fourteen percent is adopted as the cutoff to identify Luminal A and B breast cancers in Europe [7] but not widely accepted in North America [29]. A promising Ki-67 index cut-off point for prognosis or treatment response prediction is lacking because of unreproducibility and analytical bias among different laboratories [30]. The clinical utility of Ki-67 index as a prognostic marker might be more apparent if it were considered within more narrowly defined tumor subgroups.

In order to get more information on Luminal B/HER2-negative breast cancer, we have attempted to identify prognostic factors for early relapse, as well as to define an appropriate Ki-67 index cutoff in our center which might predict early relapse. It is also important to at least add some data about breast cancer prognosis in Eastern countries and specifically in China, since etiologies and genetic background might lead to different form one area of the world to another.

Patients and methods

Patients

This retrospective study has been approved by the Ethical Committees of Shanghai Ruijin Hospital, whose results do not effect the treatment decision of any patient enrolled. All the patients provided their written informed consents to participant this study before the clinical and pathological data were collected. Using the Electronic Medical History Administration System V2.0 and database from Comprehensive Breast Health Center, Shanghai Ruijin Hospital, we collected information on consecutive breast cancer patients undergoing breast surgery between January 2009 and December 2011. Only Luminal B/HER2-negative breast cancer patients were included. Data on each patient's past medical history, current disease, surgical information, pathological results. and pathologic staging examinations (chest film/CT scan, upper abdominal ultrasonography, bone scan, etc.) were retrieved. Latest follow-up was at the end of June, 2013.

Evaluation of ER, PR, HER2, Ki-67 index status

Tumors were classified histologically according to the World Health Organization Classification of Tumors [31]. Tumor staging was assessed according to American Joint Committee on Cancer (AJCC) Cancer Staging Handbook [32].

Histological grades and all biological features were evaluated based on the invasive components. Histological grade was evaluated according to Elston and Ellis scoring system [33]. We used a revised technique involves semiquantitative evaluation of three morphological features: the percentage of tubule formation, the degree of nuclear pleomorphism and an accurate mitotic count using a defined field area. A numerical scoring system was used and the overall grade is derived from a summation of individual scores for the three variables; three grades of differentiation were used. For tubule formation, 1 = >75% of the tumor area was composed of definite tubules, 2 = 10 to 75% of the area showed tubule formation, 3 = <10% of the area showed tubule formation. As to nuclear pleomorphism, 1 = Small, regular uniform cells, 2 = Moderate increase in size and variability, 3 = Marked variation. For mitotic counts, since we used Nikon Labophot microscope with ×40 objective, and a field area of 0.152 mm^2, 1 = 0–5 mitoses per 10 fields, 2 = 6–10 mitoses per 10 fields, 3 = ≥ 11 mitoses per 10 fields. To obtain the overall tumor grade, the scores for each category were added together, giving a possible total of 3–9. Tumor grade was then allocated as 3–5 points: grade I, well-differentiated; 6–7 points: grade II, moderately differentiated; 8–9 points: grade III, poorly differentiated.

IHC staining of ER, PR, HER2 and Ki-67 was routinely carried out by using Ventana BenchMark XT system (Ventana Medical Systems, Tucson, AZ) in our hospital. All procedures were performed automatically in the BenchMark. IHC staining was performed on 4-μm slices of formalin-fixed paraffin-embedded (FFPE) tissue sections with primary antibodies against ER (SP1, 1:100, Dako, Denmark), PR (PgR 636, 1:100, Dako, Denmark), HER2 (4B5,Roche, Switzerland), Ki67(MIB-1, 1:100, Dako, Denmark). The tissue sections were incubated with primary antibody of ER, PR and Ki67 for 32 minutes at 42°C and of HER2 for 16 minutes at 42°C. Sections were counterstained with hematoxylin.

A Fluorescence in situ hybridization (FISH) test for HER2 gene amplification was routinely ordered when HER2 was IHC 2+. FISH was performed using the PathVysion HER-2 DNA FISH Kit, (Vysis Inc, Downers Grove, IL) according to the manufacturer's instructions. Acid pretreatment and protease digestion were performed (Vysis paraffin pretreatment kit; Vysis Inc), followed by standard saline citrate (SSC) and formamide denaturation (72°C 5 minutes). After dehydration, the HER2/CEP 17 probe mixer was added. Slides were incubated in a moist chamber overnight at 37°C under a coverslip. On the following day, slides were washed in a stringency buffer (SSC, NP40), air-dried in the dark and incubated with 4,6 diamidino-2-phenylindole (DAPI) for nuclear identification.

The cutoff for ER positivity and PR positivity was 1% positive tumor cells with nuclear staining [34]. Positive for HER2 was either IHC HER2 3+_(defined as uniform intense membrane staining of >30% of invasive tumor cells) or FISH amplified (ratio of HER2 to CEP17 of >2.2) [35]. The Ki-67 index was expressed as the percentage of positively nuclear staining cells among at least 1000 invasive cells in the area scored. Staining intensity was not relevant [36].

Follow-up and Statistical Analysis

Breast cancer relapse was defined as the first proven invasive local/contralateral breast, regional, or distant recurrence in any site [37]. First relapse would be biopsied if it was technically available but the biopsy was not compulsive. Recurrence and metastasis could be diagnosed base on clinical manifestation, physical examinations and radiographic images. Only invasive tumor recurrences were counted as a relapse and a recurrence with only in situ tumor was not counted as a relapse.

Follow-up and events were censored if they occurred beyond 2 years after diagnosis. The analysis thus focused exclusively on early relapse.

Chi-Square test was employed for categorized variables (Fisher's exact test when the Chi-square test was unavailable). Survival curves were plotted by Kaplan-Meier method. Log-rank test was used to determine the associations between individual variables and survival, logistic regression modeling to examine the association of tumor features with PR negativity and Cox proportional hazards regression analyses to identify significant prognostic factors in Luminal B/HER2-negative breast cancer. Statistical analyses were carried out in SPSS version 16.0(SPSS, Inc., Chicago, IL).

Results

PR status was identified as negative in tumors from 101 of 398 patients (25.4%). One hundred and ninety-nine patients expressed

PR with >1% to <20% of positive cells(50.0%), and all of which had weak to moderate staining intensity of PR. Conversely, the other 98 patients(24.6%) with staining percentage of PR-positive cells greater than 20% mostly had moderate to strong intensity. Patient and tumor characteristics of this cohort are summarized in Table 1 according to PR status.

The Ki-67 index was dichotomized to high (>30% immunoreactive cells) and low (≤30% immunoreactive cells) groups by using the median value of the Ki-67 index immunoreactivity as the cut-off point. One hundred and sixty-four of 398 patients (41.2%) were identified as Ki-67 index-high.

Treatment information was available in 348 patients. Generally, 198 patients received chemotherapy while another 150 patients did not. Chemotherapy regimens were given according to physicians' preference, including EC (Epirubicin 100 mg/m2 IV day 1, Cyclophosphamide 600 mg/m2 IV day 1, cycled every 21 days for 4 cycles), EC-T(Epirubicin 100 mg/m2 IV day 1, Cyclophosphamide 600 mg/m2 IV day 1, cycled every 21 days for 4 cycles followed by Docetaxel 100 mg/m2 IV on day 1, cycled every 21 days for 4 cycles), TEC (Docetaxel 75 mg/m2 IV day 1, Epirubicin 75 mg/m2 IV day 1, Cyclophosphamide 600 mg/m2 IV day 1, cycled every 21 days for 6 cycles), and TC (Docetaxel 75 mg/m2 IV day 1, Cyclophosphamide 600 mg/m2 IV day 1, cycled every 21 days for 4 cycles).

Associations of PR status with patient and tumor characteristics

There was no correlation between PR and patient age ($p = .195$) or menstruation status ($p = .100$) (Table 1). PR negativity was associated with higher grade tumors ($p < .001$) and higher Ki-67 index ($p = .010$); PR-negative tumors received more chemotherapy ($p = .009$). In multivariable logistic regression modeling which included trial cohort and selected by tumor features, tumor grade was strongly associated with PR negativity (p<.001) (Table 2).

A significant correlation was identified between PR expression and Ki-67 index by Spearman Rank correlation. Luminal B/HER2- patients with PR negativity were more likely to have a Ki-67 index higher than 30% (r = −.138, p = .006).

Table 1. Association of patient and tumor characteristics with PR status.

Characteristics	Luminal B, HER2-, PR+	Luminal B, HER2-, PR−	*P*-value	Cases available (n)
Age (y/o), mean (±SD)	55.2(±12.8)	55.7(±12.4)	.195	398
Menstruation status			.100	398
Premenopausal	126(42.4%)	33(32.7%)		
Postmenopausal	171(57.6%)	68(67.3%)		
Histology			.835	398
IDC	273(91.9%)	92(91.1%)		
Non-IDC	24(8.1%)	9(8.9%)		
Tumor size (cm)			.280	393
≤2	188(63.7%)	56(57.1%)		
>2	107(36.3%)	42(42.9%)		
Positive ALN numbers			.784	392
0	177(60.6%)	64(64.0%)		
1~3	71(24.3%)	21(21.0%)		
≥4	44(15.1%)	15(15.0%)		
Tumor grade			<.001	394
G2	190(64.8%)	39(38.6%)		
G3	76(25.9%)	51(50.5%)		
others	27(9.3%)	11 (10.9%)		
Ki-67 labeling index			.010	398
High	111(37.4%)	53(52.5%)		
Low	186(62.6%)	48(47.5%)		
Breast surgery			1.000	398
Mastectomy	248(83.5%)	84(83.2%)		
BCS	49 (16.5%)	17(16.8%)		
Chemotherapy			.009	348
Yes	137(52.7%)	61(69.3%)		
No	123(47.3%)	27(30.7%)		
Radiation Therapy			.615	363
Yes	88(32.3%)	34(37.8%)		
No	180(67.7%)	61(62.2%)		

Abbreviation: IDC = infiltrating ductal carcinoma, ALN = axillary lymph node, ER = Estrogen receptor, PR = progesterone receptor, BCS = breast conserving surgery.

Table 2. Multivariable logistic regression model for PR negativity.

Characteristics	Estimate± SE	Odds Ratio (95%CI)	P-value
Grade III (vs. Grade II)	1.223±.264	3.396 (2.023–5.700)	<.001
High Ki-67 index (vs. low Ki-67 index)	.471±.251	1.601 (.979, 2.618)	.061

DFS and OS by PR status

At a median follow-up of 28 months (range 5.7–50.1 months), 17 patients (4.9%) had relapses, 7 in PR-positive group (2.4%) and 10 in PR-negative group (9.9%). Eight patients died due to breast cancer (2.0%). Among 17 patients with relapses, 6 patients had locoregional recurrences, 2 had contralateral breast cancers, and 9 had distant metastases. All the locoregional recurrence lesions and contralateral breast lesions were proven by using either fine needle aspiration or core needle biopsy. For the 9 patients with distant metastasis, the first metastatic lesion was biopsied in 4 patients (2 liver metastasis, 2 lung metastasis). The other 5 patients were diagnosed as metastatic breast caner based on clinical and radiographic findings.

Information on 265 patients was available for Kaplan-Meier analysis. The 2-year DFS was 97.7% in the PR-positive group and 90.4% in the PR-negative group (Log-rank p = .002) (Figure 1A) in Kaplan-Meier analysis. A poorer 2-year OS was also detected in PR-negative group (99.6%%Vs 94.8%, respectively; Log-rank p = .002). (Figure 1B)

DFS and OS by Ki-67 labeling index

High Ki-67 index was significantly associated with poorer 2-year DFS (98.0%Vs 92.4% Log-rank p = .013; Figure 2A) in Kaplan-Meier analysis. However, No significant overall survival difference was detected between the high Ki-67 index group and the low Ki-67 index group (98.3% Vs 97.0%, Log-rank p = .233) (Figure 2B).

Multivariate analysis of DFS

In univariate models, axillary lymph node status was the only insignificant covariate (Table 3). PR negativity (HR = 4.04, 95% CI 1.54–10.60; p = .005) and high Ki-67 index (HR = 3.45, 95% CI 1.22–9.80; p = .020) were both risk factors for early relapse in Luminal B/HER2-negative patients.

Since axillary lymph node status is a standard reported characteristic, it was included in the multivariate Cox proportional Hazards regression model. Results from the final multivariate Cox regression model are presented in Table 3. PR negativity was the only prognosis factor, resulting in an increased risk of relapse (HR = 4.031, 95% CI 1.293–12.574; p = .016).

One representative case

One representative patient was a 48 year-old female, diagnosed as infiltrating ductal carcinoma in Dec 2009. She received modified radical mastectomy. The pathology report showed IDC grade III, tumor size 1.5 cm, ALN 0/14, ER 10%+, PR−, HER2-, Ki-67 50%+. After 4 courses of TC (Docetaxel+Cyclophosphamide) chemotherapy, she received tamoxifen as adjuvant endocrine

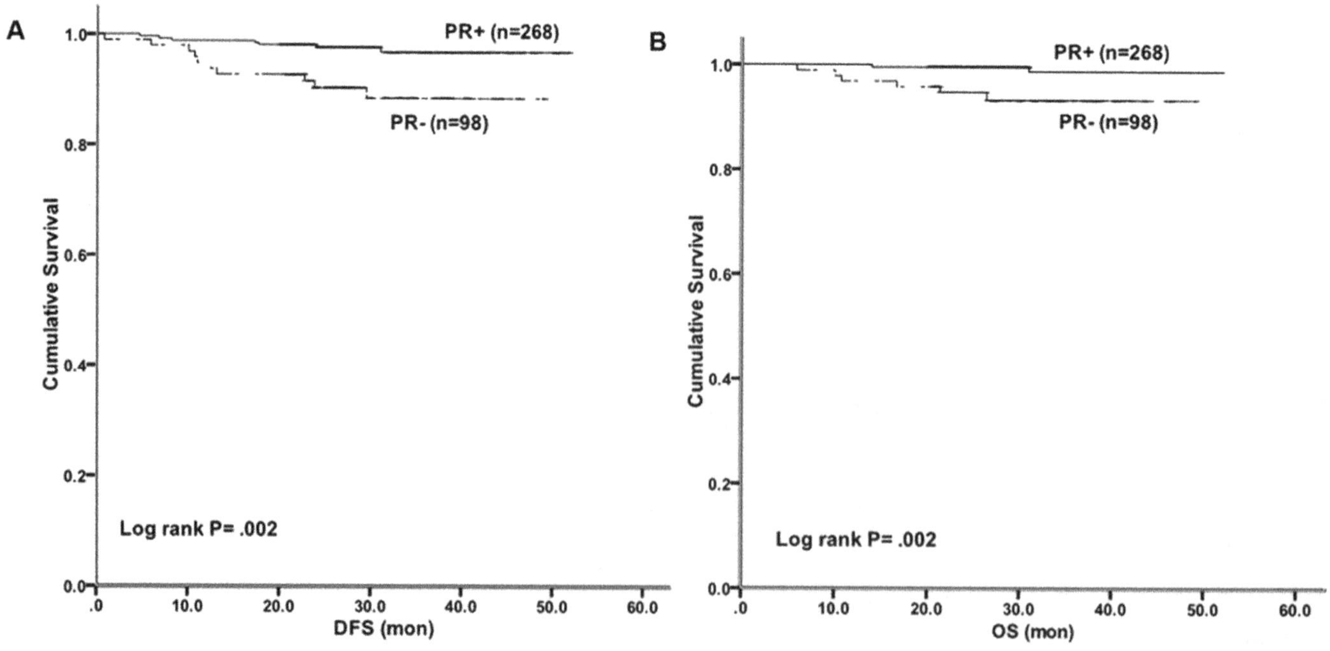

Figure 1. Disease-free survival and overall survival by PR status among Luminal B/HER2- patients. (A) The 2-year DFS was significantly better in the PR-positive group than in the PR-negative group (97.7% Vs 90.4%, Log-rank p = .002). (B) A poorer 2-year OS was also detected in PR-negative group (99.6% Vs 94.8%, Log-rank p = .002).

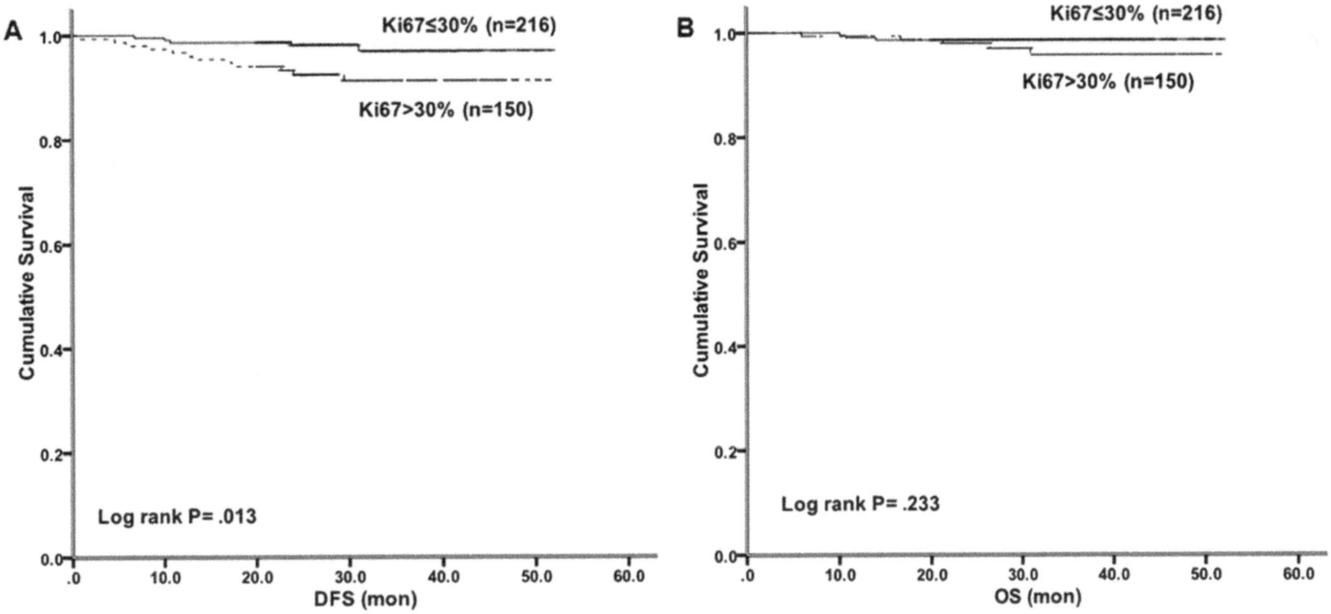

Figure 2. Disease-free survival and overall survival by high/low Ki-67 index among Luminal B/HER2- patients. (A) A significantly better 2-year DFS was detected in the high Ki-67 index group when compared to the low Ki-67 index group (98.0%Vs 92.4%, Log-rank p = .013). (B) No significant overall survival difference was detected between the high Ki-67 index group and the low Ki-67 index group (98.3% Vs 97.0%, Log-rank p = .233).

therapy. However, in Oct 2010, she received a abdominal CT scan due to abdominal discomfort, which suggested liver metastasis. Then, a CT-guided liver biopsy was done and the pathology report showed liver metastasis originated from breast cancer, ER-, PR−, HER2-, Ki-67 20%. She died after failing three lines of salvage chemotherapy in Sept, 2011. The images were showed in Fig. 3.

Discussion

It is widely accepted that clinical factors combined with pathological characteristics and gene expression profiles provide useful prognostic information for the different breast cancer subtypes. However, Luminal B breast cancer, as one of the five intrinsic subtypes, still represents a heterogeneous disease, with distinct prognoses. Only one study has focused on Luminal B/HER2-negative breast cancer despite its tendency to early relapse [15]. Although the St. Gallen consensus recommends endocrine therapy±chemotherapy for the Luminal B/HER2-negative subtype [7], this subtype remains relative insensitivity to both treatments. In this study, we attempted to identify prognostic factors for early relapse in this subgroup.

PR is an estrogen-regulated gene, and its synthesis in normal breast and cancer cells requires estrogen and ER and PR expression represents a functional PR pathway [38]. PR-negative breast cancers are more frequent in postmenopausal patients [39], patients with a high BMI [40] and a high glucose intake [41]. This could be a result of loss of ovarian function in the elderly, causing insufficient levels of estrogen to transcribe PR [42].

In the 394 patients whose grade information was available, none had a grade I tumor, while in 38 patients, grade could not be established since they had non-infiltrating ductal carcinoma or micro-invasion. High tumor grade in present study is independently related to PR negativity after adjusting tumor size, axillary lymph node status, tumor histology. High Ki-67 index is also found significantly associated to PR status in Chi-square text and still has borderline meaning after multivariate logistic regression. Thus, we believe PR negativity in luminal B/HER2 negative breast cancer might suggest more aggressive tumor biology. Retrospective analysis showed that PR status did not affect decision making of surgery or radiation therapy. However, more chemotherapy was prescribed for those with PR negative luminal B/HER2 negative breast cancer.

Data are somewhat conflicting regarding the prognostic value of PR. According to an analysis by Bardou [22], PR negativity was an independent predictive marker for tamoxifen resistance and breast cancer relapse. Otherwise a meta-analysis by Early Breast Cancer Trialists' Collaborative Group (EGCTCG) found tamoxifen improves relapse-free survival in case of ER positive tumors, regardless of PR status [23]. More recently, a retrospective analysis by Cancello also identified PR negativity as high risk of relapse in luminal B breast cancer [26]. Our analysis showed that higher risk of early relapse was linked to PR negativity in luminal B/HER2 negative breast cancer in spite that chemotherapy and endocrine therapy was already employed. Several preclinical studies suggested that molecular crosstalk between ER and growth factor signaling pathways causes down-regulation of PR, activation of membrane initiated steroid signaling and tamoxifen resistance [43–45]. It is also observed that three times as many ER positive/PR negative tumors as ER positive/PR positive tumors expressed HER-1, which is associated with a higher likelihood of recurrence [46]. This crosstalk may explain the bad outcome of PR negative patients in our study.

Ki-67 index, a proliferation associated marker, has been widely accepted as a prognostic factor. Several studies suggested that higher values of Ki-67 index indicate a worse prognosis [27,28]. Different methods were employed to identify Ki-67 index cut points for specific endpoints, such as median/mean value, ROC curves, or subpopulation treatment effect pattern plots (STEPP) analysis [8,47,48]. Instead of using any cut point as previously

Table 3. Multivariate Cox proportional Hazards regression model results in Luminal B/HER2-negative tumors.

	Univariate		Multivariate	
	HR (95% CI)	P value	HR (95% CI)	P value
PR				
Positive	1.000		1.00	
Negative	4.04 (1.54–10.60)	.005	3.91 (1.29–11.88)	.016
Ki-67				
Low	1.000		1.00	
High	3.45 (1.22–9.80)	.020	2.54 (.79–8.20)	.119
ALN				
0	1.000		1.00	
1–3	.22 (.03–1.67)	.142	.23 (.03–1.79)	.160
≥4	1.93 (.54–6.83)	.309	2.34 (.63–8.66)	.204
Chemotherapy				
No	1.000		1.00	
Yes	9.40 (1.23–71.9)	.031	7.79 (0.99–60.77)	.050

Abbreviation: PR = progesterone receptor, Ki-67 = Ki-67 labeling index, ALN = axillary lymph node.

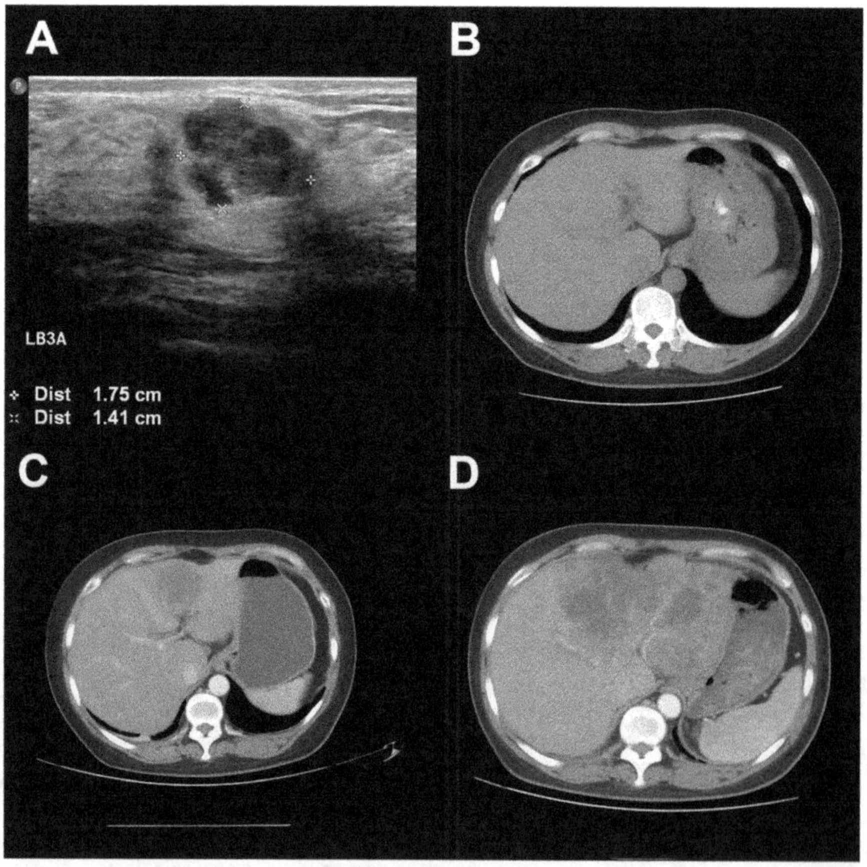

Figure 3. Representitive images of one patients with PR negative breast cancer. (A) Ultrasonography of the primary breast tumor before surgery (Dec, 2009). (B) No metastatic lesion showed on abdominal CT scan before surgery(Dec, 2009). (C) Liver metastasis confirmed by core needle biopsy 10 months after the surgery (Oct, 2010). (D) Last abdominal CT scan shortly before the patient died, which suggested no response to chemotherapy (Sept, 2011).

published, we chose median value of Ki-67 labeling index in our study population– 30% as cut-off point in case of reproducibility and analytical bias among different laboratories. Patients with high Ki-67 index (>30%) had more frequency having PR negative breast cancer according to logistic regression results and more risk of early relapse as univariate COX regression analysis presented but not multivariate models.

Despite of a median 28-month follow-up, PR might already show its prognostic value in luminal B/HER2 negative breast cancer and high Ki-67 index may also be an early relapse related factor. We also notice that the latest 2013 St Gallen Consensus employed high PR expression (>20%) to define a Luminal A subtype further [49]. Since all the patients in this study received surgery and adjuvant chemotherapy before 2013, the treatment strategies were given based on both tumor burden and intrinsic breast cancer subtypes, whose definition was from 2011 St. Gallen Consensus. Therefore, we did not use the new definition of Luminal B tumors in order to avoid bias in this retrospective study. Our results were also in line with that PR negativity was an unfavorable feature of breast cancer biology. However, previous data suggested that risk of death continues for an additional 10–15 years after diagnosis in HR positive/HER2 negative breast cancer [23,50]. Therefore, longer follow-up period is warranted to identify whether PR status or Ki-67 index could still be a prognostic factor.

Conclusion

PR status is a prognostic factor of early relapse in luminal B/HER2 negative breast cancer and high Ki-67 index may also suggest increased risk of early relapse. Therefore, PR status and Ki-67 index should be taken into account when discussing more aggressive treatment with specific luminal B/HER2 negative breast cancer patients.

Author Contributions

Conceived and designed the experiments: YZ LZ JW XC KS. Performed the experiments: YZ LZ JW XC OH XF JH YL WC KS. Analyzed the data: YZ LZ JW WC KS. Contributed reagents/materials/analysis tools: YZ LZ JW XC OH XF JH YL WC KS. Wrote the paper: YZ LZ KS.

References

1. Chen W, Zheng R, Zhang S, Zhao P, Li G, et al. (2013) Report of incidence and mortality in China cancer registries, 2009. Chin J Cancer Res 25: 10–21.
2. Sotiriou C, Pusztai L (2009) Gene-expression signatures in breast cancer. N Engl J Med 360: 790–800.
3. Perou CM, Sorlie T, Eisen MB, van de Rijn M, Jeffrey SS, et al. (2000) Molecular portraits of human breast tumours. Nature 406: 747–752.
4. Sorlie T, Perou CM, Tibshirani R, Aas T, Geisler S, et al. (2001) Gene expression patterns of breast carcinomas distinguish tumor subclasses with clinical implications. Proc Natl Acad Sci U S A 98: 10869–10874.
5. Mauriac L, Keshaviah A, Debled M, Mouridsen H, Forbes JF, et al. (2007) Predictors of early relapse in postmenopausal women with hormone receptor-positive breast cancer in the BIG 1–98 trial. Ann Oncol 18: 859–867.
6. Dowsett M, Allred C, Knox J, Quinn E, Salter J, et al. (2008) Relationship between quantitative estrogen and progesterone receptor expression and human epidermal growth factor receptor 2 (HER-2) status with recurrence in the Arimidex, Tamoxifen, Alone or in Combination trial. J Clin Oncol 26: 1059–1065.
7. Goldhirsch A, Wood WC, Coates AS, Gelber RD, Thurlimann B, et al. (2011) Strategies for subtypes–dealing with the diversity of breast cancer: highlights of the St. Gallen International Expert Consensus on the Primary Therapy of Early Breast Cancer 2011. Ann Oncol 22: 1736–1747.
8. Cheang MC, Chia SK, Voduc D, Gao D, Leung S, et al. (2009) Ki67 index, HER2 status, and prognosis of patients with luminal B breast cancer. J Natl Cancer Inst 101: 736–750.
9. Hugh J, Hanson J, Cheang MC, Nielsen TO, Perou CM, et al. (2009) Breast cancer subtypes and response to docetaxel in node-positive breast cancer: use of an immunohistochemical definition in the BCIRG 001 trial. J Clin Oncol 27: 1168–1176.
10. Cuzick J, Dowsett M, Pineda S, Wale C, Salter J, et al. (2011) Prognostic value of a combined estrogen receptor, progesterone receptor, Ki-67, and human epidermal growth factor receptor 2 immunohistochemical score and comparison with the Genomic Health recurrence score in early breast cancer. J Clin Oncol 29: 4273–4278.
11. Sorlie T, Tibshirani R, Parker J, Hastie T, Marron JS, et al. (2003) Repeated observation of breast tumor subtypes in independent gene expression data sets. Proc Natl Acad Sci U S A 100: 8418–8423.
12. Brenton JD, Carey LA, Ahmed AA, Caldas C (2005) Molecular classification and molecular forecasting of breast cancer: ready for clinical application? J Clin Oncol 23: 7350–7360.
13. Hu Z, Fan C, Oh DS, Marron JS, He X, et al. (2006) The molecular portraits of breast tumors are conserved across microarray platforms. BMC Genomics 7: 96.
14. Perou CM, Jeffrey SS, van de Rijn M, Rees CA, Eisen MB, et al. (1999) Distinctive gene expression patterns in human mammary epithelial cells and breast cancers. Proc Natl Acad Sci U S A 96: 9212–9217.
15. Tran B, Bedard PL (2011) Luminal-B breast cancer and novel therapeutic targets. Breast Cancer Res 13: 221.
16. Rouzier R, Perou CM, Symmans WF, Ibrahim N, Cristofanilli M, et al. (2005) Breast cancer molecular subtypes respond differently to preoperative chemotherapy. Clin Cancer Res 11: 5678–5685.
17. Carey LA, Dees EC, Sawyer L, Gatti L, Moore DT, et al. (2007) The triple negative paradox: primary tumor chemosensitivity of breast cancer subtypes. Clin Cancer Res 13: 2329–2334.
18. Esserman L, Perou C, Cheang M, DeMichele A, Carey L, et al. (2009) Breast cancer molecular profiles and tumor response of neoadjuvant doxorubicin and paclitaxel: the I-SPY TRIAL (CALGB 150007/150012, ACRIN 6657) [abstract]. J Clin Oncol 27:LBA515.
19. de Ronde JJ, Hannemann J, Halfwerk H, Mulder L, Straver ME, et al. (2010) Concordance of clinical and molecular breast cancer subtyping in the context of preoperative chemotherapy response. Breast Cancer Res Treat 119: 119–126.
20. Bhargava R, Beriwal S, Dabbs DJ, Ozbek U, Soran A, et al. (2010) Immunohistochemical surrogate markers of breast cancer molecular classes predicts response to neoadjuvant chemotherapy: a single institutional experience with 359 cases. Cancer 116: 1431–1439.
21. Conneely OM, Jericevic BM, Lydon JP (2003) Progesterone receptors in mammary gland development and tumorigenesis. J Mammary Gland Biol Neoplasia 8: 205–214.
22. Bardou VJ, Arpino G, Elledge RM, Osborne CK, Clark GM (2003) Progesterone receptor status significantly improves outcome prediction over estrogen receptor status alone for adjuvant endocrine therapy in two large breast cancer databases. J Clin Oncol 21: 1973–1979.
23. Davies C, Godwin J, Gray R, Clarke M, Cutter D, et al. (2011) Relevance of breast cancer hormone receptors and other factors to the efficacy of adjuvant tamoxifen: patient-level meta-analysis of randomised trials. Lancet 378: 771–784.
24. Dowsett M, Houghton J, Iden C, Salter J, Farndon J, et al. (2006) Benefit from adjuvant tamoxifen therapy in primary breast cancer patients according oestrogen receptor, progesterone receptor, EGF receptor and HER2 status. Ann Oncol 17: 818–826.
25. Stendahl M, Ryden L, Nordenskjold B, Jonsson PE, Landberg G, et al. (2006) High progesterone receptor expression correlates to the effect of adjuvant tamoxifen in premenopausal breast cancer patients. Clin Cancer Res 12: 4614–4618.
26. Cancello G, Maisonneuve P, Rotmensz N, Viale G, Mastropasqua MG, et al. (2013) Progesterone receptor loss identifies Luminal B breast cancer subgroups at higher risk of relapse. Ann Oncol 24: 661–668.
27. Trihia H, Murray S, Price K, Gelber RD, Golouh R, et al. (2003) Ki-67 expression in breast carcinoma: its association with grading systems, clinical parameters, and other prognostic factors–a surrogate marker? Cancer 97: 1321–1331.
28. de Azambuja E, Cardoso F, de Castro G, Jr., Colozza M, Mano MS, et al. (2007) Ki-67 as prognostic marker in early breast cancer: a meta-analysis of published studies involving 12,155 patients. Br J Cancer 96: 1504–1513.
29. Harris L, Fritsche H, Mennel R, Norton L, Ravdin P, et al. (2007) American Society of Clinical Oncology 2007 update of recommendations for the use of tumor markers in breast cancer. J Clin Oncol 25: 5287–5312.
30. Dowsett M, Nielsen TO, A'Hern R, Bartlett J, Coombes RC, et al. (2011) Assessment of Ki67 in Breast Cancer: Recommendations from the International Ki67 in Breast Cancer Working Group. JNCI Journal of the National Cancer Institute 103: 1656–1664.
31. Tavassoli F, Devilee P (2003) Pathology and genetics of tumors of the breast and female genital organs. Lyon, France: IARC Press. pp. 13–48.
32. Edge S, Byrd D, Compton C (2009) AJCC Cancer Staging Handbook: From the AJCC Cancer Staging Manual. 7th edition. New York: Springer.
33. Elston CW, Ellis IO (1991) Pathological prognostic factors in breast cancer. I. The value of histological grade in breast cancer: experience from a large study with long-term follow-up. Histopathology 19: 403–410.
34. Hammond ME, Hayes DF, Dowsett M, Allred DC, Hagerty KL, et al. (2010) American Society of Clinical Oncology/College Of American Pathologists

guideline recommendations for immunohistochemical testing of estrogen and progesterone receptors in breast cancer. J Clin Oncol 28: 2784–2795.
35. Wolff AC, Hammond ME, Schwartz JN, Hagerty KL, Allred DC, et al. (2007) American Society of Clinical Oncology/College of American Pathologists guideline recommendations for human epidermal growth factor receptor 2 testing in breast cancer. J Clin Oncol 25: 118–145.
36. Dowsett M, Nielsen TO, A'Hern R, Bartlett J, Coombes RC, et al. (2011) Assessment of Ki67 in breast cancer: recommendations from the International Ki67 in Breast Cancer working group. J Natl Cancer Inst 103: 1656–1664.
37. Hudis CA, Barlow WE, Costantino JP, Gray RJ, Pritchard KI, et al. (2007) Proposal for standardized definitions for efficacy end points in adjuvant breast cancer trials: the STEEP system. J Clin Oncol 25: 2127–2132.
38. Jacobsen BM, Schittone SA, Richer JK, Horwitz KB (2005) Progesterone-independent effects of human progesterone receptors (PRs) in estrogen receptor-positive breast cancer: PR isoform-specific gene regulation and tumor biology. Mol Endocrinol 19: 574–587.
39. Yu KD, Liu GY, Di GH, Wu J, Lu JS, et al. (2007) Progesterone receptor status provides predictive value for adjuvant endocrine therapy in older estrogen receptor-positive breast cancer patients. Breast 16: 307–315.
40. Suzuki R, Orsini N, Saji S, Key TJ, Wolk A (2009) Body weight and incidence of breast cancer defined by estrogen and progesterone receptor status–a meta-analysis. Int J Cancer 124: 698–712.
41. Larsson SC, Bergkvist L, Wolk A (2009) Glycemic load, glycemic index and breast cancer risk in a prospective cohort of Swedish women. Int J Cancer 125: 153–157.
42. Thakkar JP, Mehta DG (2011) A review of an unfavorable subset of breast cancer: estrogen receptor positive progesterone receptor negative. Oncologist 16: 276–285.
43. Cui X, Schiff R, Arpino G, Osborne CK, Lee AV (2005) Biology of progesterone receptor loss in breast cancer and its implications for endocrine therapy. J Clin Oncol 23: 7721–7735.
44. Osborne CK, Shou J, Massarweh S, Schiff R (2005) Crosstalk between estrogen receptor and growth factor receptor pathways as a cause for endocrine therapy resistance in breast cancer. Clin Cancer Res 11: 865s–870s.
45. Zhang Y, Su H, Rahimi M, Tochihara R, Tang C (2009) EGFRvIII-induced estrogen-independence, tamoxifen-resistance phenotype correlates with PgR expression and modulation of apoptotic molecules in breast cancer. Int J Cancer 125: 2021–2028.
46. Arpino G, Weiss H, Lee AV, Schiff R, De Placido S, et al. (2005) Estrogen receptor-positive, progesterone receptor-negative breast cancer: association with growth factor receptor expression and tamoxifen resistance. J Natl Cancer Inst 97: 1254–1261.
47. Viale G, Regan MM, Mastropasqua MG, Maffini F, Maiorano E, et al. (2008) Predictive value of tumor Ki-67 expression in two randomized trials of adjuvant chemoendocrine therapy for node-negative breast cancer. J Natl Cancer Inst 100: 207–212.
48. Denkert C, Blohmer J, Mülle B, Eidtmann H, Eiermann W, et al. Ki67 levels in pretherapeutic core biopsies as predictive and prognostic parameters in the neoadjuvant GeparTrio trial [Abstract]. Cancer Res. 2012; 72(24 Suppl):Ab-Abstract nr S4-5.
49. Goldhirsch A, Winer EP, Coates AS, Gelber RD, Piccart-Gebhart M, et al. (2013) Personalizing the treatment of women with early breast cancer: highlights of the St Gallen International Expert Consensus on the Primary Therapy of Early Breast Cancer 2013. Ann Oncol 9:2206–2223.
50. Esserman LJ, Moore DH, Tsing PJ, Chu PW, Yau C, et al. (2011) Biologic markers determine both the risk and the timing of recurrence in breast cancer. Breast Cancer Res Treat 129: 607–616.

14

Downregulation of Ras Association Domain Family Member 6 (RASSF6) Underlies the Treatment Resistance of Highly Metastatic Nasopharyngeal Carcinoma Cells

Ying-Ying Liang[1], Ming-Yuan Chen[2], Yi-Jun Hua[2], Shi Chen[3], Li-Sheng Zheng[1], Xue Cao[1], Li-Xia Peng[1], Ping Xie[1], Bi-Jun Huang[1], Rui Sun[2], Lin Wang[2], Yan-Qun Xiang[2], Xiang Guo[2], Chao-Nan Qian[1,2]*

1 State Key Laboratory of Oncology in South China and Collaborative Innovation Center for Cancer Medicine, Sun Yat-sen University Cancer Center, Guangzhou, China, **2** Department of Nasopharyngeal Carcinoma, Sun Yat-sen University Cancer Center, Guangzhou, China, **3** Department of Gastroesophageal surgery, The Sixth Affliated Hospital (Gastrointestinal and Anal Hospital), Sun Yat-sen University, GuangZhou, China

Abstract

Radiation and cisplatin-based chemotherapy are major treatments for nasopharyngeal carcinoma (NPC). However, a major impediment for further improving the cure rate is the development of treatment resistance with an undetermined molecular mechanism in metastatic NPC cells. Our established, highly metastatic NPC cells have been reported to be more resistant to cisplatin chemotherapy. In the present study, we found that Ras association domain family member 6 (RASSF6) was downregulated in highly metastatic cells but upregulated in low metastatic cells in comparison to their parental cell line. Ectopic-expression of RASSF6 enhanced the sensitivity of highly metastatic NPC cells to cisplatin or radiation by enhancing apoptosis. RASSF6 depletion conversely reduced treatment sensitivity by decreasing the apoptosis rate. Over-expression of RASSF6 in highly metastatic NPC cells could enhance the phosphorylation of JNK when exposed to cisplatin or radiation treatment, while knocking down RASSF6 in low metastatic NPC cells could reduce the level of phospho-JNK when exposed to the same treatments. The activation of JNK signaling by RASSF6 and its subsequent sensitivity to apoptosis in NPC cells could be inhibited by applying the JNK inhibitor SP600125. In conclusion, the downregulation of RASSF6 in highly metastatic NPC cells contributed to their treatment resistance, and over-expression of RASSF6 conferred treatment sensitivity to highly metastatic NPC cells by activating JNK signaling. RASSF6 could be a valuable molecular marker for identifying sensitive metastatic NPC tumors during cisplatin treatment or radiotherapy.

Editor: Sai Wah Tsao, The University of Hong Kong, China

Funding: This work was supported by grants from the National Natural Science Foundation of China (No. 81030043 and No. 81272340) for these authors: Chao-Nan Qian, Li-Xia Peng, Shi Chen, Ying-Ying Liang, and Xue Cao. The funders had no role in study design, data collection and analysis, decision to publish, or preparation of the manuscript.

Competing Interests: The authors have declared that no competing interests exist.

* Email: qianchn@sysucc.org.cn

Introduction

Nasopharyngeal carcinoma (NPC) is a common malignancy in southern China and south-east Asia that has the highest metastasis rate among head and neck cancers [1,2]. NPC is relatively sensitive to radiation therapy and chemotherapy. For those newly diagnosed with loco-regional advanced NPC, which accounts for approximately 70% of cases, concurrent chemo-radiotherapy is the standard for care, while cisplatin-base chemotherapy is the first-line chemotherapy regimen. However, distant metastasis will eventually occur in approximately 20% of NPC patients after the standard treatment [3–5]. Metastatic lesions of this particular malignancy are more frequently resistant to further chemotherapy or radiation therapy due to undetermined mechanisms. As a consequence, distant metastasis is currently the main reason for treatment failure in NPC [3–5].

Numerous efforts have been applied to disclose the mechanisms that underlie the resistance of cancer cells to cisplatin-based chemotherapy or radiotherapy. The known mechanisms include defects in the DNA repair pathways, the promotion of cell survival signals, or decreased drug accumulation inside cancer cells [6–8]. Our recent efforts to explore the sensitivity factors for cisplatin treatment in NPC cells have revealed that asparagine synthetase, matrix metalloproteinase 19, and eIF3a confer cisplatin sensitivity to NPC cells [9,10]. However, to our knowledge, no study has reported the promotion of cisplatin sensitivity in highly metastatic NPC cells.

Ras association family members (RASSFs) are a group of ten mammalian proteins that can directly bind to the Ras oncoprotein, and accumulating evidence has suggested that apoptosis promotion is a common characteristic of the RASSF family [11–15]. It has been reported that RASSF1A overcomes resistance to interferons [16], and RASSF1C is linked to DNA damage through activation of JNK signaling [17]. RASSF6 is similar to other RASSFs and is also linked to DNA repair [15,18]. The relationship between RASSF6 and the DNA damage treatment response, however, has not been investigated.

In our previous study, we isolated a highly metastatic NPC cellular clone, S18, and a low metastatic clone, S26, from the parental NPC cell line CNE-2 [19]. It has been reported that S18 is more resistant to cisplatin treatment then its parental CNE-2 line and the low metastatic S26 clone [20]. Interestingly, our preliminary screening in the present study found that RASSF6 was the only member of the RASSF family that was remarkably upregulated in low metastatic S26 cells. We therefore hypothesized that RASSF6 could confer sensitivity to treatment in highly metastatic NPC cells. Our further explorations confirmed that restoring RASSF6 could induce treatment sensitivity in highly metastatic cells and that RASSF6 depletion could increase treatment resistance in low metastatic cells. The influence of RASSF6 in NPC cells partially depended on the regulation of apoptosis through the activation of JNK signaling because inhibition of the JNK pathway reduced the effect caused by RASSF6. Our study demonstrated that RASSF6 plays an important role in the cellular response to cisplatin and radiation treatment; therefore, RASSF6 could be used as a potential biomarker of NPC for predicting treatment response.

Materials and Methods

Ethics statement

The study was approved by the Ethics Committee of Sun-yat sen University Cancer Center. As all samples used in this study were anonymous and collected from patients for routine pathology use, no informed consent (written or verbal) was obtained for use of retrospective tissue samples from the patients in this study.

Cell lines and culture

The human NPC cell lines/clones CNE-2, S26, and S18 (S26 and S18 were isolated from the parental line CNE-2 by limiting dilution method, as previously described [19]), and SUNE-1 and 5-8F (from the parental line SUNE-1 [21]) were maintained in DMEM (Invitrogen, CA) containing 10% fetal bovine serum (Invitrogen) in a humidified atmosphere with 5% CO_2 at 37°C.

Lentiviral transduction studies

A RASSF6 expression construct was generated by subcloning PCR-amplified, full-length human RASSF6 cDNA into the pCDH-CMV-MCS-EF1-RFP plasmid. Cells stably expressing either the RASSF6 short hairpin RNA (shRNA) or a scrambled, non-target shRNA were established using the LV3 plasmid according to the manufacturer's instructions. The targets of the RASSF6 shRNA-1 are 5′- GAACAAAGACGACTAAAGA-3′ and shRNA-3: 5′- GGAATTTGACGATCTCTAT-3′. Retroviral production and infection were performed as previously described [22], and stable cell lines were selected using 5 μg/ml puromycin for 7 days.

Quantitative real-time PCR (qPCR)

Total RNA was extracted from cultured cells using TRIzol reagent (Invitrogen) according to the manufacturer's instructions and was reverse-transcribed using a cDNA Synthesis Kit (Takara, CA). Real-time qPCR was performed using a SYBR Green PCR Kit (Bio-Rad, CA), and expression of the target gene was normalized to endogenous levels of GAPDH. The relative mRNA levels were shown as the value of 2ΔCt. The PCR primer sequences that were used for amplification were as follows: GAPDH forward, 5′- AAGGTCATCCCTGAGCTGAA -3′; GAPDH reverse, 5′- TGACAAAGTGGTCGTTGAGG -3′; RASSF6 forward, 5′- GGGGGAATTTGACGATCTCT -3′; RASSF6 reverse, 5′- TAGAGCACTGGGGAGTCTGG -3′; RASSF1 forward 5′- GGACGGTTCTTACACAGGCT-3′; RASSF1 reverse 5′-CACCACCAAGAACTTTCGCA -3′; RASSF2 forward 5′-GCCAGAATTTACAGCTCCGG -3′; RASSF2 reverse 5′- GAACTTTGGGCACAGTCAGG-3′; RASSF3 forward 5′-ACCCACAGTTACCTCAGCAA -3′; RASSF3 reverse 5′-CACTTCCCCGACAGTGTTTG -3′; RASSF4 forward 5′-AGGCTGAGAGTTCCACAGAC -3′; RASSF4 reverse 5′- TCACATTGGTCACGGATCCA-3′; RASSF5 forward 5′- CTCTCCAGAAAGCACCCTCA-3′; and RASSF5 reverse 5′- CACTCAGTTTCATGCCCAGG-3′. The experiments were performed in triplicate.

Cell viability assays

The cytotoxicities of cisplatin and radiation were determined using MTS assays (Cell Titer 96 Aqueous One Solution Cell Proliferation Assay solution; Promega, WI) and colony formation assays. For the MTS assay, cells were harvested and cultured in 96-well plates at a density of 2000 cells/well. Twenty four hours later, various concentration of cisplatin was added and the cells were incubated for 48 hours for drug treatment. For radiation treatment, the cells were treated with radiation at various dose 12 hours after plating the cells and then incubated for another 72 hours. The viable cells were then stained with MTS followed by determination of the OD490 using a microplate reader. For the colony formation assay, cells were plated at 500 cells per well in a 6-well plate (Corning, NY) for 24 hours and then radiated at various doses. Two weeks later, the cells were washed with phosphate buffered saline (PBS), fixed with methanol, and stained with crystal violet.

Apoptosis assays

After treatment of the cells with cisplatin (48 hours) or radiation (72 hours), the floating and adherent cells were harvested, washed with PBS, and stained with Annexin-V-phycoerythrin (or Annexin-V-FITC) and 7-AAD (BD Biosciences, NJ) for 15 minutes at room temperature. The cells were then subjected to flow cytometry analysis (Beckman Coulter, Cytomics FC500, CA).

Immunoblotting

Immunoblotting was performed according to the standard methods as described previously [22]. Briefly, cells were harvested, lysed on ice, and centrifuged (10,000 g for 30 min at 4°C) to remove debris. Supernatants were collected, and 50–100 g of total protein of each sample was subjected to SDS–PAGE/Western blotting. The blots were incubated with primary antibodies overnight at 4°C, followed by incubation with HRP-conjugated secondary antibodies (Promega) for 1 hour at room temperature. Finally, the signals were detected using an ECL system.

Antibodies and chemical drugs

The antibodies that were used for Western blotting were as follows: RASSF6 (HPA037711, Sigma, CA); and human cleaved PARP (#6525), caspase 3 (#9662), SAPK/JNK (#9258), phospho-SAPK/JNK (#4668), c-Jun (#9165), phospho-c-Jun (Ser63, #9261), phospho-c-Jun (Ser73, #3270), ERK (#4780), phosphor-ERK1/2 (#5726), p38 (#8690), phosphor-p38 (#4511), β-actin (#4970), and GAPDH (#2118) were obtained from Cell Signaling Technology (BSN). SP600125 was purchased from Sigma and dissolved in 100% dimethyl sulfoxide (DMSO) at a concentration of 20 mM for storage.

Statistical analyses

All statistical analyses were performed using the SPSS 17.0 statistical software package. Data from three independent experiments were presented as the mean values and standard deviations. The differences between two groups were evaluated using Student's t-test, and differences among three groups were evaluated using analysis of variance (ANOVA). *P* value <0.05 was considered to be statistically significant.

Results

Downregulation of RASSF6 in highly metastatic NPC cells correlates with resistance to treatment sensitivity

Highly metastatic S18 cells have been found to be more resistant to cisplatin treatment [20]. In the present study, we evaluated the radiotherapy sensitivities of S18, S26, and their parental line CNE-2. S18 cells displayed the lowest amount of irradiation-induced cell inhibition among the three cell lines, as shown using the MTS and colony formation assays (Figure 1A and 1B).

Then, the expression profile of the RASSF family in these three cell lines was analyzed. RASSF7~10 belong to the N-terminal RASSFs and display different characteristics from the C-terminal RASSF1-6; therefore, we focused on RASSF1-6 in the present study. Compared with S18, the S26 line generally had higher expression levels of RASSF1-5. Interestingly, RASSF6 showed the greatest differential expression among the three cell lines (more than a 19-fold change between S18 and S26, Figure 1C). Western blotting also showed that the protein level was higher in S26 (Figure 1D). It is well known that the majority of NPCs are sensitive to radiotherapy and chemotherapy at the beginning, and only a small portion of NPCs becomes treatment-resistant manifesting as relapsed tumors. Therefore we compared 18 samples of relapsed NPC tissues, representing treatment resistance in some extents, versus 25 primary NPC tissues collected before treatment. RASSF6 mRNA expression in relapsed tissues was significantly lower than the expression in untreated tissues (Figure 1E, $p<0.05$).

Over-expression of RASSF6 in highly metastatic NPC cells increases their sensitivity to cisplatin and radiation treatment

To assess whether RASSF6 alters the sensitivity of NPC cells toward cisplatin or radiation treatment and to determine the general role of RASSF6 in NPC cells, we compared another highly metastatic NPC cell line, 5-8F, to its parental, low metastatic cell line SUNE-1. 5-8F was more resistant to cisplatin treatment than SUNE-1(Figure S1A, IC50 of 9.94±1.86 μM in 5-8F cells *versus* IC50 of 5.92±1.09 μM in SUNE-1 cells). Compared to SUNE-1, 5-8F seemed to show no obvious different sensitivity to radiation (Figure S1B). 5-8F displayed lower RASSF6 expression compared with SUNE-1 (Figure 2A). Next, we effectively ectopically overexpressed RASSF6 in S18 and 5-8F cells (Figure 2B) and determined if the upregulation of RASSF6 would increase the sensitivity to cisplatin or radiation treatment. An MTS assay showed that the number of viable RASSF6-expressing S18 (Figure 2C upper, IC50 of 11.8±1.34 μM in S18 cells transfected with an empty vector *versus* IC50 of 6.37±0.68 μM in S18 cells with RASSF6 overexpression, $P<0.01$) and RASSF6-expressing 5-8F cells (Figure 2C bottom, IC50 of 9.85±1.04 μM in 5-8F cells transfected with an empty vector *versus* IC50 of 5.6±0.42 μM in the 5-8F cells with RASSF6 overexpression, $P<0.05$) decreased after treatment with cisplatin. Then, the cells were treated with various doses of radiation. The same dose of radiation led to a higher rate of cell death in RASSF6-transfected S18 or 5-8F cells in contrast to their respective control cells (Figure 2D). To rule out the effect of early-accelerated repopulation during radiotherapy,

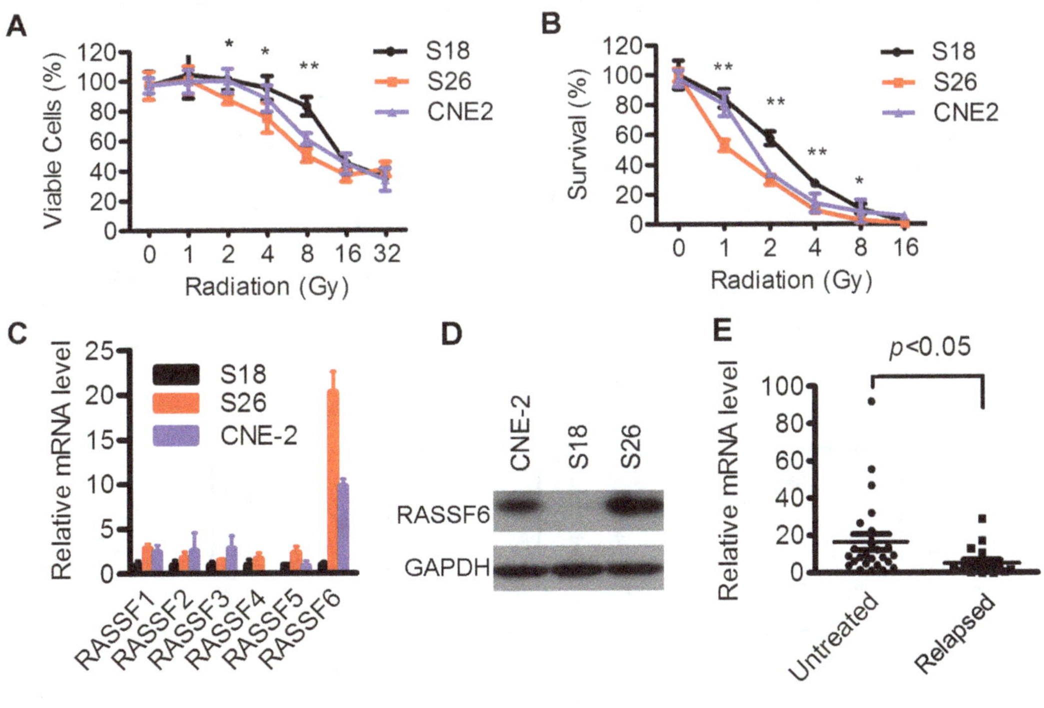

Figure 1. Characteristics of treatment sensitivity and RASSF6 expression in NPC cells and tissues. (**A, B**) CNE-2, S18, and S26 cells were treated with various doses of radiation. The viable cells were evaluated using an MTS assay (**A**); and the abilities of colony formation upon various radiation doses were compared. $*P<0.05$, $**P<0.01$, ANOVA. (**C**) mRNA expression of RASSF family members in CNE-2, S18, and S26 cells. (**D**) Western blot analysis of the RASSF6 protein level in CNE-2, S18, and S26 cells; GAPDH was used as a loading control. (**E**) RASSF6 mRNA expression levels in 18 relapsed NPC tissues (Relapsed) and 25 untreated NPC tissues (Untreated) were determined by qPCR assays. GAPDH and 18S were used as reference genes. $P<0.05$, student's t-test.

we tested for colony formation ability in these cells. Again, we found that RASSF6-transfected S18 or 5-8F cells formed fewer colonies compared to the control cells, even at low doses of radiation therapy (Figure 2E). Together, these data proved that overexpression of RASSF6 in highly metastatic NPC cells could significantly sensitize the cells to cisplatin treatment and radiotherapy.

Knockdown of RASSF6 in low metastatic NPC cells reduces their sensitivity to cisplatin and radiation treatment

We then performed the reverse experiment by knocking down RASSF6 in low metastatic S26, CNE-2 and SUNE-1 cells and determined whether the reduction in RASSF6 expression would decrease the cellular sensitivity to cisplatin or radiation treatment. As shown in Figure 3A, RASSF6 could be effectively knocked down in S26, CNE-2 and SUNE-1 cells by sh-RNAs against RASSF6. S26 cells with RASSF6 knocked down were significantly more resistant to cisplatin than those transfected with the negative control vector (Figure 3B upper, IC50 of 4.8±0.39 μM in S26 transfected with vector (NC) *versus* IC50 of 9.1±0.75 μM and 8.6±0.89 μM in S26 cells transfected with RASSF6 shRNA-1 (KD1) and shRNA-3 (KD3), respectively, $P<0.05$ for both comparisons). Consistent results were observed in CNE-2 cells (Figure 3B middle, IC50 of 5.88±0.54 μM in CNE-2 cells transfected with vector (NC) *versus* IC50 of 10.4±0.75 μM and 11.62±1.7 μM in CNE-2 cells transfected with RASSF6 shRNA 1 (KD1) and shRNA3 (KD3), respectively, $P<0.05$ for both comparisons) and SUNE-1 cells upon cisplatin treatment (Figure 3C bottom, IC50 of 6.72±0.87 μM in SUNE-1 cells transfected with vector (NC) *versus* IC50 of 10.82±1.45 μM and

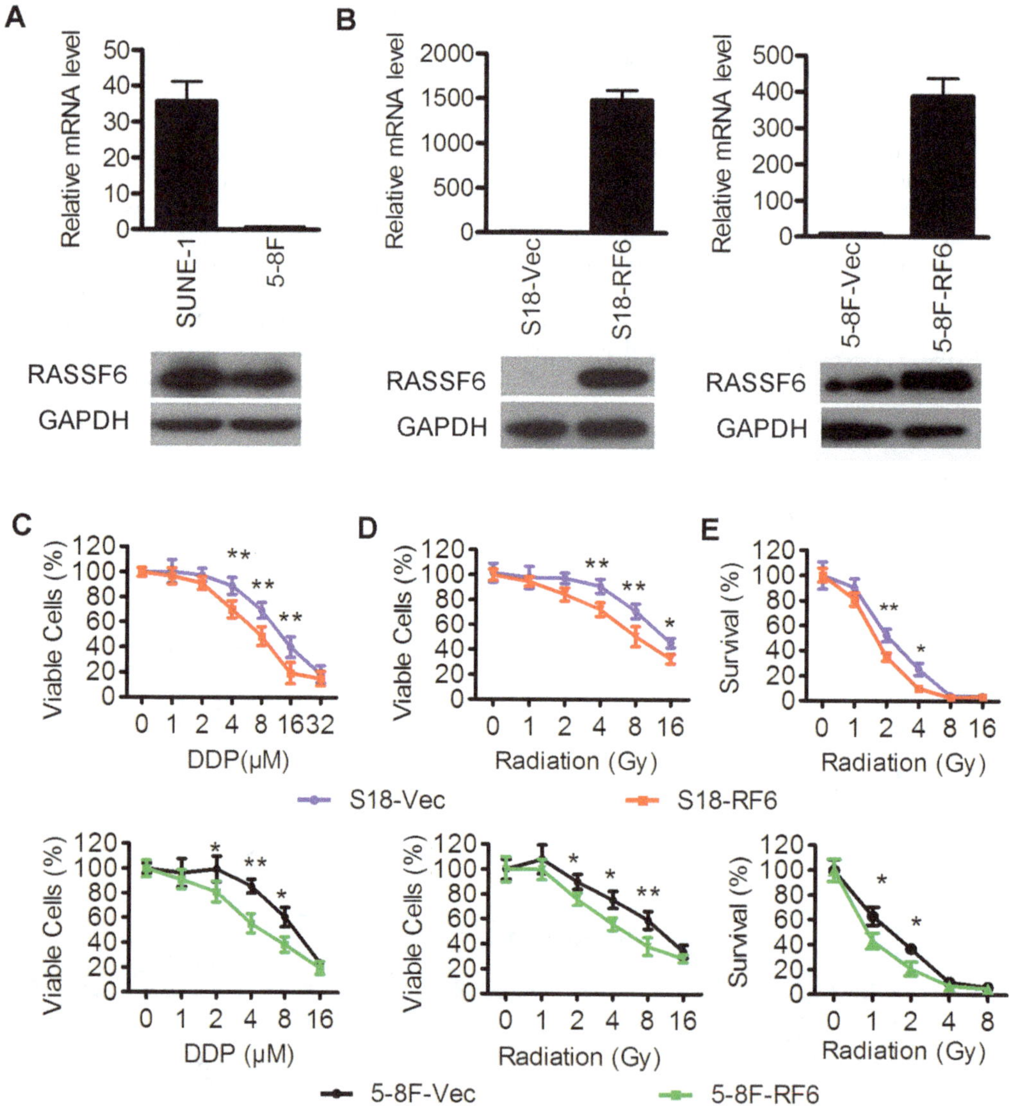

Figure 2. Overexpression of RASSF6 enhanced the sensitivities of highly metastatic NPC cells to cisplatin and radiotherapy. (A) mRNA (upper) and protein level (bottom) of RASSF6 in another highly metastatic clone, 5-8F, in contrast to its low metastatic parental line SUNE-1. **(B, C, D, E)** S18 and 5-8F cells with stable RASSF6 overexpression (RF6) or transfected with an empty vector control (Vec) were analyzed for: **(B)** RASSF6 mRNA (upper) and protein (lower) levels; **(C)** the response to various doses of cisplatin (DDP) treatment using MTS assays; **(D)** the response to various doses of radiation treatment using MTS assays; and **(E)** the ability for colony formation upon various radiation doses. *$P<0.05$, **$P<0.01$, Student's t test.

9.1±1.13 μM in SUNE-1 cells transfected with RASSF6 shRNA 1 (KD1) and shRNA3 (KD3), respectively, $P<0.05$ for both comparisons). After irradiation, more viable cells were detected in the S26,CNE-2 and SUNE-1 cells with RASSF6 stably knocked down (Figure 3C). The ability of the low metastatic cells to form colonies was also enhanced after knocking down RASSF6 (Figure 3D). These data further confirmed that RASSF6 played a role in the cellular sensitivity to cisplatin and radiation treatment.

RASSF6 regulates cisplatin/radiation-induced apoptosis

Cisplatin and radiation treatment are known to exert their cytotoxicity by inducing apoptosis. RASSF6 could induce apoptosis in various cells when exposed to DNA damage treatment [15,23]. Against this background, we tested whether RASSF6 mediates the treatment response via apoptosis by comparing Annexin V/7-AAD staining and the expression of cleaved-PARP or caspase 3, both of which serve as markers for cells undergoing apoptosis. S18 and 5-8F cells overexpressing RASSF6 had significantly higher apoptosis and elevated levels of cleaved PARP and caspase-3 when exposed to cisplatin or radiation treatment than cells transfected with the empty vector (Fig. 4A and 4B, Figure S2). In contrast, knockdown of RASSF6 in S26 or SUNE-1 cells reduced cisplatin- or radiation-induced apoptosis and the expression level of cleaved PARP and caspase-3 (Fig. 4C and 4D, Figure S3).

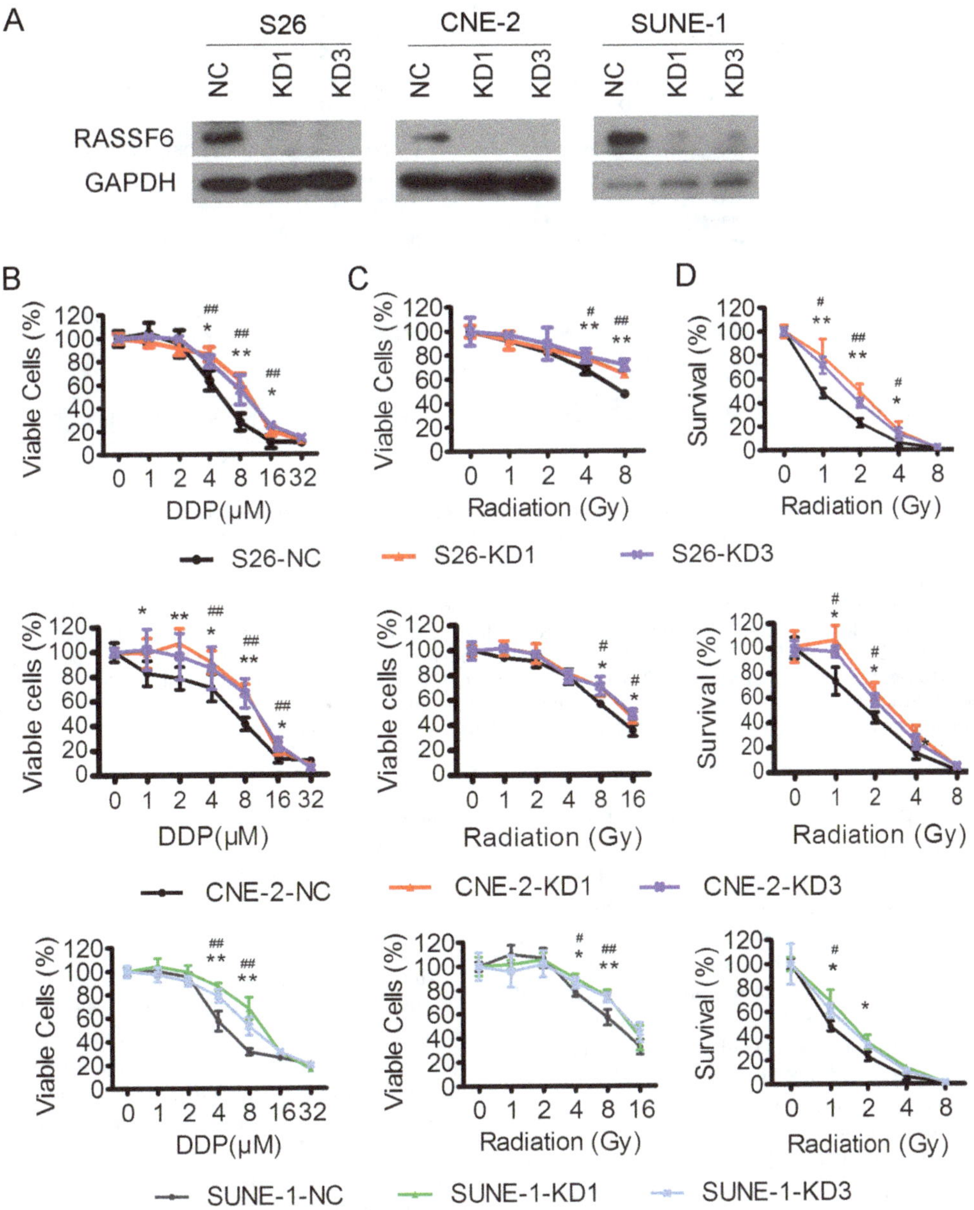

Figure 3. Depletion of RASSF6 increases the resistance of low metastatic NPC cells to cisplatin and radiotherapy. S26,CNE-2 and SUNE-1 cells were stably transfected with two different RASSF6 shRNAs (KD1, KD3) or a negative control sh-RNA (NC), followed by (**A**) Western blot analysis of RASSF6 expression, with GAPDH used as a loading control; (**B**) an MTS assay of the cellular response to various doses of cisplatin (DDP); (**C**) an MTS assay of the cellular response to various doses of radiation treatment; and (**D**) the abilities of colony formation upon various doses of radiation treatment. *$P<0.05$, **$P<0.01$ for KD1 cells compared with NC cells, # $P<0.05$, ##$P<0.01$ for KD3 cells compared with NC cells, Student's t test.

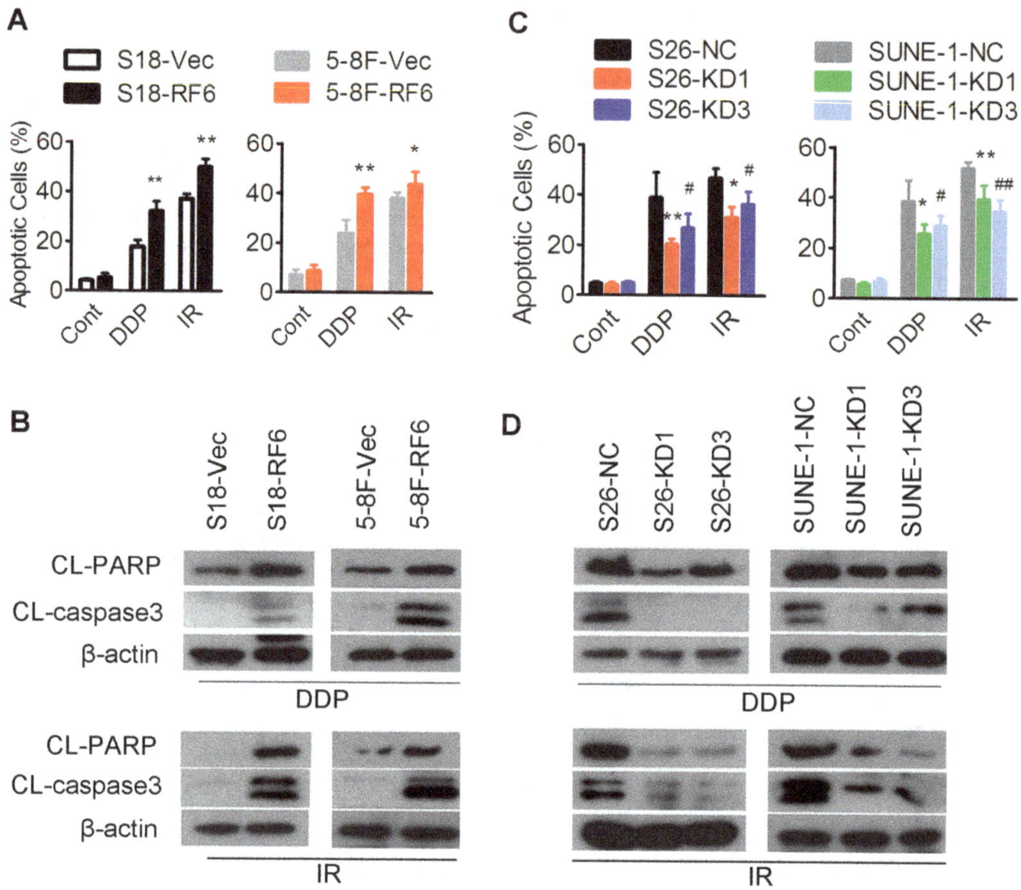

Figure 4. Upon cisplatin or radiation treatment, RASSF6 overexpression increased apoptosis, and RASSF6 depletion reduced apoptosis. (**A, B**) S18 and 5-8F cells with stable RASSF6 overexpression (RF6) or transfected with an empty vector control (Vec) were treated with the indicated doses of cisplatin (DDP, 6 μM for S18 and 8 μM for 5-8F cells), radiation (IR, 8 Gy for S18 and 5-8F cells) or not treated (Cont). Cells were collected for (**A**) flow cytometry analysis of apoptosis, *$P<0.05$, **$P<0.01$, Student's t test, and (**B**) Western blotting (upper panel for cisplatin treatment, lower panel for radiation treatment) for apoptosis-related proteins, including cleaved PARP and caspase 3, and β-actin as a loading control. (**C, D**) S26 and SUNE-1 cells stably transfected with two RASSF6 shRNAs (KD1, KD3) or with the negative control sh-RNA (NC) were treated with the indicated doses of cisplatin (DDP, 6 μM for S26 and 8 μM for SUNE-1) or radiation (IR, 8 Gy for S26 and SUNE-1) or no treated (Cont). Cells were collected for (**C**) flow cytometry analysis of apoptosis (*$P<0.05$, **$P<0.01$ for KD1 cells compared with NC cells, # $P<0.05$, ## $P<0.01$ for KD3 cells compared with NC cells, Student's t test); and (**D**) Western blotting (upper panel for cisplatin treatment, lower panel for radiation treatment) for apoptosis-related proteins, including cleaved PARP and caspase 3, and β-actin as a loading control.

RASSF6 promotes cisplatin/radiation sensitivity by activating JNK signaling

We then explored the underlying mechanism of RASSF6-promoted apoptosis. It has been reported that the RAS- MAPK signaling pathways play an important role in cellular regulation, including apoptosis caused by RASSF members. Therefore, we tested the MAPK activity in NPC cells overexpressing or depleted of RASSF6. Overexpression of RASSF6 in highly metastatic NPC cells specifically enhanced the protein level of phosphorylated JNK and C-jun (Figure 5A), but not of p38 kinase or ERK (Figure S4), when exposed to cisplatin or radiation treatment. On the other hand, phosphorylation of JNK and C-jun were inhibited in RASSF6-depleted NPC cells (Figure 5B). To confirm that the involvement of JNK signaling is essential for the RASSF6-promoted sensitivity to chemotherapy and radiotherapy in NPC cells, we applied the JNK inhibitor SP600125 to cells exposed to cisplatin or radiation treatment (Figure 5C). As expected, pharmacologic inhibition of JNK clearly suppressed the phosphorylation of c-Jun that was caused by RASSF6 and partially blocked RASSF6-promoted apoptosis (Figure 5D, Figure S5). Taken together, these results suggested that the RASSF6-promoted sensitivity to chemotherapy and radiotherapy depended on the activation of JNK signaling in NPC cells.

Discussion

Metastatic cancers are usually resistant to conventional chemotherapy and/or radiation therapy [24–26]. Successful metastasis involves the interaction of cancer cells with a compatible, organ-specific environment. The use of organ-derived molecules (e.g., P-gp, fibroblast growth factor, hepatocyte growth factor) is one important mechanism for cancer cell metastasis, and these mechanisms influence response of metastatic tumor cells to chemo-/radio-therapy [27]. Some believe that the metastatic cancer cells themselves are responsible for treatment resistance by gaining stemness characteristics within metastatic lesions [28–30]. The development of treatment resistance in a highly metastatic tumor is a complex process, and it is unrealistic to expect that any single mechanism will uncover the truth [31]. More studies are needed to investigate the conditions by which treatment resistance

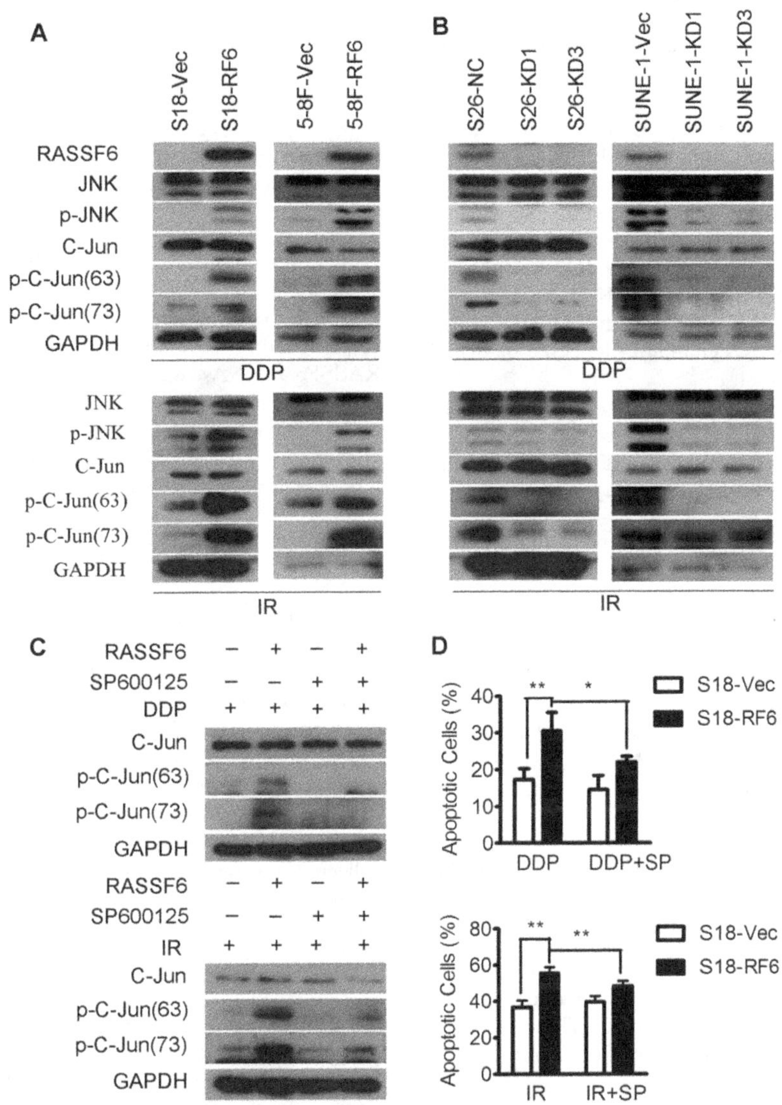

Figure 5. JNK signaling was activated by RASSF6 during the cellular response to cisplatin and radiation treatment. (**A**) S18 (left) and 5-8F (right) cells stably overexpressing RASSF6 (RF6) or transfected with an empty vector control (Vec) were treated with the indicated doses of cisplatin (upper panel, DDP, 6 μM for S18 and 8 μM for 5-8F cells) or radiation (lower panel, IR, 8 Gy for S18 and 5-8F cells). Protein was collected for Western blot analysis to evaluate the expression of RASSF6, phosphorylated JNK, total JNK, phosphorylated C-jun (ser63), phosphorylated C-jun (ser73), total C-jun, and GAPDH as a loading control. (**B**) S26 (left) and SUNE-1 (right) cells stably transfected with two RASSF6 shRNAs (KD1, KD3) or with a negative control sh-RNA (NC) were treated with the indicated doses of cisplatin (upper panel, DDP, 6 μM for S26 and 8 μM for SUNE-1 cells) or radiation (lower panel, IR, 8 Gy for S26 and SUNE-1 cells). Protein was collected for Western blot analysis of the expression of RASSF6, phosphorylated JNK, total JNK, phosphorylated C-jun (ser63), phosphorylated C-jun (ser73), total C-jun, and GAPDH as a loading control. (**C, D**) S18 cells stably overexpressing RASSF6 (RF6) or transfected with an empty vector control (Vec) were treated with cisplatin (DDP, 6 μM) or radiation (IR, 8 Gy) in the presence or absence (0.1% DMSO was used as a control) of the JNK inhibitor SP600125 (8 μM). The cells were then collected for (**C**) Western blot analysis of the expression of phosphorylated C-jun (ser63), phosphorylated C-jun (ser73), and total C-jun, with GAPDH as a loading control; and (**D**) flow cytometry analysis of apoptosis after exposure to cisplatin or radiation treatment, *$P<0.05$, **$P<0.01$, Student's t test.

is linked or not linked to metastasis and the signals or factors that may be relevant.

RASSF6 has been found to be tightly associated with tumorigenesis and functions as a tumor suppressor. RASSF6 harbors Ras-association (RA) domains in its C-terminal region that are conserved in the primary structure [18]. RASSF6 is involved in apoptosis in various cells with treatment with pro-apoptotic agents by triggering caspase-dependent and caspase-independent pathways or a Hippo-independent pathway [15,32]. RASSF6 also increases DNA repair in ultraviolet- and VP-16-treated cells [33]. We report here, for the first time, that the downregulation of RASSF6 in highly metastatic NPC cells conferred resistance to cisplatin and radiation treatment.

RAS conveys growth/stress stimuli from the cell surface to the inner cell through RAS- MAPK signaling, which mainly includes the stress-activated protein kinase/c-Jun-N-terminal kinase (JNK), p38 kinase, and extracellular signal-regulated kinase (ERK) pathways. The Ras-association domain (RA), which is a characteristic feature of the RASSF family, confers a direct binding ability to RAS. Consequently, RASSF members most likely affect the activity of MAPK pathways. In fact, some other RASSF members have been found to induce apoptosis through the inactivation of ERK [34,35] and the activation of SAPK/JNK [17]. In the present study, we observed that cisplatin or radiation treatment enhanced JNK activation in RASSF6-expressing cells. The importance of JNK activation in the cell response to anti-cancer drug and resistance development has been investigated in recent years [7]. DNA damage treatment could activate a robust apoptotic response that involves activation of the JNK pathway, but it failed to elicit JNK activation in treatment-resistant cells. Furthermore, inhibition of JNK activation partially restored the sensitivity of cancer cells to cisplatin [36–38]. Consistent with previous reports, specific inhibition of the JNK pathway in our study significantly reduced RASSF6-promoted apoptosis, which further confirmed a role for JNK signaling in RASSF6-mediated regulation of the treatment response.

Taken together, our results demonstrate that downregulation of RASSF6 was responsible for the treatment resistance of highly metastatic NPC cells and that over-expression of RASSF6 and the subsequent activation of JNK signaling conferred treatment sensitivity to NPC cells. RASSF6 could be a valuable molecule for the reversal of treatment resistance in NPC, especially for metastatic lesions.

Supporting Information

Figure S1 The response of highly metastatic 5-8F cells and low metastatic SUNE-1 cells to cisplatin and radiotherapy. 5-8F and SUNE-1cells were treated with various doses of cisplatin (**A**) or radiation (**B**). The viable cells were evaluated using an MTS assay. $^*P<0.05$, $^{**}P<0.01$, student's t-test.

Figure S2 Representative images of Annexin-V and 7-AAD double staining of high-metastatic NPC cells upon cisplatin and radiation treatment. S18 (**A**) and 5-8F cells (**B**) stably overexpressing RASSF6 (RF6) or transfected with an empty vector (Vec) were untreated (Control) or treated with the indicated doses of cisplatin (DDP, 6 μM for S18 and 8 μM for 5-8F cells) or radiation (IR, 8 Gy for S18 and 5-8F cells). The cells were then collected for flow cytometry analysis of apoptosis using Annexin-V and 7-AAD double staining.

Figure S3 Representative images of Annexin-V and 7-AAD double staining of low-metastatic NPC cells upon cisplatin and radiation treatment. S26 (**A**) and SUNE-1 cells (**B**) stably transfected with two RASSF6 shRNAs (KD1, KD3) or the negative control sh-RNA (NC) were untreated (Control) or treated with the indicated doses of cisplatin (DDP, 6 μM for S26 and 8 μM for SUNE-1 cells) or radiation (IR, 8 Gy for S26 and SUNE-1 cells). Apoptotic cells were evaluated using Annexin-V and 7-AAD double staining and flow cytometry.

Figure S4 RASSF6 regulates the response of NPC cells to cisplatin and radiation treatment independent of ERK or P38 signaling. S18 cells stably overexpressing RASSF6 (RF6) or an empty vector (Vec) and S26 cells stably transfected with two RASSF6 shRNAs (KD1, KD3) or the negative control sh-RNA (NC) were treated with cisplatin (DDP, 6 μM) or radiation (IR, 8 Gy). The whole cell lysate was collected for immunoblotting for phosphorylated ERK, total ERK, phosphorylated p38, and total p38 proteins. β-actin was used as a loading control.

Figure S5 Inhibition of JNK signaling partially blocked the RASSF6-induced apoptosis in highly metastatic NPC cells. (**A**) S18 cells stably overexpressing RASSF6 (RF6) or an empty vector (Vec) were treated with cisplatin (DDP, 6 μM) or radiation (IR, 8 Gy) in the presence or absence (0.1% DMSO was used as control) of the JNK inhibitor SP600125 (8 μM). Apoptosis was determined using flow cytometry. (**B, C**) 5-8F cells stably overexpressing RASSF6 (RF6) or transfected with an empty vector control (Vec) were treated with cisplatin (DDP, 8 μM) or radiation (IR, 8 Gy) in the presence or absence (0.1% DMSO was used as a control) of the JNK inhibitor SP600125. The cells were collected for apoptotic analysis using flow cytometry (**B**) and quantification of the apoptotic index from the triplicate experiments is shown in (**C**), $^*p<0.05$, $^{**}p<0.01$, Student's t test.

Author Contributions

Conceived and designed the experiments: YYL CNQ. Performed the experiments: YYL MYC LSZ. Analyzed the data: YYL SC. Contributed reagents/materials/analysis tools: XC BJH. Wrote the paper: YYL SC. Experiment collaboration: YJH RS LW YQX XG LXP PX.

References

1. Sarmiento MP, Mejia MB (2013) Preliminary assessment of nasopharyngeal carcinoma incidence in the Philippines: a second look at published data from four centers. Chin J Cancer.
2. Adham M, Kurniawan AN, Muhtadi AI, Roezin A, Hermani B, et al. (2012) Nasopharyngeal carcinoma in Indonesia: epidemiology, incidence, signs, and symptoms at presentation. Chin J Cancer 31: 185–196.
3. Ma BB, Hui EP, Chan AT (2008) Systemic approach to improving treatment outcome in nasopharyngeal carcinoma: current and future directions. Cancer Sci 99: 1311–1318.
4. Spratt DE, Lee N (2012) Current and emerging treatment options for nasopharyngeal carcinoma. Onco Targets Ther 5: 297–308.
5. Zhang L, Chen QY, Liu H, Tang LQ, Mai HQ (2013) Emerging treatment options for nasopharyngeal carcinoma. Drug Des Devel Ther 7: 37–52.
6. Moncharmont C, Levy A, Gilormini M, Bertrand G, Chargari C, et al. (2012) Targeting a cornerstone of radiation resistance: cancer stem cell. Cancer Lett 322: 139–147.
7. Brozovic A, Osmak M (2007) Activation of mitogen-activated protein kinases by cisplatin and their role in cisplatin-resistance. Cancer Lett 251: 1–16.
8. Burger H, Loos WJ, Eechoute K, Verweij J, Mathijssen RH, et al. (2011) Drug transporters of platinum-based anticancer agents and their clinical significance. Drug Resist Updat 14: 22–34.
9. Liu RY, Dong Z, Liu J, Zhou L, Huang W, et al. (2013) Overexpression of Asparagine Synthetase and Matrix Metalloproteinase 19 Confers Cisplatin Sensitivity in Nasopharyngeal Carcinoma Cells. Mol Cancer Ther 12: 2157–2166.
10. Liu RY, Dong Z, Liu J, Yin JY, Zhou L, et al. (2011) Role of eIF3a in regulating cisplatin sensitivity and in translational control of nucleotide excision repair of nasopharyngeal carcinoma. Oncogene 30: 4814–4823.
11. Kudo T, Ikeda M, Nishikawa M, Yang Z, Ohno K, et al. (2012) The RASSF3 candidate tumor suppressor induces apoptosis and G1-S cell-cycle arrest via p53. Cancer Res 72: 2901–2911.
12. Lock FE, Underhill-Day N, Dunwell T, Matallanas D, Cooper W, et al. (2010) The RASSF8 candidate tumor suppressor inhibits cell growth and regulates the Wnt and NF-kappaB signaling pathways. Oncogene 29: 4307–4316.
13. Akino K, Toyota M, Suzuki H, Mita H, Sasaki Y, et al. (2005) The Ras effector RASSF2 is a novel tumor-suppressor gene in human colorectal cancer. Gastroenterology 129: 156–169.
14. Thaler S, Hahnel PS, Schad A, Dammann R, Schuler M (2009) RASSF1A mediates p21Cip1/Waf1-dependent cell cycle arrest and senescence through modulation of the Raf-MEK-ERK pathway and inhibition of Akt. Cancer Res 69: 1748–1757.
15. Ikeda M, Hirabayashi S, Fujiwara N, Mori H, Kawata A, et al. (2007) Ras-association domain family protein 6 induces apoptosis via both caspase-dependent and caspase-independent pathways. Exp Cell Res 313: 1484–1495.
16. Reu FJ, Leaman DW, Maitra RR, Bae SI, Cherkassky L, et al. (2006) Expression of RASSF1A, an epigenetically silenced tumor suppressor, overcomes resistance to apoptosis induction by interferons. Cancer Res 66: 2785–2793.
17. Kitagawa D, Kajiho H, Negishi T, Ura S, Watanabe T, et al. (2006) Release of RASSF1C from the nucleus by Daxx degradation links DNA damage and SAPK/JNK activation. EMBO J 25: 3286–3297.

18. Allen NP, Donninger H, Vos MD, Eckfeld K, Hesson L, et al. (2007) RASSF6 is a novel member of the RASSF family of tumor suppressors. Oncogene 26: 6203–6211.
19. Qian CN, Berghuis B, Tsarfaty G, Bruch M, Kort EJ, et al. (2006) Preparing the "soil": the primary tumor induces vasculature reorganization in the sentinel lymph node before the arrival of metastatic cancer cells. Cancer Res 66: 10365–10376.
20. Wu MS, Wang GF, Zhao ZQ, Liang Y, Wang HB, et al. (2013) Smac mimetics in combination with TRAIL selectively target cancer stem cells in nasopharyngeal carcinoma. Mol Cancer Ther.
21. Zhang L, Song L, Ma Y, Huang B, Liang Q, et al. (2002) [Differentially expressed gene in nasopharyngeal carcinoma cell lines with various metastatic potentialities]. Zhonghua Zhong Liu Za Zhi 24: 430–434.
22. Li XJ, Ong CK, Cao Y, Xiang YQ, Shao JY, et al. (2011) Serglycin is a theranostic target in nasopharyngeal carcinoma that promotes metastasis. Cancer Res 71: 3162–3172.
23. Withanage K, Nakagawa K, Ikeda M, Kurihara H, Kudo T, et al. (2012) Expression of RASSF6 in kidney and the implication of RASSF6 and the Hippo pathway in the sorbitol-induced apoptosis in renal proximal tubular epithelial cells. J Biochem 152: 111–119.
24. Vermorken JB, Specenier P (2010) Optimal treatment for recurrent/metastatic head and neck cancer. Ann Oncol 21 Suppl 7: vii252–261.
25. O'Shaughnessy J (2005) Extending survival with chemotherapy in metastatic breast cancer. Oncologist 10 Suppl 3: 20–29.
26. el-Kamar FG, Grossbard ML, Kozuch PS (2003) Metastatic pancreatic cancer: emerging strategies in chemotherapy and palliative care. Oncologist 8: 18–34.
27. Furukawa T, Kubota T, Tanino H, Oura S, Yuasa S, et al. (2000) Chemosensitivity of breast cancer lymph node metastasis compared to the primary tumor from individual patients tested in the histoculture drug response assay. Anticancer Res 20: 3657–3658.
28. Duru N, Candas D, Jiang G, Li JJ (2013) Breast cancer adaptive resistance: HER2 and cancer stem cell repopulation in a heterogeneous tumor society. J Cancer Res Clin Oncol.
29. Ferrari P, Nicolini A, Carpi A (2013) Targeted therapies of metastatic breast cancer: relationships with cancer stem cells. Biomed Pharmacother 67: 543–555.
30. Sampieri K, Fodde R (2012) Cancer stem cells and metastasis. Semin Cancer Biol 22: 187–193.
31. Verma A, Wang H, Manavathi B, Fok JY, Mann AP, et al. (2006) Increased expression of tissue transglutaminase in pancreatic ductal adenocarcinoma and its implications in drug resistance and metastasis. Cancer Res 66: 10525–10533.
32. Ikeda M, Kawata A, Nishikawa M, Tateishi Y, Yamaguchi M, et al. (2009) Hippo pathway-dependent and -independent roles of RASSF6. Sci Signal 2: ra59.
33. Iwasa H, Kudo T, Maimaiti S, Ikeda M, Maruyama J, et al. (2013) RASSF6 tumor suppressor regulates apoptosis and cell cycle via MDM2 and p53. J Biol Chem.
34. Thaler S, Hahnel PS, Schad A, Dammann R, Schuler M (2009) RASSF1A mediates p21Cip1/Waf1-dependent cell cycle arrest and senescence through modulation of the Raf-MEK-ERK pathway and inhibition of Akt. Cancer Res 69: 1748–1757.
35. Moshnikova A, Frye J, Shay JW, Minna JD, Khokhlatchev AV (2006) The growth and tumor suppressor NORE1A is a cytoskeletal protein that suppresses growth by inhibition of the ERK pathway. J Biol Chem 281: 8143–8152.
36. Potapova O, Haghighi A, Bost F, Liu C, Birrer MJ, et al. (1997) The Jun kinase/stress-activated protein kinase pathway functions to regulate DNA repair and inhibition of the pathway sensitizes tumor cells to cisplatin. J Biol Chem 272: 14041–14044.
37. Kartalou M, Essigmann JM (2001) Mechanisms of resistance to cisplatin. Mutat Res 478: 23–43.
38. Gebauer G, Mirakhur B, Nguyen Q, Shore SK, Simpkins H, et al. (2000) Cisplatin-resistance involves the defective processing of MEKK1 in human ovarian adenocarcinoma 2008/C13 cells. Int J Oncol 16: 321–325.

Circulating Tumor Cells in Patients with Recurrent or Metastatic Head and Neck Carcinoma: Prognostic and Predictive Significance

Salvatore Grisanti[1]*, Camillo Almici[2], Francesca Consoli[1], Michela Buglione[3], Rosanna Verardi[2], Andrea Bolzoni-Villaret[4], Andrea Bianchetti[2], Chiara Ciccarese[1], Monica Mangoni[5], Laura Ferrari[1], Gianpaolo Biti[5], Mirella Marini[2], Vittorio D. Ferrari[1], Piero Nicolai[4], Stefano M. Magrini[3], Alfredo Berruti[1]

1 Medical Oncology Unit, University of Brescia and Spedali Civili Hospital, Brescia, Italy, **2** Department of Transfusion Medicine, Laboratory for Stem Cell Manipulation and Cryopreservation, Spedali Civili Hospital, Brescia, Italy, **3** Radiation Oncology Unit, University of Brescia and Spedali Civili Hospital, Brescia, Italy, **4** Otorhinolaryngology, Head and Neck Surgery Unit, University of Brescia and Spedali Civili Hospital, Brescia, Italy, **5** Department of Radiation Oncology, University of Florence, Florence, Italy

Abstract

Introduction: We investigated the frequency of detection and the prognostic and predictive significance of circulating tumor cells (CTCs) in patients with recurrent/metastatic (R/M) head and neck carcinoma (HNC) before starting systemic therapy.

Patients and methods: Using the CellSearch technology, CTCs were assessed prospectively in peripheral blood of 53 R/M-HNC patients. We performed spiking experiments to test the diagnostic performance of the CellSearch platform in identifying squamous carcinoma cells.

Results: CTCs were identified in 14 (26%) and 22 (41%) patients at baseline and at any time point, respectively. In univariate analysis ≥2 CTCs had a poorer prognostic role than 0–1 CTC. In multivariate analysis, the presence of one CTC or more was associated with a poor prognosis both in terms of progression-free survival (PFS) [Hazard Ratio (HR): 3.068, 95% confidence interval (CI): 1.53–6.13, *p* 0.002] and overall survival (OS) [HR: 3.0, 95% CI: 1.48–6.0, *p* 0.002]. A disease control after systemic therapy was obtained in 8% of CTC-positive patients as opposed to 45% in CTC-negative ones (*p* 0.03). The epidermal growth factor receptor (EGFR) expression was identified in 45% of CTC-positive patients.

Discussion: In conclusion, CTCs are detected in one out of three patients with RM-HNC. CTC detection is a strong prognostic parameter and may be predictive of treatment efficacy. The frequency of EGFR expression in CTCs seems to be lower than that expected in the primary tumor.

Editor: A. R. M. Ruhul Amin, Winship Cancer Institute of Emory University, United States of America

Funding: This work was supported in part by a grant from the Regione Lombardia Piano Sangue 2008–2010 and Piano Sangue 2010–2012, in part by a grant from the Ministero dell'Istruzione dell'Università e della Ricerca (MIUR) 2009, and in part by a donation of Mrs Marilena Bortolotti in memory of Carlo Ridon. The funders had no role in study design, data collection and analysis, decision to publish, or preparation of the manuscript.

Competing Interests: The authors have declared that no competing interests exist.

* Email: salvatore.grisanti@tin.it

Introduction

Squamous cell carcinoma of the head and neck (HNC) is the sixth most common cancer worldwide. Concomitant chemo-radiotherapy (CRT) has improved survival and organ preservation in patients with locally advanced disease [1], however treatment failure is observed in more than 50% of cases with stage III–IV tumors. The median survival of patients with persistent, recurrent or metastatic HNC is less than 12 months [2]. Salvage surgery or re-irradiation have a limited benefit at the price of a high incidence of treatment-related morbidity [3]. Systemic chemotherapy including platin-salts agents in combination with infusional fluorouracil and/or a taxane plus/minus the anti-EGFR monoclonal antibody cetuximab is frequently adopted [2–4]. Systemic therapy, however, is effective in approximately one third of patients. The characterization of the patient subset destined to have a relatively long survival and obtain benefit from therapy is crucial to tailor individually the best treatment approach and avoid unnecessary side effects. In a retrospective analysis of 390 metastatic patients treated with chemotherapy, Argiris et al. identified a set of five clinic-pathological variables (ECOG performance status, weight loss, location of the primary tumor, prior radiotherapy and tumor cell differentiation) with prognostic significance. This model was also predictive of response to chemotherapy [5], however it is not validated.

Table 1. Patients characteristics at baseline.

Characteristic		Evaluable patients ($n = 53$) n (%)
Age (years)	Median	59
	Range	20–79
	<70 years	42 (79)
	≥70 years	11 (21)
Sex	Male	42 (79)
	Female	11 (21)
Baseline ECOG performance status	0	12 (23)
	1	27 (51)
	2	13 (24)
	3	1 (2)
N. of Argiris factors	0–2	14 (26)
	≥3	39 (74)
Weight loss	<5%	29 (55)
	≥5%	24 (45)
Alcohol abuse	Yes	26 (49)
	No	27 (51)
Smoking history	Yes	46 (87)
	No	7 (13)
Anatomic distribution of primary tumor	Nasopharynx	4 (8)
	Nasal sinus	4 (8)
	Oral cavity	17 (32)
	Oropharynx	7 (13)
	Hypopharynx	4 (8)
	Larynx	15 (28)
	Cervical esophagus	2 (3)
Tumor grade	1–2	44 (83)
	3	9 (17)
Disease extent	Locally advanced	26 (49)
	Metastatic	27 (51)
No of disease sites	1	30 (56)
	2	20 (38)
	3	2 (4)
	4	1 (2)
Prior treatments for primary tumor	Surgery	32 (60)
	Radiotherapy	34 (64)
	Chemotherapy	15 (28)
N. of prior chemotherapy lines for metastatic disease	0	40 (75)
	1	7 (13)
	2	1 (2)
	3	5 (10)

Circulating tumor cells (CTCs) can provide meaningful, "realtime" information on the biology and clinical behavior of many tumors [6–9]. CTCs are very rare in the blood and, to date, the only standardized and highly reproducible assay, is the CellSearch system (Veridex, Raritan, NJ, USA) a method based on the Epithelial Cell Adhesion Molecule (EpCAM)-specific immunomagnetic separation [10]. The presence of CTCs has already been described in HNC patients, however most studies employed unstandardized systems including immunomagnetic negative separation, flow-cytometry, immunocytochemistry and RT-PCR [11–15]. Previous reports of EpCAM expression in carcinomas of the head and neck district showed that EpCAM is overexpressed in approximately 22%–75% of oropharyngeal and larynx carcinomas, in 86% of squamous cell carcinomas of the cervical esophagus and in 83%–100% of salivary glands carcinomas with different immunostaining intensities [16–17]. Further-

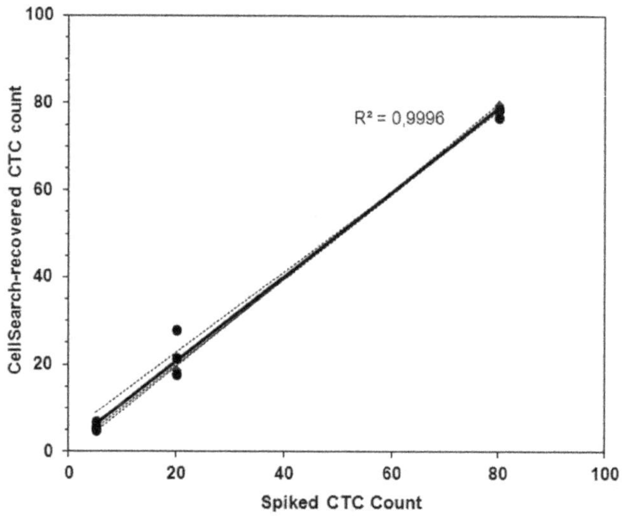

Figure 1. Recovery efficiency of known numbers of spiked A-431 cells from 7.5 mL of blood. The number of spiked cells is plotted against cells recovered by the CellSearch. The Pearson correlation value (R^2) indicates strong correlation between spiked and recovered cells.

more, CTCs have been identified by means of the CellSearch in 28%–77% of squamous cell carcinomas of the lung [6,18].

Our group conducted a multi-center prospective study to verify the presence and clinical utility of CTCs as measured by the CellSearch platform in patients with locally advanced and R/M-HNC. Previously, we reported a correlation between variation of CTCs numbers and response to chemo-radiotherapy in patients with non-metastatic HNC [19]. The current study was undertaken to demonstrate the proportion of R/M patients with detectable CTCs. Secondary aims were to provide information on 1) the prognostic significance of the presence of CTCs in this setting, 2) the role of CTCs detection in predicting treatment response and 3) the frequency of expression of EGFR in CTCs.

Patients and Methods

Ethics statement

This diagnostic observational study was conducted at three Oncology Institutions in Italy. The Institutional Ethics Review Board at the Spedali Civili of Brescia (Coordinating Centre) approved the study as part of a wider project of CTC determination in patients with solid neoplasms. However, because of the non interventional nature of the trial and because the patient's clinical management was not influenced by the study results, the other participating centers (Department of Radiotherapy Oncology, University Hospital Careggi of Florence and Department of Radiotherapy Oncology, AUSL-4 of Prato, respectively) approved the study without a formal review by the Ethics Committee Boards. All patients provided a written informed consent for diagnostic and research procedures. The present work was performed in accordance to the ethical principles for medical research involving human subjects of the Helsinki Declaration.

Study design, patients and treatments

Patient inclusion criteria were a histology-proven diagnosis of squamous carcinoma of the HN region, recurrent or metastatic disease with measurable lesions according to RECIST criteria. Exclusion criteria included poor performance status (ECOG>2) and other concomitant neoplasms. Patients were addressed to either chemotherapy or palliative care when indicated. Chemotherapy was administered as first or subsequent line for recurrent/metastatic disease. Blood for CTC detection was planned to be collected at baseline, after 3 chemotherapy cycles and at treatment completion or progression (PD). Disease status was monitored clinically and by imaging technique at the same time points. Disease control was defined as complete response (CR), partial response (PR) or stable disease (SD). Clinical variables included age, sex, ECOG performance status, weight loss, alcohol, smoking history, histology, grade of differentiation, head and neck primary sub-site, site of relapse, number of metastatic sites, previous treatment and response to chemotherapy. The Argiris prognostic score was also calculated. (Clinical data are accessible in Data S1).

Blood collection, isolation and enumeration of CTCs

Blood from HN cancer patients was drawn into 10 mL evacuated tubes which contained a cell preservative (CellSave Preservative Tubes, Veridex LLC, Raritan, NJ, USA). Blood from nine normal (ie without previous history or evidence of any neoplasm) individuals as negative controls was also drawn to confirm that CTCs do not circulate in the blood of individuals without cancer. All of them received a clinical examination to confirm absence of either neoplastic or preneoplastic lesions or inflammatory diseases of the HN district at the time of analysis. All

Table 2. CTCs prevalence in recurrent/metastatic head and neck cancer patients.

Characteristic		*n* (%)
Evaluable patients		53 (100)
CTCs+ pts at baseline		14 (26)
CTCs numbers at baseline	Median CTCs	1
	Mean CTCs ± SD	5±10
	Range	1–43
CTCs+ pts at anytime		22 (41)
N. of CTCs determinations	1	16 (31)
	2	21 (39)
	3	5 (9)
	4	11 (21)

Table 3. Univariate associations between CTCs at baseline and clinico-pathologic characteristics.

Characteristic		N. pts with ≥1CTC at baseline/total (%)	Fisher's exact test *p*
Age (years)	<70 years	13/42 (31)	.251
	≥70 years	1/11 (9)	
Sex	Male	12/42 (28)	.706
	Female	2/11 (18)	
Baseline ECOG PS	0	5/23 (22)	.547
	≥1	9/30 (30)	
Weight loss	<5%	7/29 (24)	.760
	≥5%	7/24 (29)	
Alcohol abuse	Yes	8/26 (31)	.544
	No	6/27 (22)	
Smoking history	Yes	13/46 (28)	.660
	No	1/7 (14)	
Main HN anatomical grouping	Upper HN (nasoph+nasal sinus)	2/8 (25)	.916
	Mid HN (oroph+oral cavity)	7/24 (29)	
	Lower HN (larynx+hypoph+esoph)	5/21 (24)	
Tumor grade	1–2	14/44 (32)	.092
	3	0/9 (0)	
Relapse/recurrent disease	Local	6/26 (23)	.757
	Distant	8/27 (30)	
No of sites of metastasis	1	5/30 (16)	.115
	>1	9/23 (39)	
M+ de novo vs relapsed	De novo	3/15 (20)	.732
	Relapsed	11/38 (29)	
Prior surgery for primary tumor	Yes	8/31 (26)	1.0
	No	6/22 (27)	
Prior RT for primary tumor	Yes	9/36 (25)	.748
	No	5/17 (29)	
Prior CT for primary tumor (concomitant/neoadjuvant)	Yes	4/25 (16)	.225
	No	10/28 (36)	
N. of prior CT lines for metastatic disease	0	10/40 (25)	.725
	≥1	4/13 (31)	
N. of Argiris factors	0–2	3/14 (21)	.735
	≥3	11/39 (28)	

CTC analyses were centralized at the Spedali Civili of Brescia and blood samples from peripheral participating centers were sent out by courier. Blood samples were maintained at room temperature and processed for CTC enumeration within 96 hours from collection following the manufacturer's instructions.

CellSearch assay efficiency of squamous CTCs detection

As the CellSearch system is approved by the US Food and Drug Administration (FDA) for the detection of CTCs from various adenocarcinomas [7–9], we sought to verify whether the system was also able to detect cells from squamous carcinomas. In order to estimate the accuracy of the CellSearch System in detecting CTCs in HN neoplasms, we conducted spiking experiments as previously reported [20]. Briefly, three 7.5 mL aliquots of blood from 3 normal blood donors were collected into CellSave Preservative Tubes. The three aliquots from each donor were spiked with different numbers of A-431 cells (ATCC, Rockville, MD, USA), a human squamous cell carcinoma cell line positive for both EpCAM and cytokeratins (Figure S1), to produce separate tubes with 80, 20 and 5 cells per 7.5 mL of blood. Briefly, the human A-431 cell line was cultured in flasks and subsequently harvested by trypsin treatment. Exact concentration of cells per volume (cells/μl) was determined by flow cytometry-based single platform approach using tubes containing pre-determined numbers of microbeads (TruCount, BD Biosciences, San Jose, CA, USA). Analysis was performed using a flow cytometer (FACS-Canto II, BD Biosciences, San Jose, CA, USA) by a specific gating strategy in single platform assay. After having determined the exact number of cells present in stock sample, consequent dilution was performed and final concentration of A-431 cells was confirmed applying the same counting strategy. Therefore, 80, 20 and 5 A-431 cells were spiked in triplicate in the Cell Save sample tubes. All tubes were mixed by repeated inversion and

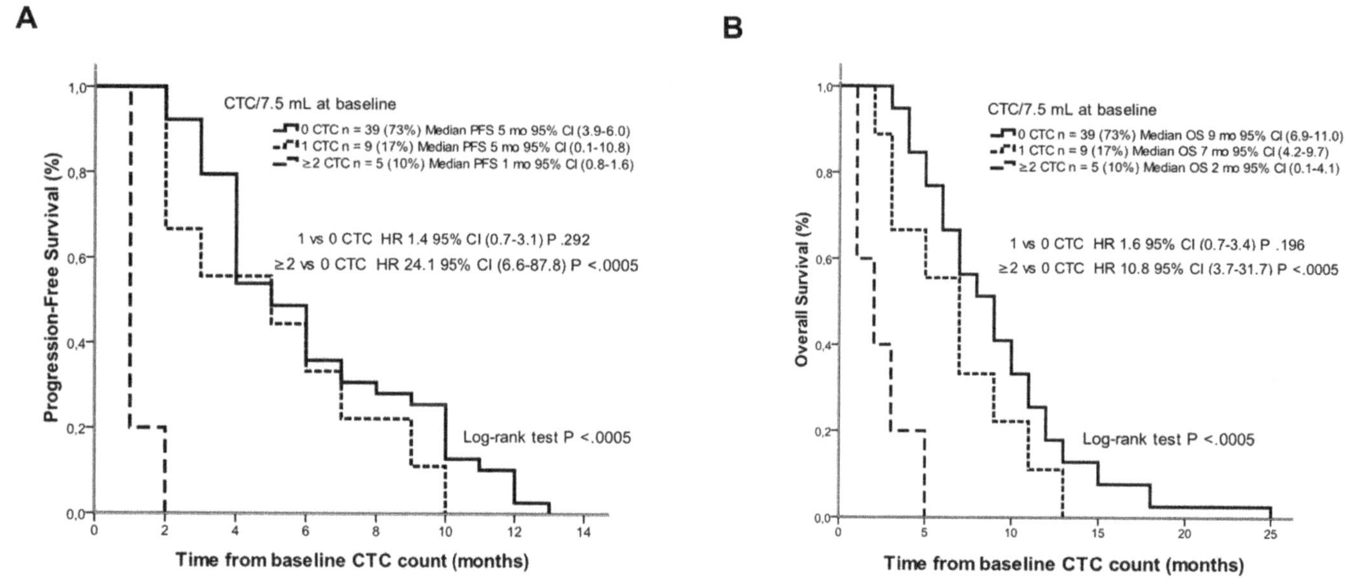

Figure 2. Kaplan-Meier curves of (A) progression-free survival and (B) overall survival in patients with 0, 1 and ≥2 CTCs.

allowed to sit overnight at room temperature. On the following day, all the nine tubes were processed and analysed by a single operator according to the manufacturer's instructions. The Pearson correlation analysis was used to establish association between CellSearch-recovered versus spiked CTC counts.

EGFR analysis on CTCs from R/M-HNC

To measure the percentage of EGFR-positive CTCs from R/M-HNC we used the commercially available CellSearch Tumor Phenotyping Reagent EGFr kit (Veridex LLC, Raritan, NJ, USA) on the fourth channel of fluorescence of the CellSearch system following the manufacturer's instructions. The analytical sensitivity

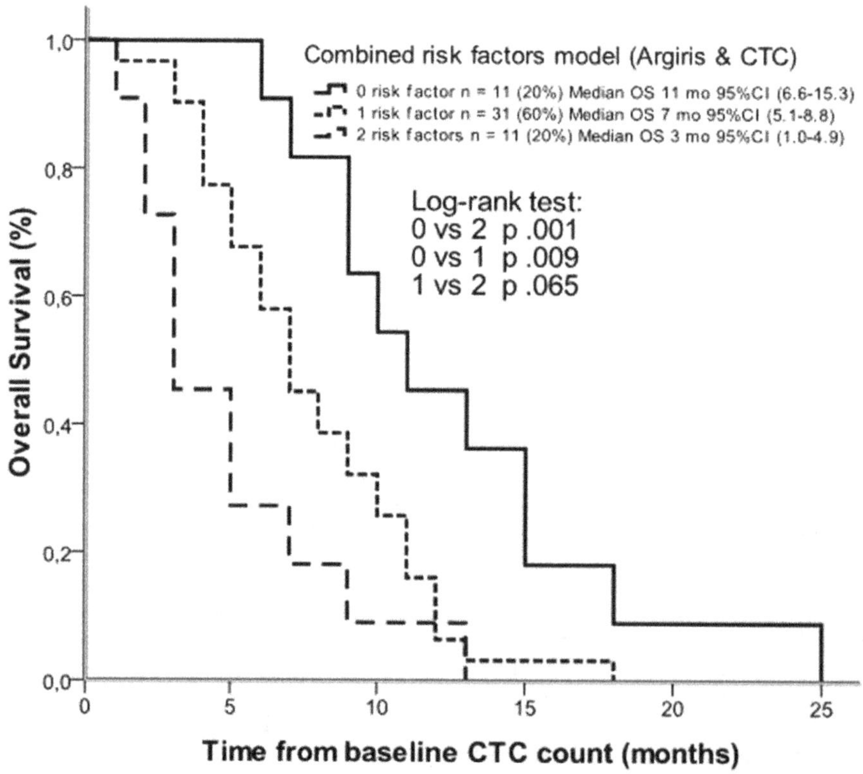

Figure 3. Kaplan-Meier estimates of overall survival according to a combined risk factors model with Argiris factors and CTCs. Continuous line indicates absence of both risk factors; small dotted line indicates the presence of only one of the two risk factors; large dotted line indicates the presence of both risk factors.

Table 4. Multivariate analysis of progression-free and overall survival.

Characteristic		PFS			OS		
		HR	95% CI	p	HR	95% CI	p
CTCs at baseline	≥1 vs 0	3.0	1.53–6.13	.002	3.0	1.48–6.02	.002
Relapse/recurrent disease	Local vs Distant	2.7	1.45–4.98	.002	2.3	1.14–4.80	.019
Argiris prognostic factors[1]	≥3 vs 0–2	-	-	-	1.3	.60–2.89	.427

[1]Argiris factors were included in the overall survival model only. Abbreviations: PFS, progression-free survival; OS, overall survival; HR, hazard ratio; CI, confidence intervals; CTCs, circulating tumor cells.

of this kit has not been reported by the manufacturer and we analysed cell lines with different (or absent) levels of expression of EGFR to test the diagnostic performance of the procedure. The CellSearch was able to correctly detect all the spiked cells from the three EGFR-positive cell lines as EGFR-positive and correctly identified the EGFR-negative cell line as EGFR-negative. (data not shown).

Statistical analysis

The primary objective of the study was to assess the frequency of CTCs in the peripheral blood of patients with RM-HNC measured by the CellSearch system. The sample size was calculated in order to reject the null hypothesis that the proportion of patients with detectable CTC was less than 5% and to provide a statistical power of 80% to demonstrate that at least 35% of patients had at least 1 CTC/7.5 mL. With a two-sided alpha of 0.05, 50 consecutive patients meeting the inclusion criteria were planned to be enrolled. Secondary objectives were to correlate the presence of CTCs with outcome endpoints and response to chemotherapy.

The relationship between categorical covariates was assessed with a Fisher's exact test. PFS and OS were defined as the time elapsed from baseline CTC analysis to the first evidence of disease progression and death or last follow-up, respectively. Survival curves were calculated with the Kaplan Meier method and compared with the log-rank (Mantel-Cox) test. Cox proportional hazard model was employed to assess the HR of progression and death both in uni- and multivariate analyses. All tests were two-sided and the $p<.05$ was considered statistically significant. Statistical analyses were conducted with the SPSS software (SPSS version 17.0, Chicago, IL, USA). The REporting of tumor MARKer Studies (REMARKS) guidelines were followed in reporting results of this study [21].

Results

Patient demographics

From January 2009 to February 2011, 57 consecutive patients were enrolled in the study. Four patients were not evaluable, two because of technical defaults of the CellSearch system and two because of lack of clinical information. The characteristics of the final 53 evaluable patients are outlined in Table 1. The vast majority of patients had a squamous cell carcinoma. Four patients had an undifferentiated carcinoma of the nasopharynx. Fifteen (28%) patients were metastatic at diagnosis and 38 had recurrent disease. Forty patients (75%) were chemotherapy-naïve. Chemotherapy was administered to 45/53 (85%) patients while 8 patients with severe comorbidities received best supportive care. Chemotherapy consisted of cisplatin monotherapy in 1 patient (2%), cisplatin plus fluorouracil in 16 (36%) patients, cisplatin, fluorouracil and paclitaxel in 21 (46%) patients, cisplatin and cetuximab in 1 patient (2%), methotrexate in 4 (9%) patients and vinorelbine in 2 (4%) patients. In the group of nine individuals selected as negative controls, median age was 51 years, 6 were males and 3 were females.

CellSearch assay efficiency of squamous CTCs detection

The approximate number of A-431 cells spiked into the blood of the three healthy donors was plotted against the number of the CellSearch-recovered cells in the samples and regression analysis using the number of observed CTCs versus the number of expected CTCs resulted in a best fit line with a slope of 1.03 (95%CI: 0.77–1.3), an intercept of −1.57 (95%CI:−13.9–10.8), and a correlation coefficient (R^2) of 0,9996 (Figure 1). The assay

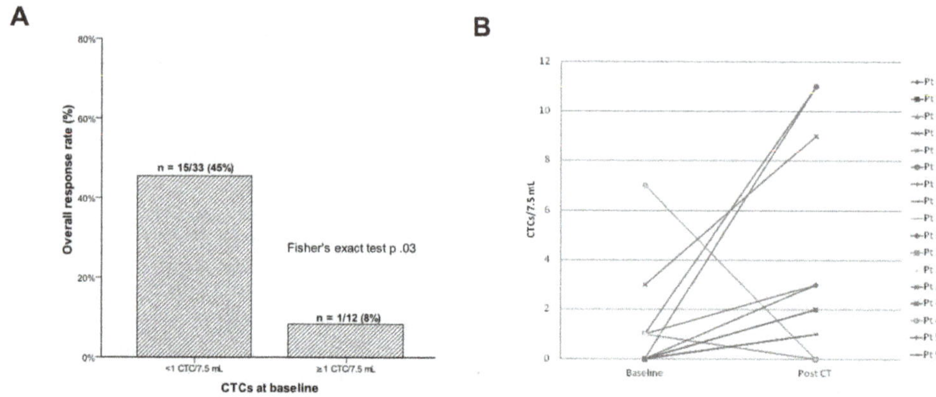

Figure 4. Association between the presence of CTCs before starting a new line of chemotherapy and response to treatment. Higher response rate is observed in CTC-negative patients at baseline (A). Dynamic variation of CTCs numbers before and after treatment in patients (n = 10) with at least two determinations and at least one CTC at any time point. CTCs changes did not correlate with tumor response (B).

efficiency of recovery was >90%, indicating that the platform was able to detect squamous cells.

CTCs assessment

Thirty-seven patients had CTC assessed at least at two time points while sixteen patients had only one sample evaluated. Twenty-two (41%) patients had detectable CTCs at least at one time point during clinical observation. In patients with detectable CTCs, median and mean CTCs values were 1 and 5 (±10 SD), respectively. We therefore used 1 CTC/7.5 mL as cutoff for subsequent analyses. At baseline, 14 (26%) patients had at least 1 CTC detected. Nine of them (64%) had 1 CTC, two (14%) had 2–10 CTCs and three (20%) more than 10 CTCs (Table 2). None of the nine normal volunteers had detectable CTCs. At univariate analysis the presence of CTCs at baseline was not related to any of the clinical variables considered. (Table 3).

Prognostic significance of CTCs in HNC patients

At the date of last follow-up (March 2012) all patients had progressed and died. In the overall population median PFS and OS from CTC analysis were 4 and 7 months, respectively. Median PFS in patients with 0, 1 and ≥2 CTCs at baseline were 5 months (95% CI 3.9–6.0), 5 months (95% CI 0.1–10.8) and 1 month (95% CI 0.8–1.6), respectively, (log-rank test $p<.0005$). Median OS in patients with 0, 1 and ≥2 CTCs at baseline were 9 months (95% CI 6.9–11.0), 7 months (95% CI 4.2–9.7) and 2 months (95% CI 0.1–4.1) respectively, (log-rank test $p<.0005$) (Figure 2A and 2B).

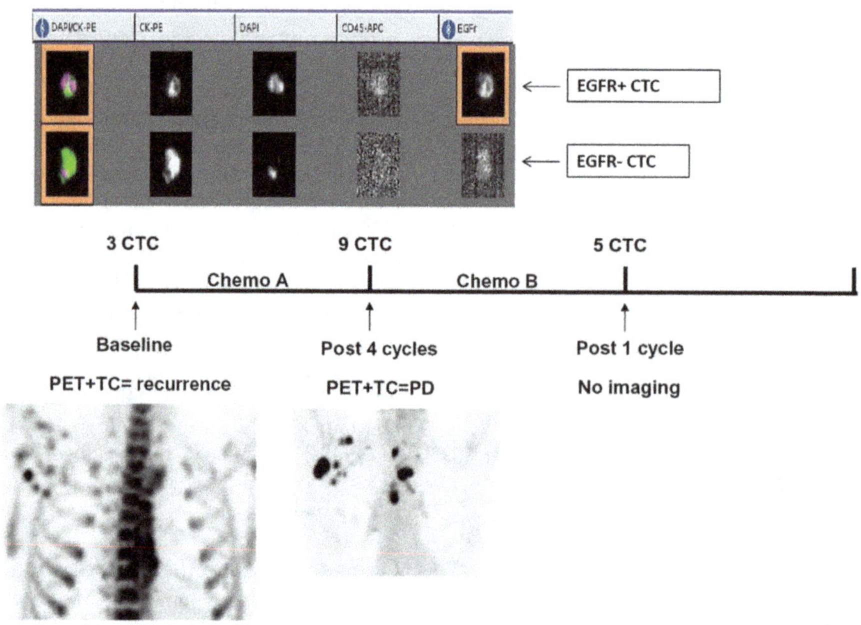

Figure 5. Example of CTCs analysis in a patient with mediastinal and axillary nodal metastases from an oropharyngeal squamous cell carcinoma. (A) the CellSearch output of baseline CTC analysis showing two CTCs with heterogeneous EGFR expression. (B) Timeline of CTC analysis and treatments. (C) Correlative imaging analysis by CT/PET at baseline and after chemotherapy. In this patient 3 CTCs were detected at baseline. After 4 cycles of a chemotherapy, CTC number rised to 9 suggesting progressive disease then confirmed by CT/PET imaging.

These results indicate that ≥2 CTCs rather than 1 CTC might be a better cutoff indicator for both PFS and OS.

Combining Argiris factors with CTC results, overall survival was better in patients with low Argiris risk and no CTC (median 11 months, 95% CI 6.6–15.3) than in patients with high Argiris risk and at least 1 CTC (median 3 months, 95% CI 1.0–4.9) (log-rank test *p* .001) (HR .22, 95% CI .09–.54). Patients with one of the 2 risk factors had an intermediate survival (median 7 months, 95% CI 5.1–8.8) (HR .52, 95% CI .26–1.0) (Figure 3).

At univariate analysis, variables with statistically significant impact on PFS and OS were the site of relapse (local vs distant) (*p* .015 and *p* .011, respectively), the Argiris prognostic factors (≥3 vs 0–2) (calculated only for OS, *p* .017) and CTCs at baseline (Table S1). At multivariate regression analysis, the covariates that maintained an independent prognostic significance both for PFS and for OS were CTCs at baseline (HR 3.0, 95% CI 1.53–6.13, *p* .002 and HR 3.0, 95% CI 1.48–6.0, *p* .002) and the site of relapse (HR 2.68, 95% CI 1.44–4.97, *p* .002 and HR 2.34, 95% CI 1.14–4.8, *p* .019), respectively (Table 4).

CTCs at baseline as predictors of response to chemotherapy and variation of CTCs number after chemotherapy

Response to chemotherapy was evaluated in 45 treated patients after 3 cycles and at treatment completion or progression. Sixteen (35%) patients obtained disease control (9 PR and 7 SD) and the remaining 29 (65%) had PD. The clinical control of the disease was mainly confined in patients with 0 CTC (15/33, 45%) while only one (8%) PR was observed in the 12 patients with detectable CTCs at baseline (p .03) (Figure 4A).

Ten out of the 14 CTC-positive patients at baseline were tested before and after chemotherapy. Of them, five had a increase, one remained stable and four had a decrease of CTCs after treatment. By contrast, seven patients without CTCs at baseline had detectable CTCs at the end of treatment (Figure 4B). As an example, Figure 5 illustrates the outcome in terms of CTCs and imaging of a patient progressing after a line of chemotherapy. Changes in CTCs levels were not found to be correlated with tumor response.

EGFR characterization of CTCs in HNSCC patients

The EGFR expression was assessed in 41 samples. Of the 22 patients with at least one CTC during clinical observation, 10 (45%) had CTCs with detectable levels of EGFR as measured with the CellSearch system and 12 (55%) had EGFR-negative CTCs. Of note, consistent heterogeneity in EGFR expression was observed intra- and intersample (Figure 5). On average, when more than one CTC was counted in 7.5 mL of blood, EGFR was expressed in 25% of the detected CTCs within the same sample. Furthermore, in 8 patients with EGFR-positive CTCs evaluated at two or more time points, EGFR was detected in 37% of the samples indicating that EGFR expression is modulated over time within the same patient.

Discussion

This study demonstrated that 26% of R/M-HNC patients at baseline conditions and 41% at any time point had ≥1 CTC. The spiking experiments performed with the EpCAM-positive cell line A-431 confirmed that the CellSearch technology can detect squamous CTCs in blood. These results are in line with recent experiences in which 16%–40% of stage III–IV HNC patients had 0–2 CTCs by the CellSearch [22,23].

The low median numbers of CTCs detected in HNC patients by the CellSearch test could reflect a true low frequency of CTCs in HNC or may be the result of an intrinsic low expression of the capture antigen, EpCAM molecule, on cancer cells surface. Alternatively it suggests the existence of epithelial-to-mesenchymal transition (EMT) phenomena with a higher number of circulating cancer cells lacking epithelial markers such as EpCAM or cytokeratins [24,25].

There is an urgent need of prognostic and predictive factors in recurrent/metastatic-HNC patients and our results showed that CTCs could serve as new independent prognostic parameter for both PFS and OS. In univariate analysis >2 CTCs had a poorer prognostic role than 0–1 CTC in patients before starting a new chemotherapy. However, this effect was observed also at any time point during clinical observation (data not shown).

The largest analysis of prognostic factors in recurrent and metastatic HNC, published by Argiris et al, identified a set of clinico-pathological factors that correlated with the patient outcome [5]. Noteworthy, in our study, after adjustment for the presence of CTCs, the Argiris criteria were no longer prognostic. By combining Argiris high risk criteria with the presence of CTCs we found a good separation in terms of survival among patients with both risk factors, one risk or none of the two. These data confirm the emerging evidence that the presence of cancer cells in the blood is *per se* associated with more aggressive features of the neoplasm, independently of the patient characteristics and the tumor stage. Another interesting aspect of our study was that there was no difference in terms of CTCs between patients with local recurrence or distant metastases. This result suggests that HNC, traditionally considered a disease with local tropism, is indeed characterized by circulation and re-circulation of cancer cells via the bloodstream regardless of the metastatic site, local or distant [26].

In our series the presence of CTCs was also predictive of chemotherapy activity. The clinical control of the disease, in fact, was mainly confined in patients with 0 CTC as opposed to their counterpart. Again, it could be hypothesized that those cancer cells that enter into the blood have acquired more aggressive features than resident cancer cells, including enhanced survival and chemoresistance [27]. Thus, the presence of CTCs before starting a new chemotherapy or their appearance during treatment could identify poor-responder patients. This interesting observation deserves confirmation.

CTCs offer the unique opportunity to monitor the changes in tumor biology over time. EGFR is overexpressed in over 90% of HNC [28] although with a wide range of expression [29]. In this work, the CellSearch was able to identify EGFR signals in 45% of patients with CTCs at any time point. These data suggest a huge discordance of EGFR expression between the primary tumor and CTCs and this could indicate a modulation of EGFR expression over time. Similar findings were already described in metastatic breast cancer patients in whom a discordance rate of 42% in terms of Her2-positivity between primary breast cancer and CTCs was observed [30]. Again, given that EMT processes induce down-regulation of epithelial markers and that EMT facilitates intravasation of cancer cells within the bloodstream [31], the presence of EGFR-negative CTCs could identify cancer cells with more proclivity to metastasize.

EGFR determination by immunohistochemistry (IHC), either in the primary or in metastatic lesions, is not required for Cetuximab prescription according to both FDA and EMEA guidelines. In the Extreme trial, response rate in the Cetuximab arm was 36%. However, neither EGFR expression by IHC nor EGFR gene copy number by FISH in the primary tumor were found to be predictive of response in two retrospective analyses [32,33]. Based on our results, evaluation of EGFR expression on CTCs could be prospectively analyzed in Cetuximab-treated patients to establish possible predictive significance.

In conclusion, this paper demonstrates for the first time that CTCs can be detected in one third of patients with RM-HNC and their presence strongly correlates with unfavorable prognosis independently of tumor and patient's characteristics. Our data also suggest a role of CTCs in predicting the treatment activity, although these results must be interpreted with caution. The clinical and therapeutic implications of CTCs in HNC and their molecular heterogeneity deserve to be further studied.

Supporting Information

Figure S1 Phenotype analysis of the A-431 squamous cell line in terms of EpCAM, cyokeratins and EGFR expression.

Table S1 Univariate analysis of progression-free and overall survival.

Data S1 (SAV)

Acknowledgments

The authors wish to thank Dr. S. Marzano, Dr. M. Spediacci and Dr. C. Polli of the Department of Radiation Oncology, ASL4, Prato, Italy for their contribution in this study. The contribution of the nursing staff and participating patients and their families is also acknowledged.

Author Contributions

Conceived and designed the experiments: SG CA MB. Performed the experiments: SG CA RV A. Bianchetti. Analyzed the data: SG FC CC CA. Contributed reagents/materials/analysis tools: RV FC MB ABV M. Mangoni LF GB VDF PN SMM M. Marini. Contributed to the writing of the manuscript: SG CA A. Berruti. Statistical analysis: SG CC A. Berruti. Administrative and financial support: M. Marini GB SMM.

References

1. Pignon JP, Le Maitre A, Bourhis J (2007) Meta-analyses of chemotherapy in head and neck (MACH-NC): an update. Int J Rad Oncol Biol Phys 69: s112–s114.
2. Vermorken JB, Specenier P (2010) Optimal treatment for recurrent/metastatic head and neck cancer. Ann Oncol 21: vii252–vii261.
3. Arnold DJ, Goodwin WJ, Weed DT, Civantos FJ (2004) Treatment of recurrent and advanced stage squamous cell carcinoma of the head and neck. Sem Radiat Oncol 14: 190–195.
4. Vermorken JB, Mesia R, Rivera F, Remenar E, Kawecki A, et al. (2008) Platinum-based chemotherapy plus cetuximab in head and neck cancer. N Engl J Med 359: 1116–1127.
5. Argiris A, Li Y, Forastiere A (2004) Prognostic factors and long-term survivorship in patients with recurrent or metastatic carcinoma of the head and neck. Cancer 101: 2222–2229.
6. Krebs MG, Sloane R, Priest L, Lancashire L, Hou JM, et al. (2011) Evaluation and prognostic significance of circulating tumor cells in patients with non-small-cell lung cancer. J Clin Oncol 29: 1556–1563.
7. Cristofanilli M, Budd GT, Ellis MJ, Stopeck A, Matera J, et al. (2004) Circulating tumor cells, disease progression, and survival in metastatic breast cancer. N Engl J Med 351: 781–791.
8. Cohen SJ, Punt CJA, Iannotti N, Saidman BH, Sabbath KD, et al. (2008). Relationship of circulating tumor cells to tumor response, progression-free survival and overall survival in patients with metastatic colorectal cancer. J Clin Oncol 26: 3213–3221.
9. De Bono JS, Scher HI, Montgomery RB, Parker C, Miller MC, et al. (2008) Circulating tumor cells predict survival benefit from treatment in metastatic castration-resistant prostate cancer. Clin Cancer Res 14: 6302–6309.
10. Mostert B, Sleijfer S, Foekens JA, Gratama JW (2009) Circulating tumor cells (CTCs): detection methods and their clinical relevance in breast cancer. Cancer Treat Rev 35: 463–474.
11. Partridge M, Brakenhoff R, Phillips E, Kulsan A, Francis R, et al. (2003) Detection of rare disseminated tumor cells identifies head and neck cancer patients at risk of treatment failure. Clin Cancer Res 9: 5287–5294.
12. Wirtschafter A, Benninger MS, Moss TJ, Umiel T, Blazoff K, et al. (2002) Micrometastatic tumor detection in patients with head and neck cancer. Arch Otolaryngol Head Neck Surg 128: 40–43.
13. Tong X, Yang L, Campbell Lang J, Zborowski M, Chalmers JJ (2007) Application of immunomagnetic cell enrichment in combination with RT-PCR for the detection of rare circulating head and neck tumor cells in human peripheral blood. Cytometry Part B (Clinical Cytometry) 72B: 310–323.
14. Jatana KR, Balasubramanian P, Lang JC, Yang L, Jatana CA, et al. (2010) Significance of circulating tumor cells in patients with squamous cell carcinoma of the head and neck. Arch Otol Head Neck Surg 136: 1274–1279.
15. Hristozova T, Konschak R, Stromberger C, Fusi A, Liu Z, et al. (2011) The presence of circulating tumor cells (CTCs) correlates with lymph node metastasis in unresectable squamous cell carcinoma of the head and neck region (SCCHN). Ann Oncol 22: 1878–1885.
16. Went PTH, Lugli A, Maier S, Bundi M, Mirlacher M, et al. (2004) Frequent EpCAM protein expression in human carcinomas. Human Pathology 35: 122–128.
17. Laimer K, Fong D, Gastl G, Obrist P, Kloss F, et al. (2008) EpCAM expression in squamous cell carcinoma of the oral cavity: frequency and relationship to clinicopathologic features. Oral Oncol 44: 72–77.
18. Tanaka F, Yoneda K, Kondo N, Hashimoto M, Takuwa T, et al. (2009) Circulating tumor cells as a diagnostic marker in primary lung cancer. Clin Cancer Res 15: 6980–6986.
19. Buglione M, Grisanti S, Almici C, Mangoni M, Polli C, et al. (2012) Circulating tumor cells in locally advanced head and neck cancer: preliminary report about their possible role in predicting response to non-surgical treatment and survival. Eur J Cancer 48: 3019–3026.
20. Allard WJ, Matera J, Miller MC, Repollet M, Connelly MC, et al. (2004) Tumor cells circulate in the peripheral blood of all major carcinomas but not in healthy subjects or patients with nonmalignant disease. Clin Cancer Res 10: 6897–6904.
21. McShane LM, Altman DG, Sauerbrei W, Taube SE, Gion, et al. (2005) Reporting recommendations for tumor markers prognostic studies (REMARK). J Natl Cancer Inst 97: 1180–1184.
22. Nichols AC, Lowes LE, Szeto CCT, Basmaji J, Dhaliwal S, et al. (2012) Detection of circulating tumor cells in advanced head and neck cancer using the cellsearch system. Head Neck 34: 1440–1444.
23. Bozec A, Ilie M, Dassonville O, Elodie L, Poissonnet G, et al. (2013) Significance of circulating tumor cell detection using the CellSearch system in patients with locally advanced head and neck squamous cell carcinoma. Eur Arch Otorhinolaryngol 270: 2745–2749.
24. Aktas B, Tewes M, Fehm T, Hauch S, Kimmig R, et al. (2009) Stem cell and epithelial-mesenchymal transition markers are frequently overexpressed in circulating tumor cells of metastatic breast cancer patients. Breast Cancer Res 11: R46. DOI: 10.1186/bcr2333.
25. Bleijerveld OB, Brakenhoff RH, Schaaij-Visser TB, Damen JM, Altelaar AF, et al. (2011) Protein signatures associated with tumor cell dissemination in head and neck cancer. J Proteomics 74: 558–566.
26. Kim MY, Oskarsson T, Acharyya S, Nguyen DX, Zhang XHF, et al. (2009) Tumor self-seeding by circulating tumor cells. Cell 139: 1315–1326.
27. Gazzaniga P, Gradilone A, Naso G, Cortesi E, Gianni W, et al. (2008) Chemoresistance profile of circulating tumor cells: toward a clinical benefit? Int J Cancer 123: 1730–1732.
28. Grandis JR, Melhem MF, Gooding WE, Day R, Holst VA, et al. (1998) Levels of TGF-a and EGFR protein in head and neck squamous cell carcinoma and patient survival. J Natl Cancer Inst 90: 824–832.
29. Ang KK, Berkey BA, Tu X, Zhang HZ, Katz R, et al. (2002) Impact of epidermal growth factor receptor expression on survival and pattern of relapse in patients with advanced head and neck carcinoma. Cancer Res 62: 7350–7356.
30. Pestrin M, Bessi S, Galardi F, Truglia M, Biggeri A, et al. (2009) Correlation of HER2 status between primary tumors and corresponding circulating tumor cells in advanced breast cancer patients. Breast Cancer Res Treat 118: 523–530.
31. Christiansen JJ, Rajasekaran AK (2006) Reassessing epithelial to mesenchymal transition as a prerequisite for carcinoma invasion and metastasis. Cancer Res 66: 8319–8326.
32. Licitra L, Storkel S, Ferr KM, Van Cutsem E, Pirker R, et al. (2013) Predictive value of epidermal growth factor receptor expression for first-line chemotherapy plus cetuximab in patients with head and neck and colorectal cancer: analysis of data from the EXTREME and CRYSTAL studies. Eur J Cancer 49: 1161–1168.
33. Licitra L, Mesia R, Rivera F, Remenar E, Hitt R, et al. (2011) Evaluation of EGFR gene copy number as a predictive biomarker for the efficacy of cetuximab in combination with chemotherapy in the first-line treatment of recurrent and/or metastatic squamous cell carcinoma of the head and neck: EXTREME study. Ann Oncol 22: 1078–1087.

16

Unilateral Cervical Nodal Metastasis is an Independent Prognostic Factor for Esophageal Squamous Cell Carcinoma Patients Undergoing Chemoradiotherapy

Peng Zhang[1☯], Mian Xi[1☯], Lei Zhao[1], Qiao-Qiao Li[1], Liru He[1], Shiliang Liu[1], Jingxian Shen[2], Meng-Zhong Liu[1]*

1 Sun Yat-sen University Cancer Center; State Key Laboratory of Oncology in South China, Collaborative Innovation Center for Cancer Medicine; Department of Radiation Oncology, Cancer Center, Sun Yat-sen University, Guangzhou, People's Republic of China, **2** Sun Yat-sen University Cancer Center; State Key Laboratory of Oncology in South China, Collaborative Innovation Center for Cancer Medicine; Imaging Diagnosis and Interventional Center, Cancer Center, Sun Yat-sen University, Guangzhou, People's Republic of China

Abstract

Purpose: To determine the prognostic significance of unilateral cervical lymph nodal metastasis (CLNM) in patients with inoperable thoracic esophageal squamous cell carcinoma (SCC) and to identify significant prognostic factors in these patients.

Patients and methods: This retrospective study involved 395 patients with inoperable esophageal SCC treated with concurrent chemoradiotherapy. The patients were classified into three groups according to their cervical lymph node status: group A, no evidence of CLNM; group B, unilateral CLNM; group C, other distant metastases. Overall survival (OS) and progression-free survival (PFS) were calculated. Significant prognostic factors were identified using univariate and multivariate analyses.

Results: The 3-year OS rates in groups A, B and C were 46.7%, 33.5% and 8.3%, respectively ($p<0.001$, log-rank test). The corresponding PFS rates were 40.7%, 26.4% and 4.7% ($p<0.001$, log-rank test). Group B had a similar prognosis to that of group A and better 3-year OS ($p=0.009$) and PFS ($p=0.006$) rates than those of group C. Multivariate analysis demonstrated that T stage, chemotherapy regimen and cervical lymph node involvement were independent prognostic factors affecting OS and PFS.

Conclusions: Compared to other distant metastases, unilateral CLNM is associated with longer OS in esophageal SCC and should be regarded as a regional disease. Sex, T stage, concurrent chemotherapy modality and cervical lymph node involvement are independent predictors of survival in esophageal SCC.

Editor: Rossella Rota, Ospedale Pediatrico Bambino Gesu', Italy

Funding: This work was supported by grants from the Natural Science Foundation of China (No. 81272487). The funders had no role in study design, data collection and analysis, decision to publish, or preparation of the manuscript.

Competing Interests: The authors have declared that no competing interests exist.

* Email: liumengzhong@126.com

☯ These authors contributed equally to this work.

Introduction

Esophageal cancer is one of the most life-threatening tumors, with a 5-year survival rate of only 17% [1]. The prognosis of patients with distant metastases is even more disappointing. However, numerous studies have shown that some patients with thoracic esophageal squamous cell carcinoma (SCC) and cervical lymph node metastasis (CLNM) could have better long-time survival than patients with visceral metastasis, which suggests that CLNM should be regarded as regional spread rather than distant metastasis [2,3,4]. The Japanese Society for Esophageal Diseases (JSED) has divided cervical nodes into four groups: cervical paraesophageal nodes, deep cervical nodes, retropharyngeal nodes and supraclavicular nodes, and involvement of the cervical paraesophageal nodes was defined as stage N1 in the case of cancers of the upper third of the esophagus [5]. Moreover, the American Joint Committee on Cancer (AJCC 7th edition) defined cervical paraesophageal nodes as regional nodes in the case of esophageal cancer [6]. According to the Chinese non-operative stage of esophageal cancer, patients with CLNM are considered to be in stage N1 (cervical esophageal cancer) or N2 (thoracic esophageal cancer) [7]. However, the prognostic significance of unilateral CLNM in esophageal cancer, if any, has not yet been explored in detail. The purpose of this study is to determine whether unilateral CLNM has an impact on the prognosis of patients with inoperable esophageal SCC and to analyze prognostic factors for esophageal SCC.

Patients and Methods

Ethics statement

This study was approved by the institutional review board (IRBs) of Cancer Center, Sun Yat-sen University. Written informed consent was obtained from all the patients in accordance with the regulations of the IRBs.

Clinical data and patient groups

We retrospectively studied 395 consecutive patients who were diagnosed with esophageal SCC and treated with concurrent chemoradiotherapy in Sun Yat-sen University Cancer Center between February 2002 and December 2011. These patients had either refused surgery or were unable to undergo surgery. The pretreatment work-up included complete history collection, physical examinations, computed tomography (CT) scans of the chest and abdomen, barium esophagography and endoscopic ultrasonography. In this study, we employed the AJCC staging system (6th edition). In all patients, the diagnosis was pathologically confirmed to be SCC. The date of last follow-up was April 1st, 2013, and the median follow-up time was 35 months (range, 10–117 months).

The 395 study patients were classified into three groups depending on the extent of regional/metastatic spread at the time of initial diagnosis: group A, no evidence of CLNM (n = 204); group B, unilateral CLNM (n = 106); and group C, other distant metastases (n = 85).

Radiotherapy and chemotherapy

External beam radiotherapy was administered using 6–10 MV X-rays. All patients received three-dimensional conformal radiotherapy at a dose of 1.8–2.0 Gy per fraction, five times a week. The patients underwent radiotherapy for 4–6 weeks, receiving a total dose of 46–70 Gy. The primary gross tumor volume (GTV) and the volume of involved lymph nodes (GTV-N) were determined. The conformal clinical target volume (CTV) included the GTV with a 3-cm margin in the craniocaudal direction and a 0.5-cm margin in the lateral and anteroposterior directions. The CTV of SCCs involving the upper third of the esophagus encompassed the right and left supraclavicular regions. In patients with unilateral CLNM, the contralateral supraclavicular fossa was included in the CTV for prophylactic purposes. The CTV for lymph nodes included the GTV-N without an additional margin. The planning target volume included the CTV with a 1-cm margin in the superior–inferior direction and a 0.5-cm margin in the lateral direction [8].

Concurrent chemotherapy was administered using regimens that mainly included cisplatin plus 5-fluorouracil and cisplatin plus docetaxel. In all, 116 patients were treated with two cycles of 60 mg/m^2 docetaxel and 80 mg/m^2 cisplatin delivered on days 1 and 22 of radiotherapy [9]. In all, 51 patients received at least four cycles of docetaxel (30 mg/m^2) and cisplatin (35 mg/m^2) per week. Another 129 patients were treated with two cycles of 60 mg/m^2 cisplatin administered on days 1 and 29 and 300 mg/m^2/24 h 5-fluorouracil administered on days 1–3 and days 29–31 [8]. The remaining 99 patients received other chemotherapy regimens such as navelbine plus cisplatin.

Statistical analysis

Overall survival (OS) and progression-free survival (PFS) were the study endpoints. OS was calculated from the day of diagnosis to the date of death or censored at the date of last follow-up. PFS was computed from the day of diagnosis to the detection of recurrent disease or to the date of death in patients without evidence of disease recurrence, censoring at the date of last follow-up. The survival analysis was performed by the Kaplan–Meier method, and differences between the curves were analyzed using the log-rank test. As categorical data, sex (male vs. female), pathological grade, tumor location (upper third vs. middle third vs. lower third), primary tumor length (<3 cm vs. ≥3 cm, ≤6 cm vs. >6 cm), clinical T stage (T1/T2 vs. T3 vs. T4), clinical M stage (M0 vs. M1), cervical lymph node involvement, radiation dose (≤ 60 Gy vs. >60 Gy) and concurrent chemotherapy (DDP+5-Fu vs. DDP+docetaxel vs. others) were included in the log-rank test. The three categories of CLNM (group A, group B, group C) were analyzed using pairwise comparison, and the p value was set at 0.017 (0.05/3) according to Hochberg's step-up procedure [10]. Multivariate analyses using the Cox proportional hazards model were used to calculate the hazard ratio and to test independent significance by backward elimination of non-significant explanatory variables. The criterion for statistical significance was set at $\alpha = 0.05$, and p values were determined from two-sided tests. All statistical analyses were performed using SPSS 16.0 software (SPSS Inc., Chicago, IL).

Results

Patients and clinicopathological features

The demographic and clinical data of the patients are shown in Table 1. Of the 395 patients, 316 were men (80.0%), and 79 were women (20.0%). The median age of the patients was 58 years (range, 35–75 years). The primary tumors were located in the upper third of the esophagus in 154 patients (39.0%), in the middle third in 206 patients (52.2%) and in the lower third in 35 patients (8.8%). According to the AJCC staging system (6th edition), 43 patients were diagnosed with stage I/II disease, and 161 patients were diagnosed with stage III disease. The remaining 191 patients were found to have stage IV disease. Of these 191 patients, 106 had unilateral CLNM, 33 had bilateral CLNM and 52 had other distant metastases.

Influence of cervical lymph node involvement on survival

By April, 2013, 235 of the 395 study patients had died. The 3-year OS rates in groups A, B and C were 46.7%, 33.5% and 8.3%, respectively ($p<0.001$; Fig. 1). The corresponding PFS rates were 40.7%, 26.4% and 4.7% ($p<0.001$; Fig. 2). The OS and PFS have been shown in Table 2. The 3-year OS rate was significantly higher in patients with CLNM than in patients with distant organ metastasis ($p = 0.027$). The laterality of CLNM did not have a significant impact on OS ($p = 0.626$) or PFS ($p = 0.945$). We next performed pairwise comparisons among the three groups. Group A and group B had a similar 3-year OS ($p = 0.162$) and PFS ($p = 0.064$). Group B had significantly better 3-year OS ($p = 0.009$) and PFS ($p = 0.006$) rates than those of group C. Group A had significantly better 3-year OS ($p<0.001$) and PFS ($p<0.001$) rates than those of group C.

Patients with unilateral CLNM were further divided into three groups depending on the location of the primary SCC: (1) upper third of the thoracic esophagus (n = 41); (2) middle third of the thoracic esophagus (n = 58); and (3) lower third of the thoracic esophagus (n = 7). The 3-year OS rates were 39.7%, 28.9% and 19.0% while the 3-year PFS rates were 32.5%, 21.5% and 19.0%

Table 1. Demographic and pathological characteristics of the study population.

Characteristic	No. of patients	
Age (years)		
Median	58	
Range	35–75	
Sex		
Male	316	(80.0%)
Female	79	(20.0%)
Pathological grade		
Well differentiated	36	(9.1%)
Moderately differentiated	178	(45.1%)
Poorly/undifferentiated	97	(24.6%)
Unknown	84	(21.2%)
Location		
Upper third	154	(39.0%)
Middle third	206	(52.2%)
Lower third	35	(8.8%)
Primary tumor length		
Median (cm)	6.0	
<3 cm	21	(5.3%)
≥3 cm, ≤6 cm	220	(55.7%)
>6 cm	154	(39.0%)
T stage		
T1–T2	54	(13.7%)
T3	184	(46.6%)
T4	157	(39.7%)
M stage		
M0	204	(51.6%)
M1a	62	(15.7%)
M1b	129	(32.7%)
Stage		
I–II	43	(10.9%)
III	161	(40.8%)
IV	191	(48.4%)
Cervical nodal involvement		
CLNM (–)	204	(51.6%)
Unilateral CLNM	106	(26.8%)
Other M	85	(21.5%)
Radiation dose (Gy)		
≤60	314	(79.5%)
>60	81	(20.5%)
Concurrent chemotherapy		
PDD+5-Fu	129	(32.7%)
PDD+Docetaxel	167	(42.3%)
Others	99	(25.0%)

in patients with SSC of the upper, middle and lower thirds of the thoracic esophagus, respectively.

Prognostic analysis

Table 3 shows the results of univariate analyses for each prognostic factor, namely, sex, pathological grade, primary esophageal tumor location, tumor length, clinical T stage, cervical lymph node involvement, clinical M stage, radiation dose and

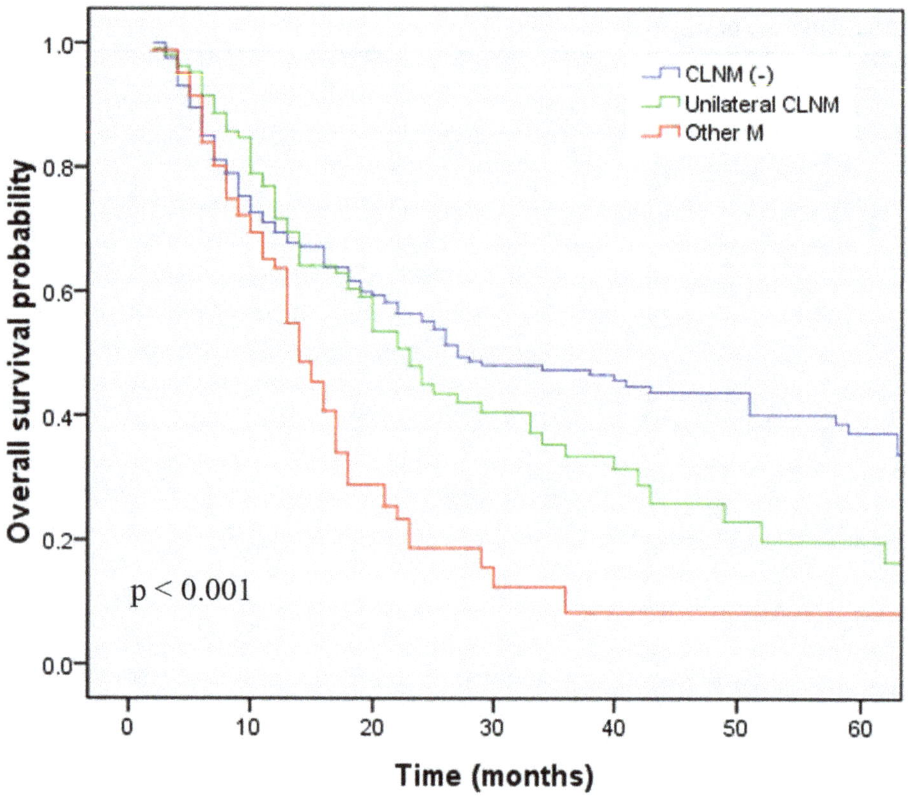

Figure 1. Overall survival in patients with different extents of cervical lymph node involvement.

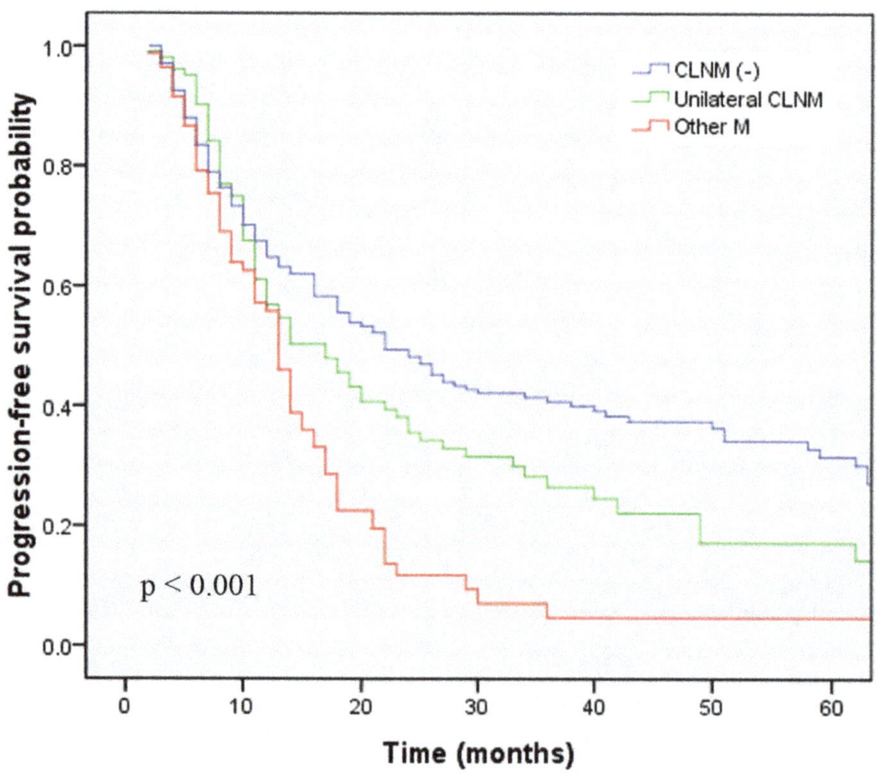

Figure 2. Progression-free survival in patients with different extents of cervical lymph node involvement.

Table 2. OS and PFS of esophageal SCC patients according to cervical lymph node involvement.

Group	No.	3 y OS	Median	95% CI	3 y PFS	Median	95% CI
			OS (m)			PFS (m)	
Group A	204	46.7%	34.0	13.1–54.9	40.7%	28.0	7.3–48.4
Group B	106	33.5%	27.0	13.2–40.8	26.4%	20.0	13.8–26.2
Group C	85	8.3%	23.0	18.9–27.1	4.7%	17.0	11.8–22.2

concurrent chemotherapy regimen. Univariate analysis showed that sex ($p<0.001$), primary tumor location ($p=0.009$), tumor length ($p=0.008$), clinical T stage ($p=0.001$), clinical M stage ($p=0.001$), cervical lymph node involvement ($p<0.001$) and concurrent chemotherapy regimen ($p=0.009$) had a significant impact on OS. SCC of the upper third of the esophagus, female sex and the cisplatin plus docetaxel regimen were associated with significantly better OS than SCC of the middle or lower third of the esophagus, male sex and other chemotherapy regimens, respectively (Table 3).

To identify independent prognostic factors, the factors that were found to be significant on univariate analysis were subjected to multivariate analysis. Because there is a duplication between the M stage and cervical lymph node involvement, only cervical lymph node involvement was entered into the multivariate analysis. Multivariate analysis revealed that clinical T stage ($p=0.005$), cervical lymph node involvement ($p<0.001$) and chemotherapy regimen ($p<0.001$) were independent factors affecting OS in esophageal SCC patients. Clinical T stage ($p=0.010$), cervical lymph node involvement ($p<0.001$) and chemotherapy regimen ($p=0.002$) were independent factors affecting PFS in esophageal SCC patients (Table 4).

Discussion

CLNM is common among esophageal SCC patients [8,11]. Li et al. reported the pattern of thoracic SCC lymph node metastases after three-field esophagectomy, the rates of CLNM in patients with upper, middle and lower thoracic tumors were 41.6%, 33.3% and 36.4%, respectively [11]. The prognosis of patients with CLNM from stage IVa/IVb esophageal cancer is not uniform. Furthermore, patients with CLNM have significantly better survival rates than patients with solid-organ metastases [8,12,13]. Liu et al. compared SCC patients with enlarged cervical paraesophageal lymph nodes without any other metastatic cervical lymph nodes (CPLNM) and those with enlargement of any other cervical lymph nodes apart from the cervical paraesophageal lymph nodes (OCLNM) [8]. They concluded that CPLNM could be considered as regional spread in patients with upper thoracic SCC, which is consistent with the AJCC staging system (7th edition) [6]. The above results suggest that the prognosis of esophageal cancer patients with CLNM might be better than that of patients with distant metastases. However, the prognostic significance of unilateral CLNM in terms of survival has not yet been explored in detail.

Effects of unilateral CLNM vs. other metastases on OS

To our knowledge, this is the first large-scale study to investigate the prognosis of SCC patients with unilateral CLNM. In nasopharyngeal carcinoma patients, unilateral CLNM has been associated with better distant metastasis–free survival rates than bilateral CLNM on univariate analysis [14]. In our study, we found that the 3-year OS rate was better in patients with CLNM (29.7%) than in patients with distant organ metastases (5.7%, $p=0.027$), which is consistent with the results reported by Nomura et al. [15]. Nomura et al. reported that the 3-year OS rates of esophageal cancer in stages III, IVa and IVb were 37.1%, 34.2% and 9.1%, respectively. Furthermore, the survival curve for stage IVa was significantly better than the curve for stage IVb [15]. In the current study, we divided our patients into three groups (group A, group B and group C). Survival rates significantly differed between the three groups (3-year OS: $p<0.001$; 3-year PFS: $p<0.001$). We next performed post hoc pairwise comparisons among the three groups. Heo et al. compared four post hoc multiple

Table 3. Univariate analyses demonstrating factors associated with OS and PFS.

Factor	No.	OS	PFS
		p value	*p* value
Sex		<0.001	0.006
Male	316		
Female	79		
Pathological grade		0.372	0.938
Well differentiated	36		
Moderately differentiated	178		
Poorly/undifferentiated	97		
Unknown	84		
Location		0.009	0.067
Upper third	154		
Middle third	206		
Lower third	35		
Primary tumor length		0.008	0.002
<3 cm	21		
≥3 cm, ≤6 cm	220		
>6 cm	154		
Clinical T classification		0.001	0.004
T1–T2	54		
T3	184		
T4	157		
Clinical M stage		0.001	<0.001
M0	204		
M1	191		
Cervical nodal involvement		<0.001	<0.001
CLNM (–)	204		
Unilateral CLNM	106		
Other M	85		
Radiation dose (Gy)		0.945	0.465
≤60 Gy	314		
>60 Gy	81		
Concurrent chemotherapy		<0.001	0.001
DDP+5-Fu	129		
DDP+Docetaxel	167		
Others	99		

pairwise testing procedures, and concluded that the Hochberg procedure has a low false discovery rate and the highest correct decision rate among the four pairwise methods. We therefore adopted the Hochberg step-up method in the pairwise comparison, and the p value of the pairwise comparisons was set at 0.017 (0.05/3) [10]. The pairwise comparisons showed that unilateral CLNM (group B) had a similar prognosis to that of patients with regional disease (group A), and had a better prognosis than that of patients with other distant metastases (group C). This suggests that some patients with M1a disease, according to the 6th edition of the AJCC staging system (thoracic esophageal cancer patients with unilateral CLNM) can be staged as having regional disease. Both the JSED guidelines and the Chinese clinical non-operative staging of esophageal cancer consider CLNM as regional disease; however, neither have analyzed this prognostic factor in these patients in as much detail as we did [6,7]. Thus, our results complement these clinical staging systems.

We consider that the similarity in the prognoses of thoracic esophageal carcinoma patients with unilateral CLNM and patients with regional disease is chiefly attributable to the fact that in the case of unilateral CLNM, the target for radiotherapy is one contiguous area [16,17]. The radiation fields may not cover all tumor lesions satisfactorily in patients with other distant metastases. Furthermore, patients with unilateral CLNM may be in an earlier stage than patients with other distant metastases. Skip metastasis may be another reason influencing prognosis. Unilateral CLNM is more likely to be a skip metastasis. Prenzel et al. reported that skip metastases are associated with better 5-year survival rates and are more common in patients with cancer of the middle and upper thirds of the esophagus [18].

Table 4. Multivariate analysis of factors influencing OS and PFS in esophageal SCC.

Endpoints	Variable	*P* value	HR	95% CI for HR
OS	Sex	0.002	0.615	0.450–0.840
	Location	0.071	1.214	0.983–1.499
	Tumor length	0.268	1.146	0.900–1.460
	T stage	0.005	1.248	1.070–1.455
	Cervical nodal involvement	<0.001	1.520	1.282–1.801
	Chemotherapy	<0.001	0.737	0.621–0.873
PFS	Sex	0.102	0.792	0.599–1.048
	Tumor length	0.145	1.183	0.944–1.482
	T stage	0.010	1.203	1.046–1.384
	Cervical nodal involvement	<0.001	1.495	1.277–1.750
	Chemotherapy	0.002	0.780	0.665–0.915

Abbreviations: 95% CI, 95% confidence interval; HR, hazards ratio; OS, overall survival; PFS, progression-free survival; SCC, squamous cell carcinoma.

Significant prognostic factors

In the current study, univariate analysis showed that pathological grade did not significantly influence the OS and PFS of patients with advanced SCC, which is in accordance with the AJCC staging system (7th edition) [6]. However, inconsistent with this staging system, the prognosis of patients with primary tumors located in the upper third of the esophagus was better than that of patients with tumors located in the lower two-thirds. This may be due in part to differences in treatment strategies: all patients enrolled in the 7th staging system received surgery. Among the 4628 patients enrolled in the study of the 7th staging system, only 177 (4.1%) had cancer of the upper third of the esophagus [19].

In our study, radiation dose was not a significant factor on univariate analysis, which suggests that high radiation doses do not increase OS or PFS in advanced SCC patients. This result is consistent with the results of Radiation Therapy Oncology Group (RTOG) 9405 [20]. RTOG 9405 has concluded that a higher radiation dose did not result in higher survival or better locoregional control in M0 patients. The authors did not determine the reason for this lack of benefit in the high-dose arm; however, they supposed that considerable prolongation of the treatment time and the administration of a low dose of 5-FU because of toxicity may have contributed, at least in part, to this result [20].

Primary tumor length was not a significant factor on multivariate analysis. It seems that the prognostic significance of tumor length is lower in advanced-stage patients than in early-stage patients. Yendamuri et al. reported that esophageal tumor length is independently associated with long-term survival, but is not statistically significant in stage III patients [21].

Female patients had an obviously better prognosis than did male patients in our study. A previous study has revealed that female esophageal cancer patients have a survival advantage [22]. The T stage of the primary lesion also affect the prognosis. In our study, T1/2 patients had a higher survival rate than did T3 patients, and the prognosis of T3 patients was better than that of T4 patients. Increasing depth of tumor invasion is associated with the presence of lymphatic dissemination, and thus leads to an unfavorable prognosis [23]. Analysis of the PFS rates revealed the same results.

Chemotherapy regimen was a significant independent predictor of prognosis in esophageal SCC, and cisplatin plus docetaxel was the most effective regimen for concurrent chemoradiotherapy. No phase III clinical trial has thus far confirmed this result. However, van Hagen et al. reported that the rate of complete pathological response was a relatively satisfactory 49% in patients who received preoperative chemoradiotherapy for esophageal or junctional SCC [24]. The chemotherapy regimen used in their study was carboplatin plus paclitaxel (50 mg/m^2).

Limitations

There are several limitations of our study. First, it was a single-institution retrospective study. Second, only SCCs were included in this study because differences in morbidity and treatment strategies between different histological types may have affected the results obtained. Finally, staging was based on radiological studies. However, the specificity and accuracy of CT for detecting nodal metastases are 96.7% and 76.6%, respectively, and these values are similar to those for positron emission tomography; nodal enlargement of >10 mm is considered indicative of cancerous involvement [25]. Therefore, our results should be further evaluated in other large cohorts.

Conclusion

In summary, we have shown that SCC patients with unilateral CLNM have a long-term survival advantage over those with other distant metastases. Unilateral CLNM can be regarded as regional disease in SCCs. The current study also revealed that clinical T stage, cervical lymph node involvement and concurrent chemotherapy modality were independently associated with the prognosis of patients with esophageal SCC.

Author Contributions

Conceived and designed the experiments: M-ZL PZ MX. Performed the experiments: LZ. Analyzed the data: Q-QL SL. Contributed reagents/materials/analysis tools: LH JS. Wrote the paper: PZ MX.

References

1. Siegel R, Naishadham D, Jemal A (2013) Cancer Statistics, 2013. CA Cancer J Clin 63: 11–30.
2. Shimada H, Shiratori T, Okazumi S, Matsubara H, Nabeya Y, et al. (2007) Surgical outcome of patients with thoracic esophageal cancer positive for cervical lymph nodes. Hepatogastroenterology. 54(73): 100–103.
3. Tong DK, Kwong DL, Law S, Wong KH, Wong J (2008) Cervical nodal metastasis from intrathoracic esophageal squamous cell carcinoma is not necessarily an incurable disease. J Gastrointest Surg. 12(10): 1638–45.
4. Kato H, Igaki H, Tachimori Y, Watanabe H, Tsubosa Y, et al. (2000) Assessment of Cervical Lymph Node Metastasis in the Staging of Thoracic Esophageal Carcinoma. J Surg Oncol. 74(4): 282–5.
5. Isono K, Uchida Y, Watanabe H (2004) Guidelines for clinical and pathologic. studies on carcinoma of the esophagus, ninth edition. Esophagus. 1: 61–88.
6. Rice TW, Blackstone EH, Rusch VW (2011) 7th edition of the AJCC cancer staging manual: esophagus and esophagogastric junction. Ann Surg Oncol. 17: 1721–4.
7. Chinese expert group of nonoperative esophageal cancer staging (2010) Standard clinical staging of nonoperative therapy of esophageal cancer (Draft). Chin J Radiat Oncol. 19(3): 179–180.
8. Liu H, Lu L, Zhu Q, Hao Y, Mo Y, et al. (2011) Cervical nodal metastases of unresectable thoracic esophageal squamous cell carcinoma Characteristics of long-term survivors after concurrent chemoradiotherapy. Radiother Oncol. 99(2): 181–6.
9. Li QQ, Liu MZ, Hu YH, Liu H, He ZY, et al. (2010) Definitive concomitant chemoradiotherapy with docetaxel and cisplatin in squamous esophageal carcinoma. Dis Esophagus. 23: 253–9.
10. Heo M, Andrew C (2013) Leon Comparison of Post Hoc Multiple Pairwise Testing Procedures as Applied to Small k-Group Logrank Tests. International Journal of Statistics in Medical Research. 2: 104–116.
11. Li H, Zhang Y, Cai H, Xiang J (2007) Pattern of lymph node metastases in patients with squamous cell carcinoma of the thoracic esophagus who underwent three-field lymphadenectomy. Eur Surg Res. 39(1): 1–6.
12. Christie NA, Rice TW, DeCamp MM, Goldblum JR, Adelstein DJ, et al. (1999) M1a/M1b esophageal carcinoma: clinical relevance. J Thorac Cardiovasc Surg. 118(5): 900–7.
13. Eloubeidi MA, Desmond R, Arguedas MR, Reed CE, Wilcox CM (2002) Prognostic factors for the survival of patients with esophageal carcinoma in the U.S.: the importance of tumor length and lymph node status. Cancer. 95(7): 1434–43.
14. Li WF, Sun Y, Mao YP, Chen L, Chen YY, et al. (2013) Proposed lymph node staging system using the international consensus guidelines for lymph node levels is predictive for nasopharyngeal carcinoma patients from endemic areas treated with intensity modulated radiation therapy. Int J Radiat Oncol Biol Phys. 86(2): 249–56.
15. Nomura M, Shitara K, Kodaira T, Hatooka S, Mizota A, et al. (2012) Prognostic impact of the 6th and 7th American Joint Committee on Cancer TNM staging systems on esophageal cancer patients treated with chemoradiotherapy. Int J Radiat Oncol Biol Phys. 82(2): 946–52.
16. Huang W, Li B, Gong H, Yu J, Sun H, et al. (2010) Pattern of lymph node metastases and its implication in radiotherapeutic clinical target volume in patients with thoracic esophageal squamous cell carcinoma: A report of 1077 cases. Radiother Oncol. 95(2): 229–33.
17. Chen J, Liu S, Pan J, Zheng X, Zhu K, et al. (2009) The pattern and prevalence of lymphatic spread in thoracic oesophageal squamous cell carcinoma. Eur J Cardiothorac Surg. 36(3): 480–6.
18. Prenzel KL, Bollschweiler E, Schröder W, Mönig SP, Drebber U, et al. (2010) Prognostic relevance of skip metastases in esophageal cancer. Ann Thorac Surg. 90(5): 1662–7.
19. Chen LQ (2008) Defining AJCC/UICC Esophageal Cancer TNM Staging 7th Edition (2009). Chin J Clin Thorac Cardiovasc Surg. 15: 52–55.
20. Minsky BD, Pajak TF, Ginsberg RJ, Pisansky TM, Martenson J, et al. (2002) INT 0123 (Radiation Therapy Oncology Group 94-05) Phase III trial of combined-modality therapy for esophageal cancer: high-dose versus standard-dose radiationtherapy. J Clin Oncol. 20(5): 1167–74.
21. Yendamuri S, Swisher SG, Correa AM, Hofstetter W, Ajani JA, et al. (2009) Esophageal tumor length is independently associated with long-term survival. Cancer. 115(3): 508–16.
22. Micheli A, Mariotto A, Giorgi Rossi A, Gatta G, Muti P (1998) The prognostic role of gender in survival of adult cancer patients. Eur J Cancer. 34(14): 2271–8.
23. Rice TW, Zuccaro G Jr, Adelstein DJ, Rybicki LA, Blackstone EH, et al. (1998) Esophageal carcinoma: Depth of tumor invasion is predictive of regional lymph node status. Ann Thorac Surg. 65: 787–792.
24. Van Hagen P, Hulshof MC, van Lanschot JJ, Steyerberg EW, van Berge Henegouwen MI, et al. (2012) Preoperative chemoradiotherapy for esophageal or junctional cancer. N Engl J Med. 366(22): 2074–84.
25. Kim K, Park SJ, Kim BT, Lee KS, Shim YM (2001) Evaluation of lymph node metastases in squamous cell carcinoma of the esophagus with positron emission tomography. Ann Thorac Surg. 71(1): 290–4.

17

Muscle Atrophy in Response to Cytotoxic Chemotherapy is Dependent on Intact Glucocorticoid Signaling in Skeletal Muscle

Theodore P. Braun[1,2], Marek Szumowski[1], Peter R. Levasseur[1], Aaron J. Grossberg[5], XinXia Zhu[1], Anupriya Agarwal[3,4], Daniel L. Marks[1]*

1 Papé Family Pediatric Research Institute, Oregon Health & Science University, Portland, Oregon, United States of America, **2** MD/PhD Program, Oregon Health & Science University, Portland, Oregon, United States of America, **3** Knight Cancer Institute, Oregon Health & Science University, Portland, Oregon, United States of America, **4** Division of Hematology & Medical Oncology, Oregon Health & Science University, Portland, Oregon, United States of America, **5** Department of Internal Medicine, Providence St. Vincent Medical Center, Portland, Oregon, United States of America

Abstract

Cancer cachexia is a syndrome of weight loss that results from the selective depletion of skeletal muscle mass and contributes significantly to cancer morbidity and mortality. The driver of skeletal muscle atrophy in cancer cachexia is systemic inflammation arising from both the cancer and cancer treatment. While the importance of tumor derived inflammation is well described, the mechanism by which cytotoxic chemotherapy contributes to cancer cachexia is relatively unexplored. We found that the administration of chemotherapy to mice produces a rapid inflammatory response. This drives activation of the hypothalamic-pituitary-adrenal axis, which increases the circulating level of corticosterone, the predominant endogenous glucocorticoid in rodents. Additionally, chemotherapy administration results in a significant loss of skeletal muscle mass 18 hours after administration with a concurrent induction of genes involved with the ubiquitin proteasome and autophagy lysosome systems. However, in mice lacking glucocorticoid receptor expression in skeletal muscle, chemotherapy-induced muscle atrophy is completely blocked. This demonstrates that cytotoxic chemotherapy elicits significant muscle atrophy driven by the production of endogenous glucocorticoids. Further, it argues that pharmacotherapy targeting the glucocorticoid receptor, given in concert with chemotherapy, is a viable therapeutic strategy in the treatment of cancer cachexia.

Editor: Antonio Musaro, University of Rome La Sapienza, Italy

Funding: Funding provided by National Institutes of Health (NIH) DK 70333 and Canadian Institutes of Health Research 200948 to DLM; NIH DK 084646, Rubenstein Radiation Research Scholarship, the AMA Foundation and the Portland ARCS Chapter to TPB. The funders had no role in study design, data collection and analysis, decision to publish, or preparation of the manuscript.

Competing Interests: The authors have declared that no competing interests exist.

* Email: marksd@ohsu.edu

Introduction

Cachexia is a progressive syndrome of weight loss that complicates numerous chronic diseases. Marked by a significant loss of skeletal muscle mass, the presence of cachexia is an independent predictor of mortality in multiple disease states [1,2]. It is estimated that cachexia is directly responsible for 20% of cancer deaths [3]. Further, declining performance status often precludes more aggressive and potentially curative anti-neoplastic treatment. Numerous preclinical studies have investigated the mechanism by which cancer produces muscle atrophy [4–6]. However, relatively few studies have explored the contribution of cancer treatment to the development of cachexia [7].

Systemic inflammation is a common uniting feature of all conditions in which cachexia is present [8]. Inflammatory cytokines are present at increased levels in cancer patients and are believed to convey the catabolic signal via at least two distinct mechanisms [9,10]. Cytokines act directly on skeletal myocytes to induce muscle atrophy via the engagement of surface receptors and the activation of NFκB [6,11]. Additionally, inflammatory cytokines activate the hypothalamic-pituitary-adrenal (HPA) axis, resulting in the release of endogenous glucocorticoids [12]. Recently it has become clear that a major component of muscle atrophy in response to systemic inflammation occurs as the result of HPA axis activation by cytokines resulting in the release of glucocorticoids from the adrenal gland [4,13]. Engagement of the glucocorticoid receptor within the myocyte induces a transcriptional program that leads to the proteasomal degradation of myofibrillar protein. Irrespective of the extracellular origin of the catabolic signal, muscle atrophy occurs via a concerted series of intracellular events culminating in the activation of the ubiquitin-proteasome and autophagy-lysosome systems [14,15].

Cytotoxic chemotherapy has numerous deleterious consequences to normal tissues, including myelosupression, gastrointestinal toxicity and pulmonary toxicity. Cardiac toxicity is also a well-known side effect of anthracycline chemotherapy and has been the subject of numerous investigations. Anthracyclines produce their biologic activity principally via interaction with topoisomerase II and subsequent double stranded DNA breaks, defects in mitochondrial biogenesis and the production of reactive oxygen [16]. The mechanisms by which cytotoxic chemotherapy affects skeletal muscle, however is less well described. Cisplatin chemotherapy produces significant muscle atrophy in mice, presumably via the activation of NFκB [7]. In addition, chemotherapy administration results in significant systemic inflammation, marked by increased levels of numerous circulating inflammatory cytokines [17]. It is unclear whether this systemic inflammation increases circulating glucocorticoids as both increases and decreases are reported after chemotherapy administration [18,19]. Therefore we investigated the role of glucocorticoids as a mediator of chemotherapy-induced muscle atrophy by administering CAF (cyclophosphamide, doxorubicin, 5-fluorouracil) chemotherapy to muscle-specific glucocorticoid receptor knockout mice (mGRKO). Our findings demonstrate that a significant component of chemotherapy-induced muscle atrophy depends on glucocorticoid signaling in skeletal muscle.

Methods

Ethics Statement

This study was carried out in strict accordance with the recommendations in the Guide for the Care and Use of Laboratory Animals of the National Institutes of Health. The protocol was approved by the Institutional Animal Care and Use Committee of Oregon Health and Science University (Protocol Number: ISO 1731). In all cases, every effort was made to minimize the suffering of experimental animals.

Animals

Wild type C57BL/6J mice and MCK Cre mice were obtained from The Jackson Laboratories (Bar Harbor, ME, USA). $GR^{Lox/Lox}$ mice were provided by L. Muglia (Washington University, St. Lois, MO, USA). All animals were maintained on a normal 12:12h light dark cycle and provided *ad libitum* access to water and food (Purina rodent diet 5001; Purina Mills, St. Louis, MO, USA). Animals were used for experimentation between 6 and 20 weeks of age, and were age, sex, and weight matched in all experiments. No effect of age, sex or weight was observed in any experiments. Mice were first given an intraperitoneal (i.p.) injection with a combination of cyclophosphamide (Baxter Healthcare Corporation, Deerfield, IL, USA), doxorubicin (Bedford Labs, Bedford, OH, USA) at concentrations of 167 mg/kg and 4 mg/kg, respectively. This was then followed by i.p. injection of 5-fluorouracil (5-FU) (American Pharmaceutical Partners, Schaumburg, IL, USA) one hour later at a concentration of 167 mg/kg, as mixing results in rapid drug precipitation [20]. Control mice were administered an equivalent volume of vehicle at these time points. Mice were euthanized by ketamine/xylazine injection. Animals sacrificed at 4 h after the second chemotherapy injection (Figure 1, Table S1) were utilized for circulating cytokine and corticosterone analysis as well as tissue cytokine expression. Animals sacrificed at 18 h were utilized for the assessment of muscle atrophy (Figure 2–5). Blood was obtained by cardiac puncture, anticoagulated with EDTA and separated by centrifugation. Plasma was stored at −80°C for further analysis. Tibialis anterior muscles were removed, frozen in isopentane/LN_2 and stored at −80°C for histologic analysis. Gastrocnemius muscles were removed and weighed. One gastrocnemius muscle was stored in RNALater (Life Technologies, Carlsbad, CA, USA) according to the manufacturers instructions. The other gastrocnemius was snap frozen in LN_2 and stored at −80°C for protein analysis.

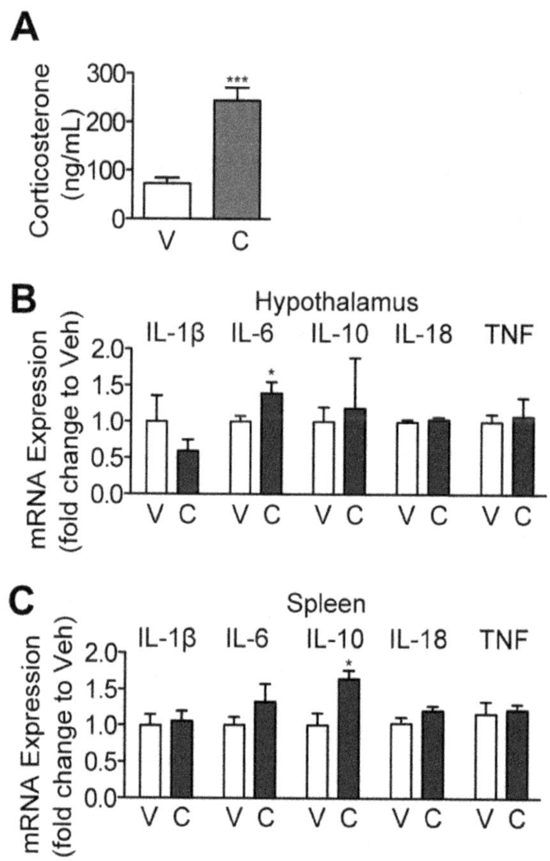

Figure 1. Chemotherapy Administration Increases Circulating Corticosterone and Induces Systemic Inflammation. Wild type mice (8–10/group) were treated with CAF chemotherapy and sacrificed 4 hours later. (A) Plasma corticosterone concentration. (B) Hypothalamic and (C) splenic inflammatory cytokine gene expression was measured by qPCR. * = $P<0.05$, and *** = $P<0.001$ vs. sham-treated mice as measured by Student's t-test. V = Vehicle, C = Chemotherapy.

Quantitative Real Time PCR

Total muscle RNA was extracted with an RNeasy fibrous tissue mini kit (Qiagen, Valencia, CA, USA) according to the manufacturer's instructions. cDNA was transcribed with Taqman reverse transcription reagents and random hexamers according to the manufacturers instructions (Life Technologies, Carlsbad, CA, USA). PCR reactions were run on an ABI 7300, with Taqman universal PCR master mix, and Taqman gene expression assays: mouse GAPDH (Mm99999915_g1), mouse *MAFbx* (Mm00499518_m1), mouse *MuRF1* (Mm01185221_m1), mouse *Foxo1* (Mm00490672_m1), Mouse *REDD1* (Mm00512504_g1), Mouse *KLF15* (Mm00517792_m1), Mouse *Mstn* (Mm01254559_m1), Mouse *Bnip3* (Mm01275600_g1), Mouse *CstL* (Mm00515597_m1), Mouse *Gabarapl1* (Mm00457880_m1), mouse TNF (Mm00443260_g1), mouse IL-10 (Mm99999062_m1), mouse IL-18 (Mm00434225_m1), mouse IL-1b (Mm01336189_m1), mouse IL-6 (Mm00446190_m1), mouse Fas (Mm00433237_m1), mouse Bax (Mm00432050_m1), mouse Bcl2 (Mm00477631_m1) (Life Technologies, Carlsbad, CA, USA). Relative expression was calculated via the delta-delta Ct method, and was normalized to vehicle treated control. Statistical analysis was performed on the normally distributed delta-Ct values.

Immunohistochemistry

Cryosections of the tibials anterior (TA) were cut in cross section at 10μm. Unfixed cryosections were blocked for 1 hour in PBS (10 mM NaPO4, 150 mM NaCl)/1% BSA/10% goat serum, and then incubated overnight in primary antibodies diluted 1:250 in PBS/1% BSA/10% goat serum. The following mouse primary antibodies were used: SC-71 for myosin IIa, BF-F3 for myosin IIb, BA-D5 for myosin I (Developmental Studies Hybridoma Bank, University of Iowa, Iowa City, Iowa, USA). Basement membrane was identified by staining with a rabbit anti-laminin antibody (Sigma, St Louis, MO, USA). Sections were washed in PBS, and incubated with the secondary antibodies diluted 1:500 in 1%BSA/10% goat serum. The following secondary antibodies were used: goat anti rabbit Alexafluor 405, goat anti mouse IgM Alexafluor 488, goat anti mouse IgG2b Alexafluor 555, and goat anti mouse IgG1 Alexafluor 633 (Life Technologies, Carlsbad, CA, USA). Sections were washed in PBS and mounted with aqua-poly mount (Polysciences, Warrington, PA, USA). Images were acquired on a Nikon Eclipse Ti confocal fluorescence microscope (Nikon Instruments Inc., Melville, NY, USA). Tiled images of entire sections were captured at ambient temperature and at 200X. Images were processed in Image J (National Institutes of Health, Bethesda, MD, USA). An evenly spaced grid was placed over the section. Fiber area was measured in fibers expressing Myosin IIb, Myosin IIa, or in those lacking expression of Myosin IIb, IIa and Myosin I (type IId/x fibers) at grid crossing points along with all adjacent fibers of the same type. Grid size was adjusted for a given fiber type such that ~100 fibers were counted per section. Representative images were selected from the same anatomic region of the TA from animals representative of the group mean fiber area.

Western Blotting

Muscles were homogenized in cell lysis buffer (Cell Signaling, Danvers, MA): 20 mM Tris pH 7.5, 150 mM NaCl, 1 mM EDTA, 1 mM EGTA 1% Triton X, 2.5 mM sodium pyrophosphate, 1 mM beta-glycerophosphate, 1 mM Sodium Orthovanadate, 1ug/mL leupeptin, and supplemented with Complete protease inhibitors (Roche, Indianapolis, IN), 1 mM PMSF (Sigma, St Louis, MO), and 5 μL/mL phosphatase inibitor cocktail II (Sigma, St Louis, MO). Samples were homogenized for 30 s using a Polytron homogenizer (Kinematica, Bohemia, NY), then were sonicated 2×10 s. Samples were then centrifuged at 13,000 RPM for 10 minutes at 4C. For western blots, 100 ug of total protein per lane was run on 10–20% gradient tris-glycine polyacrylamide gels (Life Technologies, Carlsbad, CA, USA), and transferred to Immobilon PVDF-FL membranes (Millipore, Billerica, MA). Proteins were detected using an Odyssey imaging system (Licor, Lincoln, NE). The following antibodies were used: rabbit anti-LC3b (Cell Signaling, Danvers, MA) and anti-rabbit Dylitght 680 (Cell Signaling, Danvers, MA).

Corticosterone Measurement

Plasma corticosterone levels were measured by RIA (MP Biomedicals, Solon, OH) according to the manufacturer's instructions.

Serum Cytokine Analysis

Serum cytokine levels were assessed using a multiplex magnetic bead based assay according to the manufacturers instructions (Life Technologies, Grand Island, NY). Serum levels of all cytokines on the panel are reported except for, Interleukin-13, Interleukin-1α, and Granulocyte-Macrophage Colony Stimulating Factor, which were below the limits of detection. In many cases samples fell below the lowest portion of the standard curve. When this occurred, but signal was still detectable, a value of the lowest point on the standard curve was assigned. When signal was undetectable, a zero was utilized. This analysis method resulted in data that did not follow a Gaussian distribution. Therefore, in these cases, the non-parametric Mann-Whitney test was utilized for statistical analysis of differential cytokine levels.

Statistical Analysis

Data are expressed as mean ±SEM. Statistical analysis was performed with Prism software (Version 4.0, Prism Software Corp., Irvine, CA, USA). All data were analyzed with a two-way ANOVA followed with *post hoc* analysis with a Bonferroni post-test or Students t-test as appropriate. For all analyses, significance was assigned at the level of $P<0.05$.

Results

Chemotherapy increases circulating corticosterone and systemic inflammation

To investigate whether chemotherapy induces a systemic inflammatory response, we treated wild type mice with CAF, a common chemotherapy regimen utilized in breast cancer that contains the anthracycline doxorubicin as well as the nucleoside analogue 5-fluorouracil and the alkylating agent cyclophosphamide. The mice were sacrificed 4 hours after injection and examined for evidence of inflammation as well as increases in circulating corticosterone, the predominant glucocorticoid in rodents. Chemotherapy treatment resulted in a significant increase in serum levels of corticosterone (Figure 1 A). In accordance with this, chemotherapy also induced an inflammatory response in the hypothalamus and spleen. IL-6, a known activator of the HPA axis [21], was significantly increased in expression after chemotherapy administration (Figure 1 B). In the spleen, there was a trend toward increased IL-6 expression that did not rise to the level of statistical significance (Figure 1 C). However, there was a significant increase in the expression of IL-10, which is associated with the development of cachexia [22]. We also examined circulating cytokine levels after chemotherapy administration by multiplex bead assay (Table S1). While there was a trend toward increased IL-10 levels after chemotherapy, this did not rise to the level of statistical significance. Interestingly, circulating levels of TNF and IL-5 both decreased significantly 4 h after chemotherapy administration. Collectively, these data demonstrate that the administration of chemotherapy results in significant modulation of systemic inflammatory tone and an increase in serum corticosterone levels.

Glucocorticoid signaling in skeletal muscle is required for muscle mass loss in response to chemotherapy administration

A large component of the catabolic stimulus in response to systemic inflammation is driven by increases in circulating glucocorticoids [4,12,13]. Given that CAF potently induces corticosterone, we investigated whether glucocorticoids contribute to muscle atrophy in response to chemotherapy. To address this question, we utilized muscle-specific glucocorticoid receptor knockout mice (mGRKO), which have recently been shown to resist muscle atrophy in response to tumor growth and acute inflammation [4]. Both mGRKO and $GR^{Lox/Lox}$ littermate control mice were administered CAF chemotherapy and sacrificed 18 h later. Treatment with CAF resulted in significant decrease in food intake and body weight in both genotypes of mice (Figure 2 A, B). However, while muscle mass was significantly reduced in $GR^{Lox/Lox}$ mice in response to chemotherapy, mGRKO mice were completely protected demonstrating that glucocorticoid signaling in muscle is requisite for chemotherapy-induced atrophy (Figure 2 C, D).

Chemotherapy induces genes involved in the ubiquitin-proteasome and autophagy-lysosome system in skeletal muscle via the action of glucocorticoids

Muscle atrophy occurs, at a molecular level, as the result of the proteasomal degradation of myofibrillar protein. Two muscle-specific E3 ubiquitin ligases, Muscle Atrophy F-box (MAFbx) and Muscle Ring Finger Protein 1 (MuRF1) are rapidly induced in catabolic skeletal muscle and facilitate the ubiquitination of contractile proteins [14,23]. The transcriptional regulation of these E3 ligases is complex, and includes direct regulation by the glucocorticoid receptor. Additionally, the forkhead box (Foxo) family of transcription factors, Krüpple like factor 15 (KLF15) and myostatin/SMAD signaling also play a critical role [24,25]. In response to chemotherapy administration in $GR^{Lox/Lox}$ mice, MAFbx, MuRF1 and Foxo1 expression in skeletal muscle are all increased 18 hours after chemotherapy administration (Figure 3 A). However, this response is blunted or entirely absent in mGRKO mice receiving CAF. Interestingly, KLF15 was not significantly induced by chemotherapy, despite a marked induction by exogenous glucocorticoids in other studies [4]. Regulated in Development and DNA Damage Responses 1 (REDD1), a regulator of protein synthesis was significantly induced by chemotherapy in both genotypes of mice (Figure 3 B). Despite playing a critical role in muscle atrophy in response to exogenous glucocorticoid administration, myostatin was not induced by chemotherapy administration [26].

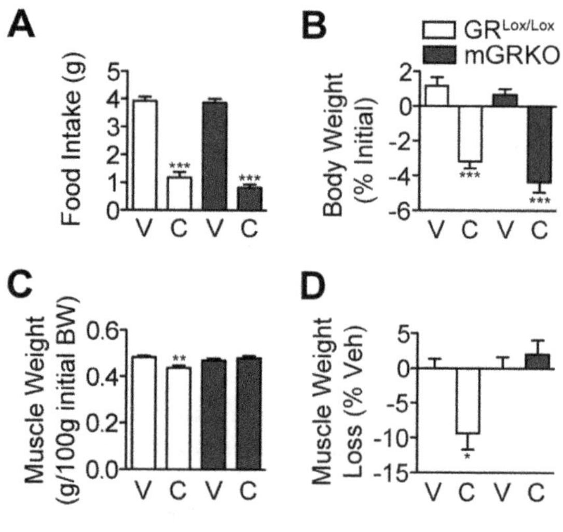

Figure 2. Chemotherapy Administration Produces Muscle Mass Loss in a Glucocorticoid-dependent Manner. $GR^{Lox/Lox}$ and mGRKO mice (n = 6–13/group) were treated with CAF chemotherapy and sacrificed 18 hours later. (A) Food intake and (B) body weight were measured. (C, D) Gastrocnemius muscle was weighed, normalized to pre-treatment body weight and presented as weight loss relative to sham-treated control mice of the same genotype. * = P<0.05, ** = P<0.01, and *** = P<0.001 vs. sham-treated mice of the same genotype as measured by two-way ANOVA with Bonferroni post-test. V = Vehicle, C = Chemotherapy.

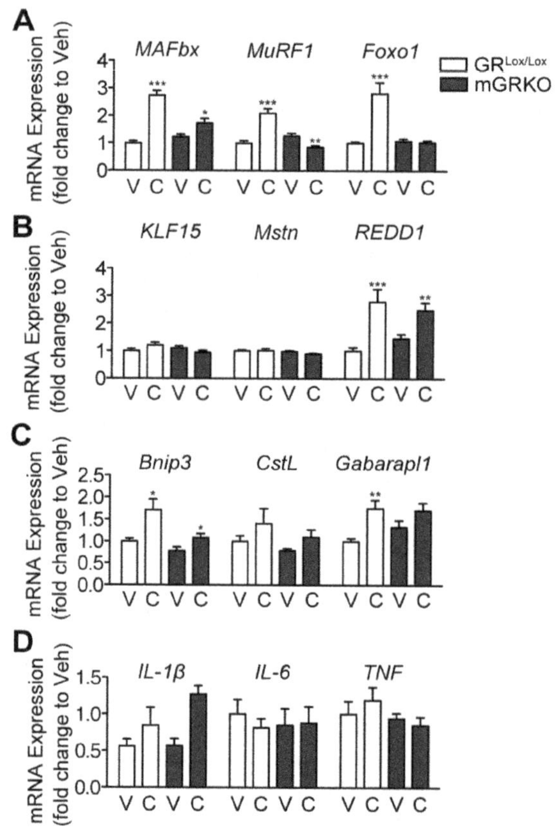

Figure 3. The Induction of Catabolic Gene Expression in Skeletal Muscle Requires Glucocorticoids. $GR^{Lox/Lox}$ and mGRKO mice (n = 6–13/group) were treated with CAF chemotherapy and sacrificed 18 hours later. (A, B, C, D) Gastrocnemius muscle gene expression was measured by quantitative real time PCR with GAPDH as an endogenous control. * = P<0.05, ** = P<0.01, and *** = P<0.001 vs. sham-treated mice of the same genotype as measured by two-way ANOVA with Bonferroni post-test. V = Vehicle, C = Chemotherapy.

It has recently become appreciated that the autophagy-lysosome system plays a fundamental role in the process of muscle atrophy [15,27]. We therefore investigated in expression of the autophagy genes BCL-2/adenovirus E1B-19kDA-interacting protein 3 (Bnip3), and GABA(A) receptor-associated protein like 1(Gabarapl1) along with the lysosomal protease Cathepsin L (CstL), which are regulated transcriptionally and consistently elevated in muscle undergoing atrophy [4,12,15]. Chemotherapy significantly induced Bnip3 and Gabapl1 $GR^{Lox/Lox}$ mice. However, this response was partially blocked in mGRKO mice, where the induction of Bnip3 by chemotherapy was significantly attenuated (Figure 3 C). We also assessed the conversion of light chain 3 B (LC3B)-I to LC3B-II, a process involving lipidation that is required for formation of autophagic vesicles. Consistent with prior work, mice treated with LPS demonstrate a significant increase in the 14 kD LC3B-II isoform (Figure S1) [28]. However, chemotherapy failed to induce a significant conversion of LC3B-I to LC3B-II in either genotype of mice, consistent with the relatively weak induction of autophagy genes relative to LPS treatment [4].

Skeletal muscle is also a known producer of inflammatory cytokines. Therefore, we investigated whether chemotherapy administration increases muscle cytokine production and whether this effect is dependent on glucocorticoid signaling. In response to chemotherapy administration, there was a significant induction of

IL-1β in the muscle of mGRKO but not in $GR^{Lox/Lox}$ mice consistent with the role of glucocorticoids as a negative regulator of inflammation (Figure 3 D). Chemotherapy failed to induce IL-6 or TNF expression in the muscle of either genotype of mouse.

Collectively, these data demonstrate that glucocorticoids are required for the induction of the catabolic program in response to chemotherapy administration. The most pronounced changes occur in genes regulating proteasomal degradation of skeletal muscle, while the effects on other pathways such as the autophagy lysosome system are relatively modest compared with other catabolic stimuli. While implicated in other forms of muscle atrophy, the transcriptional regulation of myostatin or the production of inflammatory cytokines by muscle does not occur in response to chemotherapy administration.

Muscle atrophy in response to chemotherapy is dependent on glucocorticoid signaling in skeletal muscle

To investigate the role of glucocorticoids of producing myofibrillar atrophy, tibialis anterior muscle from $GR^{Lox/Lox}$ and mGRKO mice treated with chemotherapy was cut in cross section and immunostained to delineate fiber type. A marked loss of cross sectional area was seen in the glycolytic type IIb fibers of $GR^{Lox/Lox}$ mice 18 hours after chemotherapy administration (Figure 4 A, B). However, in mGRKO mice, no loss of type IIb fiber cross sectional area was seen. While there was also a trend toward a decrease in the cross sectional area of the more oxidative type IIa and IId/x fibers in response to chemotherapy, this did not rise to the level of statistical significance. This demonstrates that the loss of skeletal muscle mass in response to chemotherapy largely arises from the atrophy of fast twitch glycolytic type IIb fibers.

Glucocorticoids contribute to induction of pro-apoptotic pathways in cardiac muscle

The MCK-Cre promoter used to generate the muscle-specific glucocorticoid receptor knockout mouse is also active in the heart, and therefore can also be utilized to assess the contribution of glucocorticoid signaling to chemotherapy-induced cardiotoxicity. We therefore examined the expression of atrophy-related genes in cardiac muscle 18 hours after chemotherapy administration (Figure 5 A). MAFbx expression was significantly increased in the hearts of animals receiving chemotherapy irrespective of genotype, while MuRF1 expression was decreased. There was a trend toward increased expression of Foxo1 in cardiac muscle from chemotherapy treated animals, however this only rose to the level of statistical significance in mGRKO mice. The expression of the mTOR regulators KLF15 and REDD1 was also examined (Figure 5 B). While the expression of KLF15 did not change in response to chemotherapy, REDD1 was significantly induced in the heart of both mGRKO mice and $GR^{Lox/Lox}$ littermates. Interestingly, there were some genotype-dependent effects on the chemotherapy-mediated induction of genes controlling autophagy in cardiac muscle (Figure 5 C).

Deletion of glucocorticoid receptor in cardiomyocytes suppressed the increase in Bnip3 and CstL brought about by chemotherapy administration.

Finally, given the extensive literature on chemotherapy-induced cardiomyocyte apoptosis, we investigated the expression of apoptotic regulators in the hearts of mGRKO mice treated with chemotherapy (Figure 5D). Cardiac expression of both Bax and Fas was increased equally by chemotherapy in mGRKO and $GR^{Lox/Lox}$ mice. The anti-apoptotic regulator Bcl2 decreased in expression as a result of chemotherapy, however, this response was significantly attenuated in mGRKO mice, where the reduction occurred to a lesser extent. Collectively these data demonstrate that, unlike skeletal muscle, the majority of the catabolic insult inflicted on cardiac muscle by chemotherapy is not conveyed by glucocorticoids. However, there is a small but significant glucocorticoid-dependent component of this process involving the regulation of genes involved in autophagy and apoptosis.

Discussion

Cytotoxic chemotherapy induces cellular damage through numerous mechanisms including the generation of oxidative stress and the induction of DNA damage. Given the well established direct effects of chemotherapy on the heart it would be reasonable to postulate an analogous direct cytotoxic effect on skeletal muscle [16]. It was therefore interesting to discover that mGRKO mice are resistant to chemotherapy-induced muscle atrophy, arguing for glucocorticoids as a critical intermediary. This demonstrates that the direct cytotoxic effects of chemotherapy on skeletal muscle are dispensable or at least not sufficient in isolation to drive the process of muscle atrophy.

The finding of localized inflammation after chemotherapy administration is consistent with an extensive literature documenting the activation of inflammatory signaling by chemotherapy. Doxorubicin exposure results in significant IL-1β production via activation of the inflammasome [17,29]. Others have reported significant increases in IL-6 after chemotherapy administration in cancer patients [30]. In addition to the direct activation of inflammatory signaling pathways, cell death and the release of intracellular damage-associated molecular patterns also likely contribute to the inflammatory response seen after the administration of chemotherapy. Potent immune activators such high mobility group box 1 (HMGB1) are released and signal via toll-like receptors to activate NFκB leading to cytokine production [31]. Interestingly, despite evidence of tissue inflammation and corticosterone release, we did not observe a significant increase in circulating inflammatory cytokines 4 hours after chemotherapy administration. It is possible that circulating cytokines may be elevated at a shorter time point after chemotherapy administration, returning to baseline after 4 hours. Alternately, chemotherapy may produce localized inflammation within the CNS leading to HPA axis activation. Although the direct action of cytokines on skeletal muscle is a well-documented mechanism of atrophy, the data presented here are consistent with a growing body of evidence demonstrating that CNS inflammation is all that is required for HPA axis activation and muscle atrophy [4,13].

A large body of evidence supports the necessity of NFκB activation in skeletal myocytes for the development of atrophy. NFκB activity is increased in response to multiple atrophic stimuli and genetic blockade of this pathway protects against atrophy in response to denervation as well as tumor growth [6]. Chemotherapy also increases NFκB DNA binding in skeletal muscle and has been proposed the driver of muscle atrophy in this setting [7]. This is seemingly at odds with our finding that glucocorticoid signaling, known to antagonize inflammatory pathways, is required for muscle atrophy in this proinflammatory state [32]. However, our results are consistent with an emerging body of literature demonstrating that under certain physiologic conditions, glucocorticoids potentiate rather than inhibit immune responses. Indeed, it appears that glucocorticoid levels within the physiologic range are permissive for a normal early immune response and only become suppressive at higher doses over longer time courses [33]. Additionally, many of the fundamental studies investigating the anti-inflammatory properties of glucocorticoids have been done

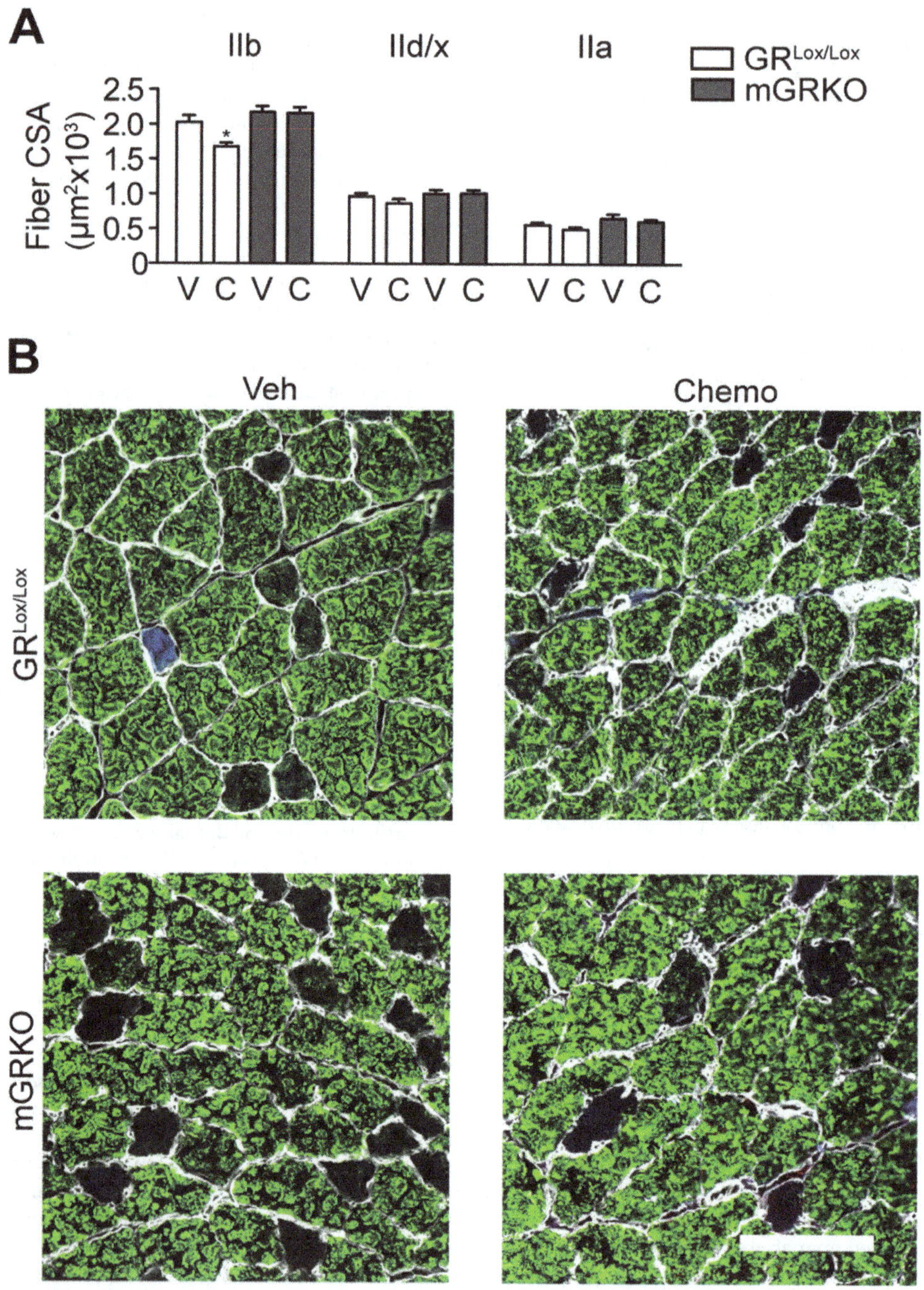

Figure 4. Chemotherapy Produces the Specific Atrophy of Type IIb Muscle Fibers That is Dependent on Glucocorticoids. GR$^{Lox/Lox}$ and mGRKO mice (n = 6–13/group) were treated with CAF chemotherapy and sacrificed 18 hours later. (A) Cryosections of tibialis anterior muscle were immunostained with antibodies to distinct myosin isoforms and the fiber cross sectional area of IIb (green), IIa (blue) and IId/x (black) fibers was measured. (B) Representative images of tibialis anterior muscles that were cut in cross section and immunostained with antibodies against laminin (white), myosin IIb (green) myosin IIa (blue). Scale bar = 100 μM.

using supraphysiologic doses of synthetic ligands with higher receptor affinity, increased half-life and altered mineralocorticoid activity when compared with endogenous glucocorticoids [34]. While a definitive understanding of the relationship between NFκB and glucocorticoid signaling in skeletal muscle awaits a detailed investigation, it is plausible that inflammatory and glucocorticoid signaling cooperatively induce the catabolic process.

The precise role of the Foxo1-MAFbx/MuRF1 axis in cardiac muscle is less clearly defined than it is in skeletal muscle. In contrast to its clearly defined role as a driver of atrophy in skeletal muscle, both MAFbx and MuRF1 are drivers of overload-induced cardiac hypertrophy [35,36]. However, others have described a catabolic role for MAFbx, where overexpression in myocardium prevents Akt-induced hypertrophy [37]. Interestingly, cardiac MAFbx expression increased after chemotherapy administration, while the expression of MuRF1 declined.

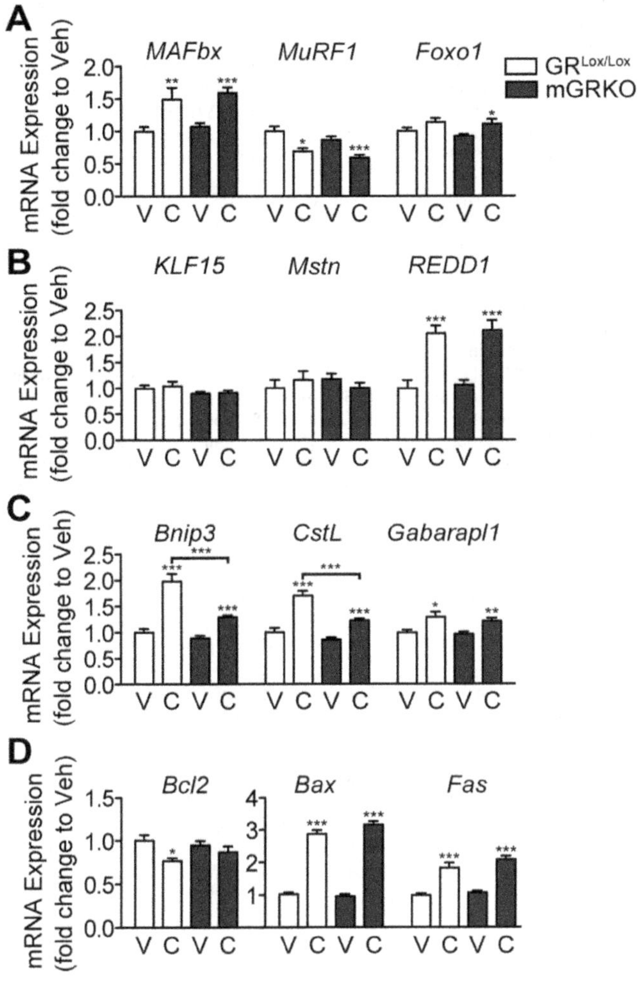

Figure 5. The Gene Expression Signature of Chemotherapy-Induced Cardiotoxicity Contains Glucocorticoid Dependent and Independent Elements. GR$^{Lox/Lox}$ and mGRKO mice (n = 6–13/group) were treated with CAF chemotherapy and sacrificed 18 hours later. (A, B, C, D) Heart gene expression was measured by quantitative real time PCR with GAPDH as an endogenous control. * = P<0.05, ** = P<0.01, and *** = P<0.001 vs. sham-treated mice of the same genotype as measured by two-way ANOVA with Bonferroni post-test. V = Vehicle, C = Chemotherapy.

Deletion of the glucocorticoid receptor from cardiac muscle failed to alter the regulation of these genes by chemotherapy. This argues that the regulation of these genes in the myocardium by chemotherapy occurs as the result of direct cytotoxicity or the regulation of an as-of-yet unknown systemic factor.

The induction of autophagy by chemotherapy has been implicated as a mediator of cardiotoxicity [38]. Our results demonstrate that this process is partially dependent on cardiac glucocorticoid signaling, as the deletion of glucocorticoid receptors in the heart attenuates the induction of genes involved in autophagy. Likewise, prior work has demonstrated that the pro-apoptotic effects of anthracycline chemotherapy on cardiomyocytes are the result of the direct interaction with cardiac topoisomerase IIb. While our results demonstrate normal induction of Bax and Fas in the absence of glucocorticoid signaling, the suppression of the anti-apoptotic gene Bcl2 by chemotherapy is attenuated when glucocorticoid signaling is blocked genetically. Given the magnitude of the suppression and the unaltered induction of pro apoptotic factors, it is unclear whether this effect alone carries physiologic significance. However, in combination with the attenuation of the induction of autophagy gene expression, it is likely that glucocorticoids contribute to the cardiotoxicity of chemotherapy.

Our findings are the first to demonstrate a role for glucocorticoids in the development of muscle atrophy after acute administration of cytotoxic chemotherapy. This finding introduces the possibility of therapeutic intervention that can be easily timed to coincide with the administration of chemotherapy. Future studies will likely evaluate the combined effects of chemotherapy and tumor growth on the development of cachexia.

Supporting Information

Figure S1 LC3B I:II Interconversion in Skeletal Muscle After CAF Chemotherapy. GR$^{Lox/Lox}$ and mGRKO mice were treated with CAF chemotherapy and sacrificed 18 hours later. Wild type mice were injected with LPS (1 mg/kg) and sacrificed 18 hours later. LC3B was detected by western blotting in muscle homogenates. Veh = Vehichle, Chemo = CAF chemotherapy.

Table S1 Circulating Cytokines After CAF Chemotherapy. Wild type mice (10/group) were treated with CAF chemotherapy and sacrificed 4 hours later. Serum cytokines were assessed by multiplex magnetic bead cytokine assay. Values presented as the mean± SEM. P values obtained via Students t-test or Mann Whitney (indicated by #) test for non-Gaussian distributions as described in the methods. Cytokines listed in bold where P<0.05.

Author Contributions

Conceived and designed the experiments: TPB MS PRL AJG XXZ AA DLM. Performed the experiments: TPB MS PRL XXZ AA. Analyzed the data: TPB MS PRL AJG XXZ AA DLM. Wrote the paper: TPB MS AJG DLM.

References

1. Tan BHL, Birdsell LA, Martin L, Baracos VE, Fearon KCH (2009) Sarcopenia in an overweight or obese patient is an adverse prognostic factor in pancreatic cancer. Clin Cancer Res 15: 6973–6979.
2. DeWys WD (1986) Weight loss and nutritional abnormalities in cancer patients: incidence, severity and significance. Clinics In Oncology 5: 251–261.
3. Tisdale MJ (2002) Cachexia in cancer patients. Nat Rev Cancer 2: 862–871.
4. Braun TP, Grossberg AJ, Krasnow SM, Levasseur PR, Szumowski M, et al. (2013) Cancer- and endotoxin-induced cachexia require intact glucocorticoid signaling in skeletal muscle. FASEB J 27: 3572–3582.
5. He WA, Berardi E, Cardillo VM, Acharyya S, Aulino P, et al. (2013) NF-κB-mediated Pax7 dysregulation in the muscle microenvironment promotes cancer cachexia. J Clin Invest 123: 4821–4835.
6. Cai D, Frantz JD, Tawa NE, Melendez PA, Oh B-C, et al. (2004) IKKbeta/NF-kappaB activation causes severe muscle wasting in mice. Cell 119: 285–298.
7. Damrauer J, Stadler M, Acharyya S, Baldwin AS (2008) Chemotherapy-induced muscle wasting: association with NF-kB and cancer cachexia. Basic Appl Myol 18: 139–148.
8. Morley JE, Thomas DR, Wilson M-MG (2006) Cachexia: pathophysiology and clinical relevance. Am J Clin Nutr 83: 735–743.
9. Richey LM, George JR, Couch ME, Kanapkey BK, Yin X, et al. (2007) Defining cancer cachexia in head and neck squamous cell carcinoma. Clin Cancer Res 13: 6561–6567.
10. Dülger H, Alici S, Sekeroğlu MR, Erkog R, Ozbek H, et al. (2004) Serum levels of leptin and proinflammatory cytokines in patients with gastrointestinal cancer. Int J Clin Pract 58: 545–549.

11. Acharyya S, Ladner KJ, Nelsen LL, Damrauer J, Reiser PJ, et al. (2004) Cancer cachexia is regulated by selective targeting of skeletal muscle gene products. J Clin Invest 114: 370–378.
12. Braun TP, Zhu X, Szumowski M, Scott GD, Grossberg AJ, et al. (2011) Central nervous system inflammation induces muscle atrophy via activation of the hypothalamic-pituitary-adrenal axis. J Exp Med 208: 2449–2463.
13. Schakman O, Dehoux M, Bouchuari S, Delaere S, Lause P, et al. (2012) Role of IGF-I and the TNFα/NF-κB pathway in the induction of muscle atrogenes by acute inflammation. Am J Physiol Endocrinol Metab 303: E729–E739.
14. Bodine SC, Latres E, Baumhueter S, Lai VK, Nunez L, et al. (2001) Identification of ubiquitin ligases required for skeletal muscle atrophy. Science 294: 1704–1708.
15. Mammucari C, Milan G, Romanello V, Masiero E, Rudolf R, et al. (2007) FoxO3 controls autophagy in skeletal muscle in vivo. Cell Metab 6: 458–471.
16. Zhang S, Liu X, Bawa-Khalfe T, Lu L-S, Lyu YL, et al. (2012) Identification of the molecular basis of doxorubicin-induced cardiotoxicity. Nat Med 18: 1639–1642.
17. Sauter KAD, Wood LJ, Wong J, Iordanov M, Magun BE (2011) Doxorubicin and daunorubicin induce processing and release of interleukin-1β through activation of the NLRP3 inflammasome. Cancer Biol Ther 11: 1008–1016.
18. Limberaki E (2011) Cortisol levels and serum antioxidant status following chemotherapy. Health 03: 512–517.
19. Morrow GR, Hickok JT, Andrews PLR, Stern RM (2002) Reduction in serum cortisol after platinum based chemotherapy for cancer: a role for the HPA axis in treatment-related nausea? Psychophysiology 39: 491–495.
20. Weymann KB, Wood LJ, Zhu X, Marks DL (2014) A role for orexin in cytotoxic chemotherapy-induced fatigue. Brain Behav Immun 37: 84–94.
21. Bethin KE, Vogt SK, Muglia LJ (2000) Interleukin-6 is an essential, corticotropin-releasing hormone-independent stimulator of the adrenal axis during immune system activation. Proc Natl Acad Sci USA 97: 9317–9322.
22. Robert F, Mills JR, Agenor A, Wang D, DiMarco S, et al. (2012) Targeting protein synthesis in a Myc/mTOR-driven model of anorexia-cachexia syndrome delays its onset and prolongs survival. Cancer Res 72: 747–756.
23. Gomes MD, Lecker SH, Jagoe RT, Navon A, Goldberg AL (2001) Atrogin-1, a muscle-specific F-box protein highly expressed during muscle atrophy. Proc Natl Acad Sci USA 98: 14440–14445.
24. Sandri M, Sandri C, Gilbert A, Skurk C, Calabria E, et al. (2004) Foxo transcription factors induce the atrophy-related ubiquitin ligase atrogin-1 and cause skeletal muscle atrophy. Cell 117: 399–412.
25. Shimizu N, Yoshikawa N, Ito N, Maruyama T, Suzuki Y, et al. (2011) Crosstalk between glucocorticoid receptor and nutritional sensor mTOR in skeletal muscle. Cell Metab 13: 170–182.
26. Gilson H, Schakman O, Combaret L, Lause P, Grobet L, et al. (2007) Myostatin gene deletion prevents glucocorticoid-induced muscle atrophy. Endocrinology 148: 452–460.
27. Masiero E, Agatea L, Mammucari C, Blaauw B, Loro E, et al. (2009) Autophagy is required to maintain muscle mass. Cell Metab 10: 507–515.
28. Doyle A, Zhang G, Abdel Fattah EA, Eissa NT, Li Y-P (2011) Toll-like receptor 4 mediates lipopolysaccharide-induced muscle catabolism via coordinate activation of ubiquitin-proteasome and autophagy-lysosome pathways. FASEB J 25: 99–110.
29. Bruchard M, Mignot G, Derangère V, Chalmin F, Chevriaux A, et al. (2013) Chemotherapy-triggered cathepsin B release in myeloid-derived suppressor cells activates the Nlrp3 inflammasome and promotes tumor growth. Nat Med 19: 57–64.
30. Janelsins MC, Mustian KM, Palesh OG, Mohile SG, Peppone LJ, et al. (2012) Differential expression of cytokines in breast cancer patients receiving different chemotherapies: implications for cognitive impairment research. Support Care Cancer 20: 831–839.
31. Apetoh L, Ghiringhelli F, Tesniere A, Obeid M, Ortiz C, et al. (2007) Toll-like receptor 4-dependent contribution of the immune system to anticancer chemotherapy and radiotherapy. Nat Med 13: 1050–1059.
32. Mukaida N, Morita M, Ishikawa Y, Rice N, Okamoto S, et al. (1994) Novel mechanism of glucocorticoid-mediated gene repression. Nuclear factor-kappa B is target for glucocorticoid-mediated interleukin 8 gene repression. J Biol Chem 269: 13289–13295.
33. Dhabhar FS, McEwen BS (1999) Enhancing versus suppressive effects of stress hormones on skin immune function. Proc Natl Acad Sci USA 96: 1059–1064.
34. Tanaka H, Hirano F, Nomura Y, Miura T, Makino Y, et al. (1994) Relative glucocorticoid potency revisited. Rheumatol Int 14: 9–12.
35. Willis MS, Ike C, Li L, Wang D-Z, Glass DJ, et al. (2007) Muscle ring finger 1, but not muscle ring finger 2, regulates cardiac hypertrophy in vivo. Circ Res 100: 456–459.
36. Usui S, Maejima Y, Pain J, Hong C, Cho J, et al. (2011) Endogenous muscle atrophy F-box mediates pressure overload-induced cardiac hypertrophy through regulation of nuclear factor-kappaB. Circ Res 109: 161–171.
37. Li H-H, Willis MS, Lockyer P, Miller N, McDonough H, et al. (2007) Atrogin-1 inhibits Akt-dependent cardiac hypertrophy in mice via ubiquitin-dependent coactivation of Forkhead proteins. J Clin Invest 117: 3211–3223.
38. Kobayashi S, Volden P, Timm D, Mao K, Xu X, et al. (2010) Transcription factor GATA4 inhibits doxorubicin-induced autophagy and cardiomyocyte death. J Biol Chem 285: 793–804.

18

Comparison of Long-Term Survival and Toxicity of Cisplatin Delivered Weekly versus Every Three Weeks Concurrently with Intensity-Modulated Radiotherapy in Nasopharyngeal Carcinoma

Chang-Juan Tao[1,2]⁹, Li Lin[1]⁹, Guan-Qun Zhou[1], Ling-Long Tang[1], Lei Chen[1], Yan-Ping Mao[1], Mu-Sheng Zeng[3], Tie-Bang Kang[3], Wei-Hua Jia[3], Jian-Yong Shao[4], Hai-Qiang Mai[5], Ai-Hua Lin[6], Jun Ma[1], Ying Sun[1]*

1 Department of Radiation Oncology, Sun Yat-sen University Cancer Center, State Key Laboratory of Oncology in South China, Collaborative Innovation Center for Cancer Medicine, Guangzhou, Guangdong Province, People's Republic of China, **2** Department of Radiation Oncology, Zhejiang Cancer Hospital, Hangzhou, Zhejiang Province, People's Republic of China, **3** Department of Experimental Research, Sun Yat-sen University Cancer Center, State Key Laboratory of Oncology in South China, Collaborative Innovation Center for Cancer Medicine, Guangzhou, Guangdong Province, People's Republic of China, **4** Department of Pathology, Sun Yat-sen University Cancer Center, State Key Laboratory of Oncology in South China, Collaborative Innovation Center for Cancer Medicine, Guangzhou, Guangdong Province, People's Republic of China, **5** Department of Nasopharyngeal Carcinoma, Sun Yat-sen University Cancer Center, State Key Laboratory of Oncology in South China, Collaborative Innovation Center for Cancer Medicine, Guangzhou, Guangdong Province, People's Republic of China, **6** Department of Medical Statistics and Epidemiology, School of Public Health, Sun Yat-sen University, Guangzhou, Guangdong Province, People's Republic of China

Abstract

Background: We aimed to compare the long-term survival outcomes and acute toxicity of cisplatin administered weekly versus every three weeks concurrently with intensity-modulated radiotherapy (IMRT) in patients with nasopharyngeal carcinoma (NPC).

Methods: This was a retrospective review of 154 patients with histologically proven, non-disseminated NPC who were treated using IMRT between January 2003 and December 2007. Seventy-three patients (47.4%) received 5–7 weeks of 30–40 mg/m^2 cisplatin weekly; 81 patients (52.6%) received two or three cycles of 80 mg/m^2 cisplatin every three weeks. IMRT was delivered at 68 Gy/30 fractions to the nasopharyngeal gross target volume and 60–66 Gy to the involved neck area.

Results: The clinical characteristics and treatment factors of the two groups were well-balanced. The median follow-up was 74 months (range, 6–123 months), and the 5-year overall survival, disease-free survival, locoregional relapse-free survival, and distant metastasis–free survival rates were 85.2% vs. 78.9% ($P=0.318$), 71.6% vs. 71.0% ($P=0.847$), 93.5% vs. 92.6% ($P=0.904$), and 80.9% vs. 80.1% ($P=0.925$) for the group treated every three weeks and weekly, respectively. Subgroup analyses indicated no significant differences in the survival rates of the two groups among patients with early- or advanced-stage disease. The incidence of acute toxicities was similar between groups.

Conclusion: IMRT with concurrent cisplatin administered weekly or every three weeks leads to similar long-term survival outcomes and acute toxicity in NPC regardless of whether patients have early- or advanced-stage disease.

Editor: Apar Kishor Ganti, University of Nebraska Medical Center, United States of America

Funding: This work was supported by grants from the National Natural Science Foundation of China (No. 8172409), the Sun Yat-Sen University Clinical Research 5010 Program (No. 2012011), the Natural Science Foundation of Guangdong Province (No. S2013010012220), the Science and Technology project of Guangzhou City, China (No. 132000507), the Health & Medical Collaborative Innovation Project of Guangzhou City, China (201400000001), and the National Science & Technology Pillar Program during the Twelfth Five-year Plan Period (2014BAI09B10). The funders had no role in study design, data collection and analysis, decision to publish, or preparation of the manuscript.

Competing Interests: The authors have declared that no competing interests exist.

* Email: sunying@sysucc.org.cn

⁹ These authors contributed equally to this work.

Introduction

Nasopharyngeal carcinoma (NPC) is highly prevalent in southern China; incidence rates range between 15 and 50 per 100,000 individuals [1]. Due to the anatomical location and radiosensitivity of NPC, radiation therapy (RT) is the mainstay treatment. According to the 7th Edition of the American Joint Commission on Cancer (AJCC) staging system [2], 60–70% of patients present with stage III–IVB disease at diagnosis [3]. Several randomized clinical trials and meta-analyses have consistently demonstrated that concurrent chemoradiotherapy

(CCRT) confers survival benefit in locoregionally advanced NPC [4–11].

The National Comprehensive Cancer Network recommends that CCRT with cisplatin (CDDP) be delivered at an intermediate dose weekly or at a high dose at 3-week intervals for stage II–IVB NPC. The Intergroup 0099 trial (INT-0099) [3] and NPC-9901 trial [5] compared concurrent CDDP (100 mg/m^2) every three weeks with RT alone; compliance to the intensive regimen was poor, and CCRT was associated with a high incidence of acute toxicity. Two other phase III clinical trials [6–7] evaluated the efficiency of CCRT with weekly CDDP (40 mg/m^2) during RT; CCRT conferred survival benefit and weekly CDDP was well-tolerated. Therefore, it is of great importance to identify the optimal administration schedule for CDDP during CCRT in patients with NPC.

To the best of our knowledge, only one study [12] has compared the dose delivery and survival outcomes of weekly CDDP versus CDDP every three weeks delivered concurrently with RT in locally advanced NPC. However, in that study, the clinical characteristics and treatment factors were unevenly distributed, and the majority of patients were treated with 3-dimensional conformal RT. Radiation technology has evolved rapidly in recent years, especially with the introduction of intensity-modulated radiotherapy (IMRT). In NPC, this treatment modality has excellent local control and less late toxicities [13]. With the widespread application of IMRT, reevaluating the survival outcomes and toxicity of concurrent weekly CDDP versus CDDP every three weeks in patients with NPC undergoing CCRT would be worthwhile.

Therefore, we aimed to compare the long-term survival outcomes and acute toxicities of weekly CDDP versus CDDP every three weeks delivered concurrently with IMRT in patients with NPC. Our results will help guide clinical CCRT treatment strategies in NPC.

Materials and Methods

Patient characteristics

Between January 2003 and December 2007, we reviewed the records of 749 patients with newly diagnosed, untreated, non-disseminated NPC who were treated using IMRT at our center. We excluded 595 patients (79.4%): 214 (28.6%) who were treated with RT only, 274 (36.6%) who received neoadjuvant chemotherapy, 86 (11.5%) who received concurrent chemotherapy using a combination of CDDP and 5-fluorouracil, and 21 (2.8%) who received concurrent chemotherapy with taxol. We included the remaining 154 patients in our retrospective study; 115 were male and 39 were female (male:female ratio, 2.95:1) and the median age was 44.0 years (range, 13–73 years). One hundred and fifty patients (97.4%) had a pathological diagnosis of World Health Organization (WHO) type II or III NPC, only one patient (0.6%) had WHO type I NPC, and three patients (1.9%) had basaloid squamous cell carcinoma. The ethics committee of Sun Yat-sen University Cancer Center approved this study. Written consent was waived because this was a retrospective study; verbal consent was obtained from the patients via telephone and documented in the informed consent form if the patient agreed to participate in this study, as was consent on behalf of the children enrolled. The Institutional Review Board approved the use of verbal consent.

All patients underwent pre-treatment evaluation, which included complete patient history, physical and neurological examination, hematological and biochemical profiles, magnetic resonance imaging (MRI) scan of the neck and nasopharynx, chest radiography, abdominal sonography, and single-photon emission computed tomography whole-body bone scans. Positron emission tomography/computed tomography (CT) was performed on 41 patients (26.6%). All patients were restaged according to the 7th edition of the AJCC staging system. The stage distribution was as follows: stage II, 40/154 (26%); stage III, 66/154 (42.8%); stage IVA, 38/154 (24.7%); stage IVB, 10/154 (6.5%). Table 1 lists the characteristics of the patient cohort.

Radiotherapy

All patients were immobilized in the supine position with a head, neck, and shoulder thermoplastic mask. We obtained two sets of images, i.e., with and without contrast, from the CT simulator for treatment planning purposes. CT was performed after administering intravenous contrast medium, and we obtained 3-mm slices from the head to 2 cm below the sternoclavicular joint. The primary tumor and upper neck above the caudal edge of the cricoid cartilage were treated by IMRT. The target volumes were delineated using a previously described institutional treatment protocol [14] in accordance with the International Commission on Radiation Units and Measurements reports 50 and 62. The clinical target volumes (CTVs) were individually delineated based on the tumor invasion pattern [15]. The contoured images were transferred to a Corvus version 3.0 inverse IMRT planning system (Peacock; Nomos Corp., Deer Park, IL, USA). The prescribed radiation dose (as per the protocol) was total dose of 68 Gy in 30 fractions at 2.27 Gy/fraction to the planning target volume (PTV) of the primary gross tumor volume (GTV), 60–64 Gy to the nodal GTV PTV, 60 Gy to the CTV-1 PTV (i.e., high-risk regions), and 54 Gy to the CTV-2 PTV (i.e., low-risk regions) and CTV-N (i.e., neck nodal regions). Treatment was delivered by a dynamic, multileaf intensity-modulating collimator (MIMiC; Nomos Corp., Sewickley, PA, USA). A conventional anterior or anteroposterior opposing cervical technique was used for the lower neck. All patients were treated with one fraction daily over five days per week. All targets were treated simultaneously using the simultaneous integrated boost technique.

Concurrent chemotherapy

All patients were treated with CCRT; eight patients (5.2%) also received adjuvant chemotherapy using CDDP and 5-fluorouracil for two or three cycles. CCRT was initiated on the first day of RT and the choice of every three weeks or weekly CDDP was based on oncologists' opinions. Seventy-three patients (47.4%) received 30–40 mg/m^2 CDDP weekly for 5–7 planned weeks, and 81 patients (52.6%) received two or three cycles of 80 mg/m^2 CDDP every three weeks. In both groups, 5-hydroxytryptamine 3 antagonists and dexamethasone were administered as antiemetic prophylaxis.

Follow-up

The duration of follow-up was calculated from the first day of treatment to either the day of death or day of the last follow-up. Patients were examined at least every three months during the first two years, and every six months thereafter until death. At every follow-up, we assessed disease status with complete physical examination, nasopharyngoscopy, hematological and biochemical profiles, chest radiography, abdominal ultrasonography, and CT/MRI scans of the nasopharynx and cervical region. Acute toxicities were scored according to the Common Terminology Criteria for Adverse Events v3.0 (CTCAE v3.0).

Statistical analysis

We used Statistical Package for the Social Sciences version 16.0 (SPSS, Chicago, IL, USA) for statistical analysis. We compared

Table 1. Clinical characteristics of patients.

Characteristic	Weekly cisplatin (n = 73)	Cisplatin every three weeks (n = 81)	P*
Age (years)			.351
≤50	52	63	
>50	21	18	
≤18	0	3	.247
>18	73	78	
Sex			.581
Male	56	59	
Female	17	22	
Histology			.116
WHO I	1	0	
WHO II	7	3	
WHO III	65	75	
BSCC	0	3	
T classification†			.651
T1	7	13	
T2	17	17	
T3	31	30	
T4	18	21	
N classification†			.538
N0	14	13	
N1	42	55	
N2	12	8	
N3	5	5	
Staging†			.939
II	18	22	
III	33	33	
IVA	17	21	
IVB	5	5	
OTT (days)			.554
Median	43	44	
SD	4.3	4.0	
Response rate			.258
CR	60	61	
PR	11	19	

WHO: World Health Organization; BSCC: basaloid squamous cell carcinoma; CR: complete response; PR: partial response; SD: standard deviation; OTT: overall treatment time.
*P-values were calculated using the chi-square test (or Fisher's exact test) and Mann–Whitney U test.
†According to the 7th AJCC/International Union against Cancer staging system.

and analyzed the clinical characteristics and toxicity rates of the two treatment groups using the chi-square test (or Fisher's exact test, if indicated). Overall treatment time and cumulative CDDP dose were compared using the Mann–Whitney U test. All events were measured from the start of treatment. The following end points (time to the first defined event) were assessed: overall survival (OS), disease-free survival (DFS), locoregional relapse–free survival (LRRFS), distant metastasis–free survival (DMFS). Actuarial rates were calculated using the Kaplan–Meier method [16]. Multivariate analyses using the Cox proportional hazards model

Table 2. Acute toxicity according to CTCAE v3.0.

Toxicity	Weekly cisplatin (n = 73)					Every three week cisplatin (n = 81)					P*
	Grade0	Grade1	Grade2	Grade3	Grade4	Grade0	Grade1	Grade2	Grade3	Grade4	
Hematological											
Leucopenia	30	17	20	5	1	23	28	25	5	0	0.312
Anemia	58	9	4	2	0	61	17	3	0	0	0.233
Thrombocytopenia	62	4	2	3	2	74	2	2	2	1	0.583
Non-hematological											
Dermatitis	0	59	13	1	0	0	54	24	3	0	0.121
Mucositis	0	29	21	23	0	0	23	34	23	1	0.139
Dysphagia	29	33	8	3	0	31	32	13	5	0	0.715
Nausea/Vomiting	32	24	17	0	0	36	27	15	3	0	0.295
Xerostomia	15	27	31	0	0	11	31	39	0	0	0.498
Ototoxicity	52	19	2	0	0	57	23	1	0	0	0.767
Neurotoxicity	70	2	1	0	0	77	3	1	0	0	0.632

*P-values were calculated with the chi-square test (or Fisher's exact test, if indicated).

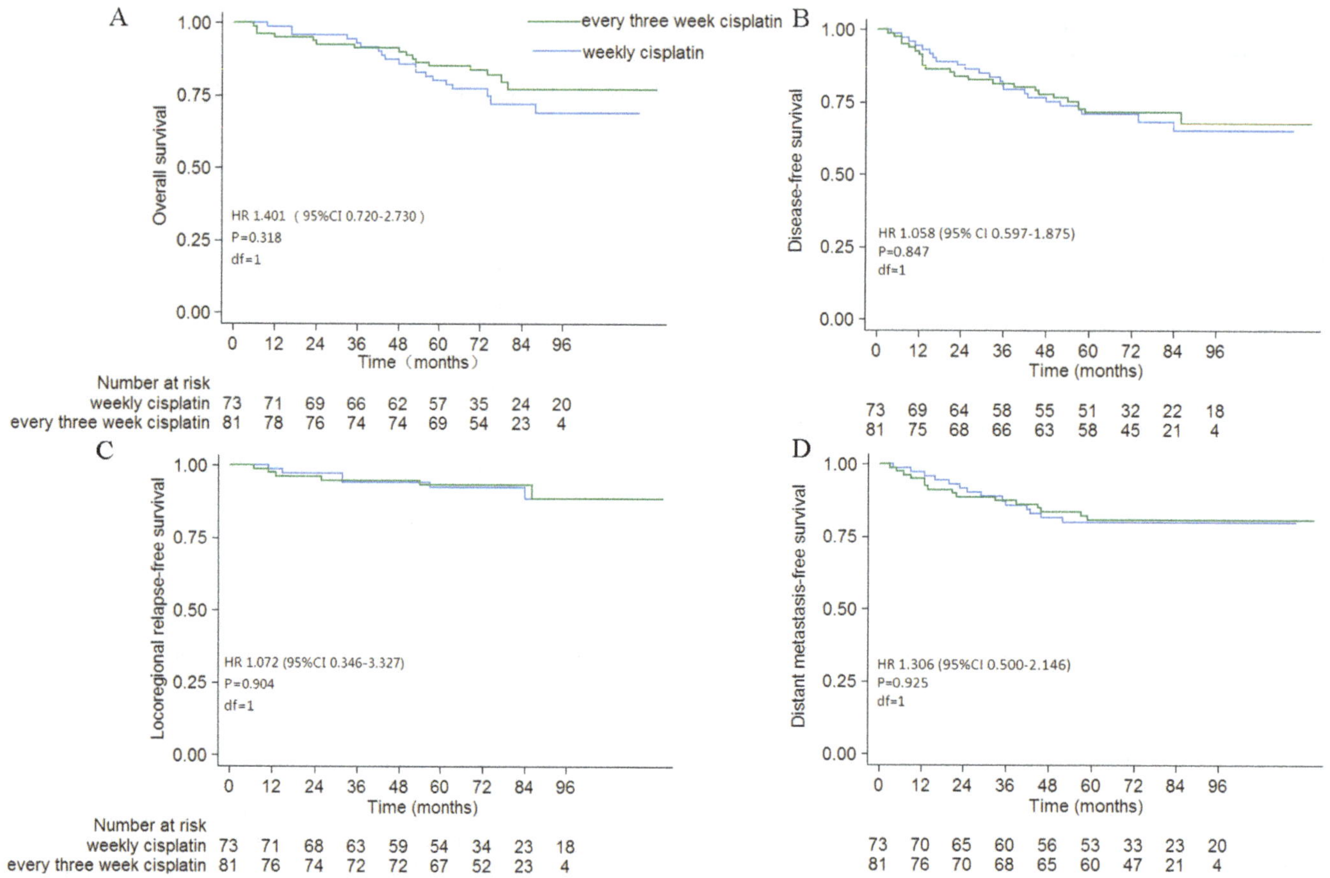

Figure 1. Survival curves for patients with NPC. (A) OS, (B) DFS, (C) LRRFS, and (D) DMFS. Hazard ratios (HRs) were calculated with an unadjusted Cox proportional hazards model; *P*-values were calculated with the unadjusted log-rank test.

were used to test for independent significance using backward elimination of insignificant explanatory variables of different parameters [17]. Host factors (age and sex) were included as covariates in all tests. The criterion for statistical significance was set at $a = 0.05$ and *P*-values were determined using 2-sided tests.

Results

Patient characteristics

Both groups were well-balanced in terms of baseline demographic and clinical characteristics and treatment factors (Table 1). Tumor response was evaluated via endoscopy and MRI scans of the neck and nasopharynx at three months after RT. The composite overall response rate for the primary site and neck region was 97.3% and 98.7% for the weekly and every three week CDDP group, respectively ($P = 0.258$).

Treatment compliance and acute toxicities

All 154 patients tolerated the treatment well and completed the prescribed dose of RT. The median overall treatment time was 43 days in the weekly group and 44 days in the every three weeks group ($P = 0.554$). In the weekly group, 66 patients (90.4%) received at least five weeks of CDDP and only four patients (5.5%) received seven weeks of CDDP. In the every three weeks group, 72 patients (88.9%) completed two cycles of CDDP and five patients (6.2%) received three cycles of CDDP. The median cumulative dose received during concurrent CCRT was 180 and 160 mg/m^2 CDDP for the weekly and every three weeks group, respectively ($P = 0.10$). Reductions in the number of chemotherapy cycles were mostly due to patient refusal, severe mucositis, or prolonged severe leucopenia.

Systemic toxicities were similar in both groups (Table 2). No treatment-related deaths were observed in either cohort. The most commonly recorded non-hematological adverse event was grade 3–4 mucositis in 23 patients (31.5%) in the weekly group and 24 patients (29.6%) in the every three weeks group ($P = 0.139$). The most common hematological adverse event was grade 3–4 leucopenia in six patients (8.2%) in the weekly group and five patients (6.2%) in the every three weeks group ($P = 0.312$).

Patterns of failure and survival rates

The overall median follow-up time was 74 months (range, 6–123 months). Twelve of the 154 patients (7.8%) developed locoregional relapse. There was distant metastasis in 29/154 patients (18.8%), and 35/154 patients (22.7%) died. The sites of relapse were local in 7/154 patients (4.5%), regional in 7/154 patients (4.5%), and both local and regional in 2/154 patients (1.3%). Three patients (1.9%) experienced both locoregional and distant failure.

The overall 5-year OS, DFS, LRRFS, and DMFS rates were 82.3%, 71.3%, 93.1%, and 80.5%, respectively. The 5-year OS, DFS, LRRFS, and DMFS rates were not significantly different between the two treatment groups (every three weeks vs. weekly: OS = 85.2% vs. 78.9%, $P = 0.318$; DFS = 71.6% vs. 71.0%, $P = 0.847$; LRRFS = 93.5% vs. 92.6%, $P = 0.904$; DMFS = 80.9%

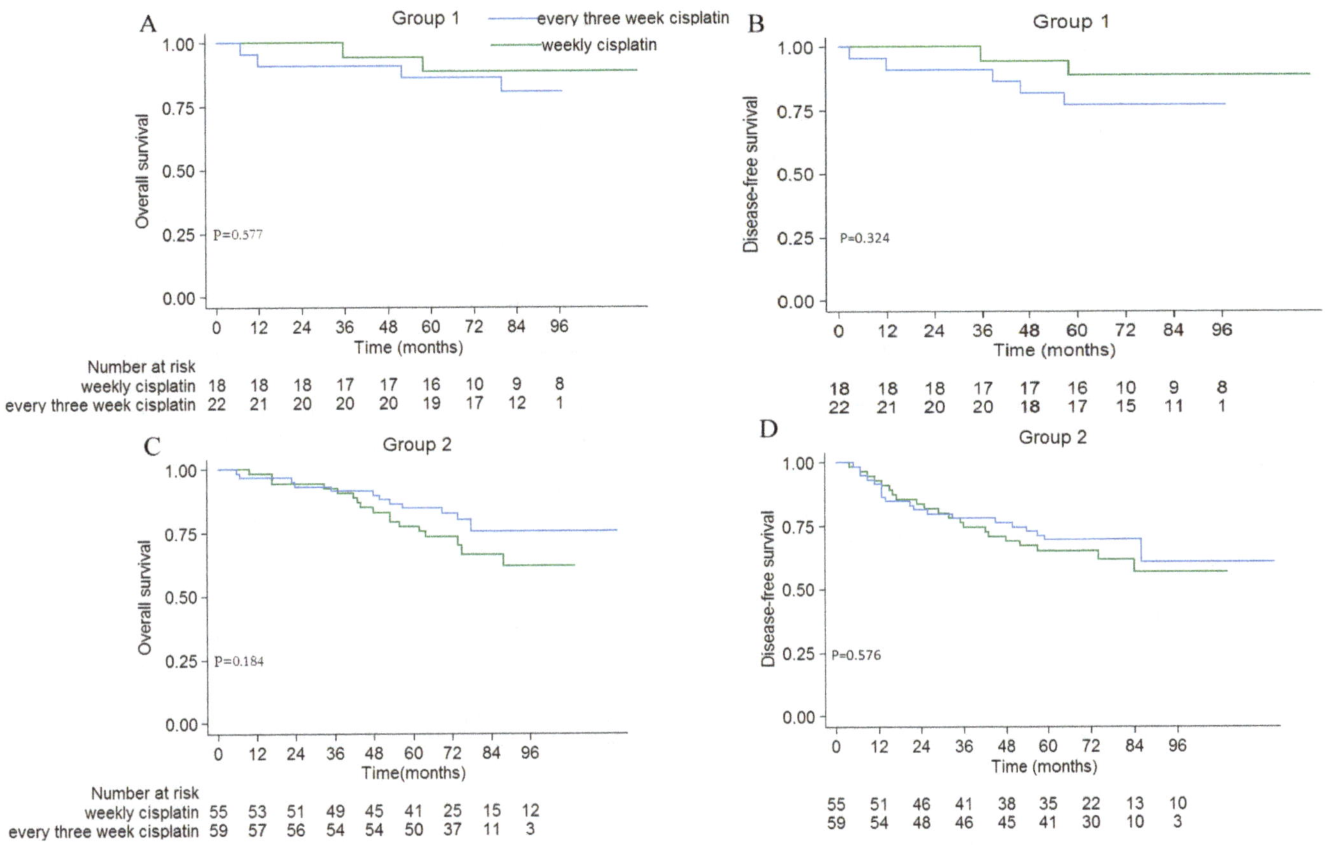

Figure 2. OS and DFS curves for NPC patients stratified by clinical stage. Group 1: patients with stage II disease; Group 2: patients with stage III–IVB disease. *P*-values were calculated with the unadjusted log-rank test.

vs. 80.1%, $P = 0.925$; Fig. 1). The 5-year OS and DFS rates for patients with early- or advanced-stage disease in the two treatment groups were not significantly different (Fig. 2).

Prognostic factors

Univariate analysis revealed that age and N classification were significant prognostic factors for OS ($P = 0.009$ and 0.011, respectively). The 5-year OS rate for patients who received

Table 3. Summary of multivariate analysis of prognostic factors in the 154 patients.

End point	HR (95% CI)	*P*-value[†]
OS		
Age,>50 years vs. ≤50 years	2.809 (1.404–5.620)	0.004
N classification (N0–1 vs. N2–3)	2.830 (1.388–5.767)	0.004
Chemotherapy regimen, weekly vs. every three weeks	0.862 (0.428–1.738)	0.679
DFS		
N classification (N0–1 vs. N2–3)	2.241 (1.213–4.141)	0.010
Chemotherapy regimen, weekly vs. every three weeks	1.099 (0.604–2.001)	0.757
DMFS		
N classification (N0–1 vs. N2–3)	2.752 (1.271–5.961)	0.010
Chemotherapy regimen, weekly vs. every three weeks	1.331 (0.607–2.917)	0.475
LRRFS		
Chemotherapy regimen, weekly vs. every three weeks	1.280 (0.382–4.288)	0.689

HR: hazard ratio; CI: confidence interval; OS: overall survival; DFS: disease-free survival; DMFS: distant metastasis-free survival; LRRFS: locoregional relapse-free survival.
[†]P-values were calculated using an adjusted Cox proportional hazards regression model adjusted for age (>50 years vs. ≤50 years), sex (male vs. female), T classification (T1–2 vs. T3–4), N classification (N0–1 vs. N2–3), chemotherapy regimen, (weekly vs. every three weeks) and cumulative cisplatin dose, (≥160 mg/m2 vs. <160 mg/m2). Only variables that were significantly associated with survival are presented except for the chemotherapy regimen.

cumulative CDDP≥160 mg/m^2 was 84.1% compared to 73.3% for patients who received cumulative CDDP<160 mg/m^2 ($P=0.175$).

Multivariate analysis was performed to adjust for various prognostic factors. The following parameters were included in the Cox proportional hazards model by backward elimination of insignificant explanatory variables: age (>50 years vs. ≤50 years), sex, T classification (T1–2 vs. T3–4), N classification (N0–1 vs. N2–3), concurrent chemotherapy regimen (CDDP weekly vs. every three weeks), and cumulative CDDP dose (≥160 mg/m^2 vs. <160 mg/m^2). Multivariate analysis demonstrated that the CCRT regimen was not a significant prognostic factor for any end point. Age and N classification were significant predictive factors for OS; furthermore, N classification was the only significant prognostic factor for DFS and DMFS (Table 3).

Discussion

NPC is a highly chemosensitive tumor and CCRT has long been a standard treatment option for locoregionally advanced NPC. Treatment regimens delivering medium doses of CDDP weekly or high CDDP doses every three weeks have been evaluated. Weekly medium doses are efficient and simple to administer, especially for outpatients; high doses every three weeks are more effective for reducing distant metastasis, but may lead to more severe acute toxicities [4–7].

In this retrospective study, we observed that CDDP-based (both weekly and every three weeks) CCRT led to similar long-term survival outcomes and acute toxicities in patients with NPC receiving IMRT regardless of whether the patients had early- or advanced-stage disease. Our results are in agreement with that of Jagdis et al. [12], which showed that 40 mg/m^2 CDDP weekly and 100 mg/m^2 CDDP every three weeks had similar deliverability, toxicity profiles, and comparable survival outcomes in locally advanced NPC.

In our study, the overall 5-year OS, DFS, LRRFS, and DMFS rates were 82.3%, 71.3%, 93.1%, and 80.5%, respectively. CDDP delivered both weekly or every three weeks concurrently with IMRT achieved excellent OS. Distant metastasis was the predominant mode of failure. One approach to improving the strategy tested in this study would be changing the sequence to induction–concurrent, as substantially better tolerance and compliance rates have been reported for induction–concurrent regimens [18]. The meta-analysis by OuYang et al. in 2013 [19] also showed that neoadjuvant chemotherapy effectively enhances OS and reduces the rate of distant metastasis in NPC.

With respect to dose delivery, both treatment groups achieved similar cumulative dose intensities; however, a low proportion of patients completed seven weeks of weekly CDDP or three cycles of every three week CDDP. The compliance rates in the present study are lower than that of previously published trials [4–7]. This may be because the weekly CDDP regimen was mostly administered to outpatients and the regimen given every three weeks was mainly administered to inpatients at our center. Poor outpatient compliance and inadequate numbers of inpatient beds led to delays in administering chemotherapy, which often resulted in patients missing the final cycle of chemotherapy.

We adopted an every three week CDDP dose of 80 mg/m^2 in our study, which was effective with low toxicity. The INT-0099 regimen is widely used, where 100 mg/m^2 CDDP is administered on days 1, 22, and 43 with radical RT, given its impressive results compared to RT alone when treating NPC. Regrettably, only 63% of patients in the chemoradiation arm of INT-0099 completed all three cycles of concurrent chemotherapy as planned. Ho et al. [20] compared the dose intensity and toxicity of CDDP administered weekly and every three weeks concurrently to 52 patients with locally advanced squamous head and neck cancer. They found that 100 mg/m^2 CDDP every three weeks with RT was less well tolerated than 40 mg/m^2 CDDP weekly or 80 mg/m^2 CDDP every three weeks and resulted in fewer patients achieving a cumulative dose of >200 mg/m^2. Therefore, the optimal CDDP dose in CCRT regimes for NPC warrants further exploration.

The dose intensity of CDDP is an important prognostic factor in NPC patients receiving CCRT [21–22]. Using pooled data from three prospective trials (in which most patients were treated with conventional RT), Loong et al. [21] explored the prognostic significance of the total CDDP dose delivered during CCRT and reported that patients with stage II or III NPC who received more than five weeks of 40 mg/m^2 CDDP weekly had significantly better OS than patients who received less than five weeks. In our study, a cumulative dose of ≥160 mg/m^2 led to obviously better OS, although the difference was not significant (84.1% vs. 73.3%, $P=0.175$); this may be related to the small number of patients who received a cumulative dose of <160 mg/m^2. Additionally, the use of IMRT has improved the long-term outcome for patients with NPC, which may render detection of the survival benefit of a higher total CDDP dose difficult.

The toxicity profiles of both groups were similar. However, there was a slightly higher incidence of grade 3–4 hematological toxicity and oropharyngeal mucositis in the weekly CDDP group, although the difference was not significant. The main reasons for this observation may be the inadequate monitoring of blood counts and poor oral care in outpatients in the weekly CDDP group. It is worth noting that there was a lower incidence of grade 3–4 dermatitis, dysphagia, and gastrointestinal reactions in patients who received CDDP weekly even though they received a relatively high median cumulative dose.

To our knowledge, this is the first single-institution study to review the difference between CDDP administered weekly and every three weeks concurrently with IMRT in NPC. The principal limitation of this study is its retrospective nature. However, the clinical characteristics of the patients in the two groups were well-balanced, which may reduce potential selection bias. To derive a definitive conclusion, a randomized phase II study of CCRT with CDDP administered every three weeks versus weekly in patients with locally advanced NPC is ongoing in Korea. The findings of this study will aid in the standardization of CCRT regimens for NPC.

Conclusions

IMRT in conjunction with concurrent CDDP chemotherapy administered weekly or every three weeks leads to similar long-term survival outcomes and acute toxicities in NPC regardless of whether the patient has early- or advanced-stage disease. The results of this study require further validation in prospective, multi-center controlled trials.

Author Contributions

Conceived and designed the experiments: C-JT LL YS. Performed the experiments: C-JT LL YS G-QZ L-LT LC Y-PM M-SZ T-BK W-HJ J-YS H-QM JM. Analyzed the data: C-JT LL YS A-HL. Contributed reagents/materials/analysis tools: H-QM A-HL JM. Wrote the paper: C-JT LL YS G-QZ.

References

1. Jemal A, Bray F, Center MM, Ferlay J, Ward E, et al. (2011) Global cancer statistics. CA Cancer J Clin 61: 69–90.
2. Edge SB, Byrd DR, Compton CC, Fritz AG, Greene FL, et al. (2009) American Joint Committee on Cancer Manual for Staging of Cancer [M]. 7th ed. Philadelphia: JB Lippincott. 649 p.
3. Chen L, Mao YP, Xie FY, Liu LZ, Sun Y, et al. (2012) The seventh edition of the UICC/AJCC staging system for nasopharyngeal carcinoma is prognostically useful for patients treated with intensity-modulated radiotherapy from an endemic area in China. Radiat Oncol Biol Phys 104: 331–337.
4. Al-Sarraf M, LeBlanc M, Giri PG, Fu KK, Cooper J, et al. (1998) Chemoradiotherapy versus radiotherapy in patients with advanced nasopharyngeal cancer: phase III randomized Intergroup Study 0099. J Clin Oncol 16: 1310–1317.
5. Lee AW, Lau WH, Tung SY, Chua DT, Chappell R, et al. (2005) Preliminary results of a randomized study on therapeutic gain by concurrent chemotherapy for regionally-advanced nasopharyngeal carcinoma: NPC-9901 trial by the Hong Kong Nasopharyngeal Cancer Study Group. J Clin Oncol 23: 6966–6975.
6. Lee AW, Tung SY, Chua DT, Ngan RK, Chappell R, et al. (2010) Randomized trial of radiotherapy plus concurrent-adjuvant chemotherapy vs. radiotherapy alone for regionally advanced nasopharyngeal carcinoma. J Natl Cancer Inst 102: 1188–1198.
7. Chen Y, Sun Y, Liang SB, Zong JF, Li WF, et al. (2013) Progress report of a randomized trial comparing long-term survival and late toxicity of concurrent chemoradiotherapy with adjuvant chemotherapy versus radiotherapy alone in patients with stage III to IVB nasopharyngeal carcinoma from endemic regions of China. Cancer 119: 2230–2238.
8. Chan AT, Leung SF, Ngan RK, Teo PM, Lau WH, et al. (2005) Overall survival after concurrent cisplatin-radiotherapy compared with radiotherapy alone in locoregionally advanced nasopharyngeal carcinoma. J Natl Cancer Inst 97: 536–539.
9. Lin JC, Jan JS, Hsu CY, Liang WM, Jiang RS, et al. (2003) Phase III study of concurrent chemoradiotherapy versus radiotherapy alone for advanced nasopharyngeal carcinoma: positive effect on overall and progression-free survival. J Clin Oncol 21: 631–637.
10. Chen L, Hu CS, Chen XZ, Hu GQ, Cheng ZB, et al. (2012) Concurrent chemoradiotherapy plus adjuvant chemotherapy versus concurrent chemoradiotherapy alone in patients with locoregionally advanced nasopharyngeal carcinoma: a phase 3 multicentre randomised controlled trial. Lancet Oncol 13: 163–171.
11. Baujat B, Audry H, Bourhis J, Chan AT, Onat H, et al. (2006) Chemotherapy in locally advanced nasopharyngeal carcinoma: an individual data meta-analysis of eight randomized trials and 1753 patients. Int J Radiat Oncol Biol Phys 64: 47–56.
12. Jagdis A, Laskin J, Hao D, Hay J, Wu J, et al. (2012) Dose delivery analysis of weekly versus 3-weekly cisplatin concurrent with radiation therapy for locally advanced nasopharyngeal carcinoma (NPC). Am J Clin Oncol Oct 29.
13. Peng G, Wang T, Yang KY, Zhang S, Zhang T, et al. (2012) A prospective, randomized study comparing outcomes and toxicities of intensity-modulated radiotherapy vs. conventional two-dimensional radiotherapy for the treatment of nasopharyngeal carcinoma. Radiother Oncol 104: 286–293.
14. Zhao C, Han F, Lu LX, Huang SM, Lin CG, et al. (2004) Intensity modulated radiotherapy for local-regional advanced nasopharyngeal carcinoma. Ai Zheng 23: 1532–1537.
15. Liang S, Sun Y, Liu L, Chen Y, Chen L, et al. (2009) Extension of local disease in nasopharyngeal carcinoma detected by magnetic resonance imaging: improvement of clinical target volume delineation. Int J Radiat Oncol Biol Phys 75: 742–750.
16. Kaplan EL, Meier P (1958) Nonparametric estimation from incomplete observation. J Am Stat Assoc 53: 457–481.
17. Cox DR (1972) Regression models and life tables. J R Stat Soc B 34: 187–220.
18. Lee AWM, Ng WT, Chan OSH, Sze HCK (2012) If concurrent-adjuvant chemoradiotherapy is beneficial for locoregionally advanced nasopharyngeal carcinoma, would changing the sequence to induction-concurrent achieve better outcome? J Radiat Oncol 1: 107–115.
19. OuYang PY, Xie C, Mao YP, Zhang Y, Liang XX, et al. (2013) Significant efficacies of neoadjuvant and adjuvant chemotherapy for nasopharyngeal carcinoma by meta-analysis of published literature-based randomized, controlled trials. Ann Oncol 24: 2136–2146.
20. Ho KF, Swindell R, Brammer CV (2008) Dose intensity comparison between weekly and 3-weekly Cisplatin delivered concurrently with radical radiotherapy for head and neck cancer: A retrospective comparison from New Cross Hospital, Wolverhampton, UK. Acta Oncol 47: 1513–1518.
21. Loong HH, Ma BB, Leung SF, Mo F, Hui EP, et al. (2012) Prognostic significance of the total dose of cisplatin administered during concurrent chemoradiotherapy in patients with locoregionally advanced nasopharyngeal carcinoma. Radiother Oncol 104: 300–304.
22. Chen QY, Wen YF, Guo L, Liu H, Huang PY, et al. (2011) Concurrent chemoradiotherapy vs radiotherapy alone in stage II nasopharyngeal carcinoma: phase III randomized trial. J Natl Cancer Inst 103: 1761–1770.

Chemotherapy Enhances Cross-Presentation of Nuclear Tumor Antigens

Chidozie C. Anyaegbu[1,2], Richard A. Lake[1,2], Kathy Heel[3], Bruce W. Robinson[1,2], Scott A. Fisher[1,2]*

1 National Centre for Asbestos Related Diseases (NCARD), QEII Medical Centre, Nedlands, Western Australia, 2 School of Medicine and Pharmacology, University of Western Australia, QEII Medical Centre, Nedlands, Western Australia, 3 School of Pathology and Laboratory Medicine, University of Western Australia, QEII Medical Centre, Nedlands, Western Australia

Abstract

Cross-presentation of tumor antigen is essential for efficient priming of naïve CD8$^+$ T lymphocytes and induction of effective anti-tumor immunity. We hypothesized that the subcellular location of a tumor antigen could affect the efficiency of cross-presentation, and hence the outcome of anti-tumor responses to that antigen. We compared cross-presentation of a nominal antigen expressed in the nuclear, secretory, or cytoplasmic compartments of B16 melanoma tumors. All tumors expressed similar levels of the antigen. The antigen was cross-presented from all compartments but when the concentration was low, nuclear antigen was less efficiently cross-presented than antigen from other cellular locations. The efficiency of cross-presentation of the nuclear antigen was improved following chemotherapy-induced tumor cell apoptosis and this correlated with an increase in the proportion of effector CTL. These data demonstrate that chemotherapy improves nuclear tumor antigen cross-presentation and could be important for anti-cancer immunotherapies that target nuclear antigens.

Editor: Ryan M. Teague, Saint Louis University School of Medicine, United States of America

Funding: This work was funded by grants from the National Health and Medical Research Council of Australia and the Insurance Commission of Western Australia. The funding bodies had no role in the study design, data collection and analysis, decision to publish, or preparation of the manuscript.

Competing Interests: The authors have declared that no competing interests exist.

* Email: scott.fisher@uwa.edu.au

Introduction

Recognition of tumor antigen by specific T cells is a necessary prerequisite for the induction of effective anti-tumor immune responses [1]. This is initiated by *cross-presentation*, a phenomenon where professional antigen presenting cells (APC) such as dendritic cells (DC) capture, process, and present exogenous antigens through the class I pathway [2]. Cross priming of naïve CD8 T cells by professional APC invokes a program leading to tumor specific-cytotoxic T lymphocytes (CTL) which proliferate and traffic to the tumor site where they ultimately attack and destroy tumor cells [3]. The efficiency of cross-priming has been shown to be influenced by the level of APC activation and maturation status [4], as well as the properties of cross-presented antigen itself. Factors such as antigen dose [5], type (modified self-antigen or mutated tumor neoantigen) [6], source (whether the antigen was derived from live or apoptotic cells) [7,8], location of the antigenic determinant (epitope) within the tumor protein [9], and subcellular location within tumor cells [10,11] can affect cross-priming efficiency. With respect to location, while some studies have shown that the cytoplasm is the main source of antigen, they typically compared the secretory, cell-membrane, and cytoplasmic compartments, but did not assess the contribution of nuclear antigen. Many of the tumor-associated antigen (TAAs) currently targeted in anti-tumor immunotherapy, such as survivin, MAGE-A10, and WT1, are predominantly expressed in the nucleus [12–14]. Moreover, several clinical studies have correlated the nuclear localization of different TAAs with poor clinical outcome in a variety of cancer types [15–20]. Therefore, it is important to understand the relative availability for cross-presentation of antigens in the nuclear compartment compared to other cellular compartments. We hypothesized that nuclear localization of an antigen would limit cross-presentation and hence cross priming of naïve CD8 T cells because APCs would not be able to access nuclear antigen as easily as antigen from other cellular locations. Furthermore, since apoptosis is known to cause nuclear degradation [21,22] and extracellular release of nuclear contents [23], we reasoned that apoptosis-inducing chemotherapy would improve the efficiency of cross-presentation of nuclear antigens.

To address these questions, we developed a murine tumor model of cross presentation in which MHC mismatch between the tumor cell and model antigen precludes direct antigen presentation. We engineered H2-K^b B16 tumors to differentially express a model tumor antigen (influenza HA H2-K^d restricted CL4 epitope expressed in frame with EGFP) in the secretory, cytoplasmic, or nuclear compartments, and compared their potential to induce proliferation of H-2K^d restricted CL4-specific CD8$^+$ T cells *in vivo* as a measure of antigen cross presentation. We then investigated the capacity of the tumor apoptosis-inducing chemotherapy agent, gemcitabine [24], to improve cross-presentation. Here, we show that nuclear antigen is not cross-presented as efficiently as its cytoplasmic and secreted counterparts, and that gemcitabine induced tumor cell apoptosis could reverses this, boosting nuclear antigen cross-presentation to equivalent levels *in vivo*, which correlated with an increase in the proportion of effector CL4-specific CTL.

Materials and Methods

Mice

Female, C57BL/6 (H-2^b) x BALB/c (H-2^d) F_1 mice (H-2^{bxd}), and Clone 4 (CL4) TCR transgenic mice, whose $CD8^+$ T cells express TCRs that specifically recognize the H-2^d restricted 'CL4' epitope (IYSTVASSL; residues 518–526) of influenza haemagglutinin (HA) protein [25], were obtained from the Animal Resource Centre (Canning Vale, Perth, Australia). All mice were used at seven to ten weeks of age, and maintained under standard conditions (M-block Animal Facility, Queen Elizabeth II Medical Centre, The University of Western Australia; UWA, Perth, Australia). Animal experiments were approved by The University of Western Australia Animal Ethics Committee (RA/3/100/1016), and conducted in accordance with the Australian National Health and Medical Research Council's Code of Practice for the Use of Animals for Scientific Purposes.

Tumor cell line and subcutaneous transplantation

B16.F10 (H-2^b) melanoma tumor cell line (ATCC, Manassas, VA; CRL-6475) was used in all experiments. Tumor cells were maintained in RPMI-1640 (Invitrogen Life Technologies, Mulgrave, Australia) supplemented with 10% Fetal Calf Serum (FCS; Invitrogen Life Technologies), 50 μg/mL gentamicin (David Bull Labs, Kewdale, Australia), 60 μg/mL penicillin (CSL, Melbourne, Australia) 20 mM HEPES (Sigma Aldrich, Sydney, Australia) and 0.05 mM 2-mercaptoethanol (pH 7.2; Merck, Kilsyth, Australia). 5×10^5 viable B16 cells in 100 μL PBS were inoculated subcutaneously (s.c.) into the lower right flank of recipient F_1 mice. Tumor size was measured across two dimensions at least three times weekly with microcalipers. Mice were euthanized via Penthrane inhalation (Abbot Laboratories, USA) and death confirmed by cervical dislocation when tumors reached 100 mm^2 as per animal ethics approval.

Generation of gene constructs targeting model antigen to distinct subcellular compartments

The secretory gene construct (sec-EGFP-CL4) was generated by attaching the H-$2K^b$ -derived endoplasmic reticulum (ER) signal peptide (MVPCTLLLLLAAALAPTQTRAV) to the amino-terminus of enhanced Green Fluorescent Protein (EGFP). A truncated version of the ER signal peptide (underlined sequence) was used to generate the cytoplasmic construct (cyto-EGFP-CL4), while the Simian Virus 40 T-antigen (SV40 T-Ag) nuclear localisation signal (MPKKKRKV), was used to generate the nuclear construct (nuc-EGFP-CL4). The following amino acid sequence QVGIYSTVASSLSELEKD was fused to the carboxyl-terminus of EGFP in all three constructs. This sequence encodes the CL4 epitope (underlined; the MHC Class I restricted region of Influenza haemagglutinin protein) preceded, and followed by, short spacer sequences to ensure that antigen presentation required cytosolic processing. All gene constructs were generated using PCR primers. Resulting PCR products were cloned into pCR4Blunt-TOPO (Zero Blunt PCR Cloning Kit; Invitrogen Life Technologies), and subcloned into pLenti6/V5-GW.blasticidin lentiviral vector, using BamH1/Xho1 cohesive ligation, for introduction into B16 cells. Sequence integrity of all clones was confirmed by DNA sequencing.

Stable lentiviral transduction of B16 tumor cells with gene constructs

To generate lentivirus for integrating gene constructs into B16 target cells, 293FT lentiviral producer cells (Invitrogen Life Technologies) were co-transfected, using Lipofectamine™ 2000 transfection reagent (Invitrogen Life Technologies), with pHIV-PV-VSVG lentiviral packaging plasmid and pLenti6/V5-GW.blasticidin expression vector containing sec-EGFP-CL4, cyto-EGFP-CL4, or nuc-EGFP-CL4 gene constructs. Transfected 293FT cells were cultured in DMEM (Invitrogen Life Technologies) containing FCS (10%), L-glutamine (2 mM), non-essential amino acids (NEAA, 0.1 mM), penicillin (100 U/ml), and streptomycin (100 mg/ml). Lentivirus-containing supernatant was harvested after a 72-hour incubation, and added neat to a fresh culture of B16 cells. Stably transduced B16 cell were generated using blasticidin antibiotic selection (10 μg/mL in RPMI-1640, Invitrogen Life Technologies, for 10–12 days). Stable EGFP positive cells were sorted to a purity of >98% using BD Influx™ cell sorter (Becton Dickinson, San Jose, USA), and clonal populations expressing EGFP-CL4 protein in secretory (B16.Sec), cytoplasmic (B16.Cyto), or nuclear (B16.Nuc) subcellular compartments isolated by limiting dilution assay.

Preparation of whole cell lysates and secretory fractions for EGFP ELISA assay

Whole cell lysates were extracted from each cell line by resuspending 5×10^6 tumor cells in 500 μL of radio immunoprecipitation assay (RIPA) lysis buffer (150 mM sodium chloride; 1.0% Triton X-100; 0.1% sodium dodecyl sulphate; 50 mM Tris, pH 8.0; 1/100 dilution Protease Inhibitor Cocktail (P8340, Sigma Aldrich) and 0.5% sodium deoxycholate) and incubating for 30 minutes at 4°C. Cell debris was removed by centrifugation (500×g for 10 mins) and supernatants containing whole cell extracts gently transferred to a fresh tube. To generate secretory fractions, each cell line was seeded at 1×10^6 cells/10 cm cell-culture dish. Following a 24-hour incubation, supernatant containing secretory fraction was harvested and concentrated using the Amicon Ultra-15 centrifugal 10 kDa filter device (Merck Millipore, Massachusetts, USA). Protein concentrations were determined by Bradford assay. EGFP-CL4 levels in cell lysates and fractions were then quantified using GFP ELISA assay kit (Cell Biolabs Inc. San Diego, USA), as per manufacturer's instructions.

Confocal microscopy

EGFP expressing B16 cells were cultured on glass coverslips and fixed with 4% paraformaldehyde. Cell nuclei were counterstained with Hoechst 33342 nuclear envelope marker (Invitrogen Life Technologies), and confocal microscopy performed using a Nikon A1Si spectral detector confocal system (Nikon, Melville, USA). Imaging was performed with a 60× oil immersion objective lens. For each cell line, at least 10 single plane images of representative cells (optical slice =0.125 μm) were recorded. Images were analysed using the NIS-C Elements software (Nikon).

Acquisition and analysis of ImageStream imaging flow cytometry data

The ImageStreamX imaging flow cytometer (Amnis, Seattle, USA) was used to confirm the differential expression of EGFP-CL4 antigen in respective B16 tumor cell lines. Briefly, each cell line was counter-stained with Hoechst 33342 nuclear marker and 10,000 cells acquired for analysis. Cell populations were hierarchically gated for single cells that expressed both EGFP and Hoechst 33342 as previously described [26]. Following acquisition,

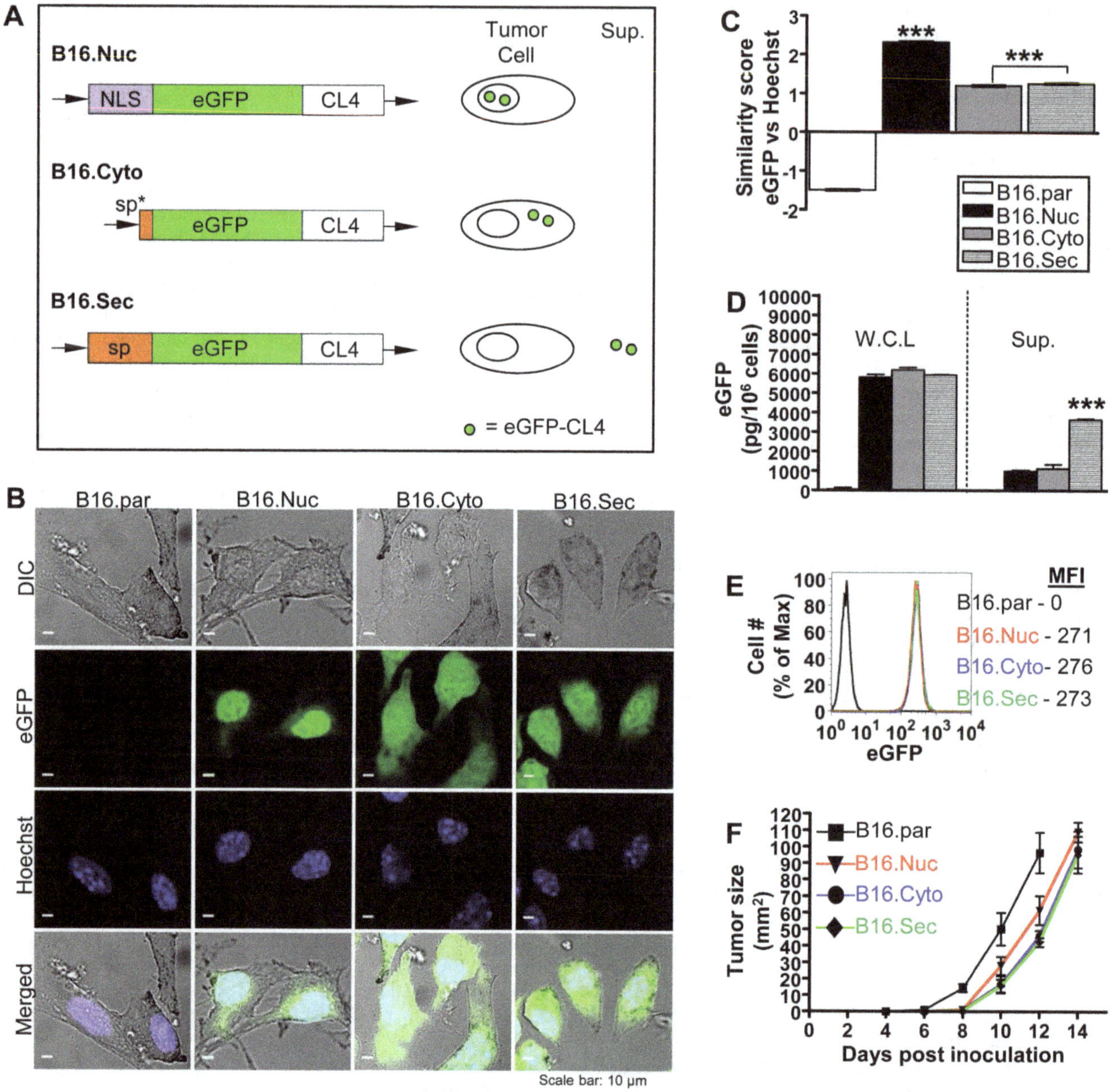

Figure 1. Schematic illustration and characterization of B16 tumor cells expressing differentially localized antigen. (A) Schematic depiction of gene constructs used to generate B16 parental (B16.par) tumors expressing EGFP-CL4 recombinant protein in secretory (B16.Sec), nuclear (B16.Nuc), or cytoplasmic (B16.Cyto) cellular compartments. (B) Confocal fluorescence microscopy demonstrated targeted expression of EGFP-CL4 in distinct subcellular compartments within respective tumors (magnification, ×60). (C) Quantitative imaging flow cytometry confirmed confocal microscopy observations. (D) EGFP ELISA was used to compare the amount of EGFP present in whole cell lysates (W.C.L) and supernatants (Sup.) of respective tumors. A standard curve of recombinant EGFP protein was used to calculate the amount of EGFP. A representative experiment is shown out of two independent ELISAs in triplicates ± SEM. (E) Relative intensity and stability of EGFP expression was determined by live-cell flow cytometry. Mean fluorescent intensities (MFI) are shown in figure. (F) *In vivo* growth pattern of respective tumors after s.c. inoculation in F1 mice. Data are means of 10 mice from two independent experiments. ***$p<0.001$. One-way ANOVA, followed by a Bonferroni post-test.

the relationship between EGFP and nuclear images was analysed using the "Similarity" feature of the IDEAS software (Amnis) [26]. The similarity score provides a measure of the degree of nuclear localisation of EGFP by comparing a log-transformed Pearson's correlation coefficient between the pixel values of two image pairs. Cells with a high similarity score exhibit strong correlation between images (i.e. EGFP is predominantly nuclear located), while cells with a low similarity score exhibit no correlation between images (i.e. EGFP is predominantly located within the cytoplasm).

MTT assay

The metabolic activity (sensitivity) of B16 tumors after exposure to gemcitabine (Gem) was determined using the MTT [3-(4,5-dimethylthiazo-2-yl)-2,5-diphenyltetrazolium bromide] colorimetric assay (Sigma-Aldrich), according to manufacturer's protocol. Briefly, 24 h after seeding tumor cells to 96-well flat-bottomed

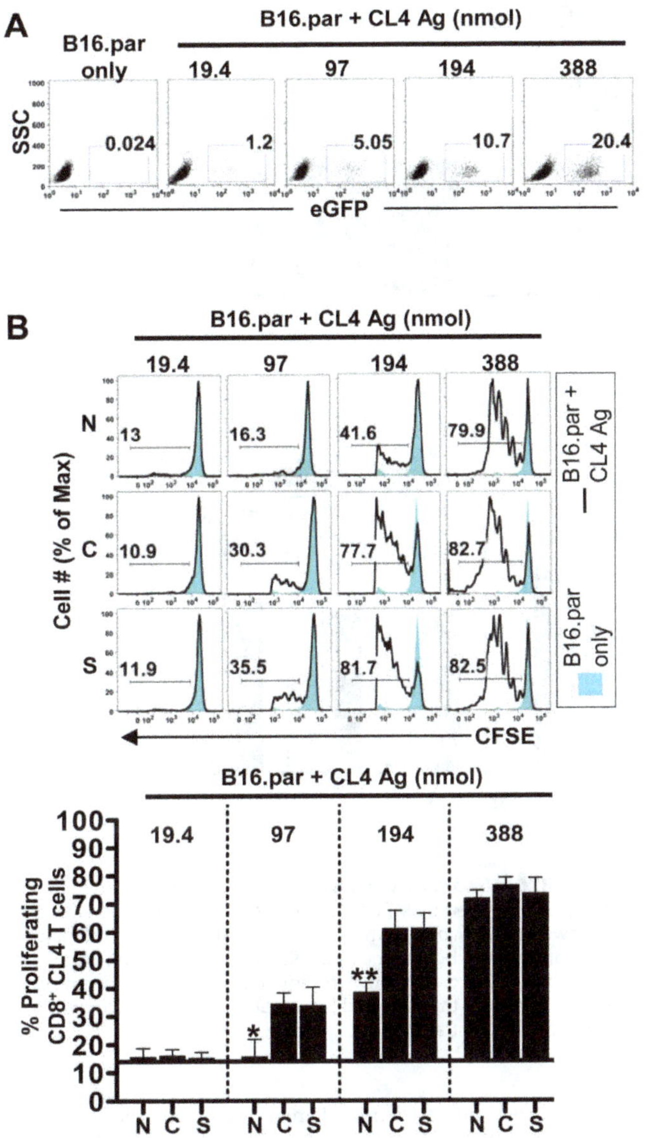

Figure 2. Nuclear localized tumor antigen was not cross-presented as efficiently as cytoplasmic and secretory counterparts. (A) The EGFP-CL4 antigen expression profile of B16 parental cells (B16 par.) or, B16 par. mixed with 1 (19.4), 5 (97), 10 (194), or 20% (388 nmol) of B16.Nuc (N), B16.Cyto (C), or B16.Sec (S) CL4 antigen-containing cells, was confirmed on the day of tumor inoculation by flow cytometry. For simplicity, Figure 2A only shows the profile of B16.Nuc mixtures, as they were not different to B16.Cyto or B16.Sec (B) CFSE-labelled CL4-specific CD8+ T cells were intravenously injected into F1 mice bearing 8-day-old subcutaneous tumors, and the proliferation of these T cells in the tumour draining lymph node examined on day 11 post-tumor inoculation by flow cytometry. Data are representative of two independent experiments, each involving five mice per group. Bars begin at the Mean ± SEM baseline proliferation for B16 parental cells.

tissue culture plates (1×10^3 cells/well), serially diluted concentrations of Gem were added to wells. Following incubation (37°C in 5% CO_2) for a further 48 h, 50 µL MTT solution (0.1 mg/well) was added and plates incubated for a further 4 hrs. Resulting formazan crystals were solubilized using dimethyl sulfoxide (DMSO, 100 µL/well; Sigma-Aldrich), and absorbance measured at 570 nm (Victor^{TM} plate reader, PerkinElmer, Massachusetts, USA). All experiments were performed in triplicate.

Carboxyfluorescein diacetate succinimidyl ester (CFSE)-based in vivo T cell proliferation assay

The CFSE-based T cell proliferation assay, originally described by Lyons and Parish [27], was used as an indirect measure of antigen cross-presentation. We used the mixing strategy of inoculating F_1 mice with B16 parental cells mixed with B16.Nuc, B16.Cyto, or B16.Sec in different proportions, because a high CL4 antigen dose could saturate the proliferation of CL4-TCR transgenic T cells, and this has the potential to mask differences in cross-presentation. Homogenized single cell suspensions from spleens and lymph nodes [28] of naïve CL4 mice were labelled with CFSE (Molecular Probes, Invitrogen Life Technologies) as described previously [29]. Tumor-bearing F_1 mice were then intravenously (i.v.) injected with CFSE-labelled lymphoid CL4 cells (1×10^7 cells/mouse in 100 µL PBS). Seventy-two hours after adoptive transfer, F_1 mice were culled and single cell suspensions prepared from their tumor draining LN (tdLN). Samples were labelled with CD8α-ef780-APC (clone 53-6.7, eBioscience, San Diego, USA) monoclonal antibody (mAb) and acquired on a FACS Canto II flow cytometer (Becton Dickinson, San Jose, USA). Cells were first gated on live lymphocytes before gating on $CFSE^+$ $CD8^+$ cells. Five hundred thousand events were collected and analysed using FlowJo software (TreeStar, Ashland, USA).

Chemotherapy

Tumor-bearing F_1 mice were intraperitoneally (i.p.) injected with a single dose of the apoptosis-inducing chemotherapeutic deoxycytidine analogue, gemcitabine hydrochloride (GEM. Sandoz. Pyrmont, Australia) at 240 µg/g body weight, in 100 µL of saline at indicated timepoints. Mice were monitored daily for potential weight loss and other toxicities.

Statistical analysis

Data comparing differences between groups were assessed using the Student t test. Differences between growth curves were compared using ANOVA. Differences were considered significant when the P value was <0.05. Statistical analysis was conducted using GraphPad Prism 4.0 Software (San Diego, USA).

Results

Characterization of B16 tumors expressing a model tumor antigen in distinct cellular locations

To study the effect of cellular localization on tumor-specific $CD8^+$ T cell responses, we modified B16 tumor cells to express the MHC class I K^d restricted immunodominant epitope of the influenza virus HA protein, CL4, fused with EGFP, as a quantifiable model tumor antigen in nuclear (B16.Nuc), secretory (B16.Sec), or cytoplasmic (B16.Cyto) compartments (Fig. 1A). The dense nuclear expression of EGFP-CL4 in B16.Nuc, but diffuse cytoplasmic expression in B16.Cyto and B16.Sec tumors, demonstrated that antigen was successfully targeted to the intended cellular locations (Fig. 1B). These data were quantitated by imaging flow cytometry, a technique that combines the statistical power of flow cytometry with the spatial resolution of confocal microscopy. Based on the IDEAS algorithm [26], where similarity scores above 2 and below 1 indicate a high, or low degree of EGFP/nuclear co-localisation respectively, B16.Nuc had the highest EGFP/nuclear co-localisation with a mean similarity score of 2.317 (Fig. 1C). Due to the low error associated with analysing large numbers of cells (>10,000 per sample), we detected a statistically significant EGFP/nuclear co-localization

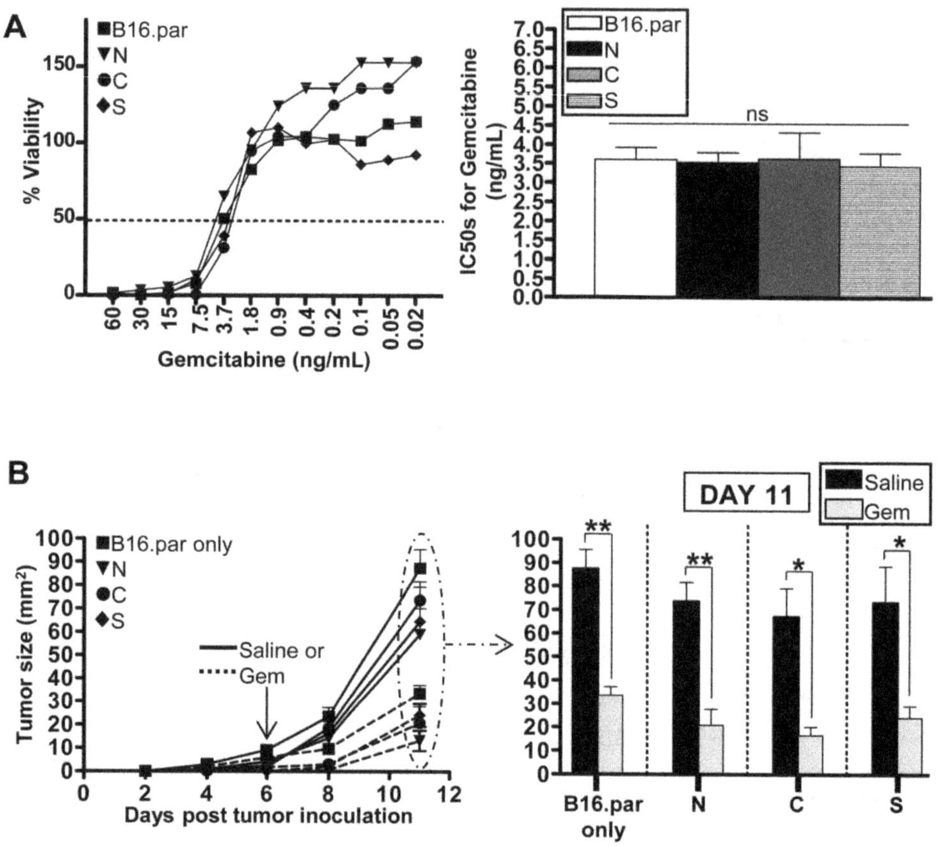

Figure 3. The apoptosis-inducing agent gemcitabine has a direct effect on B16 tumors in vitro and in vivo. (A) The relative in vitro sensitivity of B16 parental, B16.Nuc, B16.Cyto, and B16.Sec tumor cells to gemcitabine was assessed by MTT assay, after a 48 hr incubation with drug. With relevent concentrations of gemcitabine that kill 50% of respective tumors shown. (B) *In vivo* growth of B16 parental only, and B16 parental mixed with 10% (194 nmols) of B16.Sec-, Cyto-, or Nuc-CL4 antigen-containing tumors, after subcutaneous inoculation of F1 mice on day 0, and intraperitoneal administration of a single dose of gemcitabine (240 μg/g) or saline on day 6. Bar graph shows tumor sizes on day 11. For simplicity, Figure 3B only shows data from the 10% antigen concentration experiment as this was similar to that of 1 and 5%. Mean ± SEM. Six mice per group from two independent experiments. One-way ANOVA followed by a Bonferroni post test against all groups.

in B16.Sec relative to B16.Cyto (Fig. 1C). As expected, B16.Sec secreted the highest concentration of EGFP-CL4 protein into culture supernatant (Fig. 1D).

Importantly, all three tumor cell lines expressed a similar steady-state whole cell level of EGFP-CL4 protein at approximately 6000 pg per 10^6 cells, or 3.33×10^{-12} nmol of EGFP-CL4 per cell (Fig. 1D). These results were confirmed by the similar live-cell EGFP fluorescence intensities of respective tumors (Fig. 1E). This also confirmed stability of EGFP-CL4 fusion protein as the fluorescence intensities remained unchanged in long-term culture, without additional antibiotic selection, for over 50 passages (Fig. 1E). Although B16 parental tumor showed a slightly faster *in vivo* outgrowth, subsequent comparative studies confirmed that all three antigen-bearing tumors displayed a similar *in vivo* growth pattern (Fig. 1F). Taken together, these data demonstrate that B16.Nuc, B16.Cyto, and B16.Sec tumors targeted antigen to their respective cellular locations, and expressed similar levels of EGFP-CL4 fusion protein as well as *in vivo* growth pattern.

Nuclear localized tumor antigen is not cross-presented as efficiently as cytoplasmic and secretory antigen

Having generated the B16 tumors with differentially localized antigen, we proceeded to assess the impact of cellular antigen location on cross-presentation. Because our B16 tumors (H-2^b) lacked the relevant restriction element (H-2^d) for recognition by the CL4 TCR, we could rule out direct presentation of the antigen by the tumors [33] or by MHC-peptide exchange; a phenomenon described as "cross dressing" [20]. Thus in tumor-bearing C57BL/6 x BALB/C F_1 mice (H-2^{bxd}), the proliferation of adoptively transferred H-2^d restricted CL4-TCR transgenic CD8 T cells could only be induced when F1 host APCs cross-present CL4 antigen. In order to better define the threshold level of antigen that we previously reported to be required for cross-presentation [30,31] and determine whether this threshold level differed depending on the cellular location of antigen, we inoculated F_1 mice with B16 parental cells that had been mixed with either B16.Nuc, B16.Cyto, or B16.Sec tumor cells in different proportions, diluting the concentration of antigen to the doses shown in Fig. 2A. These experiments demonstrated that nuclear antigen required a twofold higher threshold concentration for cross-presentation relative to the cytoplasmic and secretory antigen; 194 nmol versus 97 nmol respectively (Fig. 2B).

Gemcitabine induces apoptosis-mediated cell death of B16 tumor cells

Since our data suggested that nuclear antigens are relatively inefficiently cross presented compared to other subcellular compartments, we hypothesised that this situation could be altered

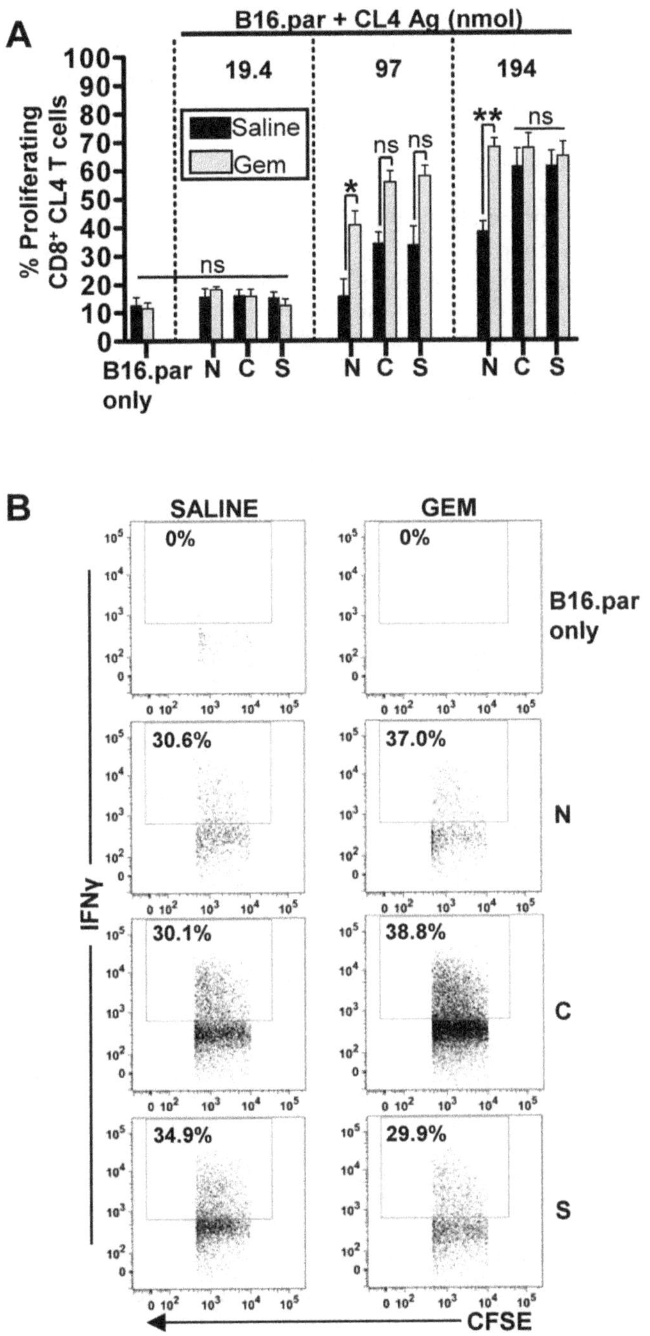

Figure 4. Gemcitabine improves the cross-presentation efficiency of nuclear localized antigen. F1 mice were inoculated on day 0 with B16 parental only (B16 only), or B16 parental mixed with 1 (19.4), 5 (97), or 10% (194 nmol), B16.Nuc (N), B16.Cyto (C), or B16.Sec (S) CL4 antigen-containing tumors, and a single dose of gemcitabine or saline administered on day 6. CFSE-labelled CL4 T cells were transferred on day 8, and the (A) proliferation and (B) Interferon gamma expression of CL4-specific CD8^{+} T cells in tumour draining lymph nodes of mice assessed on day 11. Mean ± SEM. Six mice per group from two independent experiments. One-way ANOVA followed by a Bonferroni post test against all groups. ns = not significant, *$p<0.05$, ***$p<0.001$.

by gemcitabine, an immunogenic chemotherapy agent that we previously reported to increase the availability of antigen for cross-presentation by inducing apoptotic tumor cell death [24]. Importantly, B16 parental, B16.Nuc, B16.Cyto, and B16.Sec tumors were equally sensitive to gemcitabine with an IC50 between 3 and 4 ng/ml as determined by MTT assay (Fig. 3A). This sensitivity was also observed *in vivo*, as a single i.p. injection of gemcitabine (240 µg/g) significantly retarded the outgrowth of all B16 tumors compared to saline treated mice (Fig. 3B). Thus, gemcitabine induces similar levels of apoptosis-mediated cell death on all of the B16 tumors in this model.

Gemcitabine improves cross-presentation efficiency of nuclear antigen in a dose dependent manner

After establishing the comparable sensitivity of B16 tumors to gemcitabine-mediated apoptosis, we proceeded to test whether gemcitabine could augment the cross-presentation efficiency of nuclear localized antigen and enhance cross presentation to a level similar to that seen with cytoplasmic and secreted tumor antigens. As all three tumors were similar in (i) their antigen content (Fig. 1E), (ii) were from the same parental line, (iii) grew at similar rates *in vivo* and (iv) exhibited comparable degrees of apoptosis-induced cell death, we can reasonably assume a similar amount of tumor debris following chemotherapy. Therefore, to determine if there was any change in the cross presentation of nuclear antigens following gemcitabine induced immunogenic cell death, F_1 mice were inoculated with B16 parental cells mixed with either no antigen, or 19.4, 97, or 194 nmol of CL4 antigen-containing B16.Nuc, B16.Cyto, or B16.Sec tumor cells. Tumor bearing mice were treated with gemcitabine or saline and the proliferation of adoptively transferred CL4-specific CD8^{+} T cells in tumor draining LNs of mice assessed. Compared to saline, gemcitabine doubled the cross-presentation efficiency of nuclear antigen to levels comparable to the cytoplasmic and secretory antigen, both of which demonstrated only marginal increases relative to saline treated controls, thus abrogating the difference in cross-presentation efficiency between antigens in different cellular locations (Fig. 4A). Consequently, the threshold amount of antigen required for nuclear localized antigen to be cross-presented was lowered two-fold from 194 (with saline) to 97 nmol (Fig. 4A). Interestingly, while gemcitabine doubled the cross-presentation efficiency of nuclear antigen, the proportion of CL4-specific CD8 T cells expressing IFNγ remained unchanged (Fig. 4B).

Discussion

Cross presentation is essential for the generation of effective anti-tumor immunity [3]. Tumor-specific CTL, with the capacity to destroy tumor cells, are only generated following effective cross-priming of naïve CD8 T cells by professional APC. To evaluate the efficiency of this process for different tumor compartments, we developed a murine model of tumor antigen cross-presentation, in which tumor cells differentially expressed a model antigen in either the secretory, cytoplasmic or nuclear compartments and compared their ability to induce proliferation of antigen-specific CD8 T cells as a read out of cross-presentation. We observed a significant difference in EGFP/nuclear localisation between secretory and cytoplasmic located tumor antigen. This is consistent with expression in the secretory pathway of secreted tumor antigen as secreted proteins show more nuclear co-localization than cytoplasmic proteins due to their transport through the endoplasmic reticulum, which borders the nuclear envelope [32,33]. Despite this, all tumors expressed similar levels of tumor antigen in their respective cellular compartment and grew at comparable rates *in vivo*, indicating we had developed a robust model suitable for comparing the efficacy of nuclear antigen cross-presentation versus other compartments.

Nuclear antigen is not cross-presented as efficiently as cytoplasmic or secreted antigen, but is restored following treatment with gemcitabine

Throughout this study, all tumor antigens were efficiently cross-presented when antigen concentration was sufficiently high. However, when lower tumor antigen concentrations were studied, we observed that nuclear tumor antigen was not as efficiently cross-presented, requiring at least a two-fold higher concentration relative to secreted or cytoplasmic tumor antigen to achieve similar level of CD8 T cell proliferation. We concluded that the reduced efficiency of cross-presentation was likely due to the distinct nuclear localization of tumor antigen, since all other factors, including cellular tumor antigen levels and the *in vivo* growth rates of each tumor type, were similar. However, treatment with the apoptosis inducing nucleoside analogue gemcitabine was able to restore nuclear antigen cross-presentation to levels equivalent to secreted or cytoplasmic compartments. The antigen-dose dependent nature of this improvement suggested that treatment with gemcitabine boosted the amount of antigen available for cross-presentation and thus for cross priming. While the F1 cross-presentation model precludes any assessment of tumor regression due to the inability of direct antigen presentation, the increase in the proportion of CL4 $CD8^+$ T cells associated with gemcitabine treatment and their ability to express IFNγ correlates to our earlier studies in which these CL4 cells drive an anti-tumour response against CL4 bearing tumours [25,31]. It is therefore interesting to consider whether the reduced efficacy of nuclear tumor antigen cross-presentation before gemcitabine treatment might play a crucial role in tumor development, given that tumor antigen detection is critical for effective immune surveillance that protects the host during cancer development [34]. One possible interpretation is that the relatively reduced level of nuclear antigen cross-presentation might correlate with less effective immunosurveillance, limiting recognition of nuclear antigen bearing tumors by the host immune system. This hypothesis fits with the observation that cancer patients with tumor antigen localized in the nucleus have a more aggressive disease progression than patients with the same antigen expressed in the cytoplasm, or other tumor cell compartments [15–19]. Alternatively, it might be that after gemcitabine treatment, newly synthesized antigen may not localize correctly to the nucleus, resulting in increased cytosolic antigen that led to the observed increase in cross-presentation. Importantly, the enhanced expression of nuclear tumor antigen following gemcitabine treatment has been observed in human cancers [14,35] and while the exact mechanism involved remains uncertain, it has been suggested that gemcitabine induced apoptosis promotes nuclear fragmentation [21] and such fragments may lead to the exposure of nuclear contents [23] and an increased availability of nuclear-bound tumor antigen for cross-presentation. Taken together, these data suggest that the relatively reduced cross-presentation of nuclear localized antigen can be improved by a gemcitabine-mediated, tumor apoptosis-induced, nuclear degradation and this increases the availability of these nuclear antigen for cross-presentation. Future studies will assess the key questions of antigen localization following gemcitabine treatment and also determine how effective other chemotherapy drugs are in 'exposing' nuclear tumor antigens to T cells.

Harnessing nuclear antigens to improve cancer immunotherapies

Combination chemo-immunotherapy has recently been shown to be a powerful anti-cancer strategy, provided the right combination of chemotherapy drugs and immunotherapeutic agents are used [5,36]. Therefore, the data from studies like ours have the potential to inform the planning and development of future clinical protocols. For example, since TAAs like survivin and MAGE-A10 are nuclear localized in a variety of cancer types [12,13], chemotherapy that augments the cross presentation of these antigens might boost the efficacy of survivin or MAGE-A10 vaccines. Furthermore, given the crucial role that cross-presentation also plays in thymic development of tolerance to TAAs [37], the reduced cross-presentation of nuclear localized antigen relative to cytoplasmic and secretory antigen, may result in a peripheral T cell repertoire of nuclear-TAA reactive T cells that is less tolerant than those T cells reactive to antigen from other compartments. Thus nuclear TAAs might conceivably be better targets for cancer immunotherapy. In this regard, it may be feasible to use the increased availability of nuclear antigen after chemotherapy (Fig. 4A) to 'turn tumors into their own vaccines' (reviewed in [38]). This, in turn, has the potential to enhance newly emerging immunotherapies such as anti-CTLA-4/anti-PD-1/L1 immune checkpoint blockade [39,40].

In summary, nuclear tumor antigen are relatively less well cross-presented to anti-tumor T cells than those from the cytoplasmic and secretory compartments, but this situation can be reversed by an apoptosis-inducing chemotherapy.

Acknowledgments

The authors would also like to acknowledge the facilities, and the scientific and technical assistance of staff at the UWA Animal Care Services and the National Imaging Facility at the Centre for Microscopy, Characterisation & Analysis, The University of Western Australia, a facility funded by the University, State and Commonwealth Governments.

Author Contributions

Conceived and designed the experiments: CA RAL SAF BWR KH. Performed the experiments: CA SAF KH. Analyzed the data: CA RAL KH SAF BWR. Contributed reagents/materials/analysis tools: CA RAl KH SAF BWR. Wrote the paper: CA RAL SAF BWR KH.

References

1. Steer HJ, Lake RA, Nowak AK, Robinson BW (2010) Harnessing the immune response to treat cancer. Oncogene.
2. Segura E, Villadangos JA (2011) A modular and combinatorial view of the antigen cross-presentation pathway in dendritic cells. Traffic 12: 1677–1685.
3. Kurts C, Robinson BW, Knolle PA (2010) Cross-priming in health and disease. Nat Rev Immunol 10: 403–414.
4. Nierkens S, Tel J, Janssen E, Adema GJ (2013) Antigen cross-presentation by dendritic cell subsets: one general or all sergeants? Trends Immunol 34: 361–370.
5. Lake RA, Robinson BW (2005) Immunotherapy and chemotherapy–a practical partnership. Nat Rev Cancer 5: 397–405.
6. Lennerz V, Fatho M, Gentilini C, Frye RA, Lifke A, et al. (2005) The response of autologous T cells to a human melanoma is dominated by mutated neoantigens. Proc Natl Acad Sci U S A 102: 16013–16018.
7. Brusa D, Garetto S, Chiorino G, Scatolini M, Migliore E, et al. (2008) Post-apoptotic tumors are more palatable to dendritic cells and enhance their antigen cross-presentation activity. Vaccine 26: 6422–6432.
8. Matheoud D, Perie L, Hoeffel G, Vimeux L, Parent I, et al. (2010) Cross-presentation by dendritic cells from live cells induces protective immune responses in vivo. Blood 115: 4412–4420.
9. Wolkers MC, Brouwenstijn N, Bakker AH, Toebes M, Schumacher TN (2004) Antigen bias in T cell cross-priming. Science 304: 1314–1317.
10. Shen L, Rock KL (2004) Cellular protein is the source of cross-priming antigen in vivo. Proc Natl Acad Sci U S A 101: 3035–3040.
11. Zeelenberg IS, van Maren WW, Boissonnas A, Van Hout-Kuijer MA, Den Brok MH, et al. (2011) Antigen localization controls T cell-mediated tumor immunity. J Immunol 187: 1281–1288.
12. Schultz-Thater E, Piscuoglio S, Iezzi G, Le Magnen C, Zajac P, et al. (2011) MAGE-A10 is a nuclear protein frequently expressed in high percentages of

tumor cells in lung, skin and urothelial malignancies. Int J Cancer 129: 1137–1148.

13. Andersen MH, Svane IM, Becker JC, Straten PT (2007) The universal character of the tumor-associated antigen survivin. Clin Cancer Res 13: 5991–5994.
14. Takahara A, Koido S, Ito M, Nagasaki E, Sagawa Y, et al. (2011) Gemcitabine enhances Wilms' tumor gene WT1 expression and sensitizes human pancreatic cancer cells with WT1-specific T-cell-mediated antitumor immune response. Cancer Immunol Immunother 60: 1289–1297.
15. Ingebrigtsen VA, Boye K, Tekle C, Nesland JM, Flatmark K, et al. (2012) B7-H3 expression in colorectal cancer: nuclear localization strongly predicts poor outcome in colon cancer. Int J Cancer 131: 2528–2536.
16. Lo HW, Xia W, Wei Y, Ali-Seyed M, Huang SF, et al. (2005) Novel prognostic value of nuclear epidermal growth factor receptor in breast cancer. Cancer Res 65: 338–348.
17. Tinguely M, Jenni B, Knights A, Lopes B, Korol D, et al. (2008) MAGE-C1/CT-7 expression in plasma cell myeloma: sub-cellular localization impacts on clinical outcome. Cancer Sci 99: 720–725.
18. Xia W, Wei Y, Du Y, Liu J, Chang B, et al. (2009) Nuclear expression of epidermal growth factor receptor is a novel prognostic value in patients with ovarian cancer. Mol Carcinog 48: 610–617.
19. Ralhan R, Cao J, Lim T, Macmillan C, Freeman JL, et al. (2010) EpCAM nuclear localization identifies aggressive thyroid cancer and is a marker for poor prognosis. BMC Cancer 10: 331.
20. Kitamura H, Torigoe T, Hirohashi Y, Asanuma H, Inoue R, et al. (2013) Nuclear, but not cytoplasmic, localization of survivin as a negative prognostic factor for survival in upper urinary tract urothelial carcinoma. Virchows Arch 462: 101–107.
21. Okada H, Mak TW (2004) Pathways of apoptotic and non-apoptotic death in tumour cells. Nat Rev Cancer 4: 592–603.
22. Kramer A, Liashkovich I, Oberleithner H, Ludwig S, Mazur I, et al. (2008) Apoptosis leads to a degradation of vital components of active nuclear transport and a dissociation of the nuclear lamina. Proc Natl Acad Sci U S A 105: 11236–11241.
23. Andrade R, Crisol L, Prado R, Boyano MD, Arluzea J, et al. (2010) Plasma membrane and nuclear envelope integrity during the blebbing stage of apoptosis: a time-lapse study. Biol Cell 102: 25–35.
24. Nowak AK, Lake RA, Marzo AL, Scott B, Heath WR, et al. (2003) Induction of tumor cell apoptosis in vivo increases tumor antigen cross-presentation, cross-priming rather than cross-tolerizing host tumor-specific CD8 T cells. J Immunol 170: 4905–4913.
25. Marzo AL, Lake RA, Robinson BW, Scott B (1999) T-cell receptor transgenic analysis of tumor-specific CD8 and CD4 responses in the eradication of solid tumors. Cancer Res 59: 1071–1079.
26. George TC, Fanning SL, Fitzgerald-Bocarsly P, Medeiros RB, Highfill S, et al. (2006) Quantitative measurement of nuclear translocation events using similarity analysis of multispectral cellular images obtained in flow. J Immunol Methods 311: 117–129.
27. Lyons AB, Parish CR (1994) Determination of lymphocyte division by flow cytometry. J Immunol Methods 171: 131–137.
28. Van den Broeck W, Derore A, Simoens P (2006) Anatomy and nomenclature of murine lymph nodes: Descriptive study and nomenclatory standardization in BALB/cAnNCrl mice. J Immunol Methods 312: 12–19.
29. Quah BJ, Parish CR (2010) The use of carboxyfluorescein diacetate succinimidyl ester (CFSE) to monitor lymphocyte proliferation. J Vis Exp.
30. Robinson BW, Lake RA, Nelson DJ, Scott BA, Marzo AL (1999) Cross-presentation of tumour antigens: evaluation of threshold, duration, distribution and regulation. Immunol Cell Biol 77: 552–558.
31. Marzo AL, Lake RA, Lo D, Sherman L, McWilliam A, et al. (1999) Tumor antigens are constitutively presented in the draining lymph nodes. J Immunol 162: 5838–5845.
32. Alberts B, Johnson A, Lewis J, Raff M, Roberts K, et al. (2002) Molecular Biology of the Cell. New York: Garland Science.
33. Presley JF (2005) Imaging the secretory pathway: the past and future impact of live cell optical techniques. Biochim Biophys Acta 1744: 259–272.
34. DuPage M, Mazumdar C, Schmidt LM, Cheung AF, Jacks T (2012) Expression of tumour-specific antigens underlies cancer immunoediting. Nature 482: 405–409.
35. Paroli M, Bellati F, Videtta M, Focaccetti C, Mancone C, et al. (2013) Discovery of chemotherapy-associated ovarian cancer antigens by interrogating memory T cells. Int J Cancer.
36. Lesterhuis WJ, Salmons J, Nowak AK, Rozali EN, Khong A, et al. (2013) Synergistic effect of CTLA-4 blockade and cancer chemotherapy in the induction of anti-tumor immunity. PLoS One 8: e61895.
37. Adamopoulou E, Tenzer S, Hillen N, Klug P, Rota IA, et al. (2013) Exploring the MHC-peptide matrix of central tolerance in the human thymus. Nat Commun 4: 2039.
38. van der Most RG, Currie A, Robinson BW, Lake RA (2006) Cranking the immunologic engine with chemotherapy: using context to drive tumor antigen cross-presentation towards useful antitumor immunity. Cancer Res 66: 601–604.
39. Lesterhuis WJ, Haanen JB, Punt CJ (2011) Cancer immunotherapy–revisited. Nat Rev Drug Discov 10: 591–600.
40. Rozali EN, Hato SV, Robinson BW, Lake RA, Lesterhuis WJ (2012) Programmed death ligand 2 in cancer-induced immune suppression. Clin Dev Immunol 2012: 656340.

20

miR-375 Mediated Acquired Chemo-Resistance in Cervical Cancer by Facilitating EMT

Yuanming Shen, Jiansong Zhou, Yang Li, Feng Ye, Xiaoyun Wan, Weiguo Lu, Xing Xie, Xiaodong Cheng*

Department of Gynecologic Oncology, Women's Hospital, School of Medicine, Zhejiang University, Hangzhou, China

Abstract

Acquired chemo-resistance is one of the key causal factors in cancer death. Emerging evidences suggest that miRNA and epithelial–mesenchymal transition play critical roles in the chemo-resistance in cancers. Here, we showed the association of paclitaxel-resistance with miR-375 over-expression and epithelial–mesenchymal transition inducement in cervical cancer. Using different cervical cancer cell models, we found that paclitaxel transiently induced up-regulation of miR-375 expression, proliferation inhibition, transition from epithelial to mesenchymal phenotype, and consequently impaired paclitaxel sensitivity. Forced over-expression of miR-375 may suppress Ecadherin expression by a directly targeting pathway, which led to paclitaxel resistance. Contrarily, re-expression of Ecadherin partly reversed epithelial–mesenchymal transition phenotype and miR-375 induced paclitaxel-resistance. Our findings suggest that paclitaxel-induced miR-375 over-expression facilitates epithelial–mesenchymal transition process via directly targeting Ecadherin, proliferation inhibition, and consequently results in chemo-resistance in cervical cancer cells. A reversion of miR-375 or Ecadherin expression may be a novel therapeutic approach for overcoming chemo-resistance in cervical cancer.

Editor: Zhi-Ming Zheng, National Institute of Health - National Cancer Institute, United States of America

Funding: The authors would like to acknowledge the continuous financial support from the National Natural Science Foundation of China (grant No. 81172475 and 81172474), the Natural Science Foundation of Zhejiang Province of China (grant No. Z2110056, LQ13H160005 and Y2110206). The funders had no role in study design, data collection and analysis, decision to publish, or preparation of the manuscript.

Competing Interests: The authors have declared that no competing interests exist.

* Email: chengxd@zju.edu.cn

Introduction

Emerging evidences have revealed that chemo-resistance is associated with epithelial mesenchymal transition (EMT) in cancer cells, and the acquisition of chemo-resistance in cancer cells is accompanied by a transition from an epithelial to a mesenchymal phenotype [1–3]. For instance, various drug-resistant cancers, including oxaliplatin-resistant colorectal cancer cells [4], paclitaxel-resistant ovarian cancer cells [5], and gefitinib-resistant lung cancer cells [6], present the transition from epithelial to mesenchymal phenotype along with a loss of epithelial adhesion molecule Ecadherin and a gain of mesenchymal markers such as vimentin, Ncadherin, and fibronectin. More recent studies also have shown that chemotherapy agents can facilitate the epithelial to a mesenchymal phenotypic transformation in residual surviving cancer cells which may be one of the critical steps in acquired drug resistance in cancers [7,8]. Thus, acquirement of EMT becomes a key process contributing to the malignant phenotypes of cancer cells in resistance to chemotherapy. Therefore, the intervention of EMT process has been proposed as a therapeutic approach against acquired chemo-resistance.

MicroRNAs (miRNAs) act as important gene regulators in human genomes and their aberrant expression may promote not only tumori-genesis and tumor aggressiveness but also resistance to chemotherapy [9]. More recently, the studies have revealed that miRNAs play an integral role in modulating EMT, such as miR-200s that regulates EMT through inhibiting ZEB1/2, a transcription repressor of Ecadherin [1,10,11]. We recently reported that the expression of miR-375 was reduced in cervical cancer cells [12] and enforced over-expression of miR-375 significantly inhibited proliferation and blocked G1-S cell cycle transition [13]. In another study, we further observed that miR-375 was up-regulated in paclitaxel-treated cervical cells and tissues, and forced over-expression of miR-375 decreased paclitaxel sensitivity in cervical cancer [14]. However, the precise molecular mechanism underling miR-375 regulated drug resistance remains to be explored. By the miRNA targets gene prediction, we found a binding site between miR-375 and Ecadherin 3′-UTR, which indicated that Ecadherin was a potential direct target of miR-375. Therefore, we assume that miR-375 may participate in EMT regulation and acquired paclitaxel-resistance in cervical cancer cells.

In the present study, we found for the first time that paclitaxel inhibits proliferation, induces EMT, and up-regulates miR-375 expression simultaneously in cervical cancer cells. And miR-375 over-expression directly inhibited Ecadherin expression and facilitated paclitaxel-resistance. Thus, there is a distinct positive feedback mechanism among paclitaxel, miR-375, and EMT that leads to acquired chemo-resistance phenotypes in cervical cancer cells. Such a regulatory feedback loop results in miR-375 over-expression, the epithelial to a mesenchymal phenotypic transformation, and consequently acquirement of paclitaxel-resistance. Anyway, it could be believed that a break of such a feedback loop would, at least partly, overcome chemo -resistance in cervical cancer.

Materials and Methods

Patients and samples

The samples of cancer tissue were collected from 23 cervical squamous cell carcinoma patients with FIGO (2009) stage IB_2 or IIA_2 who underwent neo-adjuvant chemotherapy followed by type III radical hysterectomy between November 1, 2008 and May 30, 2010 in Women's Hospital, School of Medicine, Zhejiang University. The collection of all samples was approved by the Ethical Committee for Clinical Research from the Women's Hospital, School of Medicine, Zhejiang University and written informed consents were obtained.

All patients underwent 2 cycles of intravenous neo-adjuvant chemotherapy (paclitaxel 135 mg/m^2 and cisplatin 75 mg/m^2, 3-week interval) before surgery. The effect of chemotherapy was evaluated according to the Response Evaluation Criteria in Solid Tumors (RECIST) [15] as previously described[14]. Of all 23 patients, mean age was 36.5 years (range 20 to 65 years), had pre- and post-chemotherapy cervical tumor samples. The specified composition of each samples were determined by an experienced pathologist.

Cell culture and EMT inducement

Two human cervical cancer cell lines, SiHa and CaSki were cultured as previously described[14]. Human recombinant TGF-β1 and EGF-β were obtained from ProSpec-Tany Techno Gene Ltd (Israel), respectively used at a final concentration of 5 ng/ml and 2 ng/ml. The cancer cell lines were seeded 1×10^5/well in 6-well plates and incubated in serum-free medium overnight, and then treated with TGF-β1 or EGF-β for 72 h respectively, to induce the EMT.

RNA Extraction and Real-Time RT-PCR

Total RNAs containing miRNAs were extracted from liquid nitrogen preserved tissues or the harvested cells using 1 ml TRIZOL reagent (Invitrogen, Carlsbad, CA, USA) following the manufacturer's instructions. cDNA was synthesized with the PrimeScript RT reagent Kit (TaKaRa Otsu, Shiga, Japan). Quantitative RT-PCR (qRT-PCR) for miRNA and mRNA was performed as described previously[14]. The sequences of all primers are given in Table 1.

Cell Proliferation Assay and MTS Assay

To determine the effect of miR-375 and paclitaxel on proliferation of cervical cell lines, the cell proliferation was determined with MTT assay and CellTrace CFSE cell proliferation assay at 24, 48, 72, 96 hours and 5 days respectively. For viability experiments, cervical cancer cells with or without 10 nM paclitaxel treatment 72 hours were plated (SiHa, 3×10^3/well in 96-well plate and 2×10^5/well in 6-well plate; CaSki, 2×10^3/well in 96-well plate and 1×10^5/well in 6-well plate) and cultured overnight. In MTT assay the absorbance of samples was measured with a spectrophotometer reader at 490 nm. CellTrace CFSE cell proliferation assay was performed by staining activated cervical cancer with CellTrace CFSE cell proliferation dye (2.5 μM) (Invitrogen) and analyze using by flow cytometry with 488 nm excitation and emission filters. An in vitro paclitaxel chemosensitivity of cervical cancer cells was evaluated using MTS assay (Promega, Madison, WI) as previously described [12]. Four replicate wells were used for each analysis, and at least three independent experiments were performed.

Western Blot Analysis

A total of 50 mg protein was separated by denaturing 8–15% SDS–polyacrylamide gel electrophoresis. Western analysis was conducted as previously described [12]. The films were analyzed by densitometry with a VersaDoc Imaging System; Model 3000 (BioRad) using Quantity One software. Analysis of variance with Bonferroni correction for multiple tests was used to determine significance. The primary antibodies used were anti-Ncadherin (1:5000), anti-Ecadherin (1:2000), anti-fibronectin (1:1000), anti-vimentin (1:1000) and anti-actin (1:2000) as an endogenous control, all from Epitomics Biotechnology (Epitomics).

Immunohistochemistry

Sections (6 μm thick) of tumor tissue were cut from paraffinised 23 couples of self-paired pre-and post-chemotherapy cervical cancer samples, and immunohistochemistry analysis and scoring were described previously[12]. The primary antibodies used for immunohistochemistry analysis were anti-Ecadherin antibody (1:1000) and anti-actin antibody as an endogenous control (1:2000), both from Epitomics Biotechnology (Epitomics).

Lentivirus construction and transfection

To generate miR-375 and Ecadherin over-expression stable transfectants, cervical cancer cells were transfected with lentiviral expressing vectors. The plasmid construction and lentivirus package were complete in GENECHEM Company. The pre-miR-375 sequences were amplified and cloned into the pGCsil-GFP vector using the following primers: (Forward) hsa-pre-miR-375-XhoI-F, ACCGCTC GAGCCCCGCGAC-GAGCCCCTCGC; (Reverse) hsa-pre-mi-R-375-MfeI-R, AC-CGCAATTGAAAAAGCCTCACGCGAGCCGAACG. The hsa-CDH1 (CDS) gene was amplified and cloned into a pGC-FU-GFP vector using the following primers: (Forward) 5′-GAGGATCCCCGGGTACCGGTCGCCAC-

Table 1. Sequences of primers for miRNAs, RNU6, and EEF1A1.

miR-375 RT	5′-GTCGTATCCAGTGCAGGGTCCGAGGTATTCGCACTGGATACGACTCACGC-3′
miR-375 forward	5′-AGCCGTTTGTTCGTTCGGCT-3′
miR-375 reverse	5′-GTGCAGGGTCCGAGGT-3′
U6 snRNA RT	5′-AACGCTTCACGAATTTGCGT-3′
U6 snRNA forward	5′-CTCGCTTCGGCAGCACA-3′
U6 snRNA reverse	5′-AACGCTTCACGAATTTGCGT-3′
EEF1A1 forward	5′-TGCGGTGGGTGTCATCAAA-3′
EEF1A1 reverse	5′-AAGAGTGGGGTGGCAGGTATTG-3′

CATGGGCCCTTGGAGCCGCAG-3′, (Reverse) 5′-TCATCCTTGTAGTCGC-TAGCGTCGTCCTCGCCGCCTCCGTACATG-3′. Viruses packaging were performed in HEK 293 T cells after the cotransfection of 20 mg pGCsil-GFP-pre-miR-375 vector or pGC-GFP-CDH1 vector with 15 mg of the packaging plasmid pHelper 1.0 Vector and 10 mg of the envelope plasmid pHelper 2.0 vector using Lipofectamine 2000. Viruses were harvested 48 h after transfection, and viral titers were determined. The titers of the viral used in this study were in the range of 5×10^{8}~2×10^{9} TU/mL.

To generate miR-375 and Ecadherin over-expression stable transfectants, cervical cancer cells were transfected with lentiviral expressing vectors as previously described [12]. An MOI = 5 was used for SiHa and MOI = 10 was used for CaSki. After 4~7 d of transfection, stable clones were selected with GFP by flow cytometry and harvested for further experimentation. An empty pGC FU-GFP-NC-LV vector was used as a negative control.

Luciferase Activity Assay

To investigate whether CDH1 expression was regulated by miR-375, a psicheck-2 dual-luciferase miRNA target expression vector (psicheck-2 -UTR vector) was used to perform the luciferase activity assay. The wild and mutant type 3′-UTR of CDH1 containing predicted miR-375 binding site was synthesized and inserted into the 3′-UTR region downstream of the firefly luciferase gene of psicheck-2 vector (psicheck-2 -UTR) using the Xho I and NotI I restriction sites. All constructs were verified by sequencing. After cotransfected with miR-375 mimics (20 uM) and reporter vectors (0.2 μg/mL), luciferase activities were measured at 24 hours using a Dual-Glo luciferase assay system (Promega). Relative luciferase activity in all figures refers to firefly luciferase activities normalized to Renilla luciferase. Values cells with empty psicheck-2 vector were set equally to 1.

Statistical Analysis

The experiments were repeated at least three times. Results are expressed as mean ± s.e.m. An independent Student's t-test or an ANOVA was used to compare continuous variables. Pearson's correlation coefficient test was used to assess the correlation between two continuous variables. $P<0.05$ was considered statistically significant.

Results

Paclitaxel induced EMT and inhibited proliferation simultaneously in cervical cancer cells

When the morphology of routinely cultured cervical cancer cells treated with or without paclitaxel were examined by microscopy, we observed that SiHa cell grew as tightly-packed "cobblestone"-like epithelial cells, whereas cells treated with paclitaxel seemed a spindle-like shape flattened and lost the majority of their cell-cell contacts. (Figure 1a) Meanwhile, the expression of Ecadherin protein was decreased (10.5%~66.6% and 43.75%~67.6% under 5 nM to 20 nM paclitaxel treatment respectively) and the expressions of Ncadherin and fibronectin protein were increased in a dose-responsive manner. (Figure 1b) Similar effects were also observed in CaSki cells. (Figure 1b, Figure S1).

Further, a transient cell proliferation inhibition induced by paclitaxel was observed by flow cytometry and MTT. SiHa and CaSki cells were routinely cultured with 10 nM paclitaxel, after 72 hours, the paclitaxel were removed and the cells were cultured with complete medium continuously, subsequently the proliferation changes in SiHa and CaSki cells before and after paclitaxel administration revealed at 24 h, 72 h, 96 h, day 5, day 7, day 14, and day 21, respectively. As showed in Figure 1c, 1d, the proliferation rate of paclitaxel treated SiHa and CaSki cells at day 7 was significantly reduced (SiHa, $p=0.002$ and $p=2.3\times10^{-5}$; CaSki, $p=3.1\times10^{-4}$ and $p=1.2\times10^{-5}$ respectively), compared with that of blank control, and restored to the levels before drug treatment at day 21. At the same time, the "cobblestone"-like morphological changes induced by paclitaxel in survived cells were also restored to normal morphology at day 21. These facts indicate that paclitaxel transiently inhibits proliferation and induces EMT simultaneously in cervical cancer cells, but all these paclitaxel-induced changes reversed after drug withdrawal.

Paclitaxel up-regulates miR-375 during inducing EMT and proliferation inhibition

We had explored miR-375 expression changing involved in paclitaxel induced EMT and proliferation inhibition in cervical cancer cells, and the clear dose dependent effect of paclitaxel on miR-375 over-expression was observed[14]. Moreover, the progressive up-regulated expression of miR-375 reached a peak at day 7 after paclitaxel administration, gradually declined after paclitaxel removed and restored to the level before drug treatment at about day 21[14]. In addition, there was a strong negative correlation between the expression of miR-375 and the relative proliferation proportion of cervical cancer cells (SiHa, $r=-0.472$, $P=1.52\times10^{-3}$; CaSki, $r=-0.835$, $P=3.03\times10^{-4}$). (Figure S2) Our data revealed that paclitaxel up-regulated miR-375 expression and inhibited proliferation simultaneously in cervical cancer cells but both paclitexel-induced changes reversed after drug withdrawal, suggesting that some of cervical cancer cells survive in paclitaxel, probably though up-regulating miR-375 expression and acquiring malignant mesenchymal phenotypes, then developing a potential to decrease proliferation and resist drug toxicity. These correlation suggest that miR-375 over-expression might have a causal role in chemotherapy induced EMT.

MiR-375 mediates EMT by directly targeting Ecadherin

By miRDB and TargetScan search programs analysis, we found a predicted binding of miR-375 with CDH1 (Ecadherin) 3′-UTR, which indicated that Ecadherin was a potential direct target of miR-375 (Figure 2c). To further ascertain that Ecadherin is a target gene of miR-375, we firstly analyze the relationship between Ecadherin and miR-375 expression in cervical cancer cells under different amounts of paclitaxel treatment. As showed in Figure 1b and Figure S2, miR-375 expression in cells was markedly unregulated in a dose dependent manner during paclitaxel-induced EMT process, as well as Ecadherin protein and miR-375 expression were reversely correlated ($r=-0.752$, $P=2.32\times10^{-4}$). Then we further used the Luciferase Activity Assay to confirm the binding of miR-375 to the 3′-UTR of Ecadherin. (Figure 2c).

To test whether the up-regulation of miR-375 contributed to paclitaxel -induced EMT, the effects of miR-375 over-expression on these events were evaluated. The expression of miR-375 was analyzed by Real-time PCR at the second week, third week and first month after pre-miRNA lentiviral stable transfection. As shown in Figure 2a and 2b, the forced over-expression of miR-375 induced EMT process in cervical cancer cells, characterized by acquisition of fibroblast-like cell morphology, suppression of Ecadherin expression (65%~69.2%), and enhancement of vimentin, Ncadherin, and fibronectin expression, similar to the effects observed in the paclitaxel treated cells.

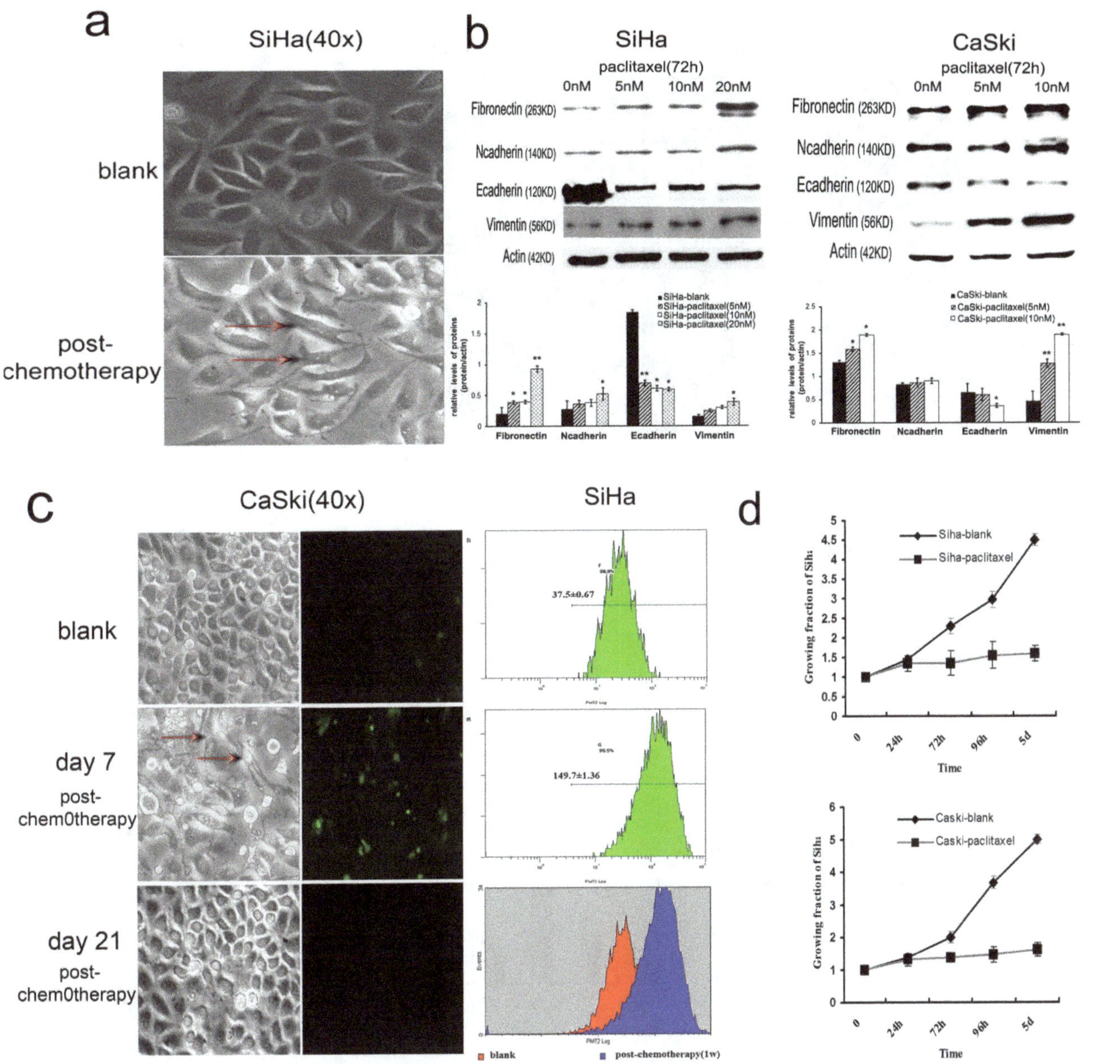

Figure 1. Paclitaxel inhibits proliferation, induces EMT, and up-regulates miR-375 expression simultaneously in cervical cancer cells. (**a**) Visible morphological changes from "cobblestone"-like to "fibroblast"-like cells was observed in SiHa after 72 h paclitaxel treatment. The representative cells with morphological changes were labeled (**b**) Immunoblotting measured the expression of Ecadherin and other EMT related proteins (vimentin, Ncadherin, and fibronectin) in cervical cancer cells (SiHa and CaSki) under different amounts (0, 5, 10, 20 nM) of paclitaxel treatment. The expression of Ecadherin protein was decreased and the expressions of vimentin, Ncadherin, and fibronectin protein were increased in cells treated with paclitaxel for 72 hours in a dose-responsive manner. All the expressions of the proteins were normalized to ß-actin and the data in bar graphs are presented as mean of triple samples from three independent experiments. All error bars indicated s.e.m. (**p≤0.01, *p≤0.05). (**c, d**) The transient cell proliferation inhibition and morphological changes induced by paclitaxel were observed. The proliferation changes in SiHa and CaSki cells after paclitaxel administration were analyzed by CellTrace CFSE cell proliferation (**c**) and MTT assay (**d**) at 24 h, 72 h, 96 h, day 5, day 7, day 14, and day 21, respectively. The proliferation rate of paclitaxel treated SiHa and CaSki cells was significantly reduced at day 7 and restored at day 21 after paclitaxel administration. The survived CaSki cells were restored into normal morphology at day 21 after paclitaxel administration.

Thus, our findings indicate that miR-375 over-expression promotes paclitaxel-induced EMT partly by directly targeting Ecadherin in cervical cancer cells.

EMT regulates the paclitaxel sensitivity but not miR-375 expression

To determine whether EMT may regulate miR-375 expression inversely, the next set of experiments was carried out. We induced EMT by TGF-β1 or EGF-β in cervical cancer cells (SiHa and CaSki) and observed the influence of EMT on paclitaxel sensitivity and miR-375 expression. Stimulated by TGF-β1 or EGF-β, cervical cancer cells underwent EMT accompanying visible morphological changes (Figure 3a), such as appearance of a spindle-like shape in cells, and EMT marker alteration, including decreased Ecadherin protein expression (28.5%~65.8% for TGF-β1 and 47.5%~67.6% for EGF-β), as well as increased

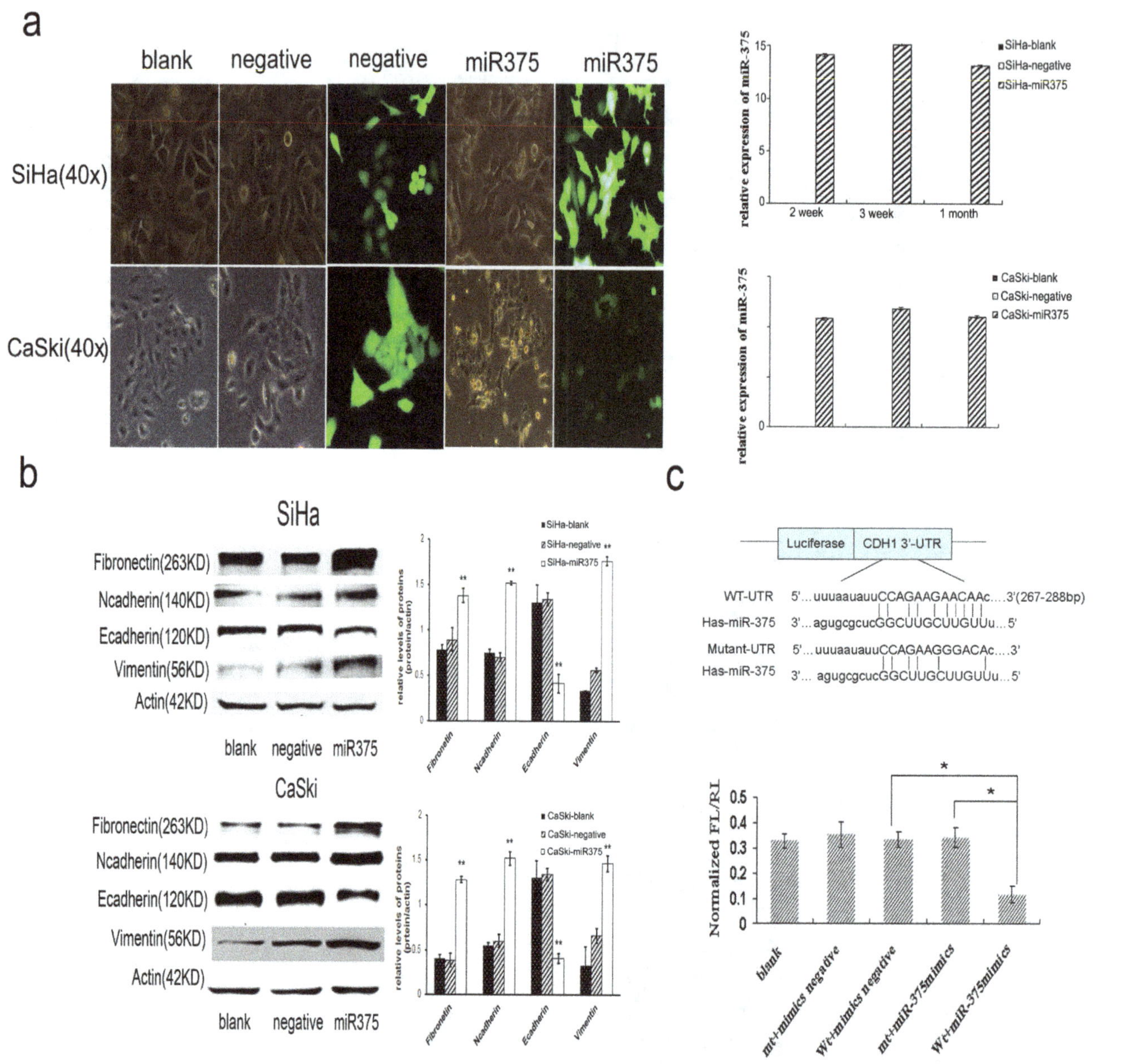

Figure 2. Conditionally over-expressed miR-375 induces EMT via targeting Ecadherin in cervical cancer cells. (a) Phase contrast images of cervical cancer cells infected with the pre-miR-375 or negative lentivirus vector and blank control. (b) Immunoblotting measurement of Ecadherin and EMT related proteins in cervical cancer tercells infected with the pre-miR-375 or negative lentivirus vector. (c) A predicted duplex formation between human CDH1 (Ecadherin) 3′-UTR and miR-375. A reduced luciferase activity was observed after cotransfection of Ecadherin 3′-UTR wild type vector with miR-375, but not mutated or empty vector ($p = 0.014$). Data in a–c were presented as the mean of triplets samples from independent experiments. All error bars indicated s.e.m. (**$p \leq 0.01$, *$p \leq 0.05$).

Ncadherin, vimentin, and fibronectin protein expression (Figure 3c). However, the expression of miR-375 was not changed during TGF-β1 or EGF-β induced EMT process in cervical cancer cells (SiHa, $p = 0.538$; CaSki $p = 0.542$) (Figure 3d).

Further, we delineated the drug sensitivity of cells undergoing EMT using MTS assay. The paclitaxel sensitivity was significantly decreased in SiHa and CaSki cells after TGF-β1 or EGF-β stimulation compared with serum-free culture controls (Figure 3b). The IC50 values were increased in SiHa and CaSki with 5 ng/ml TGF-β1 (95.81±2.53 nM and 66.66±2.32 nM respectively, SiHa, $p = 0.032$; CaSki, $p = 0.023$) or 2 ng/ml EGF-β stimulation (96.74±2.47 nM and 94.78±1.72 nM respectively, SiHa, $p = 0.038$; CaSki $p = 0.028$) compared with serum-free culture controls (24.54±1.37 nM, and 23.98±2.62 nM respectively).

Our findings indicate that TGF-β1 or EGF-β induces EMT but dose not alter miR-375 expression in cervical cancer cells, and mesenchymal cell-like cervical cancer cells induced by TGF-β1 or EGF-β are typically paclitaxel resistant. The significantly upregulated expression of miR-375 in paclitaxel treated cervical caner cells is induced by paclitaxel but not EMT.

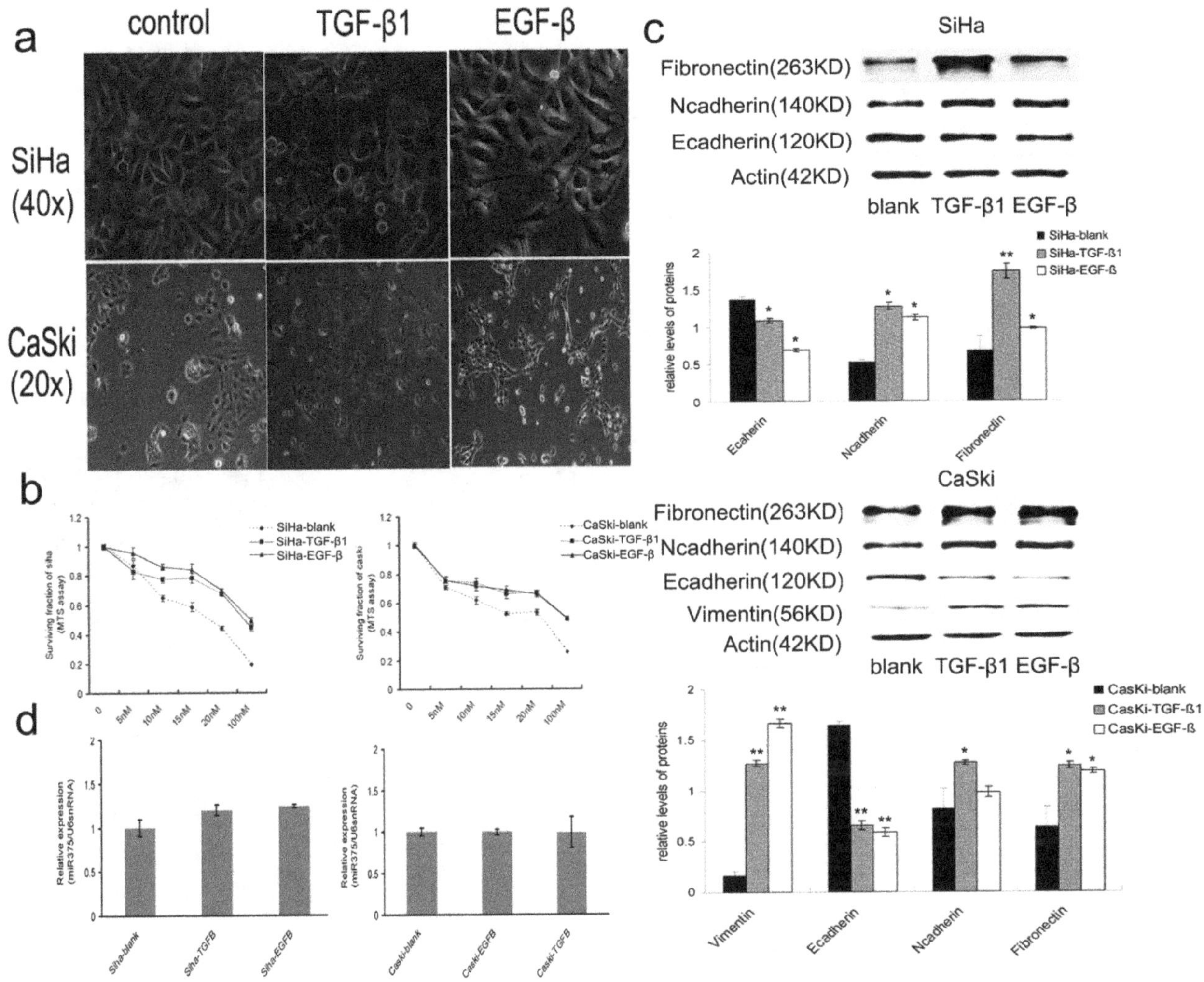

Figure 3. TGF-β1 or EGF-β induces EMT and paclitaxel resistance in cervical cells. (a) Visible morphological changes in SiHa and CaSki under TGF-β1 or EGF-β inducement. (b) MTS analysis of paclitaxel-sensitivity in cervical cancer cells. (c) Immunoblotting analysis of Ecadherin and other EMT related proteins after TGF-β1 or EGF-β induction. (d) miR-375 expression in SiHa and CaSki under TGF-β1 or EGF-β inducement. Data in b–d were presented as mean of triplets samples from independent experiments. All error bars indicated s.e.m. (**p≤0.01, *p≤0.05).

Ecadherin over-expression attenuates the ability miR-375 to mediate EMT and paclitaxel-resistance

Ecadherin is not only an important molecule in the initiation of EMT but also a hallmark for EMT and miR-375 mediates EMT by directly targeting Ecadherin.To investigate the role of Ecadherin in EMT and paclitaxel sensitivity and to test whether the up-regulation ofEcadherin can attenuates the effect of miR-375 on EMT and paclitaxel-resistance in cervical cancer cells; the Ecadherin over-expressed lentviral pGC-flag-CDH1 vector was used. We respectively transfected Ecadherin over-expressed lentviral vector and negative control into SiHa and CaSki cells with and without miR-375 over-expression, and observed that the effect of forced over-expression Ecadherin on EMT and paclitaxel-resistance. In Ecadherin over-expressing clones with and without miR-375 over-expression, there was a pronounced and significant increase in the expression of Ecadherin (Figure 4a). In cells without miR-375 over-expression, no remarkable differences of morphology and mesenchymal markers were observed in SiHa and CaSki cells after Ecadherin over-expression, which is probably because their parental cells already exhibited an epithelial phenotype. Contrarily, in cells with miR-375 over-expression, there was a transition from isolated fibroblastic cells to "cobblestone"-like epithelial cells. Meanwhile, the expressions of Ncadherin, vimentin, and fibronectin were significantly decreased after Ecadherin over-expression (Figure 4a, 4c).

The paclitaxel chemo-sensitivity was then evaluated by MTS assays. As expected, paclitaxel sensitivity was significantly increased in Ecadherin lentvirus-transfected cells with and without miR-375 overexpression compared with control cells. The IC50 values were decreased in SiHa and CaSki with Ecadherin overexpression (12.82±2.54 nM and 7.62±0.93 nM respectively, SiHa, $p = 0.043$; CaSki, $p = 0.038$) compared with negative controls (20.73±1.23 nM and 11.68±0.62 nM respectively, SiHa, $p = 0.028$; CaSki, $p = 0.021$). Moreover, the paclitaxel resistance was significantly attenuated after Ecadherin was effectively over-expressed in cervical cells with over-expressed miR-375 compared with negative control (Figure 4b). The IC50 values were decreased in SiHa and CaSki with Ecadherin and miR-375 cotransfection (22.82±3.54 nM and 13.68±0.64 nM respectively, SiHa, $p = 0.033$; CaSki, $p = 0.038$) compared with SiHa and CaSki with negative control and miR-375 cotransfection (82.83±2.23 nM and 20.31±3.01 nM respectively, SiHa, $p = 0.032$; CaSki,

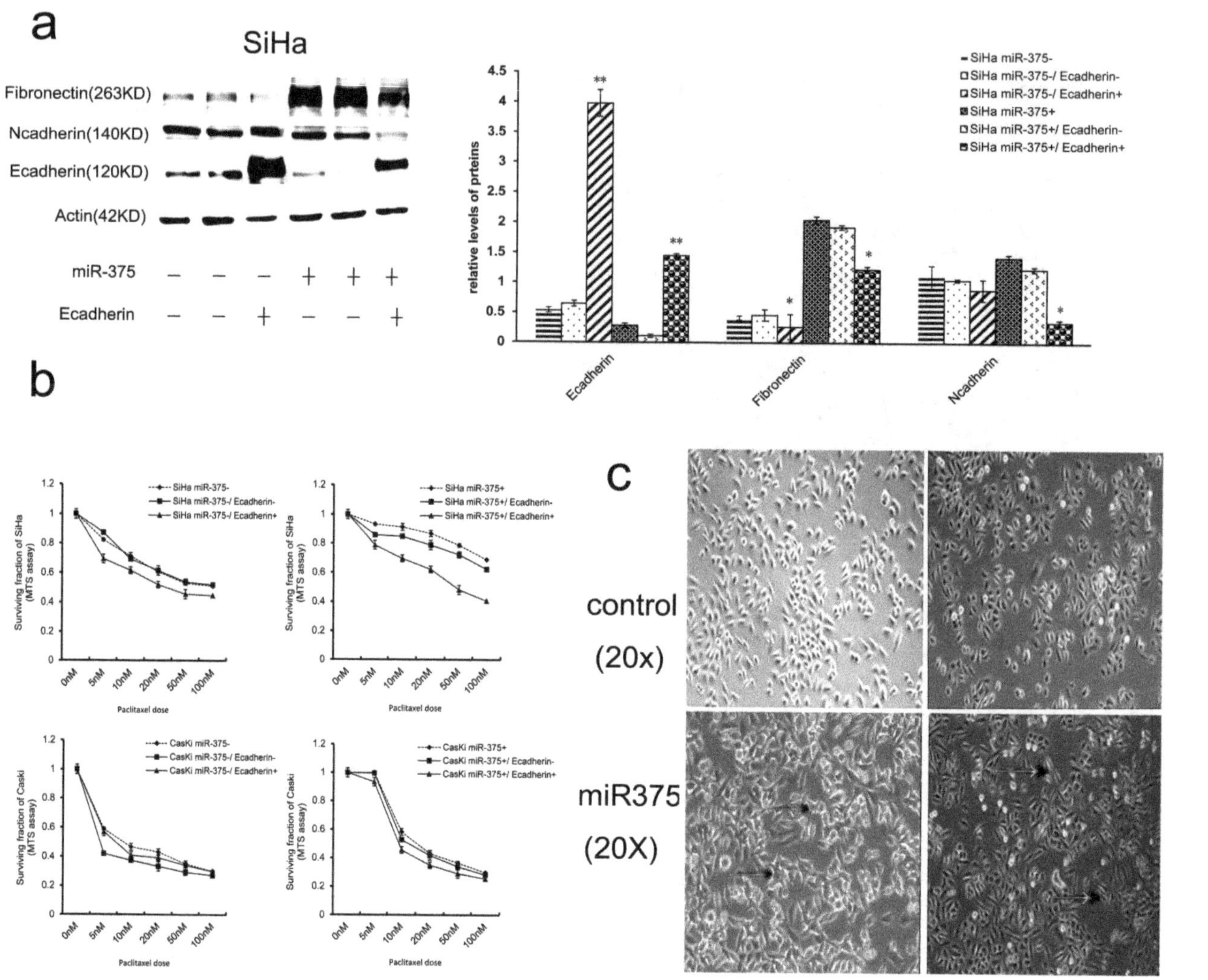

Figure 4. Forced expression of Ecadherin attenuates the ability miR-375 to mediate EMT and paclitaxel-resistance. Immunoblotting (a) and MTS (b) analysis of Ecadherin and other EMT related proteins in SiHa with and without miR-375 overexpression after the Ecadherin-expressing or negative lentivirus vector transfection. Data in (a) and (b) were presented as the mean of triplets samples from independent experiments. All error bars indicated s.e.m. (**p≤0.01, *p≤0:05). (c) Morphological changes in SiHa with and without miR-375 over-expression after the Ecadherin-expressing or negative lentivirus vector transfection. The representative cells with morphological changes had been labeled.

$p = 0.025$). Our results revealed that Ecadherin over-expression significantly enhanced paclitaxel sensitivity in cervical cancer cells with or without miR-375 over-expression, suggesting that Ecadherin over-expression dramatically enhances paclitaxel sensitivity, further, re-expression of Ecadherin reverses, at least partly, the EMT phenotype and paclitaxel-resistance mediated by miR-375 in cervical cancer cells.

miR-375 over-expression correlates with Ecadherin expression in post-chemotherapy human cervical carcinoma tissues

To establish the clinical relevance of miR-375 between Ecadherin expressions under chemotherapy effects, we assessed miR-375 and Ecadherin expression in 23 couples of self paired pre- and post-chemotherapy human cervical cancer tissues. The immunostaining for Ecadherin revealed more extensive and stronger expression in pre-chemotherapy than that in post-chemotherapy tumor tissues (Figure 5). At the same time, miR-375 was markedly upregulated (4.67 fold) in paclitaxel-treated cervical samples, Ecadherin and miR-375 expression were reversely correlated in all tissues including pre- and post-chemotherapy ($r = -0.905$, $P = 1.81 \times 10^{-3}$) (Table S1).

Of all 23 patients, 19 were chemo-sensitive and 4 chemo-resistance, the upregulated expression of miR-375 is more significantly in chemo-resistance patients when compared post-chemotherapy tissues with their self paired pre-chemotherapy tissues (6.7±2.3 fold in chemo-resistance and 4.35±0.63 fold in chemosensitive patients respectively, $p = 0.033$). But it should be noted that there is no enough power to conclude that miR-375 expression is higher in chemo-resistance patients, partially due to the small sample size for the chemo-resistance patients ($N = 4$).

Discussion

Chemo-resistance is one of the key causal factors in cancer relapses and progression. The majority of cancer cells responds well initially to chemotherapy, but eventually develops resistance following drug exposure. Emerging evidences have revealed that cancer cells undergo EMT promotes cell survival and resistance to

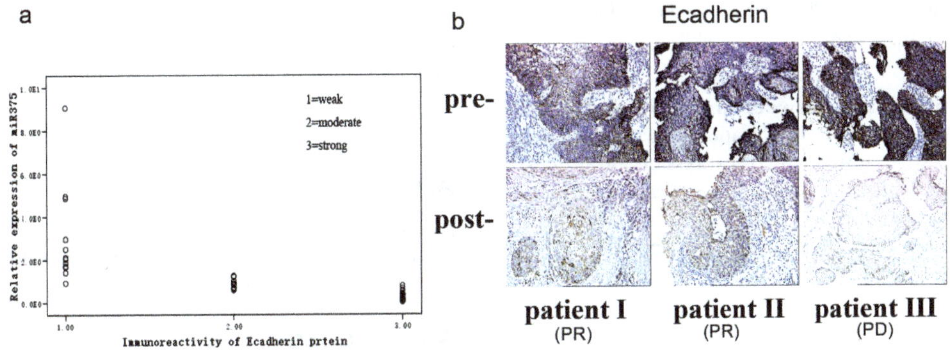

Figure 5. miR-375 over-expression correlates with Ecadherin expression in post-chemotherapy human cervical carcinoma tissues. (a) Ecadherin and miR-375 expression were reversely correlated in all tissues including pre- and post-chemotherapy ($r = -0.905$, $P = 1.81 \times 10^{-3}$). (b) Staining of human-specific Ecadherin expression in three representatives (1 PD and 2 PR) (×200). A decreased Ecadherin expression was shown in the tissues after chemotherapy ($p = 0.0023$).

chemotherapy [3]. Although it has been reported that miRNAs may play an integral role in modulating EMT [16]; however, detailed regulatory procedure remains unexplored. miR-375 was initially found to be expressed in pancreatic islet, where it regulates the secretion of insulin and metabolism of glucose [17]. Recently, miR-375 was identified as an important regulator in tumorgenesis and cancer progression; however, the precise functions of this miRNA remain largely obscure. miR-375 was identified as a tumor suppressor in most of cancers, such as gastric cancer [18,19], liver cancer [20], head and neck squamous cell carcinoma [21] and prostate cancers [22], but plays an oncogenic role in ERα-positive breast cancer [23], in lung adenocarcinoma patients [24], and in HBV positive HCC patients [25]. Thus, these conflicting reports regarding the association between miR-375 level and cancer suggested a more complex and possibly cancer specific relationship. In another study of ours, we observed the association between miR-375 over-expression and paclitaxel - resistance in cervical cancer[16]. Here, we directly link miR-375 to chemotherapy-induced EMT process in cervical cancer. We found for the first time that paclitaxel inhibits proliferation, induces EMT, and up-regulates miR-375 expression in a dose-dependent manner simultaneously in cervical cancer cells, but all these paclitaxel-induced changes reversed after drug withdrawal. Mechanistically, ectopic over-expression of miR-375 resulted in reduced Ecadherin expression and accompanied by acquired mesenchymal characteristics and chemo-resistance in cervical cancer cells. Thus, our findings suggested that paclitaxel does not eliminate all cervical cancer cells and some of residual cells can survive under drug exposure. During this procedure, those residual cervical cancer cells with up-regulated miR-375 expression probably possess a potential to acquire mesenchymal phenotypes, slow down proliferation, and resist to drug toxicity. Thus, miR-375 induced EMT might play a key role in paclitaxel resistance in cervical cancer cells. Both cell proliferation inhibition and mesenchymal phenotype have been regarded as features of dormant tumor cells that are resistant to chemotherapy [26,27]. It is possible that residual surviving cells go into the status of tumor dormancy. More importantly, those dormant-like cells escaping from killing by drug can *de novo* down-regulate miR-375 expression and reconvert proliferation after drug withdrawal. Clinically, it is those revival cells that present the progression or recurrence and consequently contribute to poor prognosis of cancer patients. There are only few reports associating miR-375 with chemo-resistance. However, recently a reduced expression of miR-375 was found in tamoxifen resistant cell lines and re-expression of miR-375 reverses both tamoxifen resistance and accompanying EMT-like properties in breast cancer [28]. This conflicting report indicated that the role of miR-375 in regulating drug-sensitivity is possibly cancer and anticancer agents' specific relationship such as in regulating tumorgenesis and cancer progression.

Previous studies showed that miRNAs regulated EMT process but EMT in turn regulated miRNA expression. For example, miR-200 family members regulate EMT, through targeting and suppressing ZEB, and they are in turn repressed in a timely correlated manner during Snail-induced EMT in MCF7 breast cancer cells [29]. To exclude the possibility that miR-375 was regulated by EMT, we examined miR-375 expression during EMT process induced by transforming growth factor-b (TGF-β) and epidermal growth factor-b (EGF-β) treatment in cervical cancer cells. Both factors are multifunctional cytokines that induce EMT in multiple cell types [30,31]. Our results showed that miR-375 was regulated only during paclitaxel induced EMT but not TGF-β and EGF induced EMT. Thus, our findings recognize that the upregulated expression of miR-375 in paclitaxel treated cervical caner cells is only induced by paclitaxel but not EMT.

Ecadherin is a calcium dependent cell adhesion molecule which plays an important role in the growth and development of cells via controlling tissue architecture and maintaining tissue integrity [32]. Recently some studies have demonstrated that reduction and/or loss of Ecadherin expression is a hallmark of the EMT process, which is required for enhancing drug resistance of cancer cells [33]. Here, we observed that Ecadherin is a direct target of miR-375 in cervical cancer cells; moreover, re-expression of Ecadherin partly reversed the EMT phenotype and paclitaxel - resistance induced by miR-375 in cervical cancer cells. These data suggest that Ecadherin is a major molecule in regulating chemo-sensitivity.

In summary, our findings for the first time, to our knowledge, suggest that paclitaxel up-regulates miR-375 expression and over-expressed miR-375 induces EMT process via directly targeting Ecadherin, proliferation inhibition, and consequently results in chemo-resistance in cervical cancer cells. A reversion of miR-375 or Ecadherin expression may be a novel therapeutic approach for overcoming chemo-resistance in cervical cancer.

Supporting Information

Figure S1 Visible morphological changes in CaSki after chemotherapy. Visible morphological changes from "cobblestone"-like to "fibroblast"-like cells were observed in CaSki after 72 h paclitaxel treatment.

Figure S2 The correlation between miR-375 and proliferation. (a) miR-375 inhibited proliferation in cervical cancer cells. (b) The progressive up-regulated expression of miR-375 reached a peak at day 7 after paclitaxel administration, gradually declined after paclitaxel removed and restored to the level before drug treatment at about day 21. (c) miR-375 expression in cells was markedly unregulated in a dose dependent manner during paclitaxel treatment.

Table S1 miR-375 over-expression correlates with Ecadherin expression in cervical cancer tissues. Staining of human-specific Ecadherin expression in paraffin embedded 23 couples of self-paired pre-and post-chemotherapy cervical cancer samples (19 chemo-sensitive, 4 chemo-resistance). Ecadherin and miR-375 expression were reversely correlated ($r = -0.905$, $P = 1.81 \times 10{-}3$).

Acknowledgments

All authors declare that the material is an original research, has not been previously published and has not been submitted for publication elsewhere while under consideration.

Author Contributions

Conceived and designed the experiments: YS XDC YL. Performed the experiments: YS JSZ. Analyzed the data: YS FY. Contributed reagents/materials/analysis tools: XYW WGL XX. Wrote the paper: YS XX XDC.

References

1. Adam L, Zhong M, Choi W, Qi W, Nicoloso M, et al. (2009) miR-200 expression regulates epithelial-to-mesenchymal transition in bladder cancer cells and reverses resistance to epidermal growth factor receptor therapy. Clin Cancer Res 15: 5060–5072.
2. Cannito S, Novo E, di Bonzo LV, Busletta C, Colombatto S, et al. (2010) Epithelial-mesenchymal transition: from molecular mechanisms, redox regulation to implications in human health and disease. Antioxid Redox Signal 12: 1383–1430.
3. Wang Z, Li Y, Ahmad A, Azmi AS, Kong D, et al. (2010) Targeting miRNAs involved in cancer stem cell and EMT regulation: An emerging concept in overcoming drug resistance. Drug Resist Updat 13: 109–118.
4. Yang AD, Fan F, Camp ER, van Buren G, Liu W, et al. (2006) Chronic oxaliplatin resistance induces epithelial-to-mesenchymal transition in colorectal cancer cell lines. Clin Cancer Res 12: 4147–4153.
5. Kajiyama H, Shibata K, Terauchi M, Yamashita M, Ino K, et al. (2007) Chemoresistance to paclitaxel induces epithelial-mesenchymal transition and enhances metastatic potential for epithelial ovarian carcinoma cells. Int J Oncol 31: 277–283.
6. Rho JK, Choi YJ, Lee JK, Ryoo BY, Na, II, et al. (2009) Epithelial to mesenchymal transition derived from repeated exposure to gefitinib determines the sensitivity to EGFR inhibitors in A549, a non-small cell lung cancer cell line. Lung Cancer 63: 219–226.
7. Dean M, Fojo T, Bates S (2005) Tumour stem cells and drug resistance. Nat Rev Cancer 5: 275–284.
8. Ranganathan AC, Zhang L, Adam AP, Aguirre-Ghiso JA (2006) Functional coupling of p38-induced up-regulation of BiP and activation of RNA-dependent protein kinase-like endoplasmic reticulum kinase to drug resistance of dormant carcinoma cells. Cancer Res 66: 1702–1711.
9. Li Y, Kong D, Wang Z, Sarkar FH (2010) Regulation of microRNAs by natural agents: an emerging field in chemoprevention and chemotherapy research. Pharm Res 27: 1027–1041.
10. Gregory PA, Bert AG, Paterson EL, Barry SC, Tsykin A, et al. (2008) The miR-200 family and miR-205 regulate epithelial to mesenchymal transition by targeting ZEB1 and SIP1. Nat Cell Biol 10: 593–601.
11. Mongroo PS, Rustgi AK (2010) The role of the miR-200 family in epithelial-mesenchymal transition. Cancer Biol Ther 10: 219–222.
12. Li Y, Wang F, Xu J, Ye F, Shen Y, et al. (2011) Progressive miRNA expression profiles in cervical carcinogenesis and identification of HPV-related target genes for miR-29. J Pathol 224: 484–495.
13. Wang F, Li Y, Zhou J, Xu J, Peng C, et al. (2011) miR-375 is down-regulated in squamous cervical cancer and inhibits cell migration and invasion via targeting transcription factor SP1. Am J Pathol 179: 2580–2588.
14. Shen Y, Wang P, Li Y, Ye F, Wang F, et al. (2013) miR-375 is upregulated in acquired paclitaxel resistance in cervical cancer. Br J Cancer.
15. Eisenhauer EA, Therasse P, Bogaerts J, Schwartz LH, Sargent D, et al. (2009) New response evaluation criteria in solid tumours: revised RECIST guideline (version 1.1). Eur J Cancer 45: 228–247.
16. Ma L, Young J, Prabhala H, Pan E, Mestdagh P, et al. (2010) miR-9, a MYC/MYCN-activated microRNA, regulates E-cadherin and cancer metastasis. Nat Cell Biol 12: 247–256.
17. Poy MN, Hausser J, Trajkovski M, Braun M, Collins S, et al. (2009) miR-375 maintains normal pancreatic alpha- and beta-cell mass. Proc Natl Acad Sci U S A 106: 5813–5818.
18. Ding L, Xu Y, Zhang W, Deng Y, Si M, et al. (2010) MiR-375 frequently downregulated in gastric cancer inhibits cell proliferation by targeting JAK2. Cell Res 20: 784–793.
19. Tsukamoto Y, Nakada C, Noguchi T, Tanigawa M, Nguyen LT, et al. (2010) MicroRNA-375 is downregulated in gastric carcinomas and regulates cell survival by targeting PDK1 and 14-3-3 zeta. Cancer Res 70: 2339–2349.
20. Liu AM, Poon RT, Luk JM (2010) MicroRNA-375 targets Hippo-signaling effector YAP in liver cancer and inhibits tumor properties. Biochem Biophys Res Commun 394: 623–627.
21. Hui AB, Lenarduzzi M, Krushel T, Waldron L, Pintilie M, et al. (2010) Comprehensive MicroRNA profiling for head and neck squamous cell carcinomas. Clin Cancer Res 16: 1129–1139.
22. Szczyrba J, Nolte E, Wach S, Kremmer E, Stohr R, et al. (2011) Downregulation of Sec23 A protein by miRNA-375 in prostate carcinoma. Mol Cancer Res 9: 791–800.
23. de Souza Rocha Simonini P, Breiling A, Gupta N, Malekpour M, Youns M, et al. (2010) Epigenetically deregulated microRNA-375 is involved in a positive feedback loop with estrogen receptor alpha in breast cancer cells. Cancer Res 70: 9175–9184.
24. Yu L, Todd NW, Xing L, Xie Y, Zhang H, et al. (2010) Early detection of lung adenocarcinoma in sputum by a panel of microRNA markers. Int J Cancer 127: 2870–2878.
25. Li LM, Hu ZB, Zhou ZX, Chen X, Liu FY, et al. (2010) Serum microRNA profiles serve as novel biomarkers for HBV infection and diagnosis of HBV-positive hepatocarcinoma. Cancer Res 70: 9798–9807.
26. Lu Z, Luo RZ, Lu Y, Zhang X, Yu Q, et al. (2008) The tumor suppressor gene ARHI regulates autophagy and tumor dormancy in human ovarian cancer cells. J Clin Invest 118: 3917–3929.
27. Yu Y, Zhu Z (2013) Cell dormancy and tumor refractory. Anticancer Agents Med Chem 13: 199–202.
28. Ward A, Balwierz A, Zhang JD, Kublbeck M, Pawitan Y, et al. (2013) Re-expression of microRNA-375 reverses both tamoxifen resistance and accompanying EMT-like properties in breast cancer. Oncogene 32: 1173–1182.
29. Moes M, Le Bechec A, Crespo I, Laurini C, Halavatyi A, et al. (2012) A novel network integrating a miRNA-203/SNAI1 feedback loop which regulates epithelial to mesenchymal transition. PLoS One 7: e35440.
30. Doerner AM, Zuraw BL (2009) TGF-beta1 induced epithelial to mesenchymal transition (EMT) in human bronchial epithelial cells is enhanced by IL-1beta but not abrogated by corticosteroids. Respir Res 10: 100.
31. Shinto O, Yashiro M, Kawajiri H, Shimizu K, Shimizu T, et al. (2010) Inhibitory effect of a TGFbeta receptor type-I inhibitor, Ki26894, on invasiveness of scirrhous gastric cancer cells. Br J Cancer 102: 844–851.
32. von Burstin J, Eser S, Paul MC, Seidler B, Brandl M, et al. (2009) E-cadherin regulates metastasis of pancreatic cancer in vivo and is suppressed by a SNAIL/HDAC1/HDAC2 repressor complex. Gastroenterology 137: 361–371, 371 e361–365.
33. Rosano L, Cianfrocca R, Spinella F, Di Castro V, Nicotra MR, et al. (2011) Acquisition of chemoresistance and EMT phenotype is linked with activation of the endothelin A receptor pathway in ovarian carcinoma cells. Clin Cancer Res 17: 2350–2360.

21

Multi-Targeted Antiangiogenic Tyrosine Kinase Inhibitors in Advanced Non-Small Cell Lung Cancer

Wenhua Liang[◑], **Xuan Wu**[◑], **Shaodong Hong**[◑], **Yaxiong Zhang, Shiyang Kang, Wenfeng Fang, Tao Qin, Yan Huang, Hongyun Zhao, Li Zhang***

Sun Yat-sen University Cancer Center, State Key Laboratory of Oncology in South China, Collaborative Innovation Center for Cancer Medicine, Guangzhou, China

Abstract

Background: Multi-targeted antiangiogenic tyrosine kinase inhibitors (MATKIs) have been studied in many randomized controlled trials (RCTs) for treatment of advanced non-small cell lung cancer (NSCLC). We seek to summarize the most up-to-date evidences and perform a timely meta-analysis.

Methods: Electronic databases were searched for eligible studies. We defined the experimental arm as MATKI-containing group and the control arm as MATKI-free group. The extracted data on objective response rates (ORR), disease control rates (DCR), progression-free survival (PFS) and overall survival (OS) were pooled. Subgroup and sensitivity analyses were conducted.

Results: Twenty phase II/III RCTs that involved a total of 10834 participants were included. Overall, MATKI-containing group was associated with significant superior ORR (OR 1.29, 95% CI 1.08 to 1.55, $P = 0.006$) and prolonged PFS (HR 0.83, 0.78 to 0.90, $P = 0.005$) compared to the MATKI-free group. However, no significant improvements in DCR (OR 1.08, 1.00 to 1.17, $P = 0.054$) or OS (HR 0.97, 0.93 to 1.01, $P = 0.106$) were observed. Subgroup analyses showed that the benefits were predominantly presented in pooled results of studies enrolling previously-treated patients, studies not limiting to enroll non-squamous NSCLC, and studies using MATKIs in combination with the control regimens as experimental therapies.

Conclusions: This up-to-date meta-analysis showed that MATKIs did increase ORR and prolong PFS, with no significant improvement in DCR and OS. The advantages of MATKIs were most prominent in patients who received a MATKI in combination with standard treatments and in patients who had previously experienced chemotherapy. We suggest further discussion as to the inclusion criteria of future studies on MATKIs regarding histology.

Editor: William B. Coleman, University of North Carolina School of Medicine, United States of America

Funding: This study was funded by the National High Technology Research and Development Program of China Molecular classification and individualized diagnosis and treatment of lung cancer (grant numbers: 2012AA02A502) and the role of monitoring circulating tumor cells and drug-resistance-associated molecular in the therapeutic prediction, evaluation and mechanism of drug-resistance in EGFR mutant advanced NSCLC patients receiving EGFR-TKI (grant numbers: Wu Jieping Funds 320.6750.1316). The funders had no role in study design, data collection and analysis, decision to publish, or preparation of the manuscript.

Competing Interests: The authors have declared that no competing interests exist.

* Email: zhangli6@mail.sysu.edu.cn

◑ These authors contributed equally to this work.

Introduction

Lung cancer is the leading cause of cancer-related mortality worldwide, with about 85% patients diagnosed with non-small cell lung cancer (NSCLC) [1]. Locally advanced or metastatic NSCLC accounts for 80% patients; for these patients the standard care is systemic chemotherapy [2]. Regardless of the emergence of new agents, however, chemotherapy provides only marginal benefit in overall survival [3].

Another treatment option is to inhibit angiogenesis, a complicated process that is regulated by cellular cues, multiple receptor-mediated signaling networks, and a number of pro- and antiangiogenic factors [4,5]. Antiangiogenic therapy is designed to minimize the acquisition of nutrients and oxygen diffusion to starve tumors. Vascular endothelial growth factor (VEGF) is a key mediator of angiogenesis which has been well studied. Currently, the only antiangiogenic agent approved for patients with NSCLC is bevacizumab, an anti-VEGF monoclonal antibody [6]. However, many other antiangiogenic agents are under clinical development.

VEGF receptor (VEGFR) also plays an important role in the pathways regarding angiogenesis. Multi-targeted antiangiogenic tyrosine kinase inhibitors (MATKIs) are novel agents that target VEGFR-dependent tumor angiogenesis and simultaneously inhibit some other key pathways, such as platelet-derived growth factor (PDGF), fibroblast growth factor (FGF), epidermal growth factor and their associate receptors. Previous studies showed that these small-molecule inhibitors are activitive in a wide variety of cancers [7]. MATKIs could fill in a unique niche for cancer therapeutics, especially in western countries where a relatively small population is suitable for receiving targeted therapies that direct known gene alterations [8]. Recently, these similar MATKIs have showed promising advantages in the treatment of advanced NSCLC [9]. A previous meta-analysis suggested that a regimen of chemotherapy in combination with MATKIs have specific advantages over chemotherapy alone in terms of PFS and ORR, but not in OS [10]. However, it involved only six randomized controlled trials (RCTs) and three agents. Since then, plenty of novel results from phase II/III RCTs have been reported. Thus, we sought to perform a timely meta-analysis to summarize all the evidence including the updated reports. In addition, the abundant data allowed us to carry out some subgroup analyses.

Methods

Search Strategy

PubMed, EMBASE, the Cochrane Library as well as the ASCO and ESMO databases from Jan 2005 to Jan 2014 were searched for eligible trials. Search terms were the combination of "non-small-cell lung cancer" with any of the following: "multitargeted antiangiogenesis tyrosine kinase inhibitors" or "sorafenib", "sunitinib", "cediranib", "vandetanib", "motesanib", "nintedanib", "pazopanib" or "axitinib". The reference lists of the included studies and recent reviews were checked manually as a supplement. No language restriction was applied.

Eligibility Criteria

In order for a study to be included in this analysis, the following criteria should be met: 1) phase II or III RCT; 2) studies that compared at least one MATKI-containing regimen to MATKI-free regimens as any line treatments in patients with advanced NSCLC; 3) studies reporting at least one response or survival endpoints. In cases of overlap reports, we included only the latest results. Trials will be excluded if they were not in accordance with the eligible criteria.

Endpoints

The major endpoints for this meta-analysis were overall survival (OS; defined as the time of randomization to the time of death), progression free survival (PFS; defined as the time of randomization to the time of disease progression or death), objective response rate (ORR, percent of patients whose best response was complete response or partial response according to the Recist 1.1 criteria) and disease control rate (DCR, percentage of patients whose best response was complete response, partial response or stable disease according to Recist 1.1 criteria), as well as adverse events (AEs).

Quality Assessment and Data Extraction

The quality of each eligible study was rated according to the JADAD score [11]. Baseline clinical characteristics, total number of enrolled patients, number of patients who showed complete response, partial response or stable disease, hazard ratio (HR) of median OS and PFS were extracted by two investigators independently. Discrepancies were discussed by the two investigators to reach consensus. In case of missing data, we contacted the primary investigators through emails.

Statistical Analysis

We defined the experimental arm as MATKI-containing group and the control arm as MATKI-free group. Pooled hazard ratios (HRs) for survival outcomes (PFS and OS) and pooled odds ratio (ORs) for dichotomous data (ORR, DCR and toxicities) with 95% confidence intervals (CI) were calculated using the Inverse Variance algorithm and Mantel-Haenszel algorithm. Heterogeneity across studies was assessed with a forest plot and the inconsistency statistic (I^2). An I^2 of 25%, 50% and 75% was considered the cutoff of mild, moderate and severe statistical heterogeneity respectively. A random-effects model was employed in case of the existence of potential heterogeneity; however, both fixed-effect and random effects model were tested. All calculations were performed using STATA 11.0 (StataA Corp, College Station, TX). Subgroup analysis was conducted according to the line of treatment (1st-line vs. 2nd-/3rd-line/maintenance), involved histological type (unselective population vs. selective population for non-squamous carcinoma), the comparison pattern (MATKI + standard treatment/standard treatment vs. MATKI/standard treatment) respectively. Interaction tests were conducted to assess the inter-subgroup differences. Sensitivity analyses were performed. Graphical funnel plots were generated to visually inspect for publication bias. The statistical methods for detecting funnel plot asymmetry were the rank correlation test of Begg and Mazumdar and the regression asymmetry test of Egger [12,13]. For all analyses, $P<0.05$ was considered statistically significant.

Results

Selection and Features of Included Studies

Six agents (vandetanib, sunitinib, cediranib, sorafenib, motesanib and nintedanib) could be analyzed while trial data for the other agents remain immature. After screening, 20 phase II/III RCTs (7 for vandetanib, 2 for sunitinib, 3 for cediranib, 5 for sorafenib, 2 for motesanib, and 1 for nintedanib) involving a total of 10834 participants [14–33]. Figure 1 showed the flow chart of study selection. The definitions of all studied endpoints were consistent among included studies. Among all studies, 10 trials enrolling patients who previously received chemotherapy while the other 10 included chemo-naïve patients. In addition, five studies limited the eligible histological type to non-squamous carcinoma [18,20,31–33]. The 2007 study by Heymach et al. [24] contained two dose groups (100 mg/d and 300 mg/d) and the 2008 study by Heymach et al. [27] contained two experimental regimens, they were therefore divided into two separate arms for all analyses. Similarly, Blumenschein's study [32] was divided into two arms: motesanib 125 mg arm and motesanib 75 mg arm respectively. Table 1 summarized the characteristics of both the included agents and studies.

Meta-analysis of the MATKI-containing Regimens versus MATKI-free Regimens

When compared to MATKI-free group, MATKI-containing group was associated with significantly superior ORR (OR 1.29, 95% CI 1.08 to 1.55, $P=0.006$; Fig. 2A) and longer PFS (HR 0.83, 95% CI 0.78 to 0.90, $P=0.005$; Fig. 2C). However, no significant improvement in DCR (OR 1.08, 95% CI 1.00 to 1.17, $P=0.054$; Fig. 2B) and OS (HR 0.97, 95% CI 0.93 to 1.01,

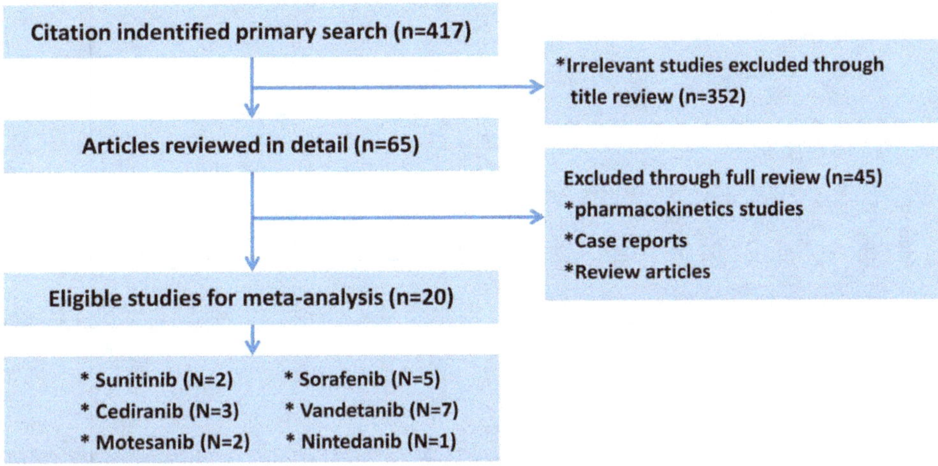

Figure 1. Flow chart of study selection.

P = 0.106; Fig. 2D) was observed. Figure 2 illustrates all results of the overall meta-analyses.

Subgroup Analyses, Sensitivity Analyses and Publication Bias

When stratifying patients according to chemotherapy history, we observed that greater benefits of MATKIs in ORR and DCR were presented in patients who failed the prior chemotherapy than those without any prior chemotherapy regarding all outcomes (2nd-/3rd-line/maintenance vs. 1st-line: ORR, OR 1.547 vs. 1.116, $P_{interaction} = 0.08$; DCR, OR 1.183 vs. 0.956, $P_{interaction} = 0.003$; PFS, HR 0.817 vs. 0.848, $P_{interaction} = 0.60$; OS, HR 0.965 vs. 0.97, $P_{interaction} = 0.92$) (greater OR indicated better ORR or DCR, while smaller HR indicated better PFS or OS). In terms of histology, the pooled results of studies that includes tumors of all histological types (not limited to non-squamous NSCLC) showed a favorable trend in comparison with studies selectively enrolled non-squamous carcinoma especially in ORR and PFS (unselective population vs. selective population: ORR, OR 1.375 vs. 1.140, $P_{interaction} = 0.33$; DCR, OR 1.077 vs. 1.081, $P_{interaction} = 0.97$; PFS, HR 0.811 vs. 0.899, $P_{interaction} = 0.21$; OS, HR 0.965 vs. 0.966, $P_{interaction} = 0.98$). We found that the studies whose experimental arms investigated regimens of adding MATKIs to the regimens in the control arm were associated with greater benefits on PFS (HR 0.798 vs. 0.998, $P_{interaction} = 0.03$). In addition, significance of DCR improvement (OR 1.095, 95% CI 1.016 to 1.180, $P = 0.018$) and OS benefits (HR 0.951, 95% CI 0.907 to 0.998, P = 0.042) were found to be statistically significant, which differed from the overall results and the results of other subgroups. Conversely, we failed to observe any benefit from studies comparing the efficacy of MATKI to the standard regimens in the control arms. All results of the subgroup analyses (including test of interaction) are illustrated in Figure 3 and were summarized in Table S1.

We conducted a sensitivity analysis by using a fixed-effects model (Table S1). We also conducted a sensitivity analysis to examine the pooled results after excluding one study by lee et al. [30] because it compared vindetanib to placebo which differed significantly from all other included trials. The conclusions regarding all outcomes were not altered in sensitivity analyses. In regard to the publication bias, no significant bias was observed in analyses of all endpoints through both Begg's test and Egger's test (P>0.05).

Discussions

The angiogenesis pathways, which play a critical role in the nourishment of both the tumors and metastatic lesions, have been targeted as a therapeutic option. Bevacizumab, a monoclonal antibody that binds to VEGF, is the only antiangiogenic drug approved for the treatment of NSCLC since it showed overall survival improvement when combined with chemotherapy [6]. An alternative approach is to shut down the VEGFR functions. Therefore, several multi-targeted tyrosine kinase inhibitors (MATKIs) that target VEGFR as well as other key pathways concerning angiogenesis and tumor proliferation are being developed. In some solid tumors, such as renal cell carcinoma and hepatocellular carcinoma, MAKTIs did reduce tumor burden and prolong overall survival [7]. Several of these agents have been evaluated in a series of phase II/III clinical trials for NSCLC patients. A previous meta-analysis suggested that regimens of chemotherapy plus MATKIs were superior to chemotherapy alone in terms of PFS and ORR, but not in OS [10]. However, this meta-analysis involved only six RCTs and three agents (sorafenib, sunitinib, and cediranib). There have been more than ten novel studies published afterwards. Thus, we believed it necessary to update the results using the new evidence and explore some novel information.

According to the current results, regimens containing sorafenib, sunitinib, cediranib, vandetanib, motesanib or nintedanib had substantial improvements for ORR and PFS outcomes, when compared with regimens free of these agents. In contrast, benefits in DCR and OS were not statistically significant. Since ORR is a part of DCR, we speculated that the underlying reason for a difference in associated benefits between ORR and DCR was that MATKIs failed to deliver any additional benefit in patients that presented primary resistance to standard treatments (chemotherapies or TKIs). This hypothesis was strengthened by our findings in the subgroup analyses: MATKIs failed to achieve any improvement when using alone. The current results could be explained by a widely accepted hypothesis that anti-angiogenic agents can transiently normalize the abnormal structure and function of tumor vessels to make it more efficient for drug delivery [34]. Therefore, MATKIs could 'rescue' those who actually

Table 1. Features of included agents and studies.

Agents	Targets	Study by Author	Year	Phase	Line	Histology Types	Regimens (Experimental arm)	Regimens (Control arm)
Sunitinib	VEGFR-1,-2,-3; PDGFRβ; c-kit; Flt-3	Socinski[14]	2010	2	1	All	Bevacizumab+TC+Sunitinib	Bevacizumab+TC
		Scagliotti [15]	2012	3	2–3	All	Erlotinib+Sunitinib	Erlotinib
Sorafenib	b-Raf; VEGFR-2, -3; PDGFRβ; Flt-3; c-kit	Spigel[16]	2011	2	2–3	All	Erlotinib+Sorafenib	Erlotinib
		Scagliotti[17]	2010	3	1	All	TC+Sorafenib	TC
		Paz-Ares[18]	2012	3	1	N-S	GP+Sorafenib	GP
		Wang[19]	2011	2	1	All	GP+Sorafenib	GP
		Molina[20]	2011	2	2	N-S	PEM+Sorafenib	PEM
Cediranib	VEGFR-1, -2, -3; PDGFR; FGFR-1; c-kit	Goss[21]	2010	2,3	1	All	TC+Cediranib	TC
		Dy[22]	2013	2	1	All	GC+Cediranib	GC
		Laurie[22]	2012	2,3	1	All	TC+Cediranib	TC
Vandetanib	VEGFR-2, -3; EGFR	Heymach[24]	2007	2	2	All	DOC+Vandetanib 100 mg	DOC
						All	DOC+Vandetanib 300 mg	DOC
		Herbst[25]	2010	3	2	All	DOC+Vandetanib 100 mg	DOC
		deBoer[26]	2011	3	2	All	PEM+Vandetanib 100 mg	PEM
		Heymach[27]	2008	2	1	All	TC+Vandetanib 300 mg	TC
						All	Vandetanib 300 mg	TC
		Natale[28]	2011	3	2	All	Vandetanib 300 mg	Erlotinib
		Natale[29]	2009	2	2	All	Vandetanib 300 mg	Gefitinib
		Lee[30]	2012	3	2	All	Vandetanib 300 mg	Placebo
Motesanib	VEGFR-1, -2, -3; PDFGR; c-kit	Scagliotti[31]	2012	3	1	N-S	TC+Motesanib	TC
		Blumenschein[32]	2011	2	1	N-S	TC+Motesanib 125 mg	TC+Beva
						N-S	TC+Motesanib 75 mg	TC+Beva
Nintedanib	VEGFR 1–3; FGFR 1–3; PDGFR α/β	Martin[33]	2013	3	2	N-S	DOC+Nintedanib	DOC

N-S, non-squamous cell carcinoma; TC, paclitaxel+carboplatin; GP, gemcitabine+cisplatin; DOC, docetaxol; PEM, pemetrxed.

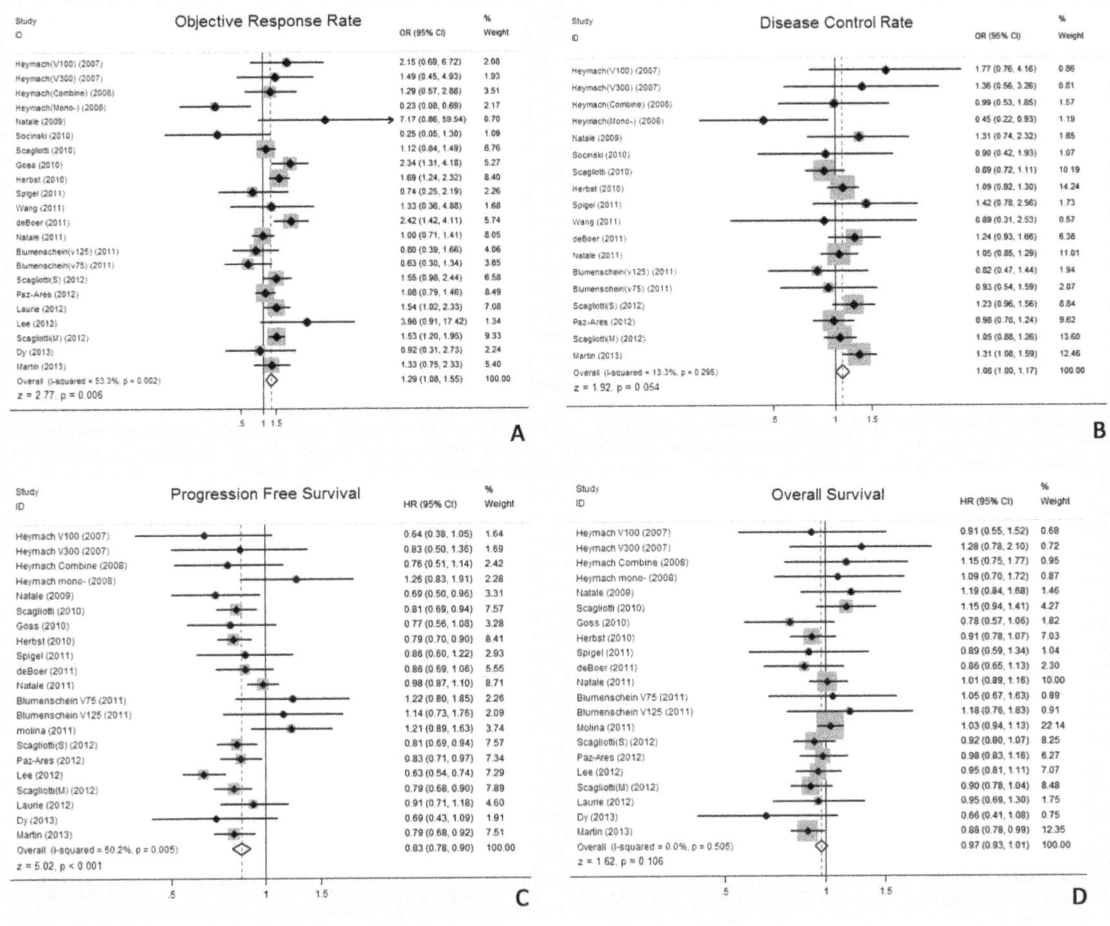

Figure 2. Meta-analyses of MATKIs-containing regimens versus MATKIs-free regimens. A, ORR; B, DCR; C, PFS; D, OS.

respond to chemotherapy but suffered from drug accessibility; this finally translated into significantly improved pooled ORR; however patients who were non-responsive remained the same status, therefore there was no significant increase in DCR. Another hypothesis derived from these results was that regulating the VEGFR pathway might play a more important role than inhibition of other targets (EGFR, PDGFR, etc) in the use of MATKIs when no selection for specific patients was conducted. It implied that MATKIs might have to work in combination with other anti-proliferative agents.

With respect to the survival outcomes, the improvement in PFS of MATKIs failed to translate into overall survival benefits. In the perspective of trial design, this might be attributed to the confounding effects from bias of the subsequent treatments. This speculation was supported by the current subgroup analyses which showed that trials studying the maintenance/2nd-line/3rd-line settings have greater magnitudes of benefits compared with those studying the 1st-line settings. This evidence highlighted the advantages of using MATKIs and highlighted the need for balancing post-trial therapies in the future studies.

Since increased risk of hemoptysis in squamous cell carcinoma was documented during the early trials, bevacizumab is only indicated for non-squamous NSCLC [35]. Similarly, part of trials on MATKIs excluded patients with squamous cell carcinoma. Through subgroup analyses, we observed that these trials did not reveal any advantages of MATKI-containing regimens over MATKI-free regimens. However, significant differences were presented when pooling the studies that recruited all histological types (including squamous cell carcinoma). It at least suggested that non-squamous NSCLC might not the targeted subpopulation that benefits most from MATKIs. An exploratory analysis revealed an increased pooled incidence of hemorrhage based on two studies including all histological types, while the incidence was similar between the groups based on the other two studies including only non-squamous NSCLC (data not shown). Although our results did not provide direct evidences, they suggested that patients with squamous cell carcinoma might benefit more from MATKI but might be associated with increased risk for hemorrhage compared with non-squamous NSCLC. However, some recent reports argued that the risk of hemorrhage among squamous NSCLC when using anti-angiogenic agents was acceptable [36]. Therefore, the inclusion criteria, in terms of histology, require further discussion for future studies on MATKIs. Of course, direct comparison of histology associated hemorrhage risk should be proposed to clarify this issue.

This is the most up-to-date comprehensive analysis to compare the MATKI-containing to MATKI-free regimens, confirming the true efficacy of MATKIs. Nevertheless, there are several limitations. Firstly, the meta-analysis might suffer from significant clinical heterogeneity. There were various chemotherapeutic

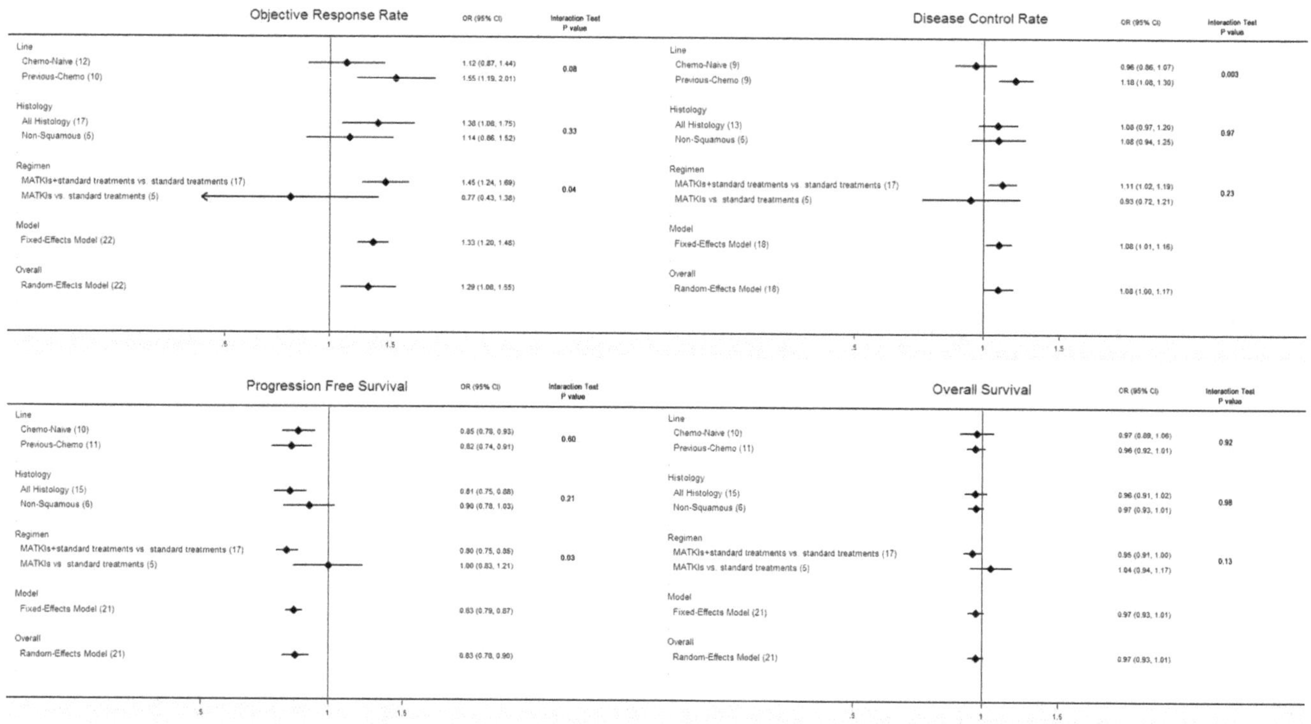

Figure 3. Subgroup analyses of each endpoint (number of studies or arms). A, ORR; B, DCR; C, PFS; D, OS.

regimens and patterns involved but we were unable to evaluate the respective effect of different MATKIs or treatment settings since current data were not sufficient to draw any solid conclusion for each subset. Secondly, only six agents were finally included in the analysis because studies on other agents were still ongoing (http://clinicaltrials.gov). Thirdly, we were unable to conduct this analysis based on individual patient data, which could definitely provide more reliable information especially in subgroup analyses. To be sure, further studies are warranted to complete the information.

In conclusion, regimens consisting of multi-targeted antiangiogenic TKIs were superior to those without these agents in terms of ORR and PFS in patients with advanced NSCLC. However, no significant benefits in DCR or OS were observed. In addition, subgroup analyses provided us some hints to improve future studies and clinical application of MATKIs.

Author Contributions

Conceived and designed the experiments: WHL XW SDH LZ. Performed the experiments: WHL XW YXZ SYK. Analyzed the data: WHL SDH WFF TQ. Contributed reagents/materials/analysis tools: WFF YH HYZ. Contributed to the writing of the manuscript: WHL XW YXZ.

References

1. Jemal A, Siegel R, Xu J, Ward E. Cancer statistics, 2010. CA Cancer J Clin 2010; 60: 277–300.
2. National Comprehensive Cancer Network. NCCN Clinical Practice Guidelines in OncologyTM. Non-Small Cell Lung Cancer. V 2.2010. http://www.nccn.org/professionals/physician gls/PDF/nscl.pdf. Accessed April 8; 2010.
3. Ramalingam S, Belani C. Systemic chemotherapy for advanced non-small cell lung cancer: recent advances and future directions. Oncologist 2008; (Suppl. 1): 5–13.
4. Ferrara N, Gerber HP, LeCouter J. The biology of VEGF and its receptors. Nat Med 2003; 9: 669–76.
5. Carmeliet P, Jain RK. Angiogenesis in cancer and other diseases. Nature 2000; 407(6801): 249–57.
6. Sandler A, Gray R, Perry MC, Brahmer J, Schiller JH, et al. Paclitaxel carboplatin alone or with bevacizumab for non-smallcell lung cancer. N Engl J Med 2006; 355: 2542–2550.
7. Ivy SP, Wick JY, Kaufman BM. An overview of small molecule inhibitors of VEGFR signaling. Nat Rev Clin Oncol 2009; 6: 569–579.
8. Dearden S, Stevens J, Wu YL, Blowers D. Mutation incidence and coincidence in non small-cell lung cancer: meta-analyses by ethnicity and histology (mutMap). Ann Oncol 2013; 24(9): 2371–6.
9. Wozniak A. Challenges in the current antiangiogenic treatment paradigm for patients with non-small cell lung cancer. Crit Rev Oncol Hematol. 2012 May; 82(2): 200–12.
10. Xiao YY, Zhan P, Yuan DM, Liu HB, Lv TF, et al. Chemotherapy plus multitargeted antiangiogenic tyrosine kinase inhibitors or chemotherapy alone in advanced NSCLC: a meta-analysis of randomized controlled trials. Eur J Clin Pharmacol 2013; 69(2): 151–9.
11. Jadad AR, Moore RA, Carroll D, Jenkinson C, Reynolds DJ, et al. Assessing the quality of reports of randomized clinical trials: is blinding necessary? Control Clin Trials 1996; 17: 1–12.
12. Egger M, Davey Smith G, Schneider M, Minder C. Bias in meta-analysis detected by a simple, graphical test. BMJ 1997; 315(7109): 629–34.
13. Begg CB, Mazumdar M. Operating characteristics of a rank correlation test for publication bias. Biometrics 1994; 50: 1088–1101.
14. Socinski MA, Scappaticci FA, Samant M, Kolb MM, Kozloff MF. Safety and efficacy of combining sunitinib with bevacizumab + paclitaxel/carboplatin in non-small cell lung cancer. J Thorac Oncol 2010; 5(3): 354–60.
15. Scagliotti GV, Krzakowski M, Szczesna A, Strausz J, Makhson A, et al. Sunitinib plus erlotinib versus placebo plus erlotinib in patients with previously treated advanced non-small-cell lung cancer: a phase III trial. J Clin Oncol 2012; 30(17): 2070–8.

16. Spigel DR, Burris HA 3rd, Greco FA, Shipley DL, Friedman EK, et al. Randomized, double-blind, placebo-controlled, phase II trial of sorafenib and erlotinib or erlotinib alone in previously treated advanced non-small-cell lung cancer. J Clin Oncol 2011; 29(18): 2582–9.
17. Scagliotti G, Novello S, von Pawel J, Reck M, Pereira JR, et al. Phase III study of carboplatin and paclitaxel alone or with sorafenib in advanced non-small-cell lung cancer. J Clin Oncol 2010; 28(11): 1835–42.
18. Paz-Ares LG, Biesma B, Heigener D, von Pawel J, Eisen T, et al. Phase III, randomized, double-blind, placebo-controlled trial of gemcitabine/cisplatin alone or with sorafenib for the first-line treatment of advanced, nonsquamous non-small-cell lung cancer. J Clin Oncol 2012; 30(25): 3084–92.
19. Wang Y, Wang L, Liu Y, Yu S, Zhang X, et al. Randomize trial of cisplatin plus gemcitabine with either sorafenib or placebo as first-line therapy for non-small cell lung cancer. [Article in Chinese] Zhongguo Fei Ai Za Zhi 2011; 14(3): 239–44.
20. Molina JR, Dy GK, Foster NR, Allen Ziegler KL, Adjei A, et al. A randomized phase II study of pemetrexed (PEM) with or without sorafenib (S) as second-line therapy in advanced non-small cell lung cancer (NSCLC) of nonsquamous histology: NCCTG N0626 study. Journal of Clinical Oncology 2011; 29 [Abstract 7513].
21. Goss GD, Arnold A, Shepherd FA, Dediu M, Ciuleanu TE, et al. Randomized, double-blind trial of carboplatin and paclitaxel with either daily oral cediranib or placebo in advanced non-small-cell lung cancer: NCIC clinical trials group BR24 study. J Clin Oncol 2010; 28(1): 49–55.
22. Dy GK, Mandrekar SJ, Nelson GD, Meyers JP, Adjei AA, et al. A randomized phase II study of gemcitabine and carboplatin with or without cediranib as first-line therapy in advanced non-small-cell lung cancer: North Central Cancer Treatment Group Study N0528. J Thorac Oncol 2013; 8(1): 79–88.
23. Laurie SA, Solomon BJ, Seymour L, Ellis PM, Goss GD, et al. A randomized double-blind trial of carboplatin plus paclitaxel (CP) with daily oral cediranib (CED), an inhibitor of vascular endothelial growth factor receptors, or placebo (PLA) in patients (pts) with previously untreated advanced non-small cell lung cancer (NSCLC): NCIC Clinical Trials Group study BR.29. J Clin Oncol 2012; 30 S:abstr 7511.
24. Heymach JV, Johnson BE, Prager D, Csada E, Roubec J, et al. Randomized, placebo-controlled phase II study of vandetanib plus docetaxel in previously treated non small-cell lung cancer. J Clin Oncol 2007; 25(27): 4270–7.
25. Herbst RS, Sun Y, Eberhardt WE, Germonpré P, Saijo N, et al. Vandetanib plus docetaxel versus docetaxel as second-line treatment for patients with advanced non-small-cell lung cancer (ZODIAC): a double-blind, randomised, phase 3 trial. Lancet Oncol 2010; 11(7): 619–26.
26. de Boer RH, Arrieta Ó, Yang CH, Gottfried M, Chan V, et al. Vandetanib plus pemetrexed for the second-line treatment of advanced non-small-cell lung cancer: a randomized, double-blind phase III trial. J Clin Oncol 2011; 29(8): 1067–74.
27. Heymach JV, Paz-Ares L, De Braud F, Sebastian M, Stewart DJ, et al. Randomized phase II study of vandetanib alone or with paclitaxel and carboplatin as first-line treatment for advanced non-small-cell lung cancer. J Clin Oncol 2008; 26(33): 5407–15.
28. Natale RB, Thongprasert S, Greco FA, Thomas M, Tsai CM, et al. Phase III trial of vandetanib compared with erlotinib in patients with previously treated advanced non-small-cell lung cancer. J Clin Oncol 2011; 29(8): 1059–66.
29. Natale RB, Bodkin D, Govindan R, Sleckman BG, Rizvi NA, et al. Vandetanib versus gefitinib in patients with advanced non-small-cell lung cancer: results from a two-part, double-blind, randomized phase ii study. J Clin Oncol 2009; 27(15): 2523–9.
30. Lee JS, Hirsh V, Park K, Qin S, Blajman CR, et al. Vandetanib Versus placebo in patients with advanced non-small-cell lung cancer after prior therapy with an epidermal growth factor receptor tyrosine kinase inhibitor: a randomized, double-blind phase III trial (ZEPHYR). J Clin Oncol 2012; 30(10): 1114–21.
31. Scagliotti GV, Vynnychenko I, Park K, Ichinose Y, Kubota K, et al. International, randomized, placebo-controlled, double-blind phase III study of motesanib plus carboplatin/paclitaxel in patients with advanced nonsquamous non-small-cell lung cancer: MONET1. J Clin Oncol 2012; 30(23): 2829–36.
32. Blumenschein GR Jr, Kabbinavar F, Menon H, Mok TS, Stephenson J, et al. A phase II, multicenter, open-label randomized study of motesanib or bevacizumab in combination with paclitaxel and carboplatin for advanced nonsquamous non-small-cell lung cancer. Ann Oncol 2011; 22(9): 2057–67.
33. Reck M, Kaiser R, Mellemgaard A, Douillard JY, Orlov S, et al. Docetaxel plus nintedanib versus docetaxel plus placebo in patients with previously treated non-small-cell lung cancer (LUME-Lung 1): a phase 3, double-blind, randomised controlled trial. Lancet Oncol 2014; 15(2): 143–55.
34. Cesca M, Bizzaro F, Zucchetti M, Giavazzi R. Tumor Delivery of Chemotherapy Combined with Inhibitors of Angiogenesis and Vascular Targeting Agents. Front Oncol 2013; 3: 259.
35. Johnson DH1, Fehrenbacher L, Novotny WF, Herbst RS, Nemunaitis JJ, et al. Randomized phase II trial comparing bevacizumab plus carboplatin and paclitaxel with carboplatin and paclitaxel alone in previously untreated locally advanced or metastatic non-small-cell lung cancer. J Clin Oncol 2004; 22(11): 2184–91.
36. Hellmann MD1, Chaft JE, Rusch V, Ginsberg MS, Finley DJ, et al. Risk of hemoptysis in patients with resected squamous cell and other high-risk lung cancers treated with adjuvant bevacizumab. Cancer Chemother Pharmacol 2013; 72(2): 453–61.

Time-Varying Pattern of Postoperative Recurrence Risk of Early-Stage (T1a-T2bN0M0) Non-Small Cell Lung Cancer (NSCLC): Results of a Single-Center Study of 994 Chinese Patients

Jian-fei Zhu[1,2¶], **Xing-yu Feng**[3¶], **Xue-wen Zhang**[4], **Ying-sheng Wen**[1], **Peng Lin**[1], **Tie-hua Rong**[1], **Ling Cai**[5*☯], **Lan-jun Zhang**[1*☯]

1 Department of Thoracic Surgery, Sun Yat-sen University Cancer Center, Guangzhou, Guangdong, China, **2** Shaanxi Provincial People's Hospital, Xi'an, Shaanxi, China, **3** Department of Gastro-pancreatic Surgery, Sun Yat-sen University Cancer Center, Guangzhou, Guangdong, China, **4** Department of Pathology, Sun Yat-sen University Cancer Center, Guangzhou, Guangdong, China, **5** Department of Radiation-Oncology, Sun Yat-sen University Cancer Center, Guangzhou, Guangdong, China

Abstract

Background: The aim of this study was to analyze the time-varying pattern of recurrence risk of early-stage (T1a-T2bN0M0) non-small cell lung cancer (NSCLC) after surgery using the hazard function and identify patients who might benefit from adjuvant chemotherapy.

Patients and Methods: This retrospective study enrolled 994 patients with early-stage NSCLC who underwent radical surgical resection between January 1999 and October 2009. Survival curves were generated using the Kaplan-Meier method, and the annual recurrence hazard was estimated using the hazard function.

Results: The median recurrence-free survival (RFS) was 8.8 years. The life table survival analysis showed that the 1-year, 3-year, 5-year and 10-year recurrence rates were 82.0%, 67.0%, 59.0% and 48.0%, respectively. Approximately 256 (25.7%) patients experienced relapse [locoregional: 32 (3.2%) and distant: 224 (22.5%)], and 162 patients died from cancer. The annual recurrence hazard curve for the entire population showed that the first major recurrence surge reached a maximum 1.6 years after surgery. The curve subsequently declined until reaching a nadir at 7.2 years. A second peak occurred at 8.8 years. An analysis of clinical-pathological factors demonstrated that this double-peaked pattern was present in several subgroups.

Conclusions: The presence of a double-peaked pattern indicates that there is a predictable temporal distribution of the recurrence hazard of early-stage NSCLC. The annual recurrence hazard may be an effective method of selecting patients at high risk of recurrence, who may benefit from adjuvant therapy.

Editor: Prasad S. Adusumilli, Memorial Sloan-Kettering Cancer Center, United States of America

Funding: This research was supported by national and provincial Science and technology projects (No. 2012AA021502 and No.2012B031800295). The funders had no role in study design, data collection and analysis, decision to publish, or preparation of the manuscript.

Competing Interests: The authors have declared that no competing interests exist.

* Email: zhanglj@sysucc.org.cn (LJZ); cailing@sysucc.org.cn (LC)

☯ These authors contributed equally to this work.

¶ JFZ and XYF also contributed equally to this work. JFZ and XYF are first authors on this work.

Introduction

Screening with low-dose computed tomography (CT) has resulted in a growing number of early-stage non-small cell lung cancer (NSCLC) diagnoses [1]. Although curative surgical resection is the current treatment of choice for early-stage NSCLC, the risk of locoregional and distant relapse remains high, at 22%–40% [2–4]. Thus, understanding the clinical course of postoperative recurrent disease is essential for guiding effective treatment.

In most studies, the risk of recurrence is analyzed using survival curves rather than hazard functions [5,6]. The hazard function, which depicts the rate of recurrence at any point in time among the remaining at-risk individuals, has been applied to provide insights into the patterns of recurrence of breast cancer [7,8] and gastric cancer [9]. The hazard function describes not only the magnitude of the recurrence rate but also how it changes over time [7,10].

To our knowledge, the present work is the first study of the temporal distribution of tumor recurrence hazard conducted with

Table 1. Kaplan-Meier postoperative survival analysis (log-rank test) according to clinical-pathological factors of patients with early-stage NSCLC.

Variable	N	Recurrence-free survival	95% CI	P
	994	8.784	8.389–9.179	
Sex				
Male	702	8.604	8.133–9.076	0.193
Female	292	9.204	8.488–9.921	
Age (years)				
≤65	680	9.179	8.713–9.646	0.010
>65	314	7.593	6.897–8.289	
Smoking history				0.037
Non-smoker[1]	429	9.267	8.685–9.848	
Smoker	565	8.400	7.866–8.935	
Initial symptoms				0.015
Examination	419	9.359	8.761–9.957	
Symptoms[2]	575	8.377	7.857–8.897	
Pathological type				0.663
Squamous cell carcinoma	319	8.859	8.259–9.214	
Non-squamous cell carcinoma	675	8.733	8.256–9.210	
Visceral pleural invasion				0.003
Present	392	8.249	7.598–8.901	
Absent	602	9.171	8.679–9.662	
Tumor diameter				<0.001
≤4.0 cm	759	9.138	8.691–9.585	
>4.0 cm	235	7.659	6.845–8.473	
Stations of resected lymph nodes				0.064
<6		8.575	8.111–9.038	
≥6		9.281	8.537–10.025	
Number of resected lymph nodes				0.022
<15	471	8.325	7.777–8.873	
≥15	523	9.265	8.700–9.830	
Lobar bronchus invasion				0.909
Present	181	8.922	7.844–10.000	
Absent	813	8.760	8.330–9.189	
Histological grade				0.012
G1+G2	631	9.111	8.619–9.602	
G3+G4	363	8.159	7.503–8.815	
CEA				<0.001
≤5 g/l	565	9.110	8.582–9.638	
>5 g/l	248	7.667	6.900–8.434	
Adjuvant chemotherapy[3]				0.321
Yes	147	8.681	8.255–9.107	
No	847	9.574	8.618–10.530	
Pathological T category				<0.001
P T1a	172	10.032	9.162–10.902	
P T1b	147	9.550	8.600–10.501	
P T2a	568	8.473	7.938–9.008	
P T2b	107	7.079	5.911–8.248	
AJCC stage				<0.001
P Ia stage	319	9.832	9.186–10.478	
P Ib stage	568	8.473	7.938–9.008	
P IIa stage	107	7.079	5.911–8.248	

[1]Non- smokers were defined as having smoked fewer than 100 cigarettes in their lifetime; [2]Common symptoms of lung cancer: cough, dyspnea, weight loss and chest pain; [3]Postoperative cisplatin-based chemotherapy.

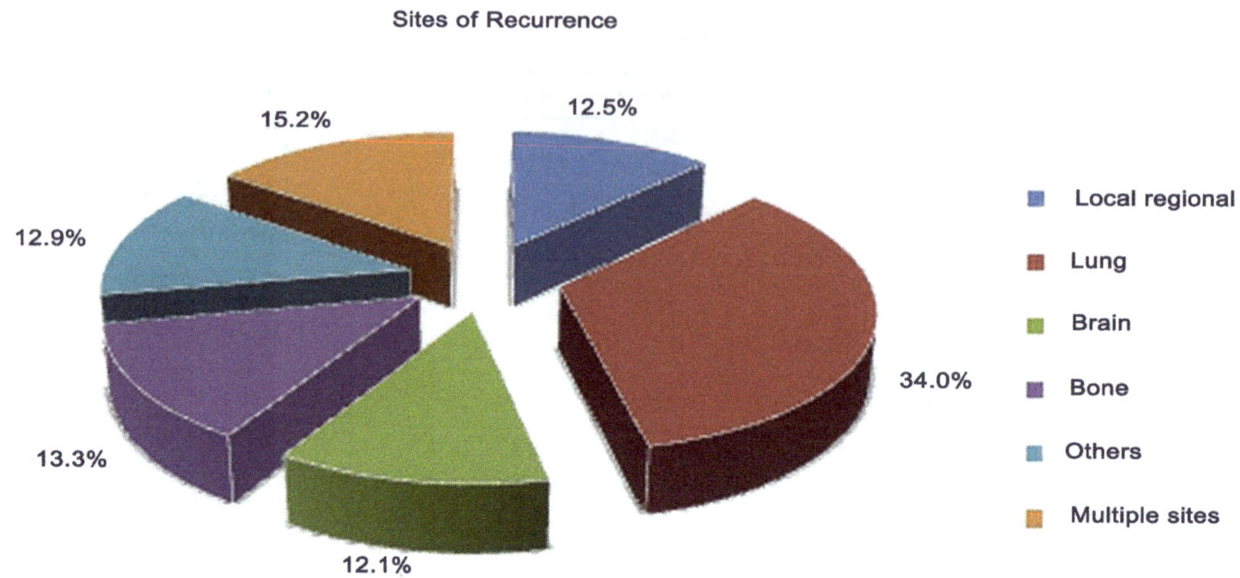

Figure 1. Relative frequencies for recurrence sites for postoperative early-stage NSCLC.

NSCLC patients. The temporal distribution of the recurrence hazard of early-stage NSCLC may shed light on the pattern of recurrence of NSCLC and may help identify patients who might benefit from adjuvant chemotherapy.

Patients and Methods

Institutional Review Board (IRB)

This study was approved by the Institutional Review Board of Sun Yat-sen University Cancer Center for the use of tumor samples and patients' clinical history.

Patients' selection

A total of 994 primary NSCLC patients who underwent radical resection at the Sun Yat-sen University Cancer Center between January 1999 and October 2009 were eligible for inclusion in this study. All patients' were staged or restaged as T1a-2bN0M0 according to the seventh edition of the International Union Against Cancer Staging System for Lung Cancer that was released in 2007 [11]. Non-smokers were defined as having smoked fewer than 100 cigarettes in their life time [12]. The cases selected for this study fulfilled the following criteria: (1) histological confirmed primary NSCLC; (2) no evidence of metastatic disease, as determined by history, physical examination and routine computed tomography (CT); (3) complete surgical resection (R0) at our cancer center; and (4) at least 3 months of follow-up information concerning disease recurrence and death. Patients who underwent non-curative resection (R1) or neo-adjuvant therapy and those who died of postoperative complications were excluded from the study.

There were 147 patients received platinum-based adjuvant chemotherapy within 4 to 8 weeks after surgical resection. Among these patients, 91 patients were in stage Ib and 56 patients in stage IIa. The average length of time between surgery and start of chemotherapy was 5.7 weeks. Among the patients who received adjuvant chemotherapy, four cycles of cisplatin (75 mg/m2) with paclitaxel or vinorelbine chemotherapy were performed in 94 (63.9%) patients and four cycles of carboplatin (an area under the curve dose of 6 mg/mL per minute over 60 minutes) with paclitaxel or vinorelbine were performed in the remaining 53 (36.1%) patients.

All participants had signed the written informed consent for their clinical records to be used in future study before starting initial treatment.

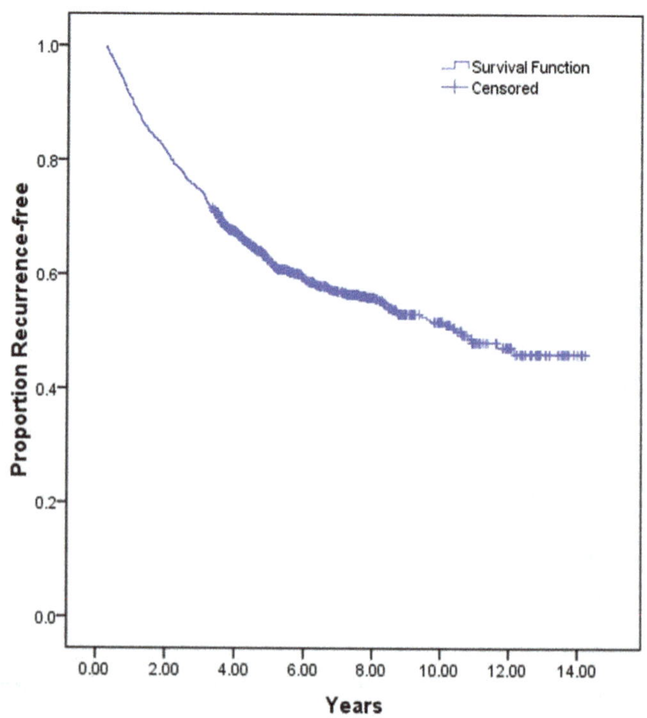

Figure 2. Recurrence-free survival for patients in early-stage NSCLC.

Table 2. Results of multivariate survival analyses of Recurrence-free survival (RFS) according to the Cox regression model.

Variable	N	RR	95% CI	P value
Tumor diameter		1.323	1.000–1.750	0.050
≤4.0 cm	759			
>4.0 cm	235			
CEA		1.414	1.131–1.768	0.002
≤5 g/l	565			
>5 g/l	248			
Number of dissected lymph nodes		0.781	0.630–0.968	0.024
<15	471			
≥15	523			
Age (years)		1.191	0.949–1.495	0.132
≤65	680			
>65	314			
Smoking history		1.003	0.795–1.264	0.983
Non-smoker	429			
Smoker	565			
Initial symptoms		1.137	0.904–1.429	0.273
Examination	419			
Symptoms	575			
Histological grade		0.824	0.655–1.036	0.097
G1+G2	631			
G3+G4	363			
Visceral pleural invasion		1.160	0.896–1.503	0.260
Present	392			
Absent	602			
Pathological T category		1.191	1.026–1.384	0.022
PT1a	172			
PT1b	147			
PT2a	568			
PT2b	107			

RR: relative risk; 95%CI: 95% confidence interval.

Definition of recurrence

Local-regional recurrences were defined as those at the surgical site, at the anastomotic or bronchial stump, or in the local-regional lymph nodes (levels 1–14, including supraclavicular). Distant recurrences were defined as hematogenous metastases within solid organs, such as the lung, liver, brain and bone. Cervical or abdominal lymph node disease was considered a distant recurrence. Recurrences were diagnosed histologically, cytologically, and radiologically. A combined recurrence was defined as the detection of both locoregional and distant recurrences either simultaneously or within 30 days [13].

Follow-up of patients

The patients were routinely followed up at the Cancer Center of Sun Yat-sen University every 3 months during the first year after surgery, every 6 months during the next 2 years and once per year thereafter. Follow-up was maintained through the retrieval of follow-up medical records stored in the outpatient department database or followed by personal contact with the patients by our professional follow-up institution, including requests for information regarding tumor recurrences and survival status. Recurrence or its absence was diagnosed by queries to the patient, chest CT, abdominal CT, bone scans, whole-brain CT/MRI or PET/CT. If a tumor had recurred, additional information, including sites of recurrence and therapy, was requested. All of the patients were contacted again in January 2013 to determine their vital status.

Statistical analysis

Recurrence-free survival (RFS) was defined as the time from surgery to the earliest occurrence of relapse (locoregional or distant) or death from cancer or cancer-related disease. Patients who were lost to follow-up were censored at the time of last contact. Patients who were alive at the end of the study were censored for the purpose of data analysis. RFS was assessed using the Kaplan-Meier method and was compared using the log-rank test. The Cox regression model was used to perform a multivariate survival analysis of all of the variables that were significant in the univariate analysis. For the graphical display of RFS, the annual hazard rates were estimated using a kernel smoothing method. A two-sided probability value of less than 0.05 was considered statistically significant. All the statistical analyses were performed using the Stata statistical software package (release 9.0; Stata

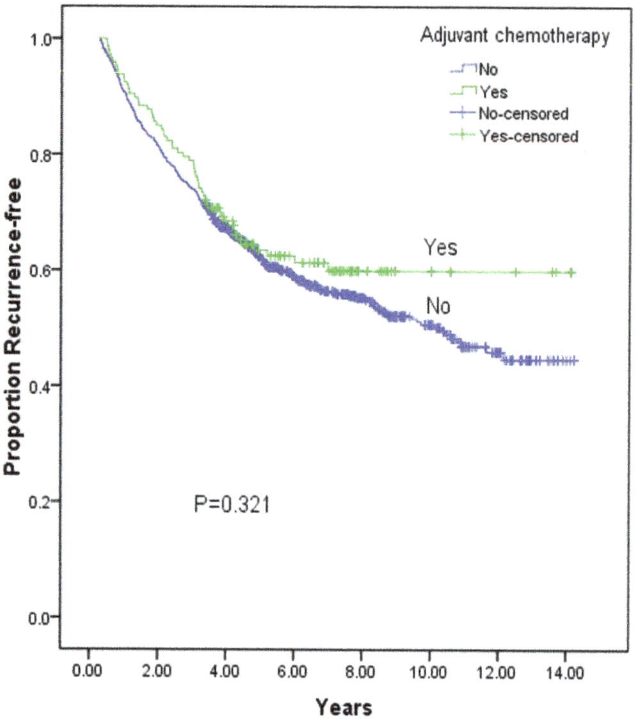

Figure 3. Recurrence-free survival for patients in early-stage NSCLC according to adjuvant chemotherapy.

Corporation, College Station, TX, USA). The relative risks (RRs) are presented with their 95% confidence intervals (CIs).

Results

Patient characteristics

A total of 994 cases satisfied the inclusion criteria and were included in this study. The clinical-pathological characteristics of the 994 patients are listed in Table 1. All of these patients received rigorous follow-up, with a median follow-up time of 6.1 years.

Overall recurrence patterns

Approximately 256 patients experienced relapse (locoregional: 32 and distant: 224). The most common sites of failure were distant (87.5%, 224/256) in this group of patients. The most common site of distant metastasis was the lung (34.0%, 87/256), followed by the bone (13.3%, 34/256) (Figure 1). Overall, 162 patients died from cancer, and approximately 576 patients remained alive at the last follow-up.

Survival analysis according to clinical-pathological factors

The survival curve for the entire population declined the most rapidly between 0.5 year and 2.5 years after surgery, with an extremely steep slope during this period. Subsequently, the entire curve continued a downward trend, albeit with a gentler slope, and it reached a virtual plateau by 10 years (Figure 2).

The median RFS was 8.8 years. The life table survival analysis showed that the 1-year, 3-year, 5-year, and 10-year recurrence rates were 82.0%, 67.0%, 59.0% and 48.0%, respectively. The univariate analysis revealed that the following variables were significantly correlated with RFS: patient age, smoking history, initial symptoms, visceral pleural invasion, tumor diameter, number of resected lymph nodes, histological grade, level of carcinoembryonic antigen (CEA), and pathological T category (Table 1). The patients who received platinum-based adjuvant chemotherapy showed a longer RFS compared with those who did not (median 9.6 years versus 8.7 years); however, this difference was not statistically significant (Table 2) (Figure 3).

When the above variables were included in the multivariate analysis, the results suggested that tumor diameter, number of lymph nodes, CEA level, and pathological T category were independent factors that affected RFS (Table 2).

Recurrence hazard analysis according to clinical-pathological factors

The annual recurrence hazard curve for the entire population showed that the first major recurrence surge peaked 1.6 years after surgery. Subsequently, the curve declined until reaching a nadir at 7.2 years. A second peak occurred at 8.8 years (Figure 4). The time-varying patterns of recurrence after surgery are listed in Table 3.

Table 3. Patterns of recurrence after surgery.

Years after surgery	n	N		Type of recurrence		
			Locoregional	Distant	Death	
0–1	90	994	7	59	24	0
1–2	91	904	8	44	39	0
2–3	70	813	7	36	27	0
3–4	70	743	4	38	28	81
4–5	41	592	4	22	15	116
5–6	19	435	1	9	9	70
6–7	13	346	1	6	6	64
7–8	4	269	0	2	2	75
8–9	9	190	0	1	8	49
9–10	3	132	0	2	1	26
≥10	8	103	0	5	3	95
	418		32	224	162	576

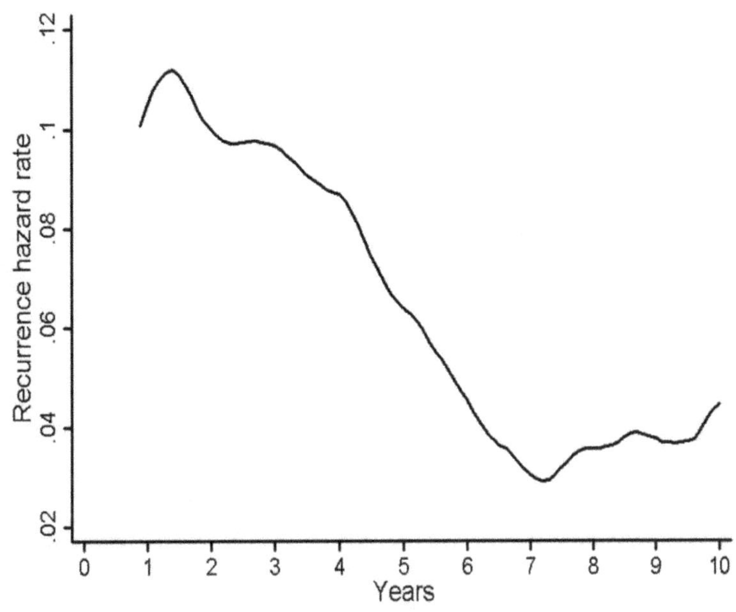

Years	1	2	3	4	5	6	7	8	9	10
	Number at risk									
	994	904	813	743	592	435	346	269	190	132

Years	1	2	3	4	5
HR (%)	9.48	10.60	9.00	10.49	7.98
CI (%)	(7.53 11.44)	(8.43 12.77)	(6.89 11.10)	(8.03 12.94)	(5.54 10.43)
Years	6	7	8	9	10
HR (%)	4.87	4.23	1.74	5.59	2.55
CI (%)	(2.68 7.05)	(1.93 6.53)	(0.03 3.45)	(1.94 9.24)	(0.00 5.44)

Figure 4. Annual recurrence hazard rates for patients in early-stage NSCLC.

The temporal distribution of the recurrence risk varied with age. The older (≥65 years) patients exhibited a relatively pronounced and variable pattern compared with the younger (<65 years) ones. The smoothed hazard plots of these two subgroups were parallel to each other, with lower hazard rates in the younger (<65 years) patients (Figure 5A). The curve of the older (≥65 years) patients increased almost linearly after 7 years.

A visual inspection of the hazard curves for different grades of histological differentiation (Figure 5B) suggested that the patients with poorly differentiated tumors exhibited earlier and higher first peaks compared with the patients with well-differentiated tumors. However, the curves of the two groups were nearly identical after 2.8 years.

The hazard rate curves of the smokers and non-smokers were virtually superimposable (Figure 5C). The first peak of the smokers was lower than that of the non-smokers. The risk of recurrence was significantly higher for the smokers than for the non-smokers after 7.5 years. A similar phenomenon was observed among the patients with visceral pleural invasion(Figure 5D). The first peak of the patients without visceral pleural invasion appeared lower and later than that of the patients with visceral pleural invasion.

The analysis according to tumor diameter (≤4.0 cm versus >4.0 cm) demonstrated that the first recurrence peak was significantly lower and later for the patients with a tumor diameter of ≤4.0 cm compared with those with a tumor diameter of >4.0 cm(Figure 5E). The curves of both subgroups tended to intersect after 5.0 years, and there was no clear second peak in either group. The analysis according to CEA level (Figure 5F) revealed that although the patients with abnormal CEA level exhibited a higher first peak, the patients with normal CEA level tended to have a greater risk of recurrence after 6.8 years compared with the patients with abnormal level of CEA.

When the hazard rate was analyzed in terms of the number of dissected mediastinal lymph nodes, a double-peaked temporal distribution of recurrence was again revealed. The smoothed hazard plots of these two subgroups were parallel to each other, and the annual recurrence hazard curve (Figure 5G) demonstrated that the patients with <15 dissected lymph nodes tended to experience more relapses at all the analyzed time periods. In terms of the stations of the dissected mediastinal lymph nodes, the patients who were dissected at <6 stations exhibited both peaks at earlier time points(Figure 5H).

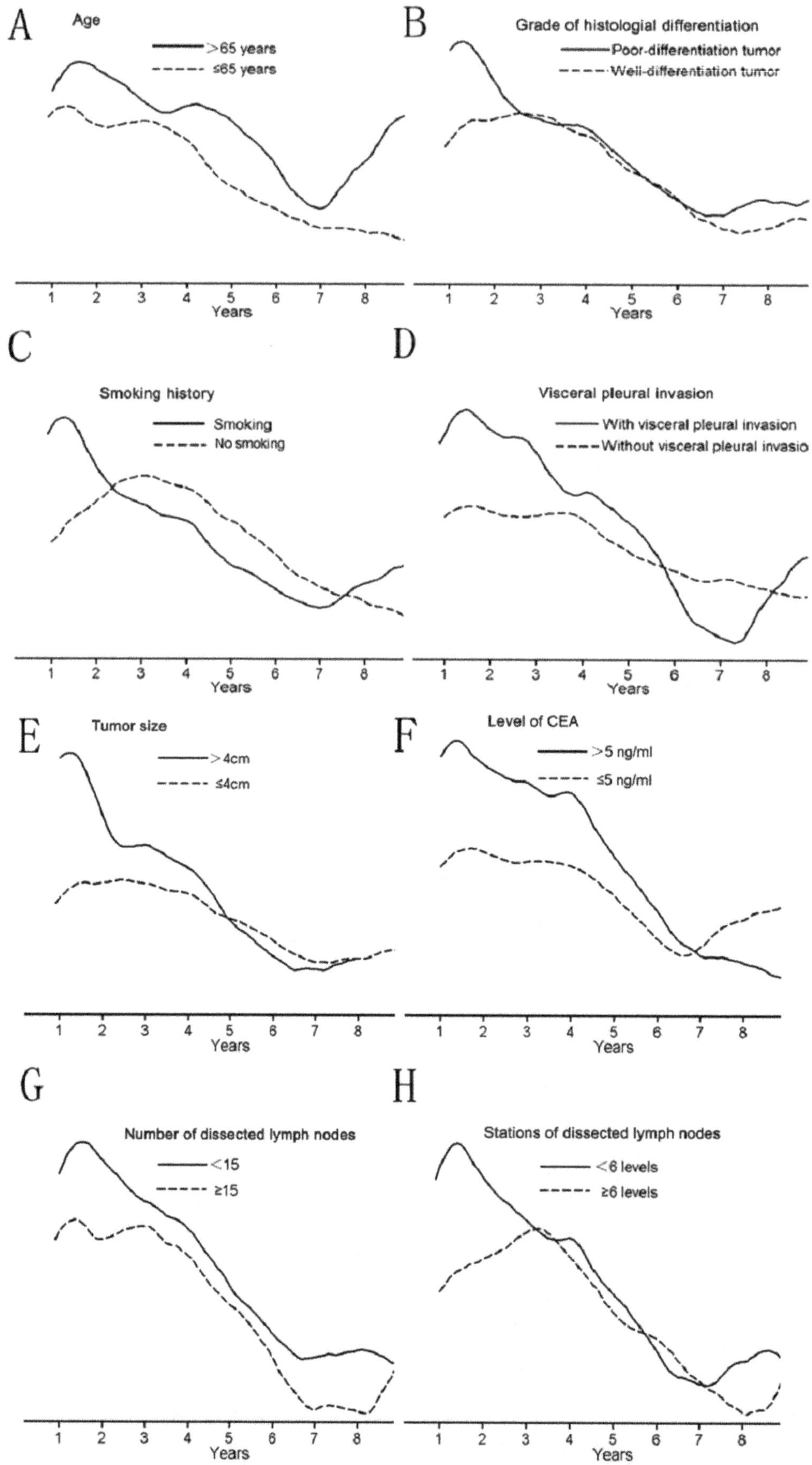
A
Age
>65 years
≤65 years
1 2 3 4 5 6 7 8
Years
B
Grade of histologial differentiation
Poor-differentiation tumor
Well-differentiation tumor
1 2 3 4 5 6 7 8
Years
C
Smoking history
Smoking
No smoking
1 2 3 4 5 6 7 8
Years
D
Visceral pleural invasion
With visceral pleural invasion
Without visceral pleural invasio
1 2 3 4 5 6 7 8
Years
E
Tumor size
>4cm
≤4cm
1 2 3 4 5 6 7 8
Years
F
Level of CEA
>5 ng/ml
≤5 ng/ml
1 2 3 4 5 6 7 8
Years
G
Number of dissected lymph nodes
<15
≥15
1 2 3 4 5 6 7 8
Years
H
Stations of dissected lymph nodes
<6 levels
≥6 levels
1 2 3 4 5 6 7 8
Years

Figure 5. Recurrence hazard rates according to clinic-pathological characteristics. A: age; B: grade of histological differentiation; C: smoking history; D: visceral pleural invasion; E: tumor diameter; F: level of CEA; G: number of dissected lymph nodes; H: stations of dissected lymph nodes.

The type of treatment also affected the shape of the curves. Compared with those without adjuvant chemotherapy, the patients who received platinum-based adjuvant chemotherapy exhibited an later major recurrence surge. The first peak of the adjuvant chemotherapy-treated subgroup was 3.5 years after surgery, and the corresponding peak of their without chemotherapy-treated counterparts occurred at 1.5 years. After 4.2 years, the curve of the patients who received adjuvant chemotherapy was lower than that of the patients without adjuvant chemotherapy, and this pattern continued for the remainder of the study period (Figure 6).

Discussion

Patients with early-stage (T1a-T2bN0M0) disease represent approximately 20%–30% of all patients with non-small cell lung cancer (NSCLC). Currently, surgery is the preferred treatment for early-stage NSCLC, and it is considered the only procedure with the potential to cure this condition [14]. However, the long-term survival of patients with early-stage NSCLC is still not optimistic. Despite surgical resection, approximately 20–40% of these patients die from local recurrence or distant metastasis within 5 years [2]. The present study is the first to demonstrate the presence of a double-peaked recurrence hazard pattern among early-stage (T1a-T2bN0M0) non-small cell lung cancer (NSCLC) patients after surgery. Our outcome of a double-peaked recurrence hazard pattern provides support for the theory of tumor dormancy [15,16], which postulates that micrometastatic foci may exist in different biologic steady states, most of which do not promote tumor growth. However, this orderly and stable process may be perturbed by surgery, which stimulates a transition from dormancy to growth, resulting in a sudden acceleration of the metastatic process and eventually leading to recurrence [17]. This phenomenon may account for the first peak of recurrence risk of malignant carcinoma after surgery.

The site of recurrence of early-stage NSCLC after surgical resection was also investigated in this study. Among patients with early-stage NSCLC, most tumors recurred as distant metastases, rather than local-regional recurrences (22.5% versus 3.2%). In early-stage NSCLC after surgical resection, the rate of distant metastasis has been reported to be between 14.0% and 23.0% [18,19], and the local-regional recurrence was 5.0% [20]. The patterns of tumor recurrence affect the therapy and survival of NSCLC patients. Based on the present study, the adjuvant treatment for early-stage NSCLC should be systemic therapy, rather than local therapy, due to the recurrence pattern of this disease.

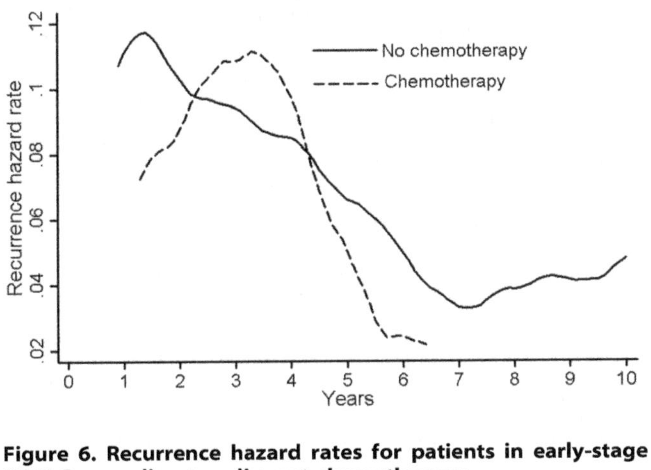

Figure 6. Recurrence hazard rates for patients in early-stage NSCLC according to adjuvant chemotherapy.

High-risk factors, include poorly differentiated tumors [21,22], vascular invasion [23], wedge resection [24], tumors >4.0 cm [25], visceral pleural involvement [26,27], and incomplete lymph node sampling (Nx) [28,29], are prognostic factors strongly associated with increased risks of recurrence and death among early-stage NSCLC patients. In our study, a double-peaked pattern was observed in a variety of patient subgroups, regardless of histological differentiation grade, tumor diameter, visceral pleural involvement or the number of dissected mediastinal lymph nodes; the patients with high-risk factors exhibited earlier and higher peaks. These factors should be considered when pondering treatment with adjuvant chemotherapy.

There is controversy concerning whether age affects the treatment and prognosis of lung cancer, particularly for patients with early lung cancer. Mery et al. [30] reported that age was an important prognostic factor for the survival of patients with stage I–II NSCLC after controlling for factors such as gender, histological type, clinical stage and type of surgery. Agarwal et al. [31] also confirmed that the mortality rate increased sharply with age in patients with stage I–II NSCLC: a one-year increase in age was associated with a nearly 6% increase in HR. However, some researchers have reported that age is not an important prognostic factor for the survival of early-stage lung cancer patients because elderly patients experience complications, organ impairment and other non-cancer-related factors [32,33]. In the current study, older (≥65 years) patients exhibited a relatively pronounced and variable pattern compared with younger (<65 years) ones. The smoothed hazard plots of these two subgroups were parallel to each other, with lower hazard rates in the younger (<65 years) patients. The curve of the older (≥65 years) patients increased almost linearly after 7.0 years. Older age (≥65 years) may be an adverse prognostic indicator in early-stage NSCLC, especially among patients who live longer than 5 years after surgery.

In the present study, we verified that the double peaks were more prominent among patients who were smokers. The primary risk factor for NSCLC is tobacco smoking, which is involved in more than 85–90% of all lung cancer-related deaths [34,35]. Although a history of smoking is well established as a risk factor for NSCLC, it remains controversial as a prognostic factor [36,37]. In our data, the hazard rate curves of the non-smokers and smokers were virtually superimposable. The smokers showed an earlier major recurrence surge, with the first peak occurring 1.2 years after surgery, while the corresponding peak for their non-smoking counterparts occurred at 3.2 years. The risk of recurrence was significantly higher for the smokers than the non-smokers after 7.5 years.

Some studies have shown that level of CEA has prognostic significance in NSCLC [38,39]. This finding was supported by our survival analysis, which showed that the risk of recurrence among patients with normal CEA level was significantly higher than that of the patients with abnormal CEA level before 7.0 years. However, the opposite pattern was observed after 7 years, indicating that the usefulness of CEA as a prognostic factor for recurrence risk may change over time. Thus, the CEA level tested before surgery may have significance for early recurrence, but not for late recurrence.

Many randomized clinical trials have reported the efficacy of platinum-based adjuvant chemotherapy after surgical resection in stage II-IIIA lung cancer [40–42]. However, the efficacy of platinum-based adjuvant chemotherapy in stage IB cancer is controversial [43,44]. Pignon et al. performed a meta-analysis of the large adjuvant trials for NSCLC conducted since 1995 (excluding CALGB 9633) [45]. Their stage IB subset analysis (1,371 patients) trended toward showing a benefit of adjuvant treatment (HR, 0.93) but failed to reach statistical significance (95% CI, 0.78–1.10). In the current study, compared with those without adjuvant chemotherapy, the patients who received platinum-based adjuvant chemotherapy exhibited a first peak that appeared lower and later. After 4.2 years, the curve of the patients who received adjuvant chemotherapy was lower than that of the patients without adjuvant chemotherapy, and this pattern continued for the remainder of the study period. The results of our study demonstrate that for early-stage NSCLC patients, platinum-based adjuvant chemotherapy may reduce and delay the recurrence hazard.

The mechanisms for recurrence and metastasis of early stage NSCLC was unclear. Driver gene mutations were associated with the carcinogenesis and response to targeted therapies and prognosis of NSCLC. Some studies had reported that identification the driver gene mutation can select patients with early-stage disease who are at high risk of recurrence [46–47]. Brock et al. [48] also confirmed that methylation of the promoter region of the cyclin-dependent kinase inhibitor 2A gene p16, the H-cadherin gene CDH13, the Ras association domain family 1 gene RASSF1A, and the adenomatous polyposis coli gene APC in patients with stage I NSCLC treated with curative intent by means of surgery is associated with early recurrence.

Previous study reported that about 5.0% non small cell lung cancer have the risk of developing metachronous second primary lung cancer [49]. The standard diagnosis of second primary lung cancer was controversial, the different histological type from that of the first tumor was considered as the key criteria to define the second lung cancer. In our study, the initial data showed about 3.54% (39/1103) patients developed second malignant tumor during the flow-up after surgical resection: 10 patients developed second primary lung cancer, and 29 patients developed the other site malignant tumor. All these patients were diagnosed as secondary malignant tumor in histological type and were excluded from the present study. However, for patients with multiple tumors after surgical resection, our study was limited to distinguish the second malignant tumor from metastatic disease.

As a retrospective study, this study has other several potential limitations. The median follow-up time of 6.1 years was not sufficiently long; 576 patients were still alive at the last follow-up. Because there were only 147 patients who received platinum-based adjuvant chemotherapy, the subgroup analysis was unable to identify patients who might benefit from adjuvant chemotherapy.

In conclusion, we confirmed the validity of a double-peaked pattern of recurrence risk of early-stage (T1a-T2bN0M0) non-small cell lung cancer. The main pattern of tumor recurrence was distant metastasis, rather than local-regional recurrence. The hazard function may be useful for selecting patients at high risk of recurrence to receive postoperative therapy, which offers the possibility of decreasing and/or delaying the recurrence hazard.

Author Contributions

Conceived and designed the experiments: LJZ LC. Performed the experiments: JFZ XYF LC. Analyzed the data: JFZ LC LJZ. Contributed reagents/materials/analysis tools: JFZ LC XWZ YSW PL THR. Contributed to the writing of the manuscript: JFZ LC LJZ.

References

1. Kovalchik SA, Tammemagi M, Berg CD, Caporaso NE, Riley TL, et al. (2013) Targeting of low-dose CT screening according to the risk of lung-cancer death. N Engl J Med 369: 245–254.
2. Kelsey CR, Marks LB, Hollis D, Hubbs JL, Ready NE, et al. (2009) Local recurrence after surgery for early stage lung cancer: an 11-year experience with 975 patients. Cancer 115: 5218–5227.
3. Chansky K, Sculier JP, Crowley JJ, Giroux D, Van Meerbeeck J, et al. (2009) The International Association for the Study of Lung Cancer Staging Project: prognostic factors and pathologic TNM stage in surgically managed non-small cell lung cancer. J Thorac Oncol 4: 792–801.
4. Detterbeck FC, Boffa DJ, Tanoue LT (2009) The new lung cancer staging system. Chest 136: 260–271.
5. Tantraworasin A, Saeteng S, Lertprasertsuke N, Arreyakajohn N, Kasemsarn C, et al. (2013) Prognostic factors of tumor recurrence in completely resected non-small cell lung cancer. Cancer Manag Res 5: 77–84.
6. Kobayashi N, Toyooka S, Soh J, Ichimura K, Yanai H, et al. (2007) Risk factors for recurrence and unfavorable prognosis in patients with stage I non-small cell lung cancer and a tumor diameter of 20 mm or less. J Thorac Oncol 2: 808–812.
7. Yin W, Di G, Zhou L, Lu J, Liu G, et al. (2009) Time-varying pattern of recurrence risk for Chinese breast cancer patients. Breast Cancer Res Treat 114: 527–535.
8. Saphner T, Tormey DC, Gray R (1996) Annual hazard rates of recurrence for breast cancer after primary therapy. J Clin Oncol 14: 2738–2746.
9. Feng XY, Chen YB, Wang W, Guan YX, Li YF, et al. (2013) Time-varying pattern of recurrence risk for gastric cancer patients. Med Oncol 30: 514.
10. Simes RJ, Zelen M (1985) Exploratory data analysis and the use of the hazard function for interpreting survival data: an investigator's primer. J Clin Oncol 3: 1418–1431.
11. Goldstraw P, Crowley J, Chansky K, Giroux DJ, Groome PA, et al. (2007) The IASLC Lung Cancer Staging Project: proposals for the revision of the TNM stage groupings in the forthcoming (seventh) edition of the TNM Classification of malignant tumours. J Thorac Oncol 2: 706–714.
12. Li C, Fang R, Sun Y, Han X, Li F, et al. (2011) Spectrum of oncogenic driver mutations in lung adenocarcinomas from East Asian never smokers. PLoS One 6: e28204.
13. Amini A, Lou F, Correa AM, Baldassarre R, Rimner A, et al. (2013) Predictors for locoregional recurrence for clinical stage III-N2 non-small cell lung cancer with nodal downstaging after induction chemotherapy and surgery. Ann Surg Oncol 20: 1934–1940.
14. Henschke CI, Yankelevitz DF, Libby DM, Pasmantier MW, Smith JP, et al. (2006) Survival of patients with stage I lung cancer detected on CT screening. N Engl J Med 355: 1763–1771.
15. Gimbrone MJ, Leapman SB, Cotran RS, Folkman J (1972) Tumor dormancy in vivo by prevention of neovascularization. J Exp Med 136: 261–276.
16. Varani J, Lovett ER, Lundy J (1981) A model of tumor cell dormancy: effects of anesthesia and surgery. J Surg Oncol 17: 9–14.
17. Demicheli R, Retsky MW, Hrushesky WJ, Baum M (2007) Tumor dormancy and surgery-driven interruption of dormancy in breast cancer: learning from failures. Nat Clin Pract Oncol 4: 699–710.
18. Al-Kattan K, Sepsas E, Fountain SW, Townsend ER (1997) Disease recurrence after resection for stage I lung cancer. Eur J Cardiothorac Surg 12: 380–384.
19. Nakagawa T, Okumura N, Ohata K, Igai H, Matsuoka T, et al. (2008) Postrecurrence survival in patients with stage I non-small cell lung cancer. Eur J Cardiothorac Surg 34: 499–504.
20. Lou F, Huang J, Sima CS, Dycoco J, Rusch V, et al. (2013) Patterns of recurrence and second primary lung cancer in early-stage lung cancer survivors followed with routine computed tomography surveillance. J Thorac Cardiovasc Surg 145: 75–81, 81–82.
21. Sun Z, Aubry MC, Deschamps C, Marks RS, Okuno SH, et al. (2006) Histologic grade is an independent prognostic factor for survival in non-small cell lung cancer: an analysis of 5018 hospital- and 712 population-based cases. J Thorac Cardiovasc Surg 131: 1014–1020.
22. Jones DR, Daniel TM, Denlinger CE, Rundall BK, Smolkin ME, et al. (2006) Stage IB nonsmall cell lung cancers: are they all the same? Ann Thorac Surg 81: 1958–1962, 1962.
23. Shimada Y, Saji H, Yoshida K, Kakihana M, Honda H, et al. (2012) Pathological vascular invasion and tumor differentiation predict cancer

recurrence in stage IA non-small-cell lung cancer after complete surgical resection. J Thorac Oncol 7: 1263–1270.
24. Ou SH, Zell JA, Ziogas A, Anton-Culver H (2008) Prognostic significance of the non-size-based AJCC T2 descriptors: visceral pleura invasion, hilar atelectasis, or obstructive pneumonitis in stage IB non-small cell lung cancer is dependent on tumor size. Chest 133: 662–669.
25. Ou SH, Zell JA, Ziogas A, Anton-Culver H (2007) Prognostic factors for survival of stage I nonsmall cell lung cancer patients : a population-based analysis of 19,702 stage I patients in the California Cancer Registry from 1989 to 2003. Cancer 110: 1532–1541.
26. Shimizu K, Yoshida J, Nagai K, Nishimura M, Ishii G, et al. (2005) Visceral pleural invasion is an invasive and aggressive indicator of non-small cell lung cancer. J Thorac Cardiovasc Surg 130: 160–165.
27. Nakagawa T, Okumura N, Kokado Y, Miyoshi K, Matsuoka T, et al. (2007) Clinical relevance of intraoperative pleural lavage cytology in non-small cell lung cancer. Ann Thorac Surg 83: 204–208.
28. Park SY, Lee JG, Kim J, Byun GE, Bae MK, et al. (2013) Efficacy of platinum-based adjuvant chemotherapy in T2aN0 stage IB non-small cell lung cancer. J Cardiothorac Surg 8: 151.
29. Wang WL, Shen-Tu Y, Wang ZQ (2011) Prognostic Factors for Survival of Stage IB Upper Lobe Non-small Cell Lung Cancer Patients: A Retrospective Study in Shanghai, China. Chin J Cancer Res 23: 265–270.
30. Mery CM, Pappas AN, Bueno R, Colson YL, Linden P, et al. (2005) Similar long-term survival of elderly patients with non-small cell lung cancer treated with lobectomy or wedge resection within the surveillance, epidemiology, and end results database. Chest 128: 237–245.
31. Agarwal M, Brahmanday G, Chmielewski GW, Welsh RJ, Ravikrishnan KP (2010) Age, tumor size, type of surgery, and gender predict survival in early stage (stage I and II) non-small cell lung cancer after surgical resection. Lung Cancer 68: 398–402.
32. Yamamoto K, Padilla AJ, Calvo MV, Garcia-Zarza A, Pastor GJ, et al. (2003) Surgical results of stage I non-small cell lung cancer: comparison between elderly and younger patients. Eur J Cardiothorac Surg 23: 21–25.
33. Janssen-Heijnen ML, Houterman S, Lemmens VE, Louwman MW, Maas HA, et al. (2005) Prognostic impact of increasing age and co-morbidity in cancer patients: a population-based approach. Crit Rev Oncol Hematol 55: 231–240.
34. Secretan B, Straif K, Baan R, Grosse Y, El GF, et al. (2009) A review of human carcinogens–Part E: tobacco, areca nut, alcohol, coal smoke, and salted fish. Lancet Oncol 10: 1033–1034.
35. Doll R, Peto R (1976) Mortality in relation to smoking: 20 years' observations on male British doctors. Br Med J 2: 1525–1536.
36. Maeda R, Yoshida J, Ishii G, Hishida T, Nishimura M, et al. (2011) Poor prognostic factors in patients with stage IB non-small cell lung cancer according to the seventh edition TNM classification. Chest 139: 855–861.
37. Jin Y, Zhao L, Peng F (2013) Prognostic impact of serum albumin levels on the recurrence of stage I non-small cell lung cancer. Clinics (Sao Paulo) 68: 686–693.
38. Molina R, Filella X, Auge JM, Fuentes R, Bover I, et al. (2003) Tumor markers (CEA, CA 125, CYFRA 21–1, SCC and NSE) in patients with non-small cell lung cancer as an aid in histological diagnosis and prognosis. Comparison with the main clinical and pathological prognostic factors. Tumour Biol 24: 209–218.
39. Gaspar MJ, Diez M, Rodriguez A, Ratia T, Martin DA, et al. (2003) Clinical value of CEA and CA125 regarding relapse and metastasis in resectable non-small cell lung cancer. Anticancer Res 23: 3427–3432.
40. Arriagada R, Bergman B, Dunant A, Le Chevalier T, Pignon JP, et al. (2004) Cisplatin-based adjuvant chemotherapy in patients with completely resected non-small-cell lung cancer. N Engl J Med 350: 351–360.
41. Winton T, Livingston R, Johnson D, Rigas J, Johnston M, et al. (2005) Vinorelbine plus cisplatin vs. observation in resected non-small-cell lung cancer. N Engl J Med 352: 2589–2597.
42. Douillard JY, Rosell R, De Lena M, Carpagnano F, Ramlau R, et al. (2006) Adjuvant vinorelbine plus cisplatin versus observation in patients with completely resected stage IB-IIIA non-small-cell lung cancer (Adjuvant Navelbine International Trialist Association [ANITA]): a randomised controlled trial. Lancet Oncol 7: 719–727.
43. Kato H, Ichinose Y, Ohta M, Hata E, Tsubota N, et al. (2004) A randomized trial of adjuvant chemotherapy with uracil-tegafur for adenocarcinoma of the lung. N Engl J Med 350: 1713–1721.
44. Strauss GM, Herndon JN, Maddaus MA, Johnstone DW, Johnson EA, et al. (2008) Adjuvant paclitaxel plus carboplatin compared with observation in stage IB non-small-cell lung cancer: CALGB 9633 with the Cancer and Leukemia Group B, Radiation Therapy Oncology Group, and North Central Cancer Treatment Group Study Groups. J Clin Oncol 26: 5043–5051.
45. Pignon JP, Tribodet H, Scagliotti GV, Douillard JY, Shepherd FA, et al. (2008) Lung adjuvant cisplatin evaluation: a pooled analysis by the LACE Collaborative Group. J Clin Oncol 26: 3552–3559.
46. Kratz JR, He J, Van Den Eeden SK, Zhu ZH, Gao W, et al. (2012) A practical molecular assay to predict survival in resected non-squamous, non-small-cell lung cancer: development and international validation studies. Lancet 379: 823–832.
47. Zhu ZH, Sun BY, Ma Y, Shao JY, Long H, et al. (2009) Three immunomarker support vector machines-based prognostic classifiers for stage IB non-small-cell lung cancer. J Clin Oncol 27: 1091–1099.
48. Brock MV, Hooker CM, Ota-Machida E, Han Y, Guo M, et al. (2008) DNA methylation markers and early recurrence in stage I lung cancer. N Engl J Med 358: 1118–1128.
49. Ishigaki T, Yoshimasu T, Oura S, Ota F, Nakamura R, et al. (2013) Surgical treatment for metachronous second primary lung cancer after radical resection of primary lung cancer. Ann Thorac Cardiovasc Surg 19: 341–344.

The Prognostic Value of Excision Repair Cross-Complementation Group 1 (ERCC1) in Patients with Small Cell Lung Cancer (SCLC) Receiving Platinum-Based Chemotherapy

Yanlong Yang[1], Xiuping Luo[2], Nuo Yang[1], Ronghao Feng[2], Lei Xian[1]*

1 Department of Cardiothoracic Surgery, The First Affiliated Hospital of Guangxi Medical University, Nanning, Guangxi Zhuang Autonomous Region, China, 2 Department of Chemotherapy, The Affiliated Tumor Hospital of Guangxi Medical University, Nanning, Guangxi Zhuang Autonomous Region, China

Abstract

Recently, the correlation between the efficacy of platinum-based chemotherapy and ERCC1 expression in patients with SCLC has attracted wide-spread attention, and a lot of investigations have been conducted, whereas conflicting results were presented. Therefore, we performed the present meta-analysis of eligible studies to derive a more precise evaluation of the association between ERCC1 expression and the clinical outcome in SCLC patients receiving platinum-based chemotherapy. A literature search for relevant studies was conducted in the electronic databases of PubMed, EMBASE and Web of Science. The inclusive criteria were SCLC patients treated by platinum-based chemotherapy, and evaluated the relationship between ERCC1 expression and the clinical outcomes [including overall response rate (ORR), overall survival (OS) or progression-free survival (PFS)]. Odds ratio (OR) or hazard ratio (HR) with 95% confidence interval (CI) was calculated to assess the risk. A total of nine studies including 1129 patients were included in final analysis. Our analysis indicated that positive/high ERCC1 expression was associated with unfavorable OS (HR = 1.18, 95%CI = 1.02–1.37) and PFS (HR = 1.46, 95%CI = 1.14–1.88). Subgroup analysis according to disease stage suggested the significant relationship was found in limited stage (LS-SCLC), but not in extensive stage (ES-SCLC). However, no significant association was found between ERCC1 expression and ORR. Our analysis suggested ERCC1 expression may be a prognostic factor in SCLC patients receiving platinum-based chemotherapy, especially for LS-SCLC.

Editor: Qing-Yi Wei, Duke Cancer Institute, United States of America

Funding: The authors have no support or funding to report.

Competing Interests: The authors have declared that no competing interests exist.

* Email: xianlei59@163.com

These authors contributed equally to this work.

Introduction

Lung cancer is a common malignancy and has been a leading cause of mortality and a burden of health finance cost worldwide [1]. It has been reported by the International Agency for Research on Cancer for 2008 that a total of 1.6 million individuals were diagnosed as lung cancer and approximately 1.4 million died from the disease, making it the first leading cause of cancer mortality in men and second in women throughout the world [2]. Accounting for around 14% of lung cancer new cases in the Europe, USA, and Korea, small cell lung cancer (SCLC) is the most aggressive subtype of lung cancer and is characterized by rapid growth and early dissemination [3–6]. Most of the SCLC cases (70%–80%) are diagnosed at an extensive stage (ES-SCLC) and only a small number of SCLC patients are found to be limited to the thorax (LS-SCLC) [7]. In fact, the median survival time is 14 to 20 months for LS-SCLC and 7 to 10 months for ES-SCLC [8]. The standard treatment for patients with limited stage is a combination of chest radiation and chemotherapy on the basis of etoposide and cisplatin. For patients with extensive stage, platinum-based combination chemotherapy has considered to be the main treatment. However, the emergence of drug resistance and the high rate of relapse of the neoplastic disease often lead to poor prognosis for SCLC patients, in spite of its initial high response to the chemotherapy [3–7,9,10]. A growing number of evidence suggests that biological markers may contribute greatly to the efficacy of chemotherapy; ERCC1 is one of the most notable biomarkers among them.

ERCC1 enzyme belongs to nucleotide excision repair (NER) system which has the ability of repairing DNA adducts and other DNA helix-distorting lesions [11], including platinum intra-strand DNA adducts, and it is considered to be related to resistance to platinum-based chemotherapy via reducing platinum-induced DNA damage [12–21]. Platinum mainly acts by binding to DNA and forming bulky DNA adducts, which caused inter-strand and intra-strand cross-link generation, as well as DNA-protein cross-links, resulting in inhibition of cell growth and apoptosis of targeted cells unless repaired. ERCC1 enzyme involved in

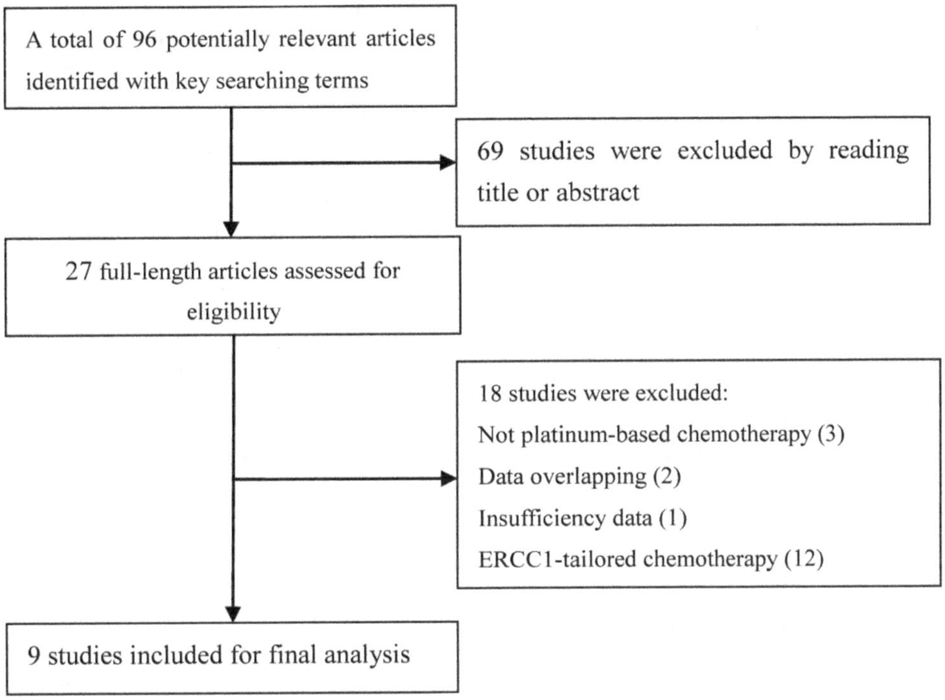

Figure 1. Flow diagram of the literature search in this meta-analysis.

recognizing and removing platinum-induced intra-strand adducts in DNA, and was reported to be a biomarker of resistance to platinum-based chemotherapy in patients with bladder, ovarian, colorectal, gastric, esophageal, and lung cancer [12–21].

The correlation between the efficacy of platinum-based chemotherapy in SCLC and ERCC1 expression has attracted wide-spread attention, and a lot of investigations have been conducted, whereas conflicting results were presented. Kim et al. [22] and Smit et al. [23] reported that there was no significant association between ERCC1 expression and overall response rate (ORR), progression-free survival (PFS) or overall survival (OS). On the other hand, Karachaliou et al [24] and Ceppi et al [21] demonstrated that low/negative expression of ERCC1 was related to longer OS. The relationship between ERCC1 expression and the clinical outcomes in SCLC patients receiving platinum-based chemotherapy thus remains unknown. Hence, we performed the present meta-analysis of all eligible investigations to derive a more precise evaluation of the association between ERCC1 level and the clinical outcomes (ORR, OS and PFS) in SCLC patients receiving platinum-based chemotherapy.

Materials and Methods

Search strategy

With the following terms combined: ("Excision Repair Cross-Complementation Group 1" or "ERCC1") and ("small cell lung cancer" or SCLC or "neoplasm, lung") and ("platinum" or "cisplatin" or "carboplatin" or "oxaliplatin"), we searched potentially relevant publications in online databases of PubMed, EMBASE and Web of Science for all years up until May 31, 2014. Only the papers written in English language were included. In addition, we also conducted an additional manual search on the basis of references.

Inclusion and Exclusion Criteria

Eligibility criteria were as follows: (1) human-based studies; (2) pathologically confirmed SCLC receiving platinum-based regimens; (3) full-text written in English; (4) to evaluate the association between ERCC1expression and clinical outcomes, i.e. overall response rate (ORR), overall survival (OS) or progression-free survival (PFS). Exclusion criteria were as follows: (1) patients younger than 18 years old; (2) studies without necessary data to extract ORR, OS or PFS; (3) For overlapping data, the studies with small sample sizes or insufficient information were excluded.

Data extraction and synthesis

Two independent researchers (X.P. Luo and Y.L. Yang) reviewed the included studies and extracted the following data: the first author, publication year, original country, ethnicity, sample size, age of patients, disease stage, chemotherapy regimens, detection method of ERCC1expression, distribution of high/positive ERCC1 expression in patients, and clinical outcomes. Any disagreement between the investigators was resolved through discussions until a consensus was reached.

Quality assessment

The quality of the methodology of the included studies was assessed by the Newcastle-Ottawa scale (NOS) recommended by the Cochrane Non-Randomized Studies Methods Working Group [25]. Studies with five or more stars were defined as high quality studies. Quality assessment was performed by two investigators (Y.L. Yang and L. Xian) independently. Disagreements were resolved by discussion.

Statistical analysis

The odds ratios (ORs) with corresponding 95% confidence intervals (CIs) were employed to estimate the association between ERCC1 status and the ORR to platinum-based chemotherapy in

Table 1. Baseline characteristics of studies included in the meta-analysis.

Study	Year	Country	Ethnicity	No. of cases	Mean/median age	Stage	Therapy	Methods	Threshold	High expression (%)	Outcome
Ceppi[21]	2008	Italy	Caucasian	85	63(43–81)	LS, ES	Cisplatin/carboplatin and etoposide	RT-PCR	0.5	50.6	ORR,OS
Lee[10]	2008	Korea	Asian	77	61(41–76)	LS, ES	Platinum-based doublets	IHC	H-score = 2	22.1	ORR,OS
Kim[22]	2009	Japan	Asian	130	67(28–83)	ES, LS	Platinum-based combination	IHC	10%	27.7	ORR,OS
Skov[33]	2010	Denmark	Caucasian	186	68 (47–93)	LS, ES	Platinum-based combination	IHC	H-score >0	9.1	OS
Smit[23]	2011	NR	Mixed	323	NR	ES	Platinum-based combination	IHC	H-score =25	27.7	OS
Lee[32]	2012	Korea	Asian	111	65 (44–80)	LS, ES	Platinum-based doublets	IHC	H-score = 2	44.1	ORR,OS
Sereno[34]	2012	Spain	Caucasian	76	62(43–81)	LS, ES	Etoposide-cisplatin, carboplatin-etoposide	RT-PCR	0.1	54.7	ORR,PFS
Sodja[35]	2012	Slovenia	Caucasian	77	59 (42–77)	LS, ES	Platinum-based doublets	IHC	50%	51.9	ORR,OS,PFS
Karachaliou[24]	2013	Greece	Caucasian	64	63 (33–78)	LS	Cisplatin-etoposide.	RT-PCR	Median(11.49)	50.0	OS,PFS

Abbreviations: NR, not reported; **LS,** limited stage; **ES,** extensive stage; **IHC,** immunohistochemistry; RT-**PCR,** reverse transcription-polymerase chain reaction; **PFS,** progression-free survival; **ORR,** objective response rate; **OS,** overall survival.

SCLC patients. The hazard ratios (HRs) and their corresponding 95% CIs were used to evaluate the relationship between ERCC1 expression and OS and PFS in SCLC patients treated by platinum-based chemotherapy. When the direct HRs and their 95% CIs were not provided in studies, the indirect estimates by Tierney's method were applied [26]. Heterogeneity among studies was evaluated by Q test and I^2 metric [27]. In the presence of heterogeneity between studies (p<0.1 for Q test, or I^2>50%), the pooled OR/HR was calculated using a random-effect model [28]; otherwise, the fixed-effect model was applied [29]. Subgroup analyses by ethnicity (Asian/Caucasian), stage of SCLC (LS/ES), and detection method (IHC/RT-PCR) were also conducted. Sensitivity analysis was performed to assess the stability of results. Each study was excluded one at a time to determine the magnitude of influence on the overall summary estimate. Publication bias was tested by funnel plots qualitatively and estimated by Begg's test and Egger's test quantitatively [30,31]. All statistical analyses were performed by software of STATA version 11.2 (StataCorp, College Station, TX, USA).

Results

Eligible studies

The present work followed the guidelines for systematic reviews and meta-analyses (PRISMA) (Checklist S1). Details for the literature search were presented in Figure 1 and Figure S1. A number of 96 potentially relevant articles were yielded in the initial search with the searching terms. After reading the titles and abstracts, 27 potential articles were assessed for eligibility. However, 18 studies were further excluded because of the following reasons: not platinum-based chemotherapy (n = 3); data overlapping (n = 2); insufficiency data (n = 1); ERCC1-tailored chemotherapy (n = 12). Thus, nine studies including 1129 patients were included in meta-analysis [10,21–24,32–35]. All nine studies were assessed by the NOS quality scale and were scored highly (with five stars or more). The quality score of 9 eligible studies can be found in Table S1.

The characteristics of included publications were detailed in Table 1. The nine studies were published between 2008 and 2013. There were three studies conducted in Asian patients [10,22,32], five studies conducted in Caucasian patients [21,24,33–35], and one study conducted in mixed race [23]. The sample sizes of all the included studies ranged from 64 to 323. As shown in Table 1, in nine independent studies, one study focused on LS-SCLC [24], one study focused on ES-SCLC [23], and seven studies focused on both stage [10,21,32–35]. Of all eligible studies, three studies employed reverse transcription-polymerase chain reaction (RT-PCR) as detecting method [21,24,34] and the other six studies employed immunohistochemistry (IHC) [10,22,23,32,33,35].

Objective response rate

The association between ERCC1 expression and the response to platinum-based chemotherapy was explored in six studies containing 533 SCLC patients [10,21,22,32,34,35]. And the result indicated that ERCC1 expression was not significantly associated with the ORR in SCLC patients receiving platinum-based chemotherapy (OR = 0.93, 95% CI = 0.61–1.41, I^2 = 16.1%, P = 0.31 for heterogeneity; Table 2, Figure. 2).

Subgroup analyses according to ethnicity and disease stage were also performed in this meta-analysis. Of the six studies reporting the data on ORR, three studies [10,22,32] consisted of 318 patients were conducted among Asians and the other three studies [21,34,35] containing 215 patients were performed among Caucasians. Subgroup analysis based on ethnicity indicated that

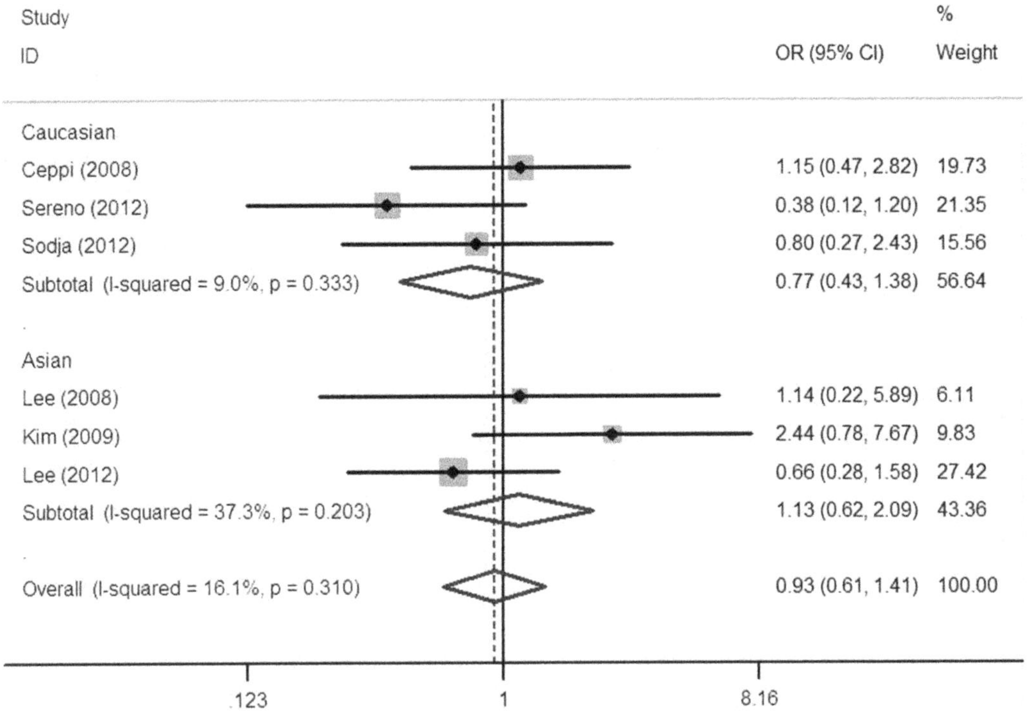

Figure 2. Forest plot for the association between ERCC1 level and objective response rate (ORR) in SCLC patients receiving platinum-based chemotherapy.

ERCC1 expression was not related to the ORR to platinum-based chemotherapy for SCLC patients both among Asian (OR = 1.13, 95%CI = 0.62–2.09, I^2 = 37.3%, P = 0.20 for heterogeneity) (Table 2) and Caucasian population (OR = 0.77, 95%CI = 0.43–1.38, I^2 = 9.0%, P = 0.33 for heterogeneity) (Table 2). Three studies focused on limited stage [21,32,35], Three studies focused on extensive stage [21,32,35]. Subgroup analysis on the basis of disease stage suggested that ERCC1 expression was not associated with the ORR to platinum-based chemotherapy in limited stage (OR = 1.66, 95%CI = 0.61–4.48, I^2 = 21.0%, P = 0.28 for heterogeneity) or extensive stage (OR = 0.67, 95%CI = 0.35–1.29, I^2 = 39.9%, P = 0.19 for heterogeneity). According to ERCC1 detection method, both IHC and RT-PCR groups did not show significant association between the expression of ERCC1 and the ORR in patients with SCLC (Table 2).

Overall survival

A total of eight studies [10,21–24,32,33,35] composed of 1053 patients reported the data on overall survival (OS). Overall, the pooled analysis showed that positive/high ERCC1 expression was significantly associated with shorter OS for SCLC patients receiving platinum-based chemotherapy (HR = 1.18, 95% CI = 1.02–1.37, I^2 = 19.8%, P = 0.27 for heterogeneity; Table 2, Figure 3). Of the eight studies reporting the data on OS, three studies [10,22,32] were conducted in Asian patients, four studies [21,24,33,35] were conducted in Caucasians and one study [23] was conducted in mixed ethnicity. In the stratified analysis according to ethnicity, our analysis indicated that ERCC1 expression was related to OS in Caucasian population (HR = 1.25, 95% CI = 1.01–1.53, I^2 = 0.0%, P = 0.41 for heterogeneity; Table 2), but not in Asian population (HR = 1.25, 95% CI = 0.96–1.63, I^2 = 47.4%, P = 0.13 for heterogeneity; Table 2). Five studies [10,21,24,32,35] focused on limited stage, Four studies [10,23,32,35] focused on extensive stage. Subgroup analysis based on disease stage suggested that the patients with positive/high ERCC1 expression would have shorter OS for limited stage (positive/high vs. negative/low: HR = 1.54, 95% CI = 1.21–1.96, I^2 = 38.2%, P = 0.17 for heterogeneity; Table 2, Figure 4), but not for extensive stage (positive/high vs. negative/low: HR = 0.96, 95% CI = 0.74–1.24, I^2 = 0.0%, P = 0.74 for heterogeneity; Table 2). We then focused on ERCC1 detection method, only two studies [21,24] using RT-PCR showed a significant association between the expression of ERCC1 and the OS in patients with SCLC (HR = 1.37, 95% CI = 1.06–1.78, I^2 = 0.0%, P = 0.74 for heterogeneity; Table 2).

Progression-free survival

The association of ERCC1 expression and PFS was explored in three studies [24,34,35] composed of 217 SCLC patients. The summarized analysis showed that positive/high ERCC1 expression was associated with unfavorable PFS for SCLC patients receiving platinum-based chemotherapy (HR = 1.46, 95% CI = 1.14–1.88, I^2 = 15.1%, P = 0.31 for heterogeneity; Table 2, Figure 5). In the stratified analysis according to disease stage, significant association between ERCC1 expression and PFS was found in limited stage (HR = 1.39, 95% CI = 1.01–1.91, I^2 = 0.0%, P = 0.55 for heterogeneity; Table 2), but not in extensive stage (HR = 1.02, 95% CI = 0.55–1.89; Table 2). The subgroup analysis of the ERCC1 detection methods indicated that the expression of ERCC1 was significantly associated with the PFS in the two studies [24,34] using RT-PCR as the detection method (HR = 1.63, 95% CI = 1.00–2.63, I^2 = 53.1%, P = 0.14 for heterogeneity; Table 2).

Table 2. Meta-analysis results about ERCC1 expression and ORR, OS and PFS in SCLC patients who received platinum-based chemotherapy.

	ORR				OS				PFS			
	Study (No. of patients)	Model	OR(95%CI)	I^2,P	Study (No. of patients)	Model	HR(95%CI)	I^2,P	Study (No. of patients)	Model	HR(95%CI)	I^2,P
Overall	6(533)	F	0.93(0.61–1.41)	16.1%,0.31	8(1053)	F	1.18(1.02–1.37)	19.8%,0.27	3(217)	F	1.46(1.14–1.88)	15.1%,0.31
Ethnicity												
Asian	3(318)	F	1.13(0.62–2.09)	37.3%,0.20	3(318)	F	1.25(0.96–1.63)	47.4%,0.13	/	/	/	/
Caucasian	3(215)	F	0.77(0.43–1.38)	9.0%,0.33	4(412)	F	1.25(1.01–1.53)	0%,0.41	/	/	/	/
Stage												
LS	3(106)	F	1.66(0.61–4.48)	21.0%,0.28	5(210)	F	1.54(1.21–1.96)	38.2%,0.17	2(96)	R	1.39(1.01–1.91)	0.0%,0.55
ES	3(167)	F	0.67(0.35–1.29)	39.9%,0.19	4(487)	F	0.96(0.74–1.24)	0.0%,0.74	1(45)	/	1.02(0.55–1.89)	/
Detection method												
IHC	4(395)	F	1.05(0.671,1.78)	11.7%,0.33	6(886)	F	1.10(0.91,1.31)	24.4%,0.24	1(77)	/	1.32(0.82.2.15)	/
RT-PCR	2(138)	R	0.71(0.24,2.05)	54.3%,0.139	2(167)	F	1.37(1.06,1.78)	0.0%,0.74	2(140)	R	1.63(1.00,2.63)	53.1%,0.14

Abbreviations: ERCC1, excision repair cross complementation group 1; **SCLC**, small cell lung cancer; **LS**, limited stage; **ES**, extensive stage; **R**, random model; **F**, fixed model; **ORR**, objective response rate; **OS**, overall survival; **PFS**, progression-free survival.

Sensitivity analysis

In the sensitivity analysis, the influence of each study on the pooled OR/HR was examined by repeating the meta-analysis while omitting each study one at a time. When the study by Karachaliou et al. [24] was excluded, the relationship between ERCC1 expression and OS in overall SCLC patients showed no significant association (HR = 1.14, 95% CI = 0.97–1.35, $I^2 = 24.7\%$, P = 0.23 for heterogeneity), indicating the study by Karachaliou et al.may affect the OS in overall patients. Except for OS, the analysis results suggested that no individual study significantly affected the pooled OR/HR in ORR and PFS.

Publication bias

Visual inspection of the funnel plot did not show any evidence of obvious asymmetry in three comparisons (figure not shown). Also, no significant bias was indicated by the Begg's and Egger's test (ORR: $P_{Begg} = 0.71$, $P_{Egger} = 0.78$; OS: $P_{Begg} = 0.05$, $P_{Egger} = 0.14$; PFS: $P_{Begg} = 0.30$, $P_{Egger} = 0.44$).

Discussion

In the present meta-analysis, our analysis indicated that SCLC patients with positive/high ERCC1 expression were significantly associated with shorter OS and PFS, especially in LS-SCLC. Hoverer, no significant association between ERCC1 expression and ORR was observed.

Previous meta-analysis by Hubner et al. [36] has reported that ERCC1 expression was not associated with OS for SCLC patients receiving platinum-based chemotherapy. In the stratified analysis according to stage, they found ERCC1 expression was associated with OS in LS-SCLC, but not in ES-SCLC. In the present study, we observed that positive/high ERCC1 expression was related to shorter OS and PFS. In subgroup analysis by stage, we found high/positive ERCC1 was associated with worse OS and PFS in LS-SCLC, but not in ES-SCLC. We think it is necessary to update the meta-analysis and make a more comprehensive estimation of the association between ERCC1 expression and the efficacy of platinum-based chemotherapy for the following reasons. Firstly, compared with the study by Hubner et al., which containing 292 patients from five studies, our analysis included larger sample size of 1129 patients from 9 studies, with which the reliability was largely enhanced. Besides, Hubner et al only evaluated the relationship between ERCC1 expression and OS; in the present analysis, we employed ORR, OS and PFS as primary parameters to comprehensively examine the relationship between ERCC1 expression and clinical outcomes of platinum-based chemotherapy. As we all know, a low ORR indicates tumor resistance to the chemotherapeutic regimen and a short OS and PFS suggest a poor prognosis. Thus, including all three parameters could make a comprehensive assessment. However, our analysis did not find the significant association between ERCC1 expression and ORR.

The weight of the study by Karachaliou et al. [24] is considerable in figures 3(21.25%), 4 (56.92%) and 5(54.83%). We think three possible reasons should be acknowledged. First of all, the sample size is relatively larger. A total of 64 LS-SCLC patients were included. In the comparison of OS in LS-SCLC (figure 4), and PFS in overall patients (figure 5), the patients' number in this study account for 30.5% and 29.5% in overall patients, respectively. Secondly, the study by Karachaliou et al is highly homogeneous. All included samples were LS-SCLC, they all received first line cisplatin-etoposide doublet. In other studies, most of studies received all kinds of platinum-based doublets and may be biased by imbalances between studies regarding fist-, second- and later-lines of treatment. At last, the HRs we obtained

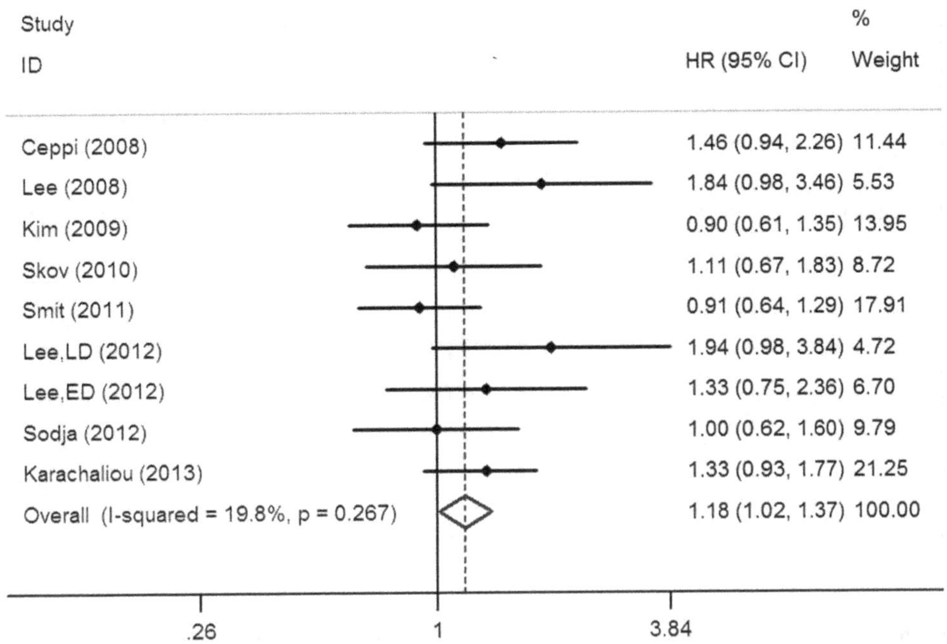

Figure 3. Forest plot for the association between ERCC1 level and overall survival (OS) in SCLC patients receiving platinum-based chemotherapy.

from this study were multivariate-adjusted results. In the sensitivity analysis, when the study by Karachaliou et al was removed in each comparison, except for the overall OS, the HR for OS in LS-SCLC and the overall PFS did not changed (for overall OS, HR = 1.14, 95% CI = 0.97–1.35; for OS in LS-SCLC, HR = 1.87, 95% CI = 1.29–2.71; for overall PFS, HR = 1.63, 95% CI = 1.12–2.36, respectively). As many study found the ERCC1 expression was more likely to be a prognostic factor in limited stage-SCLC, it was not surprise that the HR in overall OS was not significant when the study by Karachaliou et al (all included samples were LS-SCLC) was removed. Generally, the result of our study was stable and reliable.

Why the significant association between positive/high ERCC1 expression and shorter OS and PFS was mainly found in patients with LS-SCLC? Firstly, the possibility is that disease progression from the limited to the extensive stage leads to a potential transcriptional deregulation of ERCC1 for SCLC patients [21]. In the study by Kang et al., who found when compared with primary

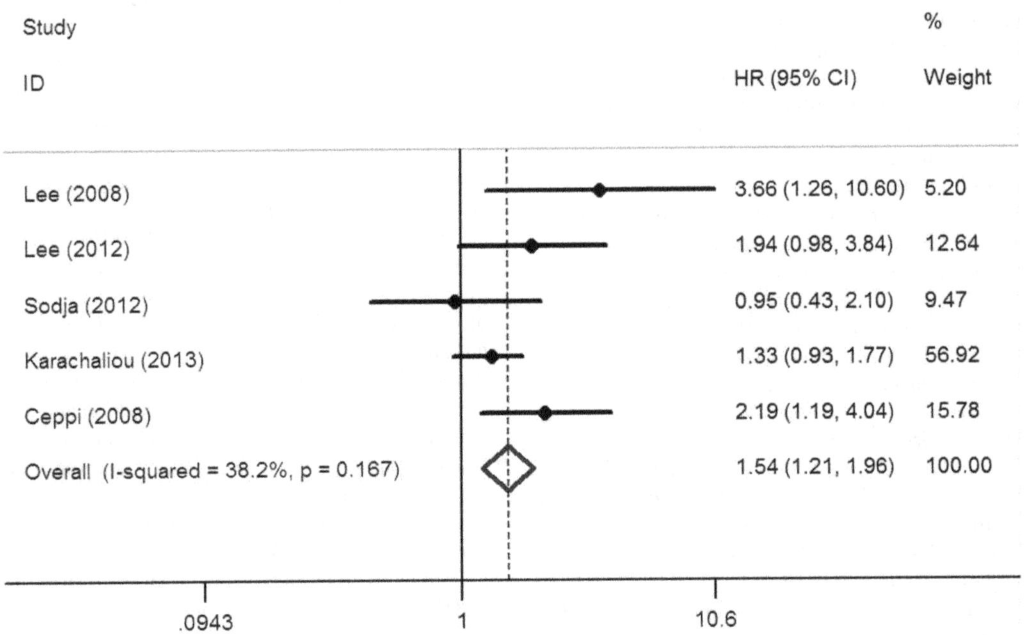

Figure 4. Forest plot for the association between ERCC1 level and overall survival (OS) in LS-SCLC patients receiving platinum-based chemotherapy.

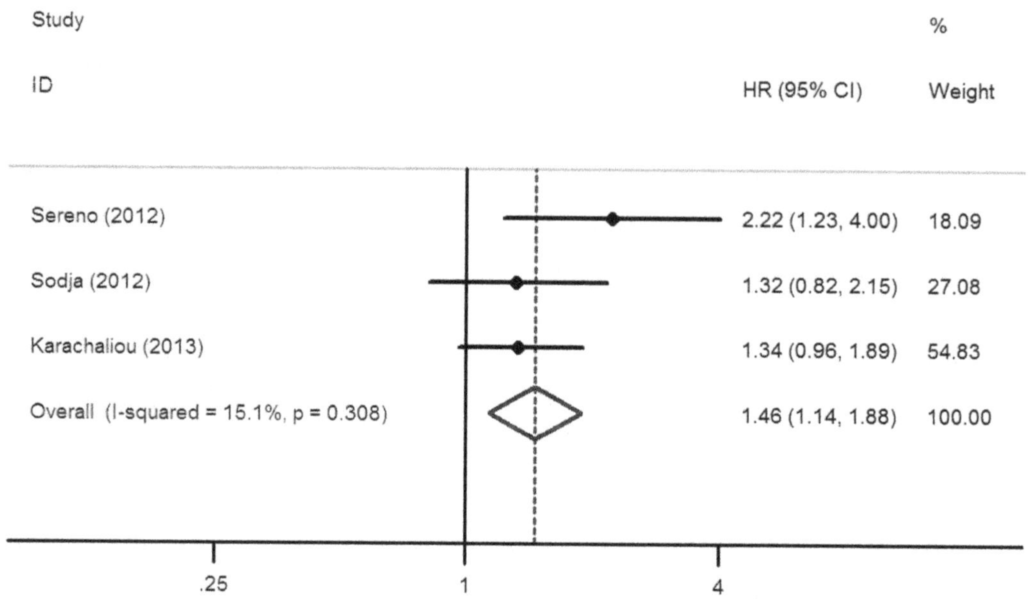

Figure 5. Forest plot for the association between ERCC1 level and progression free survival (PFS) in SCLC patients receiving platinum-based chemotherapy.

tumors in NSCLC, ERCC1 expression was upregulated in metastatic lymph nodes [37]. Besides, the expression of ERCC1 would be induced by platinum. In human lung adenocarcinoma cell line A549, up-regulation of ERCC1 expression could be induced by low-dose cisplatin [38]; in metastatic colorectal cancer, after oxaliplatin-based first-line chemotherapy, ERCC1 expression was upregulatedin [39]. Also, the standard treatment for patients with LS-SCLC is a combination of concurrent thoracic irradiation and chemotherapy with etoposide and cisplatin whereas for patients with ES-SCLC, chemotherapy is the main method. ERCC1 is related to radiation-induced DNA damage in a few in-vitro studies, although the mechanism is not well known [40,41]. Thus, this could probably be the consequence of expression levels up-regulation resulting in radiotherapy. At last, patients with high expression of ERCC1 might benefit from alternative strategies such as incorporation of different sequencing of chemoradiotherapy and new chemotherapeutic agents [3–5], which may lead to false positive. However, the specific regulatory mechanism need to be further investigated in the future.

It was meaningful to identify more efficacy biomarkers for SCLC, especially for ES-SCLC. Many biomarkers have been evaluated, for example, multidrug resistance-associated proteins such as multidrug resistance protein 1 (P-glycoprotein; MDR1), multidrug resistance-associated protein1 (MRP1) and 2 (MRP2), major vault protein (MVP), topoisomerases II (topo II) [42], and serum markers such as lactate dehydrogenase (LDH), neuron-specific enolase (NSE) [43]and so on. Nowadays, circulating tumour cells (CTCs) has also emerged as a potential predictive and prognostic factor for SCLC [44]. As the predictive and prognostic role of a single biomarker is limited, to detect more relevant biomarkers as a combination would be more efficient.

However, a clinical value of the findings obtained by our meta-analysis remains questionable. Friboulet L. et al. was unable to validate the predictive effect of immunostaining for ERCC1 protein by three independent trails [IALT, Cancer and Leukemia Group B (CALGB) 9633, and National Cancer Institute of Canada Clinical Trials Group JBR.10 trials] [45]. This may have arisen from assessment of ERCC1 expression in clinical samples is complicated by the existence of 4 functionally distinct protein isoforms (201, 202, 203, and 204); on the other hand, current available antibodies used to evaluate ERCC1 expression do not have adequate discrimination. In our study, the included studies detected ERCC1 by different method: three studies detected ERCC1 expression in transcriptional level by RT-PCR, and six studies determined at protein level by IHC. In addition, the detecting tools and the cutoff values for ERCC1 expression were different from each other. Friboulet's study also supported the evidence that the ERCC1-202 isoform is the sole one endowed with ERCC1 activity in DNA repair pathways and might support as an accurate predictor of cisplatin benefit in patients with NSCLC [45]. Further studies were wanted to elucidate the predict role of ERCC1-202 isoform in platinum-based chemotherapy.

Several limitations should be addressed when interpreting the result of our meta-analysis. First, the individual studies included in our study differed obviously in the study design, such as ERCC1 detection method, patient selection and chemotherapeutic protocols. Our meta-analysis may be biased by sex, age, smoking status, different detection method for ERCC1, specific platinum-based drug employed (e.g., cisplatin, carboplatin, or oxaliplatin), and the imbalances between studies regarding fist-, second- and later-lines of treatment, which could influence the homogeneity among the individual studies. Secondly, apart from the chemotherapy, some studies also had surgery or radiotherapy, while the others did not have the therapy. Thirdly, due to lack of sufficient data regarding confounding factors, such as sex, age and smoking status from the original studies, we did not perform stratified analysis to evaluate the effects of these confounding factors on the predictive effect of ERCC1 for SCLC patients. Besides, the sample size in our analysis was not large enough. Only six studies including 533 patients investigated the relationship between ERCC1 expression and ORR, and three studies including 217 patients evaluated the PFS, such limited sample size still could not draw a robust conclusion and need to be interpreted with caution, Finally, potential publication bias may remain because the databases we searched and resources we processed were limited and the publications written not in English or with negative results which failed to be published were failed to be included in the present analysis.

In conclusion, this meta-analysis provided the evidence that SCLC patients with positive/high ERCC1 would have worse OS and PFS, especially in patients with LS-SCLC. Therefore, ERCC1 might act as a valuable marker of prognosis in patients with SCLC treated by platinum-based chemotherapy. However, considering the limitations and confounds of the present study, our conclusions need to be interpreted with caution. Large prospective studies with strict designed methodology are warranted to further investigated the prognostic role of ERCC1 in SCLC patients receiving platinum-based treatment.

Supporting Information

Figure S1 PRISMA flow diagram.

Table S1 Quality assessment of eligible studies with Newcastle-Ottawa Scale.

Checklist S1 PRISMA checklist.

Author Contributions

Conceived and designed the experiments: YY XL LX. Performed the experiments: YY XL. Analyzed the data: YY XL NY RF. Contributed reagents/materials/analysis tools: LX. Wrote the paper: YY XL NY LX. Involved in revising the manuscript critically for important intellectual content: NY.

References

1. Jemal A, Siegel R, Xu J, Ward E (2010) Cancer statistics, 2010. CA Cancer J Clin 60: 277–300.
2. Jemal A, Bary F, Center MM, Ferlay J, Ward E, et al. (2011) Global cancer statistics. CA Cancer J Clin 61: 69–90.
3. Jackman DM, Johnson BE (2005) Small-cell lung cancer. Lancet 366: 1385–1396.
4. Sandler AB (2003) Chemotherapy for small cell lung cancer. Semin Oncol 30: 9–25.
5. Spira A, Ettinger DS (2004) Multidisciplinary management of lung cancer. N Engl J Med 350: 379–392.
6. Shin HR, Jung KW, Won YJ, Park JG (2004) 2002 annual report of the Korea Central Cancer Registry: based on registered data from 139 hospitals. Cancer Res Treat 36: 103–114.
7. Govindan R, Page N, Morgensztern D, Read W, Tierney R, et al. (2006) Changing epidemiology of small-cell lung cancer in the United States over the last 30 years: analysis of the surveillance, epidemiologic, and end results database. J Clin Oncol 24: 4539–4544.
8. Thatcher N, Faivre-Finn C, Lorigan P (2005) Management of small-cell lung cancer. Ann Oncol 16 Suppl 2: ii235–239.
9. Jemal A, Siegel R, Ward E, Murray T, Xu J, et al. (2007) Cancer statistics, 2007. CA Cancer J Clin 57: 43–66.
10. Lee HW, Han JH, Kim JH, Lee MH, Jeong SH, et al. (2008) Expression of excision repair cross-complementation group 1 protein predicts poor outcome in patients with small cell lung cancer. Lung Cancer 59: 95–104.
11. de Laat WL, Jaspers NG, Hoeijmakers JH (1999) Molecular mechanism of nucleotide excision repair. Genes Dev 13: 768–785.
12. Kwon HC, Roh MS, Oh SY, Kim SH, Kim MC, et al. (2007) Prognostic value of expression of ERCC1, thymidylate synthase, and glutathione S-transferase P1 for 5-fluorouracil/oxaliplatin chemotherapy in advanced gastric cancer. Ann Oncol 18: 504–509.
13. Kawashima A, Nakayama M, Kakuta Y, Abe T, Hatano K, et al. (2011) Excision repair cross-complementing group 1 may predict the efficacy of chemoradiation therapy for muscle-invasive bladder cancer. Clin Cancer Res 17: 2561–2569.
14. Scheil-Bertram S, Tylus-Schaaf P, du Bois A, Harter P, Oppitz M, et al. (2010) Excision repair cross-complementation group 1 protein overexpression as a predictor of poor survival for high-grade serous ovarian adenocarcinoma. Gynecol Oncol 119: 325–331.
15. Kim SH, Kwon HC, Oh SY, Lee DM, Lee S, et al. (2009) Prognostic value of ERCC1, thymidylate synthase, and glutathione S-transferase pi for 5-FU/oxaliplatin chemotherapy in advanced colorectal cancer. Am J Clin Oncol 32: 38–43.
16. Bellmunt J, Paz-Ares L, Cuello M, Cecere FL, Albiol S, et al. (2007) Gene expression of ERCC1 as a novel prognostic marker in advanced bladder cancer patients receiving cisplatin-based chemotherapy. Ann Oncol 18: 522–528.
17. Joshi MB, Shirota Y, Danenberg KD, Conlon DH, Salonga DS, et al. (2005) High gene expression of TS1, GSTP1, and ERCC1 are risk factors for survival in patients treated with trimodality therapy for esophageal cancer. Clin Cancer Res 11: 2215–2221.
18. Kim MK, Cho KJ, Kwon GY, Park SI, Kim YH, et al. (2008) ERCC1 predicting chemoradiation resistance and poor outcome in oesophageal cancer. Eur J Cancer 44: 54–60.
19. Simon GR, Sharma S, Cantor A, Smith P, Bepler G (2005) ERCC1 expression is a predictor of survival in resected patients with non-small cell lung cancer. Chest 127: 978–983.
20. Cobo M, Isla D, Massuti B, Montes A, Sanchez JM, et al. (2007) Customizing cisplatin based on quantitative excision repair cross-complementing 1 mRNA expression: a phase III trial in non-small-cell lung cancer. J Clin Oncol 25: 2747–2754.
21. Ceppi P, Longo M, Volante M, Novello S, Cappia S, et al. (2008) Excision repair cross complementing-1 and topoisomerase IIalpha gene expression in small-cell lung cancer patients treated with platinum and etoposide: a retrospective study. J Thorac Oncol 3: 583–589.
22. Kim YH, Ishii G, Goto K, Ota S, Kubota K, et al. (2009) Expression of breast cancer resistance protein is associated with a poor clinical outcome in patients with small-cell lung cancer. Lung Cancer 65: 105–111.
23. Smit EF, Socinski MA, Mullaney BP, Myrand SP, Scagliotti GV, et al. (2012) Biomarker analysis in a phase III study of pemetrexed-carboplatin versus etoposide-carboplatin in chemonaive patients with extensive-stage small-cell lung cancer. Ann Oncol 23: 1723–1729.
24. Karachaliou N, Papadaki C, Lagoudaki E, Trypaki M, Sfakianaki M, et al. (2013) Predictive value of BRCA1, ERCC1, ATP7B, PKM2, TOPOI, TOPOmicron-IIA, TOPOIIB and C-MYC genes in patients with small cell lung cancer (SCLC) who received first line therapy with cisplatin and etoposide. PLoS One 8: e74611.
25. Wells GA, Shea B, O'Connell D, Peterson J, Welch V, et al. (2003) The Newcastle–Ottawa Scale (NOS) for assessing the quality of nonrandomised studies in meta-analyses. Available: http://wwwohrica/programs/clinicalepidemiology/oxfordasp. Accessed 2013 May 5
26. Tierney JF, Stewart LA, Ghersi D, Burdett S, Sydes MR (2007) Practical methods for incorporating summary time-to-event data into meta-analysis. Trials 8: 16.
27. Higgins JP, Thompson SG, Deeks JJ, Altman DG (2003) Measuring inconsistency in meta-analyses. BMJ 327: 557–560.
28. DerSimonian R, Laird N (1986) Meta-analysis in clinical trials. Control Clin Trials 7: 177–188.
29. Mantel N, Haenszel W (1959) Statistical aspects of the analysis of data from retrospective studies of disease. J Natl Cancer Inst 22: 719–748.
30. Begg CB, Mazumdar M (1994) Operating characteristics of a rank correlation test for publication bias. Biometrics 50: 1088–1101.
31. Egger M, Davey Smith G, Schneider M, Minder C (1997) Bias in meta-analysis detected by a simple, graphical test. BMJ 315: 629–634.
32. Lee GW, Go SI, Cho YJ, Jeong YY, Kim HC, et al. (2012) Hypoxia-inducible factor-1alpha and excision repair cross-complementing 1 in patients with small cell lung cancer who received front-line platinum-based chemotherapy: a retrospective study. J Thorac Oncol 7: 528–534.
33. Skov BG, Holm B, Erreboe A, Skov T, Mellemgaard A (2010) ERCC1 and Ki67 in small cell lung carcinoma and other neuroendocrine tumors of the lung: distribution and impact on survival. J Thorac Oncol 5: 453–459.
34. Sereno M, Cejas P, Moreno V, Belda-Iniesta C, Lopez R, et al. (2012) ERCC1 and topoisomerase I expression in small cell lung cancer: prognostic and predictive implications. Int J Oncol 40: 2104–2110.
35. Sodja E, Knez L, Kern I, Ovcaricek T, Sadikov A, et al. (2012) Impact of ERCC1 expression on treatment outcome in small-cell lung cancer patients treated with platinum-based chemotherapy. Eur J Cancer 48: 3378–3385.
36. Hubner RA, Riley RD, Billingham LJ, Popat S (2011) Excision repair cross-complementation group 1 (ERCC1) status and lung cancer outcomes: a meta-analysis of published studies and recommendations. PLoS One 6: e25164.
37. Kang CH, Jang BG, Kim DW, Chung DH, Kim YT, et al. (2009) Differences in the expression profiles of excision repair crosscomplementation group 1, x-ray repair crosscomplementation group 1, and betaIII-tubulin between primary non-small cell lung cancer and metastatic lymph nodes and the significance in mid-term survival. J Thorac Oncol 4: 1307–1312.
38. Xia Y, Hu C, Zhang M, Yang H, Zhou D, et al. (2007) [Relationship between ERCC1 expression and cisplatin intervention in human lung adenocarcinoma cell lines]. Zhongguo Fei Ai Za Zhi 10: 362–365.

39. Baba H, Watanabe M, Okabe H, Miyamoto Y, Sakamoto Y, et al. (2012) Upregulation of ERCC1 and DPD expressions after oxaliplatin-based first-line chemotherapy for metastatic colorectal cancer. Br J Cancer 107: 1950–1955.
40. Murray D, Rosenberg E (1996) The importance of the ERCC1/ERCC4[XPF] complex for hypoxic-cell radioresistance does not appear to derive from its participation in the nucleotide excision repair pathway. Mutat Res 364: 217–226.
41. Murray D, Vallee-Lucic L, Rosenberg E, Andersson B (2002) Sensitivity of nucleotide excision repair-deficient human cells to ionizing radiation and cyclophosphamide. Anticancer Res 22: 21–26.
42. Knez L, Sodja E, Kern I, Kosnik M, Cufer T (2011) Predictive value of multidrug resistance proteins, topoisomerases II and ERCC1 in small cell lung cancer: a systematic review. Lung Cancer 72: 271–279.
43. Wang X, Jiang R, Li K (2014) Prognostic significance of pretreatment laboratory parameters in combined small-cell lung cancer. Cell Biochem Biophys 69: 633–640.
44. Normanno N, Rossi A, Morabito A, Signoriello S, Bevilacqua S, et al. (2014) Prognostic value of circulating tumor cells' reduction in patients with extensive small-cell lung cancer. Lung Cancer 85: 314–319.
45. Friboulet L, Olaussen KA, Pignon JP, Shepherd FA, Tsao MS, et al. (2013) ERCC1 isoform expression and DNA repair in non-small-cell lung cancer. N Engl J Med 368: 1101–1110.

24

Tissue MicroRNAs as Predictors of Outcome in Patients with Metastatic Colorectal Cancer Treated with First Line Capecitabine and Oxaliplatin with or without Bevacizumab

Mogens K. Boisen[1]*, Christian Dehlendorff[2], Dorte Linnemann[3], Boye S. Nielsen[4], Jim S. Larsen[5], Kell Østerlind[6], Svend E. Nielsen[7], Line S. Tarpgaard[8], Camilla Qvortrup[8], Per Pfeiffer[8], Niels H. Holländer[9], Nina Keldsen[10], Torben F. Hansen[11], Brita B. Jensen[12,13], Estrid V. S. Høgdall[3], Benny V. Jensen[1], Julia S. Johansen[1,14]

1 Department of Oncology, Herlev University Hospital, Herlev, Denmark, **2** Statistics, Bioinformatics and Registry, Danish Cancer Society Research Center, Copenhagen, Denmark, **3** Department of Pathology, Herlev University Hospital, Herlev, Denmark, **4** Bioneer, Hørsholm, Denmark, **5** Department of Oncology, Roskilde Hospital, Roskilde, Denmark, **6** Department of Oncology, Rigshospitalet, Copenhagen, Denmark, **7** Department of Oncology and Palliation, Hillerød Hospital, Hillerød, Denmark, **8** Department of Oncology, Odense University Hospital, Odense, Denmark, **9** Department of Oncology, Næstved Hospital, Næstved, Denmark, **10** Department of Oncology, Herning Hospital, Herning, Denmark, **11** Department of Oncology, Vejle Hospital, Vejle, Denmark, **12** Department of Medicine, Queen Ingrid Hospital, Nuuk, Greenland, **13** Department of Oncology, Sydvestjysk Hospital, Esbjerg, Denmark, **14** Department of Medicine, Herlev University Hospital, Herlev, Denmark

Abstract

Purpose: We tested the hypothesis that expression of microRNAs (miRNAs) in cancer tissue can predict effectiveness of bevacizumab added to capecitabine and oxaliplatin (CAPEOX) in patients with metastatic colorectal cancer (mCRC).

Experimental Design: Patients with mCRC treated with first line CAPEOX and bevacizumab (CAPEOXBEV): screening (n = 212) and validation (n = 121) cohorts, or CAPEOX alone: control cohort (n = 127), were identified retrospectively and archival primary tumor samples were collected. Expression of 754 miRNAs was analyzed in the screening cohort using polymerase chain reaction (PCR) arrays and expression levels were related to time to disease progression (TTP) and overall survival (OS). Significant miRNAs from the screening study were analyzed in all three cohorts using custom PCR arrays. *In situ* hybridization (ISH) was done for selected miRNAs.

Results: In the screening study, 26 miRNAs were significantly correlated with outcome in multivariate analyses. Twenty-two miRNAs were selected for further study. Higher miR-664-3p expression and lower miR-455-5p expression were predictive of improved outcome in the CAPEOXBEV cohorts and showed a significant interaction with bevacizumab effectiveness. The effects were strongest for OS. Both miRNAs showed high expression in stromal cells. Higher expression of miR-196b-5p and miR-592 predicted improved outcome regardless of bevacizumab treatment, with similar effect estimates in all three cohorts.

Conclusions: We have identified potentially predictive miRNAs for bevacizumab effectiveness and additional miRNAs that could be related to chemotherapy effectiveness or prognosis in patients with mCRC. Our findings need further validation in large cohorts, preferably from completed randomized trials.

Editor: Ratna B. Ray, Saint Louis University, United States of America

Funding: This study was supported by an unrestricted grant from Roche Denmark (www.roche.dk), the Herlev Hospital Research Foundation (www.herlevhospital.dk), and a proof-of-concept grant from the Technical University of Denmark (www.dtu.dk). All grants were given to MKB alone, or to both MKB and JSJ. The funders had no role in study design, data collection and analysis, decision to publish, or preparation of the manuscript.

Competing Interests: The authors have read the journal's policy and the authors of this manuscript have the following competing interests: BVJ: Roche, consultant/advisory role; SEN: Roche, consultant/advisory role; PP: Roche, consultant/advisory role; JSJ: Roche, honoraria and research funding; MKB: Roche, research funding. JSJ and MKB are co-inventors on a patent-application related to the mentioned miRNAs. Patent application info: Name "Micrornas for prediction of treatment efficacy and prognosis of cancer patients"; Application number "PCT/DK2013/050015". BSN is employed by a commercial company (Bioneer).

* Email: mogens.karsboel.boisen@regionh.dk

Introduction

Colorectal cancer (CRC) is a leading cause of cancer-related mortality worldwide [1]. Most deaths occur as a result of the development of metastatic CRC (mCRC). Standard of care for patients with mCRC who cannot undergo radical resection of metastases is system chemotherapy with or without a targeted agent [2]. Bevacizumab is a monoclonal antibody that binds the ligand 'vascular endothelial growth factor' (VEGF-A) and thereby inhibits the ability of cancers to produce new blood vessels from existing vessels, a process called angiogenesis. Bevacizumab has demonstrated efficacy in patients with mCRC when used in combination with standard chemotherapy but the benefit is modest when used unselectively and bevacizumab adds significant toxicity and cost to the treatment [3–7]. Therefore, the identification of predictive biomarkers for bevacizumab has become a major goal of biomarker research in patients with mCRC. Due to its widespread adoption as a standard first- or second line treatment [8], the ability to individualize bevacizumab treatment would have a great impact on clinical practice. Numerous studies have investigated potential biomarkers in the form of RNA, DNA, or protein [9,10]. None has made it into the clinic. Currently, no commercially available test can identify patients who will benefit from bevacizumab.

MicroRNAs (miRNAs) are small, ~22 nucleotides long, non-coding RNAs involved in post-transcriptional regulation of gene expression. They have been intensely investigated as biomarkers in patients with cancer because their expression levels are dysregulated in cancer cells, they can influence cancer behavior, and they are relatively resistant to degradation in commonly used sampling media [11–16]. Several studies have identified dysregulation of miRNAs in CRC tumor tissue and in blood samples from patients with CRC; and some of the identified miRNAs were also associated with prognostic factors like depth of invasion, stage, and lymph node metastases [17]. Furthermore, important molecular features in CRC such as micro-satellite instability (MSI) and *BRAF* mutational status have been shown to be associated with distinct miRNA expression patterns [18]. Hence, there is a strong rationale for investigating the potential utility of miRNA expression as a predictive or prognostic biomarker in patients with CRC. To date, no published study has explored the predictive value of miRNA expression for bevacizumab effectiveness in a comprehensive manner.

We aimed to identify miRNAs that were predictive of outcome in patients with mCRC treated with first line capecitabine and oxaliplatin with and without bevacizumab (CAPEOXBEV/CAPEOX) and to identify which of these miRNAs could be predictive for the effect of bevacizumab-addition to chemotherapy.

Methods

Study design

A screening study using an array approach was performed on primary CRC tissue samples from patients treated with CAPEOXBEV (screening cohort) to identify candidate miRNAs with expression levels related to outcome. Thereafter, the expression levels of the identified candidate miRNAs were measured using a more precise method with duplicate determinations in three cohorts: a subgroup of the screening cohort; a validation cohort, which was an independent group of patients treated with CAPEOXBEV; and a control cohort, consisting of patients treated with CAPEOX alone.

Patients, data extraction, and end points

The BETmiRC (Bevacizumab Tissue microRNAs in Colorectal cancer) study retrospectively included patients with mCRC treated with first line CAPEOXBEV in 10 Danish hospitals from 2006 to 2011,and patients treated with first line CAPEOX at Herlev Hospital or in a randomized study from 2003 to 2006 [19], before bevacizumab was approved, as previously described [20].The end points time to disease progression (TTP) and overall survival (OS) were measured from initiation of treatment to disease progression or death from any cause, respectively (detailed definition in File S1). Vital status was updated July 5, 2013.

Tissue samples

Formalin-fixed paraffin-embedded (FFPE) tissue blocks containing samples from primary tumors were retrieved using the National Pathology Registry. Control samples from patients resected for inflammatory bowel disease were also included. An experienced gastro-intestinal pathologist (DL) selected which tissue blocks to retrieve and scored the blocks for tumor cell percentage. Three 10-µm sections were cut from each block without micro- or macro-dissection and the sections were placed in sterile Eppendorf tubes. All tissue samples were collected prior to any systemic treatment or radiotherapy.

MiRNA expression analysis

RNA was purified using the miRNeasy FFPE Kit (Qiagen, Hilden, Germany) using the manufacturer's instructions. The purification order was randomized for the validation and control cohort samples. The non-human miRNA ath-miR-159a was added to each sample before cDNA synthesis as a spike-in control.

The TaqMan Human MicroRNA array A and B Cards Set v3.0 (Applied Biosystems) was used to quantify expression of 754 human miRNAs with single determinations in the screening study. In the subsequent study of the reduced screening-, validation-, and control cohorts, miRNA expression was measured using TaqMan Custom LDA cards (Applied Biosystems) profiling 22 selected miRNAs in duplicate with 8 samples on each card. The 22 miRNAs were selected from the screening study and the micro-fluidic cards were pre-configured from the manufacturer according to our specifications. Samples were analyzed in a randomized order on the Custom LDA cards.

The instructions and reagents from the manufacturer were used in all steps (https://www.products.appliedbiosystems.com). All RNA purification- and miRNA expression studies were performed by AROS Applied Biotechnology (Aarhus, Denmark). The company was blinded to all clinical information.

MiRNA *in situ* hybridization

In situ hybridization (ISH) was performed using double-FAM (carboxyfluorescein) labeled locked nucleic acid (LNA [21]) probes (Exiqon, Vedbæk, Denmark) for miR-185-5p, miR-455-5p, miR-592, miR-664-3p, miR-21-5p, and miR-126-3p, as previously described [22]. All ISH studies were performed by Bioneer (Hørsholm, Denmark).

Statistical analysis

No sample size calculation was done prior to study initiation. We aimed for the greatest sample size possible and equal sizes of the three cohorts.

MiRNA expression analyses – screening study. Raw cycle threshold (C_t) for each miRNA was checked for outliers and data were corrected using spike-in values. In a univariate selection method, the expression of each miRNA was related to TTP and

Table 1. Patient and sample characteristics.

	Clinical CAPEOXBEV cohort	Clinical CAPEOX cohort	Screening cohort (LDA A+B card)	Screening cohort (cLDA)	Validation cohort (cLDA)	CAPEOXBEV included vs. not-included *P*	CAPEOX cohort (cLDA)	CAPEOX included vs. not-included *P*
Treatment start years, range	2006–2011	2003–2006	2006–2010	2006–2010	2007–2011		2003–2006	
Number of patients	623	211	203	155	121		127	
Age, median (range)	65 (22–84)	63 (36–85)	65 (37–84)	65 (40–84)	67 (22–82)	0.27	62 (36–82)	0.24
Sex, female (%)	281 (45%)	77 (36%)	111 (55%)	83 (54%)	40 (33%)	0.75	45 (35%)	0.66
Primary tumor location						0.15		0.45
Cecum, ascending colon	133 (21%)	37 (18%)	52 (26%)	38 (25%)	23 (19%)		26 (20%)	
Right flexure, transverse colon	60 (10%)	16 (8%)	15 (7%)	11 (7%)	7 (6%)		8 (6%)	
Left flexure, descending colon	33 (5%)	12 (6%)	9 (4%)	6 (4%)	7 (6%)		9 (7%)	
Sigmoid colon	192 (31%)	62 (29%)	70 (34%)	56 (36%)	38 (31%)		37 (29%)	
Rectum	205 (33%)	84 (40%)	57 (28%)	44 (28%)	46 (38%)		47 (37%)	
Primary tumor resected	319 (51%)	157 (74%)	186 (92%)	148 (95%)	84 (69%)	**<0.0001**	116 (91%)	**<0.0001**
Number of metastatic sites						**0.004**		1.00
1	198 (32%)	71 (34%)	74 (36%)	63 (41%)	42 (35%)		42 (33%)	
>1	425 (68%)	140 (66%)	129 (64%)	92 (59%)	79 (65%)		85 (67%)	
No. of first line cycles, median (range)	7 (1–46)	6 (1–16)*	7 (1–46)	7 (1–46)	7 (1–23)	0.25	6 (1–15)*	0.92
Treated with irinotecan	357 (58%)*	105 (64%)*	117 (58%)	95 (61%)	76 (63%)	0.05	64 (72%)	0.29
Performance status						**0.04**		0.32
0	260 (61%)	81 (50%)	93 (61%)	75 (65%)	60 (71%)		48 (48%)	
1	138 (32%)	66 (41%)	52 (34%)	37 (32%)	19 (22%)		39 (39%)	
≥2	27 (6%)	15 (9%)	8 (5%)	3 (3%)	6 (7%)		12 (12%)	
Missing	198	49	50	40	36		28	
Prior adjuvant treatment, no. (%)	57 (9%)	37 (18%)	28 (14%)	22 (14%)	13 (11%)	**0.008**	26 (20%)	0.20
TTP events				130 (84%)	98 (81%)		115 (91%)	
Median time to disease progression	8.6 mo	7.6 mo	9.2 mo	9.5 mo	8.3 mo	**0.04**	8.4 mo	0.27
OS events				130 (84%)	93 (77%)		125 (98%)	
Median overall survival	16.1 mo	15.2 mo	19.0 mo	25.0 mo	21.9 mo	**<0.0001**	16.4 mo	0.12
Sample type								
Resection	–	–	–	146 (94%)	83 (69%)		115 (91%)	
Biopsy	–	–	–	9 (6%)	38 (31%)		12 (9%)	
Tumor cell percentage, median (range)	–	–	–	30 (2–70)	30 (5–70)		30 (5–70)	

Table 1. Cont.

	Clinical CAPEOXBEV cohort	Clinical CAPEOX cohort	Screening cohort (LDA A+B card)	Screening cohort (cLDA)	Validation cohort (cLDA)	CAPEOXBEV included vs. not-included	CAPEOX cohort (cLDA)	CAPEOX included vs. not-included
						P		*P*
cLDA mean C_t, median (1/3. quartile)	–	–	–	19.9 (19.5/20.9)	20.8 (20.0/22.0)		20.7 (20.3/21.7)	

* Data were missing for some patients; ranges and percentages are based on the patients with available data.

OS using a Cox proportional hazards (CPH) model [23,24]. Candidate miRNAs were included in a multivariate CPH model adjusted for age, sex, histology, number of metastatic sites, primary tumor location, and prior adjuvant treatment, which was simplified using a backwards elimination procedure based upon Akaike's Information Criterion [25]. The analysis was then repeated for data sets normalized using quantile- and mean normalization. Finally, 22 miRNAs were selected for further study based primarily on their performance in the multivariate analyses. The number of miRNAs to include in the second study was chosen pragmatically as it allowed for duplicate measurements on the custom platform.

MiRNA expression analyses – screening-, validation-, and control cohorts. Mean C_t of the duplicate measurements was calculated and transformed to 40-C_t. If one of the two measurements was undetermined, the C_t of the other measurement was used. In each of the three cohorts, expression of the 22 miRNAs was related to TTP and OS using CPH models with adjustment for age, sex, primary tumor location, prior adjuvant treatment, and number of metastatic sites. Results were reported as hazard ratios (HR) per inter-quartile range increase in expression level with 95% confidence intervals (CI).The possible interaction between miRNA expression level and bevacizumab treatment effect was tested in the three cohorts combined using a likelihood ratio test.

Since outcome for the patients treated with bevacizumab differed greatly depending on primary tumor location [20], we also performed the interaction analyses for proximal and distal primary cancers separately.

$P<0.05$ was considered statistically significant and no formal corrections for multiple comparisons were made. The statistical software packages R [26] (www.r-project.org) and GraphPad Prism 5 (GraphPad Software, Inc) were used for all analyses.

Target prediction

In silico predicted gene targets for selected miRNAs were identified using the open-access DIANA-microT-CDS tool (http://www.microrna.gr/microT-CDS) [27].

Ethics

The study was approved by the Regional Scientific Ethics Committee of the Capital Region of Denmark (http://www.regionh.dk/vek, approval number: H-1-2010-081). Since this retrospective study would not have any influence on treatment and since most of the participants were deceased, written consent was not obtained, and this was approved by the ethics committee.

Reporting of the results was prepared according to the REMARK guidelines [28,29].

Further details are described in File S1.

Results

MiRNA expression was measured in 460 FFPE samples. The number of samples in each cohort was: screening cohort = 212, reduced screening cohort = 155, validation cohort = 121, and control cohort = 127 (Figure S1 in File S1).

The patients included in the reduced screening- and the validation miRNA cohorts differed from the patients not included. They were more likely to have: resected primary tumor, a single metastatic site, performance status 0, and prior adjuvant therapy. They also experienced a longer TTP and OS (Table 1). The patients in the control cohort were similar to the patients not included except for them being more likely to have had the primary tumor resected.

Table 2. Focused miRNA panel – miRNAs significantly associated with time to disease progression.

	Screening CAPEOXBEV cohort			Validation CAPEOXBEV cohort			Combined CAPEOXBEV cohort			Control CAPEOX cohort			Interaction[a]		
	n = 155			n = 121			n = 276			n = 127			all	distal	proximal
miRNA	HR[b]	95% CI	*P*	HR	95% CI	*P*	HR	95% CI	*P*	HR	95% CI	*P*	*P*	*P*	*P*
Raw expression values															
miR-15a-5p	0.88	0.73–1.06	0.19	0.73	0.54–0.98	**0.04**	0.86	0.73–1.00	0.05	1.03	0.80–1.31	0.84	0.14	0.25	0.15
miR-17-3p	0.68	0.54–0.84	**0.0005**	0.92	0.68–1.23	0.57	0.77	0.64–0.91	**0.003**	1.01	0.78–1.31	0.92	0.16	0.11	0.67
miR-193b-5p	0.82	0.70–0.95	**0.01**	0.74	0.54–1.01	0.06	0.82	0.72–0.94	**0.004**	0.92	0.77–1.10	0.34	–[c]	–	–
miR-204-5p	0.83	0.71–0.96	**0.02**	0.92	0.68–1.23	0.56	0.83	0.71–0.97	**0.02**	0.90	0.71–1.14	0.38	0.86	0.60	0.25
miR-501-5p	0.78	0.63–0.97	**0.03**	0.88	0.63–1.23	0.46	0.81	0.66–0.99	**0.04**	0.96	0.69–1.32	0.78	0.48	0.47	0.84
miR-545-3p	0.87	0.77–1.00	**0.04**	0.87	0.73–1.05	0.15	0.86	0.77–0.96	**0.005**	1.00	0.88–1.14	0.97	0.11	0.17	0.29
miR-592	0.71	0.54–0.93	**0.01**	0.80	0.62–1.01	0.06	0.77	0.67–0.90	**0.0007**	0.81	0.58–1.12	0.21	0.14	0.11	0.82
miR-664-3p	0.87	0.66–1.15	0.32	0.60	0.41–0.87	**0.007**	0.80	0.65–0.99	**0.04**	0.81	0.58–1.13	0.21	0.10	**0.04**	0.31
Mean-normalized expression values															
miR-17-3p	0.78	0.63–0.98	**0.03**	1.05	0.83–1.34	0.68	0.89	0.76–1.05	0.16	1.10	0.82–1.48	0.52	0.22	0.09	0.26
miR-155-5p	1.36	1.07–1.71	**0.01**	1.33	1.00–1.77	0.05	1.38	1.15–1.64	**0.0005**	1.05	0.79–1.38	0.74	0.05	0.18	0.18
miR-185-5p	1.45	1.17–1.80	**0.0008**	1.23	0.87–1.74	0.24	1.30	1.10–1.54	**0.003**	0.89	0.67–1.19	0.44	0.06	0.20	0.43
miR-204-5p	0.82	0.68–0.98	**0.03**	1.13	0.87–1.46	0.38	0.90	0.78–1.03	0.13	0.95	0.79–1.13	0.54	0.15	0.07	0.14
miR-449a	1.25	1.03–1.52	**0.02**	0.97	0.73–1.28	0.81	1.15	0.99–1.35	0.07	1.00	0.80–1.26	0.96	0.55	0.89	0.74

[a] Interaction tests were performed for all patients and for patients with distal (sigmoid and rectum) and proximal (cecum to descending) primary tumor location, separately.
[b] Hazard ratio is per inter-quartile range expression increase and is adjusted for age, sex, number of metastatic sites, prior adjuvant treatment and primary tumor location.
[c] miRNA was missing in >10% of samples so interaction was not tested.
Abbreviations: HR, hazard ratio; CI, confidence interval.

Table 3. Focused miRNA panel – miRNAs significantly associated with overall survival.

	Screening CAPEOXBEV cohort			Validation CAPEOXBEV cohort			Combined CAPEOXBEV cohort			Control CAPEOX cohort			Interaction[a]		
	n = 155			n = 121			n = 276			n = 127			all	distal	proximal
miRNA	HR[b]	95% CI	*P*	HR	95% CI	*P*	HR	95% CI	*P*	HR	95% CI	*P*	*P*	*P*	*P*
Raw expression values															
miR-15a-5p	0.80	0.65–0.99	**0.04**	0.87	0.66–1.16	0.34	0.81	0.69–0.97	**0.02**	1.05	0.83–1.34	0.68	0.31	0.41	0.74
miR-196b-5p	0.83	0.69–1.01	0.06	0.66	0.50–0.87	**0.003**	0.77	0.66–0.90	**0.0008**	0.78	0.62–0.98	**0.04**	0.20	0.06	0.23
miR-204-5p	0.76	0.64–0.91	**0.003**	0.88	0.66–1.18	0.38	0.77	0.64–0.93	**0.005**	1.02	0.81–1.28	0.87	0.94	0.80	0.54
miR-338-3p	0.81	0.65–1.00	**0.045**	0.93	0.70–1.24	0.63	0.85	0.72–1.01	0.07	1.01	0.80–1.27	0.92	0.52	0.40	0.68
miR-545-3p	0.85	0.74–0.98	**0.03**	0.95	0.80–1.12	0.53	0.90	0.81–1.01	0.06	1.06	0.95–1.19	0.30	0.39	0.39	0.45
miR-552	0.77	0.61–0.96	**0.02**	0.93	0.68–1.27	0.63	0.77	0.63–0.95	**0.01**	1.02	0.80–1.31	0.85	0.44	0.29	0.76
miR-592	0.69	0.69–0.92	**0.01**	0.76	0.60–0.95	**0.01**	0.73	0.62–0.86	**0.0001**	0.76	0.55–1.05	0.10	0.31	0.33	0.85
miR-664-3p	0.64	0.48–0.86	**0.003**	0.60	0.44–0.82	**0.002**	0.61	0.49–0.75	**<0.0001**	0.85	0.61–1.17	0.31	**0.02**	**0.03**	0.50
Mean-normalized expression values															
miR-1	1.01	0.77–1.32	0.96	1.19	0.84–1.69	0.32	1.08	0.87–1.32	0.49	1.36	1.02–1.82	**0.04**	0.98	0.82	0.75
miR-155-5p	1.31	1.03–1.67	**0.03**	1.21	0.91–1.61	0.19	1.23	1.03–1.47	**0.03**	0.96	0.75–1.23	0.76	0.38	0.70	0.30
miR-185-5p	1.49	1.18–1.88	**0.0008**	1.23	0.89–1.72	0.21	1.34	1.12–1.60	**0.001**	0.91	0.70–1.18	0.46	0.09	0.23	0.57
miR-196b-5p	0.89	0.67–1.18	0.43	0.70	0.51–0.96	**0.03**	0.79	0.64–0.97	**0.03**	0.73	0.58–0.93	**0.01**	0.99	0.43	0.09
miR-204-5p	0.75	0.61–0.93	**0.009**	0.95	0.70–1.28	0.71	0.85	0.72–1.01	0.06	1.01	0.85–1.21	0.89	0.43	0.61	0.40
miR-455-5p	1.19	0.95–1.49	0.14	1.27	1.03–1.56	**0.03**	1.24	1.06–1.45	**0.007**	0.99	0.85–1.15	0.91	**0.02**	0.19	0.38
miR-592	0.77	0.59–1.00	0.05	0.76	0.63–0.93	**0.007**	0.77	0.66–0.89	**0.0004**	0.71	0.53–0.96	**0.03**	0.52	0.21	0.35
miR-664-3p	0.66	0.49–0.91	**0.01**	0.55	0.39–0.79	**0.001**	0.60	0.48–0.76	**<0.0001**	0.81	0.59–1.11	0.18	**0.02**	**0.02**	0.45

[a] Interaction was tested for all patients and for patients with distal (sigmoid to rectum) and proximal (cecum to descending colon) primary tumor location separately.
[b] Hazard ratio is per inter-quartile range expression increase and is adjusted for age, sex, number of metastatic sites, prior adjuvant treatment and primary tumor location.
Abbreviations: HR, hazard ratio; CI, confidence interval.

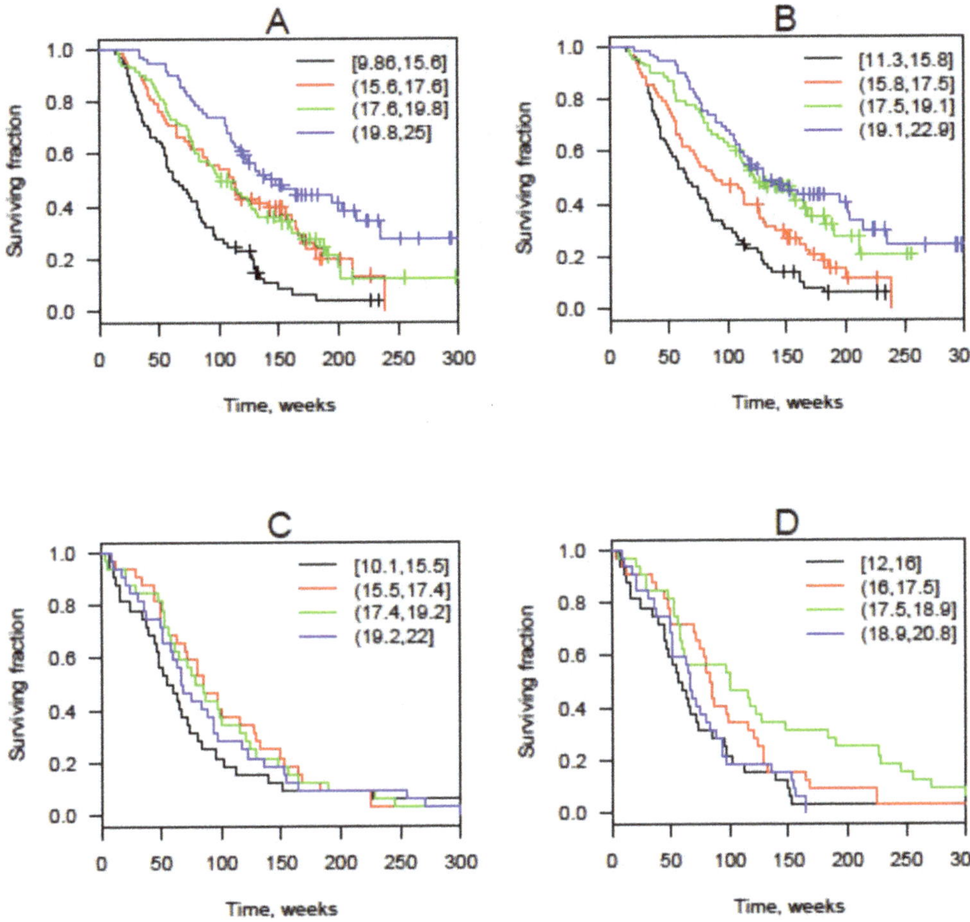

Cohort	Quartile	Raw expression HR	Raw expression 95% CI	Mean-normalized expression HR	Mean-normalized expression 95% CI
CAPEOXBEV	1	1	[reference]	1	[reference]
	2	0.50	0.34 – 0.74	0.66	0.45 – 0.98
	3	0.50	0.34 – 0.76	0.41	0.27 – 0.63
	4	0.30	0.20 – 0.46	0.34	0.23 – 0.54
CAPEOX	1	1	[reference]	1	[reference]
	2	0.75	0.42 – 1.53	0.68	0.38 – 1.25
	3	0.76	0.41 – 1.61	0.49	0.26 – 0.92
	4	0.86	0.46 – 1.70	0.98	0.59 – 1.89

Figure 1. Overall survival according to quartiles of mir-664-3p expression. Kaplan-Meier plots are shown for patients treated with CAPEOXBEV using raw (A) or mean-normalized (B) expression and patients treated with CAPEOX alone using raw (C) and mean-normalized (D) expression. Hazard ratios (HR) are unadjusted and confidence intervals (CI) are calculated using bootstrapping. The expression intervals shown in the upper right-hand corner are 40-C_t, so higher values correspond to higher expression. Black line = lowest quartile; red line = second quartile; green line = third quartile; blue line = highest quartile.

Screening study

Nine samples were identified as outliers based on a low number of miRNAs detected and these were excluded, leaving 203 samples for outcome calculations. Twenty-six miRNAs were associated with TTP or OS in multivariate analysis using raw-, quantile-normalized, or mean-normalized expression data (Table S1 in File S1). Twenty-two of these were selected for further study: miR-1, miR-15a-5p, miR-17-3p, miR-22-3p, miR-29b-3p, miR-145-3p, miR-155-5p, miR-185-5p, miR-193b-5p, miR-196b-5p, miR-204-5p, miR-214-5p, miR-338-3p, miR-382-5p, miR-449a, miR-455-5p, miR-497-5p, miR-501-5p, miR-545-3p, miR-552-3p, miR-592 and miR-664-3p.

Focused miRNA panel – miRNAs associated with TTP

Eleven miRNAs were significantly associated with TTP in either the screening- or the validation cohort, but not in both cohorts and no significant interactions were found between miRNA expression and bevacizumab effect (Table 2).

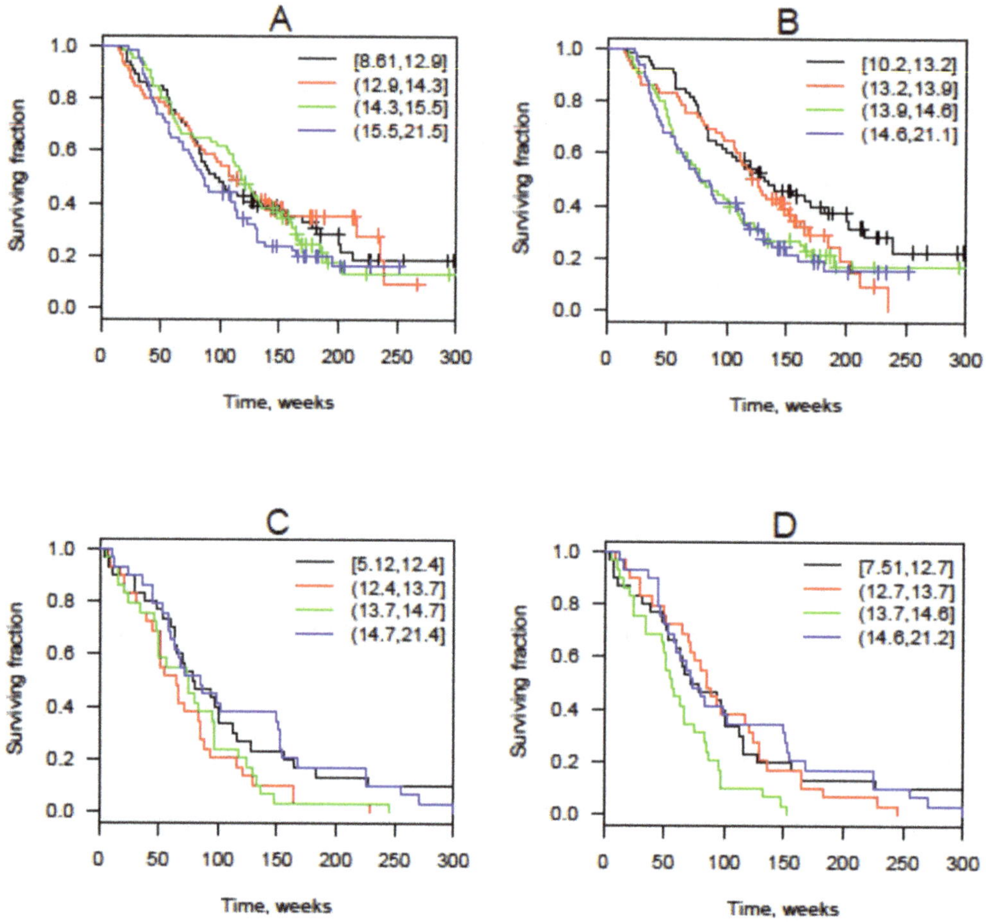

		Raw expression		Mean-normalized expression	
Cohort	Quartile	HR	95% CI	HR	95% CI
CAPEOXBEV	1	1	[reference]	1	[reference]
	2	0.89	0.59 – 1.36	1.19	0.83 – 1.70
	3	0.97	0.68 – 1.36	1.61	1.09 – 2.41
	4	1.22	0.81 – 1.75	1.71	1.13 – 2.55
CAPEOX	1	1	[reference]	1	[reference]
	2	1.70	1.01 – 2.89	1.12	0.69 – 1.79
	3	1.61	0.96 – 2.56	2.07	1.26 – 3.56
	4	1.01	0.62 – 1.65	1.01	0.62 – 1.62

Figure 2. Overall survival according to quartiles of mir-455-5p expression. Kaplan-Meier plots are shown for patients treated with CAPEOXBEV using raw (A) or mean-normalized (B) expression and patients treated with CAPEOX alone using raw (C) and mean-normalized (D) expression. Hazard ratios (HR) are unadjusted and confidence intervals (CI) are calculated using bootstrapping. The expression intervals shown in the upper right-hand corner are 40-C_t, so higher values correspond to higher expression. Black line = lowest quartile; red line = second quartile; green line = third quartile; blue line = highest quartile.

Kaplan-Meier curves for TTP according to quartiles of miR-664-3p- and miR-455-5p expression are shown in Figure S2 and S3 in File S1.

Focused miRNA panel – miRNAs associated with OS

Twelve miRNAs were significantly associated with OS in one or more of the screening-, validation- and control cohorts (Table 3). Higher miR-664-3p expression was associated with longer OS in the screening and validation cohorts using raw expression: HR 0.64 (CI 0.48–0.86) and 0.60 (CI 0.44–0.82); and normalized expression: HR 0.66 (CI 0.49–0.91) and 0.55 (CI 0.39–0.79). No association between miR-664-3p expression and OS was found in the control cohort. A significant interaction between miR-664-3p expression and bevacizumab effect was observed using both raw- and normalized expression ($P = 0.02$ and $P = 0.02$). Kaplan-Meier plots for OS according to quartiles of miR-664-3p expression are shown in Figure 1.

Higher miR-455-5p expression was associated with shorter OS in the combined bevacizumab-treated cohort when using normalized expression: HR 1.24 (CI 1.06–1.45), but not in the control

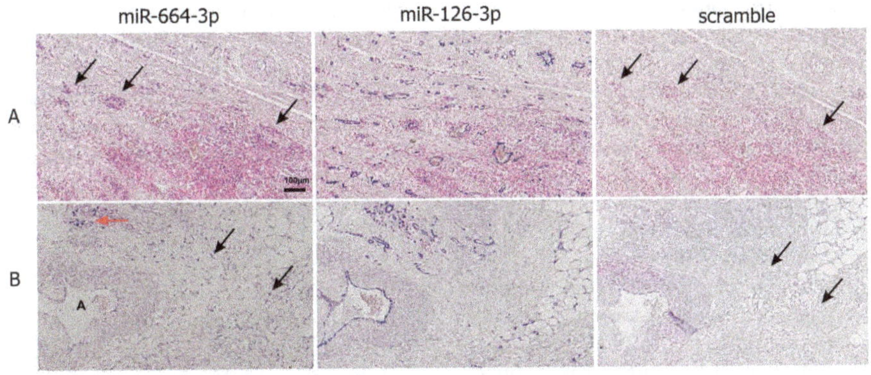

Figure 3. MiR-664-3p *in situ* hybridization (ISH). Panels A and B show examples of miR-664-3p ISH in infiltrating lymphocytes (A) and fibroblasts (B). Consecutive sections were stained with LNA probes against miR-664-3p, miR-126-3p and a scramble sequence. MiR-664-3p ISH signal is seen in infiltrating lymphocytes (A, arrows; B, red arrow) and in fibroblasts (B, black arrows), whereas no ISH signal is obtained with scramble probe. A strong ISH signal is seen in endothelial cells with the positive control probe miR-126-3p. The "A" in panel B indicates an artery.

cohort. There was a significant interaction with bevacizumab effect ($P = 0.02$). Kaplan-Meier plots for OS according to quartiles of miR-455-5p expression are shown in Figure 2.

Higher miR-592 expression was associated with longer OS in the screening- and validation cohorts using raw expression: HR 0.69 (CI 0.69–0.92) and 0.76 (CI 0.60–0.95); and in the validation cohort using normalized expression: HR 0.76 (CI 0.63–0.93), with a similar trend in the screening cohort using normalized expression: HR 0.77 (CI 0.59–1.00). Higher miR-592 expression was also associated with longer OS in the control group when using normalized expression: HR 0.71 (CI 0.53–0.96).

Higher miR-196b-5p expression was associated with longer OS using raw- and normalized expression both in the combined bevacizumab-treated cohort: HR 0.77 (CI 0.66–0.90) and 0.79 (CI 0.64–0.97); and in the control group: HR 0.78 (CI 0.62–0.98) and 0.73 (CI 0.58–0.93).

Focused miRNA panel – primary tumor location and second line outcome

In analyses stratified for primary tumor location, a significant interaction with bevacizumab effect was seen for miR-664-3p expression in the sigmoid colon and rectum group for both TTP using raw expression and for OS using raw- and normalized expression. Expression levels of all miRNAs according to primary tumor location are shown in Figure S4 in File S1.

In patients continuing bevacizumab in second line, high miR-664-3p expression was associated with longer TTP (HR 0.30, $P = 0.04$) and high miR-455-5p expression was associated with a trend towards shorter TTP (HR 2.72, $P = 0.09$), while no such associations were seen in patients that did not continue bevacizumab (Figure S5 in File S1).

MiRNA *in situ* hybridization

An intense miR-664-3p ISH signal, primarily with a cytoplasmic localization, was seen in subpopulations of tumor-infiltrating lymphocytes, fibroblasts, and endothelial cells located at the invasive border (Figure 3). A weak miR-664-3p ISH signal was seen in tumor epithelial cells, but a similar staining was observed with the scramble probe, suggesting an unspecific binding of the probe to these cells. MiR-455-5p ISH signal was found in some lymphocyte-like stromal cells in half of the samples, while tumor epithelial cells were negative (Figure S6 in File S1). No ISH signal was obtained with the probes against miR-185, miR-449a or miR-592. Positive control probes for miR-21-5p and miR-126-3p showed moderate to intense staining in fibroblasts and endothelial cells, respectively, in all cases.

Target prediction

Table S2 in File S1 shows the 20 highest ranked predicted gene targets for miR-196b-5p, miR-455-5p, miR-592, and miR-664-3p, and references published articles regarding the function and expression level of these miRNAs in cancer.

Discussion

This is the first comprehensive study of miRNAs as predictive biomarkers for bevacizumab effectiveness in CRC. Of the 22 miRNAs selected from the screening study, miR-664-3p and miR-455-5p showed the greatest potential as predictive biomarkers for bevacizumab effectiveness.

The association between miR-664-3p and OS differed significantly between patients treated with bevacizumab and patients treated with chemotherapy alone: Increasing miR-664-3p expression in primary CRC tissue was associated with longer OS in both cohorts of patients treated with bevacizumab combined with CAPEOX but not in the cohort treated with chemotherapy alone. Increasing miR-664-3p expression was also associated with longer TTP in patients treated with bevacizumab, but the interaction test was only significant in the subgroup of patients with sigmoid colon- and rectal primary tumors. We previously hypothesized that this subgroup of patients could be more likely to derive benefit from treatment with bevacizumab than patients with more proximal primary tumors [20]. MiR-664-3p expression was also higher in these patients than in patients with more proximal primary tumors (Figure S4 in File S1). In the small cohort of patients with available second line outcome data, high miR-664-3p expression was also associated with a longer TTP only in patients continuing bevacizumab, supporting a connection between miR-664-3p expression and bevacizumab effectiveness.

We observed high expression of miR-664-3p in stromal cells, including endothelial cells, which is in accordance with a role for miR-664-3p in angiogenesis. Very little data have been published about this miRNA (Table S2 in File S1). Interestingly, among the top predicted targets of miR-664-3p are neuroligin 1 (NLGN1), MDGA2, and gephyrin, which are all involved in the same synaptogenic process in the nervous system [30,31]. Recently, neuroligin and its binding partner neurexin have been shown to be widely expressed in the vascular system and involved in angiogenesis [30]. Overexpression of neuroligin 1 in endothelial cells grown in a tumorigenic environment increased angiogenesis, and knockdown of neurexin reduced fibroblast growth factor 2-induced angiogenesis [32]. In a zebra fish embryo model of angiogenesis, inhibition of VEGF-A or neuroligin caused similar magnitudes of vascular defects, but inhibition of both resulted in a more than additive anti-angiogenic effect [33]. Hypothetically, the impact of miR-664-3p expression on outcome may thus be explained by its downregulation of the neuroligin system and the resulting synergy with VEGF-A inhibition by bevacizumab.

Increasing miR-455-5p expression was associated with shorter OS in the combined bevacizumab treated cohort while no such association was observed in the cohort treated with chemotherapy alone. We identified high expression of this miRNA in lymphocyte-like cells located in the stroma around the cancer cells. MiR-455-5p has been reported to be dysregulated in cancer; however, no validated targets have been identified (Table S2 in File S1).

Increasing expression of both miR-196b-5p and miR-592 was associated with longer OS in all three cohorts, with similar effect estimates. Both these miRNAs have been shown to be downregulated in CRCs with deficient mismatch repair (dMMR) [34]. Higher miR-592 expression has been shown to be associated with improved OS in patients receiving salvage anti-EGFR treatment and higher miR-196b-5p expression has been linked to response to neo-adjuvant 5-FU and radiotherapy in patients with locally advanced rectal cancer [35,36]. MiR-592 expression has been reported to be higher in left-sided compared to right-sided CRCs [37], which we also found in our study. We could not stain our tissue sections for miR-592, but expression of both miR-592 and miR-196b-5p has previously been shown to be 2.5–3.7 fold higher in CRC epithelium than in CRC stroma [38]. The function of miR-592 has not been described. MiR-196b-5p is dysregulated in many malignancies, has been related to cancer prognosis, and targets c-myc, ERG, MEIS1, FAS, ABL1, BCL-2 and several HOX genes (Table S2 in File S1).

There are important limitations to consider regarding our results. We studied retrospectively identified cohorts from different time periods, which increases the risk of bias, since differences other than the treatments used could exist between the cohorts. We used mean expression for normalization, but since the miRNAs used for calculating the mean were related to outcome, this is sub-optimal. Even though the association with outcome for some of the miRNAs was identified in two or three independent cohorts, the predictive effect related to bevacizumab remains unvalidated. We did not correct for multiple testing, but miR-664-3p would still be significantly associated with OS in the validation cohort, even after correcting for the 22 miRNAs tested. Also, effect estimates were similar in the cohorts, indicating a non-random association. Among the strengths of our study are the large sample size, the initial comprehensive screening study, the use of three independent cohorts, and randomization of purification- and miRNA expression analysis order.

In conclusion, this is the first study to examine the potential for miRNA expression in primary tumors to predict benefit of bevacizumab in patients with mCRC. We have identified miR-664-3p and miR-455-5p as possible predictive biomarkers for bevacizumab. MiR-592 and miR-196b-5p were predictive of outcome both with and without bevacizumab and these could be prognostic biomarkers or biomarkers related to chemotherapy effectiveness. These findings need validation in independent cohorts – preferably from randomized trials and using stable miRNA normalizers –before they can be implemented in clinical decision making. Elucidation of the cellular origins and biological functions of these miRNAs is warranted.

Acknowledgments

We would like to thank: Jørgen Hansen, MD from the Department of Oncology at Aalborg Hospital, Denmark for help regarding acquisition of patient data; Mel Heeran, PhD for excellent technical assistance with the sectioning of the FFPE tissue samples; Jakob Z. Johansen, MD for inputting clinical data in the BETmiRC database; Mogens Kruhøffer, PhD, from AROS Applied Biotechnology A/S, Denmark for help with the miRNA analyses, and the Danish CancerBiobank (DCB) for biological material and for the data regarding handling and storage.

Author Contributions

Conceived and designed the experiments: MKB CD DL BSN EVSH BVJ JSJ. Analyzed the data: MKB CD DL BSN JSL KØ SEN LST CQ PP NHH NK TFH BBJ EVSH BVJ JSJ. Contributed reagents/materials/analysis tools: MKB CD DL BSN JSL KØ SEN LST CQ PP NHH NK TFH BBJ EVSH BVJ JSJ. Wrote the paper: MKB CD DL BSN JSL KØ SEN LST CQ PP NHH NK TFH BBJ EVSH BVJ JSJ.

References

1. Ferlay J, Soerjomataram I, Ervik M, Dikshit R, Eser S, et al. (2013) GLOBOCAN 2012 v1.0, Cancer Incidence and Mortality Worldwide: IARC CancerBase No. 11 [Internet]. Lyon, France: International Agency for Research on Cancer.
2. Van Cutsem E, Nordlinger B, Cervantes A, Group EGW (2010) Advanced colorectal cancer: ESMO Clinical Practice Guidelines for treatment. Ann Oncol 21 Suppl 5: v93–97.
3. Bennouna J, Sastre J, Arnold D, Osterlund P, Greil R, et al. (2013) Continuation of bevacizumab after first progression in metastatic colorectal cancer (ML18147): a randomised phase 3 trial. Lancet Oncol 14: 29–37.
4. Giantonio BJ, Catalano PJ, Meropol NJ, O'Dwyer PJ, Mitchell EP, et al. (2007) Bevacizumab in combination with oxaliplatin, fluorouracil, and leucovorin (FOLFOX4) for previously treated metastatic colorectal cancer: results from the Eastern Cooperative Oncology Group Study E3200. J Clin Oncol 25: 1539–1544.
5. Hurwitz H, Fehrenbacher L, Novotny W, Cartwright T, Hainsworth J, et al. (2004) Bevacizumab plus irinotecan, fluorouracil, and leucovorin for metastatic colorectal cancer. N Engl J Med 350: 2335–2342.
6. Hurwitz HI, Tebbutt NC, Kabbinavar F, Giantonio BJ, Guan ZZ, et al. (2013) Efficacy and safety of bevacizumab in metastatic colorectal cancer: pooled analysis from seven randomized controlled trials. Oncologist 18: 1004–1012.
7. Saltz LB, Clarke S, Diaz-Rubio E, Scheithauer W, Figer A, et al. (2008) Bevacizumab in combination with oxaliplatin-based chemotherapy as first-line therapy in metastatic colorectal cancer: a randomized phase III study. J Clin Oncol 26: 2013–2019.
8. Kopetz S, Chang GJ, Overman MJ, Eng C, Sargent DJ, et al. (2009) Improved survival in metastatic colorectal cancer is associated with adoption of hepatic resection and improved chemotherapy. J Clin Oncol 27: 3677–3683.
9. Jubb AM, Harris AL (2010) Biomarkers to predict the clinical efficacy of bevacizumab in cancer. Lancet Oncol 11: 1172–1183.
10. Lambrechts D, Lenz HJ, de Haas S, Carmeliet P, Scherer SJ (2013) Markers of response for the antiangiogenic agent bevacizumab. J Clin Oncol 31: 1219–1230.
11. Cortez MA, Bueso-Ramos C, Ferdin J, Lopez-Berestein G, Sood AK, et al. (2011) MicroRNAs in body fluids–the mix of hormones and biomarkers. Nat Rev Clin Oncol 8: 467–477.
12. Farazi TA, Spitzer JI, Morozov P, Tuschl T (2011) miRNAs in human cancer. J Pathol 223: 102–115.
13. Kong YW, Ferland-McCollough D, Jackson TJ, Bushell M (2012) microRNAs in cancer management. Lancet Oncol 13: e249–258.
14. Nana-Sinkam SP, Fabbri M, Croce CM (2010) MicroRNAs in cancer: personalizing diagnosis and therapy. Ann N Y Acad Sci 1210: 25–33.
15. Xi Y, Nakajima G, Gavin E, Morris CG, Kudo K, et al. (2007) Systematic analysis of microRNA expression of RNA extracted from fresh frozen and formalin-fixed paraffin-embedded samples. RNA 13: 1668–1674.

16. Schwarzenbach H, Nishida N, Calin GA, Pantel K (2014) Clinical relevance of circulating cell-free microRNAs in cancer. Nat Rev Clin Oncol 11: 145–156.
17. Mazeh H, Mizrahi I, Ilyayev N, Halle D, Brucher B, et al. (2013) The Diagnostic and Prognostic Role of microRNA in Colorectal Cancer - a Comprehensive review. J Cancer 4: 281–295.
18. Nosho K, Igarashi H, Nojima M, Ito M, Maruyama R, et al. (2014) Association of microRNA-31 with BRAF mutation, colorectal cancer survival and serrated pathway. Carcinogenesis 35: 776–783.
19. Qvortrup C, Jensen BV, Fokstuen T, Nielsen SE, Keldsen N, et al. (2010) A randomized study comparing short-time infusion of oxaliplatin in combination with capecitabine XELOX(30) and chronomodulated XELOX(30) as first-line therapy in patients with advanced colorectal cancer. Ann Oncol 21: 87–91.
20. Boisen MK, Johansen JS, Dehlendorff C, Larsen JS, Osterlind K, et al. (2013) Primary tumor location and bevacizumab effectiveness in patients with metastatic colorectal cancer. Ann Oncol 24: 2554–2559.
21. Braasch DA, Corey DR (2001) Locked nucleic acid (LNA): fine-tuning the recognition of DNA and RNA. Chem Biol 8: 1–7.
22. Nielsen BS, Jorgensen S, Fog JU, Sokilde R, Christensen IJ, et al. (2011) High levels of microRNA-21 in the stroma of colorectal cancers predict short disease-free survival in stage II colon cancer patients. Clin Exp Metastasis 28: 27–38.
23. Andersen PK, Gill RD (1982) Cox Regression-Model for Counting-Processes - a Large Sample Study. Annals of Statistics 10: 1100–1120.
24. Cox DR (1972) Regression Models and Life-Tables. Journal of the Royal Statistical Society Series B-Statistical Methodology 34: 187–220.
25. Sakamoto MIGKY (1986) Akaike Information Criterion Statistics: D. Reidel Publishing Company.
26. R Core Team (2013) R: A Language and Environment for Statistical Computing. R Foundation for Statistical Computing.
27. Paraskevopoulou MD, Georgakilas G, Kostoulas N, Vlachos IS, Vergoulis T, et al. (2013) DIANA-microT web server v5.0: service integration into miRNA functional analysis workflows. Nucleic Acids Res 41: W169–173.
28. McShane LM, Altman DG, Sauerbrei W, Taube SE, Gion M, et al. (2005) Reporting recommendations for tumor marker prognostic studies. J Clin Oncol 23: 9067–9072.
29. Altman DG, McShane LM, Sauerbrei W, Taube SE (2012) Reporting recommendations for tumor marker prognostic studies (REMARK): explanation and elaboration. BMC Med 10: 51.
30. Bottos A, Rissone A, Bussolino F, Arese M (2011) Neurexins and neuroligins: synapses look out of the nervous system. Cell Mol Life Sci 68: 2655–2666.
31. Lee K, Kim Y, Lee SJ, Qiang Y, Lee D, et al. (2013) MDGAs interact selectively with neuroligin-2 but not other neuroligins to regulate inhibitory synapse development. Proc Natl Acad Sci U S A 110: 336–341.
32. Bottos A, Destro E, Rissone A, Graziano S, Cordara G, et al. (2009) The synaptic proteins neurexins and neuroligins are widely expressed in the vascular system and contribute to its functions. Proc Natl Acad Sci U S A 106: 20782–20787.
33. Rissone A, Foglia E, Sangiorgio L, Cermenati S, Nicoli S, et al. (2012) The synaptic proteins beta-neurexin and neuroligin synergize with extracellular matrix-binding vascular endothelial growth factor a during zebrafish vascular development. Arterioscler Thromb Vasc Biol 32: 1563–1572.
34. Sarver AL, French AJ, Borralho PM, Thayanithy V, Oberg AL, et al. (2009) Human colon cancer profiles show differential microRNA expression depending on mismatch repair status and are characteristic of undifferentiated proliferative states. BMC Cancer 9: 401.
35. Mosakhani N, Lahti L, Borze I, Karjalainen-Lindsberg ML, Sundstrom J, et al. (2012) MicroRNA profiling predicts survival in anti-EGFR treated chemorefractory metastatic colorectal cancer patients with wild-type KRAS and BRAF. Cancer Genet 205: 545–551.
36. Svoboda M, Sana J, Fabian P, Kocakova I, Gombosova J, et al. (2012) MicroRNA expression profile associated with response to neoadjuvant chemoradiotherapy in locally advanced rectal cancer patients. Radiat Oncol 7: 195.
37. Schee K, Lorenz S, Worren MM, Gunther CC, Holden M, et al. (2013) Deep Sequencing the MicroRNA Transcriptome in Colorectal Cancer. PLoS One 8: e66165.
38. Nishida N, Nagahara M, Sato T, Mimori K, Sudo T, et al. (2012) Microarray analysis of colorectal cancer stromal tissue reveals upregulation of two oncogenic miRNA clusters. Clin Cancer Res 18: 3054–3070.

Permissions

All chapters in this book were first published in PLOS ONE, by The Public Library of Science; hereby published with permission under the Creative Commons Attribution License or equivalent. Every chapter published in this book has been scrutinized by our experts. Their significance has been extensively debated. The topics covered herein carry significant findings which will fuel the growth of the discipline. They may even be implemented as practical applications or may be referred to as a beginning point for another development.

The contributors of this book come from diverse backgrounds, making this book a truly international effort. This book will bring forth new frontiers with its revolutionizing research information and detailed analysis of the nascent developments around the world.

We would like to thank all the contributing authors for lending their expertise to make the book truly unique. They have played a crucial role in the development of this book. Without their invaluable contributions this book wouldn't have been possible. They have made vital efforts to compile up to date information on the varied aspects of this subject to make this book a valuable addition to the collection of many professionals and students.

This book was conceptualized with the vision of imparting up-to-date information and advanced data in this field. To ensure the same, a matchless editorial board was set up. Every individual on the board went through rigorous rounds of assessment to prove their worth. After which they invested a large part of their time researching and compiling the most relevant data for our readers.

The editorial board has been involved in producing this book since its inception. They have spent rigorous hours researching and exploring the diverse topics which have resulted in the successful publishing of this book. They have passed on their knowledge of decades through this book. To expedite this challenging task, the publisher supported the team at every step. A small team of assistant editors was also appointed to further simplify the editing procedure and attain best results for the readers.

Apart from the editorial board, the designing team has also invested a significant amount of their time in understanding the subject and creating the most relevant covers. They scrutinized every image to scout for the most suitable representation of the subject and create an appropriate cover for the book.

The publishing team has been an ardent support to the editorial, designing and production team. Their endless efforts to recruit the best for this project, has resulted in the accomplishment of this book. They are a veteran in the field of academics and their pool of knowledge is as vast as their experience in printing. Their expertise and guidance has proved useful at every step. Their uncompromising quality standards have made this book an exceptional effort. Their encouragement from time to time has been an inspiration for everyone.

The publisher and the editorial board hope that this book will prove to be a valuable piece of knowledge for researchers, students, practitioners and scholars across the globe.

List of Contributors

Martin Lundsgaard Hansen, Eva Fallentin and Michael Bachmann Nielsen
Department of Radiology, Rigshospitalet, Copenhagen, Denmark

Carsten Lauridsen
Department of Radiology, Rigshospitalet, Copenhagen, Denmark
Bachelor's Degree Programme in Radiography, Department of Technology, Metropolitan University College, Copenhagen, Denmark

Ian Law
Department of Clinical Physiology, Nuclear Medicine and PET, Rigshospitalet, Copenhagen, Denmark

Birgitte Federspiel
Department of Pathology, Rigshospitalet, Copenhagen, Denmark

Lene Bæksgaard
Department of Oncology, Rigshospitalet, Copenhagen, Denmark,

Lars Bo Svendsen
Department of Surgical Gastroenterology, Rigshospitalet, Copenhagen, Denmark

Lucia Perez-Carbonell, Yuji Toiyama, C. Richard Boland and Ajay Goel
Division of Gastroenterology, Department of Internal Medicine, Charles Sammons Cancer Center and Baylor Research Institute, Baylor University Medical Center, Dallas, Texas, United States of America

Francesc Balaguer and Antoni Castells
Gastroenterology Department, Hospital Clinic, CIBERehd, IDIBAPS, University of Barcelona, Barcelona, Spain

Cecilia Egoavil and Estefania Rojas
Department of Pathology, Hospital General Universitario de Alicante, Alicante, Spain

Carla Guarinos
Research Unit, Hospital General Universitario de Alicante, Alicante, Spain

Montserrat Andreu
Gastroenterology Department, Hospital del Mar, Barcelona, Spain

Xavier Llor
Department of Medicine and Cancer Center, University of Illinois at Chicago, Chicago, Illinois, United States of America

Rodrigo Jover
Unidad de Gastroenterología, Hospital General Universitario de Alicante, Alicante, Spain

Ning Li, Wei Ou, Song-liang Zhang and Si-yu Wang
Department of Thoracic Surgery, Sun Yat-sen University Cancer Center, Guangzhou, China

Lu Yang
Department of Breast Oncology, Sun Yat-sen University Cancer Center, Guangzhou, China

Liang Zhang
Department of Thoracic Surgery, Tianjin First Center Hospital, Tianjin, China

Sung Han Kim
Department of Urology, National Cancer Center, Goyang, Gyanggi, Korea

Hyung-Kook Yang
Department of Epidemiology and Statistics and Cancer Policy Branch of the National Cancer Control Research Institute, National Cancer Center, Goyang, Gyanggi, Korea

Jung Hoon Lee and Eun-Sik Lee
Department of Urology, Seoul National University Hospital, Seoul, Seoul, Korea

Dorthe Skovgaard and Andreas Kjaer
Cluster for Molecular Imaging, University of Copenhagen, Copenhagen, Denmark,
Department of Clinical Physiology, Nuclear Medicine and PET, Rigshospitalet and University Hospital of Copenhagen, Copenhagen, Denmark

Philip Hasbak
Department of Clinical Physiology, Nuclear Medicine and PET, Rigshospitalet and University Hospital of Copenhagen, Copenhagen, Denmark

Yan Du, Tong Su, Xiaojie Tan, Wenjun Chang, Hongwei Zhang and Guangwen Cao
Department of Epidemiology, Second Military Medical University, Shanghai, China

Lijun Zhao
Department of Pulmonary Medicine, Changhai Hospital, Second Military Medical University, Shanghai, China

Hiro Takahashi
Graduate School of Horticulture, Chiba University, Matsudo, Chiba, Japan
Plant Biology Research Center, Chubu University, Kasugai, Aichi, Japan
Division of Genetics, National Cancer Center Research Institute, Tokyo, Japan

Anna Takahashi
Plant Biology Research Center, Chubu University, Kasugai, Aichi, Japan

Yoko Odaka, Misuzu Okuyama, Hiromi Sakamoto and Teruhiko Yoshid
Division of Genetics, National Cancer Center Research Institute, Tokyo, Japan

Risa Ichinohe and Ayano Doi
Division of Genetics, National Cancer Center Research Institute, Tokyo, Japan
Faculty of Horticulture, Chiba University, Matsudo, Chiba, Japan

Kimie Sai, Yoshiro Saito, Nahoko Kaniwa and Haruhiro Okuda
Division of Medicinal Safety Science, National Institute of Health Sciences, Tokyo, Japan

Yasuhiro Matsumura
Division of Developmental Therapeutics, Research Center for Innovative Oncology, National Cancer Center Hospital East, Kashiwa, Chiba, Japan

Tetsuya Hamaguchi and Yasuhiro Shimada
Gastrointestinal Medical Oncology Division, National Cancer Center Hospital, Tokyo, Japan

Atsushi Ohtsu, Takayuki Yoshino and Toshihiko Doi
Department of Gastrointestinal Oncology, National Cancer Center Hospital East, Kashiwa, Chiba, Japan

Nagahiro Saijo
National Cancer Center Hospital East, Kashiwa, Chiba, Japan

Jun-ichi Sawada
Division of Functional Biochemistry and Genomics, National Institute of Health Sciences, Tokyo, Japan

Kelly N. H. Nudelman
Department of Medical and Molecular Genetics, Indiana University School of Medicine, Indianapolis, Indiana, United States of America
Training in Research for Behavioral Oncology and Cancer Control Program, Indiana University School of Nursing, Indianapolis, Indiana, United States of America
Center for Neuroimaging, Department of Radiology and Imaging Sciences, Indiana University School of Medicine, Indianapolis, Indiana, United States of America

Andrew J. Saykin
Department of Medical and Molecular Genetics, Indiana University School of Medicine, Indianapolis, Indiana, United States of America
Center for Neuroimaging, Department of Radiology and Imaging Sciences, Indiana University School of Medicine, Indianapolis, Indiana, United States of America
Indiana Alzheimer Disease Center, Indiana University School of Medicine, Indianapolis, Indiana, United States of America
Indiana University Melvin and Bren Simon Cancer Center, Indiana University School of Medicine, Indianapolis, Indiana, United States of America

Bryan P. Schneider
Department of Medical and Molecular Genetics, Indiana University School of Medicine, Indianapolis, Indiana, United States of America
Indiana University Melvin and Bren Simon Cancer Center, Indiana University School of Medicine, Indianapolis, Indiana, United States of America
Department of Medicine, Indiana University School of Medicine, Indianapolis, Indiana, United States of America

Susan K. Conroy and Dori J. Smith
Center for Neuroimaging, Department of Radiology and Imaging Sciences, Indiana University School of Medicine, Indianapolis, Indiana, United States of America

Yang Wang, John D. West and Darren P. O'Neill
Center for Neuroimaging, Department of Radiology and Imaging Sciences, Indiana University School of Medicine, Indianapolis, Indiana, United States of America
Indiana Alzheimer Disease Center, Indiana University School of Medicine, Indianapolis, Indiana, United States of America

Brenna C. McDonald
Center for Neuroimaging, Department of Radiology and Imaging Sciences, Indiana University School of Medicine, Indianapolis, Indiana, United States of America
Indiana Alzheimer Disease Center, Indiana University School of Medicine, Indianapolis, Indiana, United States of America
Indiana University Melvin and Bren Simon Cancer Center, Indiana University School of Medicine, Indianapolis, Indiana, United States of America

Qi Lin, Dexiang Zhu, Ye Wei, Li Ren, Lechi Ye, Qingyang Feng, Pingping Xu, Peng Zheng and Jianmin Xu
Department of General Surgery, Zhongshan Hospital, Fudan University, Shanghai, China

Qinghai Ye and Jia Fan
Department of Liver Surgery, Zhongshan Hospital, Fudan University, Shanghai, China

Minzhi Lv
Department of Biostatistics, School of Public Health, Fudan University, Shanghai, China

Yunyun Jiang, Filip Janku and Aung Naing
Department of Investigational Cancer Therapeutics (Phase I Clinical Trials Program), Division of Cancer Medicine, The University of Texas MD Anderson Cancer Center, Houston, Texas, United States of America

Vivek Subbiah
Department of Investigational Cancer Therapeutics (Phase I Clinical Trials Program), Division of Cancer Medicine, The University of Texas MD Anderson Cancer Center, Houston, Texas, United States of America
Department of Pediatrics, The University of Texas MD Anderson Cancer Center, Houston, Texas, United States of America

Razelle Kurzrock
Department of Investigational Cancer Therapeutics (Phase I Clinical Trials Program), Division of Cancer Medicine, The University of Texas MD Anderson Cancer Center, Houston, Texas, United States of America
Center for Personalized Cancer Therapy and Division of Hematology & Oncology, University of California San Diego - Moores Cancer Center, La Jolla, California, United States of America

Pete Anderson
Department of Pediatrics, The University of Texas MD Anderson Cancer Center, Houston, Texas, United States of America
Pediatric Hematology/Oncology/BMT, Levine Children's Hospital/Levine Cancer Institute, Charlotte, North Carolina, United States of America

Joseph A. Ludwig and Robert S. Benjamin
Department of Sarcoma Medical Oncology, The University of Texas MD Anderson Cancer Center, Houston, Texas, United States of America

Robert E. Brown
From the Department of Pathology, UT Health-Department of Pathology and Laboratory medicine, Houston, Texas, United States of America

Susan E. P. Bastian
Wine Science and Business Group, School of Agriculture, Food and Wine, Waite Campus, The University of Adelaide, PMB 1, Glen Osmond, Australia

Ker Y. Cheah
Wine Science and Business Group, School of Agriculture, Food and Wine, Waite Campus, The University of Adelaide, PMB 1, Glen Osmond, Australia,
Centre for Paediatric and Adolescent Gastroenterology, Children, Youth and Women's Health Service, North Adelaide, Australia

Gordon S. Howarth
Centre for Paediatric and Adolescent Gastroenterology, Children, Youth and Women's Health Service, North Adelaide, Australia
School of Animal and Veterinary Sciences, Roseworthy Campus, The University of Adelaide, Australia

Keren A. Bindon
The Australian Wine Research Institute, Urrbrae, Adelaide, Australia

James A. Kennedy
The Australian Wine Research Institute, Urrbrae, Adelaide, Australia
Department of Viticulture and Enology, California State University, Fresno, California, United States of America

Grégoire Mignot
INSERM, UMR866, Dijon, France
Faculté de Mé decine, Université de Bourgogne, Dijon, France

Alice Hervieu
INSERM, UMR866, Dijon, France
Faculté de Médecine, Université de Bourgogne, Dijon, France
Service de Dermatologie, Centre Hospitalier Universitaire le Bocage, Dijon, France

Lionel Apetoh and François Ghiringhelli
INSERM, UMR866, Dijon, France
Faculté de Mé decine, Université de Bourgogne, Dijon, France
Oncologie mé dicale, Centre Georges François Leclerc, Dijon, France

Pierre Vabres
Faculté de Médecine, Université de Bourgogne, Dijon, France
Service de Dermatologie, Centre Hospitalier Universitaire le Bocage, Dijon, France

Sophie Dalac, Geraldine Jeudy and Blandine Bel
Service de Dermatologie, Centre Hospitalier Universitaire le Bocage, Dijon, France

Yu Zong, Li Zhu, Jiayi Wu, Xiaosong Chen, Ou Huang, Jianrong He, Weiguo Chen, Yafen Li and Kunwei Shen
Comprehensive Breast Health Center, Shanghai Ruijin Hospital affiliated to Medical School of Shanghai Jiaotong University, Shanghai, China

Xiaochun Fei
Pathology Department, Shanghai Ruijin Hospital affiliated to Medical School of Shanghai Jiaotong University, Shanghai, China

Ying-Ying Liang, Li-Sheng Zheng, Xue Cao, Li-Xia Peng, Ping Xie and Bi-Jun Huang
State Key Laboratory of Oncology in South China and Collaborative Innovation Center for Cancer Medicine, Sun Yat-sen University Cancer Center, Guangzhou, China

Chao-Nan Qian
State Key Laboratory of Oncology in South China and Collaborative Innovation Center for Cancer Medicine, Sun Yat-sen University Cancer Center, Guangzhou, China
Department of Nasopharyngeal Carcinoma, Sun Yat-sen University Cancer Center, Guangzhou, China

Ming-Yuan Chen, Yi-Jun Hua, Rui Sun, Lin Wang, Yan-Qun Xiang and Xiang Guo
Department of Nasopharyngeal Carcinoma, Sun Yat-sen University Cancer Center, Guangzhou, China

Shi Chen
Department of Gastroesophageal surgery, The Sixth Affliated Hospital (Gastrointestinal and Anal Hospital), Sun Yat-sen University, GuangZhou, China

Salvatore Grisanti, Francesca Consoli, Chiara Ciccarese, Laura Ferrari, Vittorio D. Ferrari and Alfredo Berruti
Medical Oncology Unit, University of Brescia and Spedali Civili Hospital, Brescia, Italy

Camillo Almici, Rosanna Verardi, Mirella Marini and Andrea Bianchetti
Department of Transfusion Medicine, Laboratory for Stem Cell Manipulation and Cryopreservation, Spedali Civili Hospital, Brescia, Italy

Michela Buglione and Stefano M. Magrini
Radiation Oncology Unit, University of Brescia and Spedali Civili Hospital, Brescia, Italy

Andrea Bolzoni-Villaret and Piero Nicolai
Otorhinolaryngology, Head and Neck Surgery Unit, University of Brescia and Spedali Civili Hospital, Brescia, Italy

Monica Mangoni and Gianpaolo Biti
Department of Radiation Oncology, University of Florence, Florence, Italy

Peng Zhang, Mian Xi, Lei Zhao, Qiao-Qiao Li, Liru He, Shiliang Liu and Meng-Zhong Liu
Sun Yat-sen University Cancer Center; State Key Laboratory of Oncology in South China, Collaborative Innovation Center for Cancer Medicine; Department of Radiation Oncology, Cancer Center, Sun Yat-sen University, Guangzhou, People's Republic of China

Jingxian Shen
Sun Yat-sen University Cancer Center; State Key Laboratory of Oncology in South China, Collaborative Innovation Center for Cancer Medicine; Imaging Diagnosis and Interventional Center, Cancer Center, Sun Yat-sen University, Guangzhou, People's Republic of China

Marek Szumowski, Peter R. Levasseur, XinXia Zhu and Daniel L. Marks
Papé Family Pediatric Research Institute, Oregon Health & Science University, Portland, Oregon, United States of America

Theodore P. Braun
Papé Family Pediatric Research Institute, Oregon Health & Science University, Portland, Oregon, United States of America

MD/PhD Program, Oregon Health & Science University, Portland, Oregon, United States of America

Anupriya Agarwal
Knight Cancer Institute, Oregon Health & Science University, Portland, Oregon, United States of America
Division of Hematology & Medical Oncology, Oregon Health & Science University, Portland, Oregon, United States of America

Aaron J. Grossberg
Department of Internal Medicine, Providence St. Vincent Medical Center, Portland, Oregon, United States of America

Li Lin, Guan-Qun Zhou, Ling-Long Tang, Lei Chen, Yan-Ping Mao, Jun Ma and Ying Sun
Department of Radiation Oncology, Sun Yat-sen University Cancer Center, State Key Laboratory of Oncology in South China, Collaborative Innovation Center for Cancer Medicine, Guangzhou, Guangdong Province, People's Republic of China

Chang-Juan Tao
Department of Radiation Oncology, Sun Yat-sen University Cancer Center, State Key Laboratory of Oncology in South China, Collaborative Innovation Center for Cancer Medicine, Guangzhou, Guangdong Province, People's Republic of China
Department of Radiation Oncology, Zhejiang Cancer Hospital, Hangzhou, Zhejiang Province, People's Republic of China

Mu-Sheng Zeng, Tie-Bang Kang and Wei-Hua Jia
Department of Experimental Research, Sun Yat-sen University Cancer Center, State Key Laboratory of Oncology in South China, Collaborative Innovation Center for Cancer Medicine, Guangzhou, Guangdong Province, People's Republic of China

Jian-Yong Shao
Department of Pathology, Sun Yat-sen University Cancer Center, State Key Laboratory of Oncology in South China, Collaborative Innovation Center for Cancer Medicine, Guangzhou, Guangdong Province, People's Republic of China

Hai-Qiang Mai
Department of Nasopharyngeal Carcinoma, Sun Yat-sen University Cancer Center, State Key Laboratory of Oncology in South China, Collaborative Innovation Center for Cancer Medicine, Guangzhou, Guangdong Province, People's Republic of China

Ai-Hua Lin
Department of Medical Statistics and Epidemiology, School of Public Health, Sun Yatsen University, Guangzhou, Guangdong Province, People's Republic of China

Chidozie C. Anyaegbu, Richard A. Lake, Bruce W. Robinson and Scott A. Fisher
National Centre for Asbestos Related Diseases (NCARD), QEII Medical Centre, Nedlands, Western Australia
School of Medicine and Pharmacology, University of Western Australia, QEII Medical Centre, Nedlands, Western Australia

Kathy Heel
School of Pathology and Laboratory Medicine, University of Western Australia, QEII Medical Centre, Nedlands, Western Australia

Yuanming Shen, Jiansong Zhou, Yang Li, Feng Ye, Xiaoyun Wan, Weiguo Lu, Xing Xie, Xiaodong Cheng
Department of Gynecologic Oncology, Women's Hospital, School of Medicine, Zhejiang University, Hangzhou, China

Wenhua Liang, Xuan Wu, Shaodong Hong, Yaxiong Zhang, Shiyang Kang, Wenfeng Fang, Tao Qin, Yan Huang, Hongyun Zhao and Li Zhang
Sun Yat-sen University Cancer Center, State Key Laboratory of Oncology in South China, Collaborative Innovation Center for Cancer Medicine, Guangzhou, China

Ying-sheng Wen, Peng Lin, Tie-hua Rong and Lan-jun Zhang
Department of Thoracic Surgery, Sun Yat-sen University Cancer Center, Guangzhou, Guangdong, China

Jian-fei Zhu
Department of Thoracic Surgery, Sun Yat-sen University Cancer Center, Guangzhou, Guangdong, China
Shaanxi Provincial People's Hospital, Xi'an, Shaanxi, China

Xing-yu Feng
Department of Gastro-pancreatic Surgery, Sun Yat-sen University Cancer Center, Guangzhou, Guangdong, China

Xue-wen Zhang
Department of Pathology, Sun Yat-sen University Cancer Center, Guangzhou, Guangdong, China

Ling Cai
Department of Radiation-Oncology, Sun Yat-sen University Cancer Center, Guangzhou, Guangdong, China

Yanlong Yang, Nuo Yang and Lei Xian
Department of Cardiothoracic Surgery, The First Affiliated Hospital of Guangxi Medical University, Nanning, Guangxi Zhuang Autonomous Region, China

Xiuping Luo and Ronghao Feng
Department of Chemotherapy, The Affiliated Tumor Hospital of Guangxi Medical University, Nanning, Guangxi Zhuang Autonomous Region, China

Mogens K. Boisen
Department of Oncology, Herlev University Hospital, Herlev, Denmark

Christian Dehlendorff
Statistics, Bioinformatics and Registry, Danish Cancer Society Research Center, Copenhagen, Denmark

Dorte Linnemann
Department of Pathology, Herlev University Hospital, Herlev, Denmark

Nina Keldsen
Department of Oncology, Herning Hospital, Herning, Denmark

Brita B. Jensen
Department of Medicine, Queen Ingrid Hospital, Nuuk, Greenland
Department of Oncology, Sydvestjysk Hospital, Esbjerg, Denmark

Index

www.ingramcontent.com/pod-product-compliance
Lightning Source LLC
LaVergne TN
LVHW060543210926
848485LV00005B/1248